Clinical Neurology & Neuroanatomy
A Localization-Based Approach

Second Edition

Aaron L. Berkowitz, MD, PhD

Mc
Graw
Hill

New York Chicago San Francisco Athens London Madrid Mexico City
Milan New Delhi Singapore Sydney Toronto

Clinical Neurology & Neuroanatomy: A Localization-Based Approach, Second Edition

3 4 5 6 7 8 9   DSS   27 26 25 24

ISBN 978-1-260-45336-2
MHID 1-260-45336-7

Notice

Medicine is an ever-changing science. As new research and clinical experience broaden our knowledge, changes in treatment and drug therapy are required. The author and the publisher of this work have checked with sources believed to be reliable in their efforts to provide information that is complete and generally in accord with the standards accepted at the time of publication. However, in view of the possibility of human error or changes in medical sciences, neither the author nor the publisher nor any other party who has been involved in the preparation or publication of this work warrants that the information contained herein is in every respect accurate or complete, and they disclaim all responsibility for any errors or omissions or for the results obtained from use of the information contained in this work. Readers are encouraged to confirm the information contained herein with other sources. For example and in particular, readers are advised to check the product information sheet included in the package of each drug they plan to administer to be certain that the information contained in this work is accurate and that changes have not been made in the recommended dose or in the contraindications for administration. This recommendation is of particular importance in connection with new or infrequently used drugs.

This book was set in Minion Pro by KnowledgeWorks Global Ltd.
The editors were Timothy Y. Hiscock and Peter J. Boyle.
The production supervisor was Richard Ruzycka.
Production management was provided by Tasneem Kauser, KnowledgeWorks Global Ltd.
The cover designer was W2 Design.

This book is printed on acid-free paper.

Library of Congress Control Number: 2022934170

McGraw Hill books are available at special quantity discounts to use as premiums and sales promotions, or for use in corporate training programs. To contact a representative please visit the Contact Us pages at www.mhprofessional.com.

This book is dedicated to:

My mentors Dr. Martin A. Samuels, Dr. Allan H. Ropper, and Dr. Steven K. Feske, who through their extraordinary mentorship and teaching trained me not only in the science of Neurology, but in the art of Medicine.

The students and residents at Harvard Medical School and the Partners Neurology residency program (Boston); the residents and faculty at Hôpital Universitaire de Mirebalais, Hôpital St. Nicolas de St. Marc, and Hôpital St. Boniface (Haiti); and the students and residents at Queen Elizabeth Central Hospital and Kamuzu Central Hospital (Malawi), who through their brilliant questions and insatiable desire to learn taught me how to teach neurology.

The patients with and through whom I learned the practice of neurology and medicine, and whose courage in the face of suffering inspires us to learn more about their diseases, teach what we learn to others, and serve them and their families to the best of our abilities.

My wife Nina, whose boundless support, encouragement, and companionship have been both a sustaining force and a source of great joy.

My father (in memoriam), who instilled in me a passion for science, medicine, and service.

Contents

Foreword

So much of neurology exists only "in use". This is the neurology that is practiced in the clinics, wards, and offices of seasoned clinicians and cannot be found in large encyclopedic textbooks of neurology or smaller monographs intended for medical students. The accumulated experience of the neurologist can be distilled to a number of action items and thought processes that are challenging to articulate.

Dr. Aaron Berkowitz has written a book that occupies just this position. He has taken the transactional daily work of neurology and produced a wonderfully readable, concise, but by no means superficial book that fits well in the current pedagogic environment. One might ask whether any book on neurology is needed now that disembodied information is so easily available on the web and algorithms for various signs, symptoms, and diseases abound. But between information that is as often misleading as it is useful, and the storehouse of wisdom accumulated over a long career, sits a great body of neurological knowledge. It is this assembled knowledge that allows us to efficiently move through the workday and can be taught to students and residents during their rotations. Berkowitz's book is more than a compendium or teaching guide and is far superior to existing books of its size and scope because of the thoughtfulness with which the knowledge about diseases and neurological conditions has been assembled. He gets right down to business, addressing almost every major point that is encountered on the wards and in the clinic.

A book such as this one is more suitable for neurology than for any other branch of medicine. We still depend on the interface between our own refined clinical skills and our decisions regarding diagnosis and treatment. The pearls contained here about the meaning of particulars of the history and examination cannot be found elsewhere. The book makes a seamless transit from these data to practical wisdom about their application. The material is clear and avoids the ambiguity that clutters most other books. In doing so, it also incorporates the latest thinking from clinical trials and together, these features provide one of the best modern outlooks on the pragmatic practice of neurology.

It takes a certain outlook on pedagogy and practice to produce such a book. Dr. Berkowitz has more than succeeded, and I find myself looking at a number of the chapters over and over to reorient myself to solid teaching and practice.

Allan H. Ropper, MD
Professor of Neurology
Harvard Medical School
Boston, Massachusetts

Preface to the First Edition

There are many extraordinary neurology and neuroanatomy textbooks. Innumerable clinical pearls can be gleaned from dedicated time spent with these texts as a student, trainee, and practitioner. Yet when I was a student and then a trainee, I found that there was no single text that provided a comprehensive introduction to clinical neuroanatomy, its application to neurology, and the diagnosis and management of both common and rare neurologic diseases in one concise volume. I had wished that there was a book that could be read cover-to-cover as a student rotating through neurology, or when I was a soon-to-be neurology resident at the end of my medical internship, or as a quick reference to efficiently review topics as a neurology resident—a book in which one or more chapters could be read in a single sitting. As I began to teach neuroanatomy and neurology to students, residents, and non-neurologists, I learned that they too wished for such a book. In *Clinical Neurology & Neuroanatomy: A Localization-Based Approach*, I decided to attempt to write that book.

Some of the many essential textbooks that nearly all neurologists return to throughout training and practice include Brazis' *Localization in Clinical Neurology*, Patten's *Neurologic Differential Diagnosis*, and Blumenfeld's *Neuroanatomy through Clinical Cases* for neurologic localization and clinical neuroanatomy; Adams and Victor's *Principles of Neurology* and Bradley's *Neurology in Clinical Practice* for clinical neurology. *Clinical Neurology & Neuroanatomy: A Localization-Based Approach* is, by design, a fraction of the size of any one of these books, and is meant to provide a concise but comprehensive framework to facilitate engagement with those texts. My goal is to distill clinical neuroanatomy, clinical neurology, and their interrelations to their fundamental principles so as to explain them clearly and simply. In so doing, I hope to convey the core material essential to the practice of neurology in an efficient and easily digestible format with the depth and detail required of neurology residents and neurologists reviewing for recertification examinations, but also with sufficient clarity and brevity for medical students on neurology rotations and non-neurologists in settings where there are few or no neurologists.

In Part 1 of this book, clinically relevant neuroanatomy is presented in clinical context in order to provide a framework for neurologic localization and differential diagnosis. The diseases mentioned in localization-based discussions of differential diagnoses in Part 1 are then discussed in clinical detail with respect to their diagnosis and management in Part 2. For example, in Chapter 5, the anatomy of the spinal cord and its relation to clinical syndromes involving the spinal cord are discussed. The differential diagnosis of myelopathy is presented, but the evaluation and management of many of the diseases mentioned that can cause myelopathy are discussed in Part 2 (e.g., vascular diseases of the spinal cord are discussed in Ch. 19, infections of the spine in Ch. 20, inflammatory conditions of the spinal cord in Ch. 21). Part 1 of this book can therefore be consulted for a neuroanatomical localization-based approach to symptom evaluation, and Part 2 for the clinical features, diagnosis, and management of neurologic diseases. Certain diseases are more logically discussed directly in the context of their underlying anatomy, and where this is the case, these diseases are discussed in Part 1 (e.g., trigeminal neuralgia and Bell's palsy in Ch. 13 on the trigeminal and facial nerves; benign paroxysmal positional vertigo in Ch. 12 on the vestibular system and the approach to vertigo).

Neurology is learned by taking care of patients: thinking through localization and differential diagnosis, evaluation, and management of individual patients, and discussing these patients' cases with one's clinical teachers and colleagues. This book is of course no replacement for that experience. However, my hope is that this book will serve as a guide to and through that process.

Aaron L. Berkowitz, MD, PhD

Preface to the Second Edition

In the five years since the first edition of this book, there has been an explosion in new knowledge that directly impacts our care of patients with neurologic disease. New treatments have emerged for epilepsy, multiple sclerosis, and migraine. New diseases have been characterized (antibody-mediated syndromes), new criteria for diagnosis of existing diseases have been established (multiple sclerosis), and new categorizations of existing diseases have been created (brain tumors). New clinical trial data has transformed the treatment of acute stroke. New treatments for systemic cancer (immunotherapy and CAR T-cell therapy) have generated a new spectrum of cancer treatment-associated neurologic conditions. All of these exciting updates are included in this second edition, and still this book will likely have aspects that are out-of-date as soon as it goes to press. What other field of medicine has come so far in so short a time, and yet still has so far to go? This constant evolution is one of many aspects that makes neurology such a dynamic, engaging, and meaningful field to study and practice.

When I set out to revise this book to include all of the above developments, some colleagues said, "Well, at least you won't have to revise the neuroanatomy that doesn't change." While neuroanatomy may not change, it is vast and we are constantly learning more through study and practice. I've had the great fortune to work with students and residents whose questions have helped me learn more, deepen my understanding, and find new ways to teach. I've also been fortunate to receive feedback from readers and colleagues on topics to add, concepts to clarify, and clinical correlations to emphasize. Thanks to the incredible artistry of Craig Durant and his colleagues at Dragonfly Media. This second edition includes many new drawings of the neuroanatomical pathways as well as narrated animations available on the AccessMedicine website.

In working on this second edition, I have been fortunate to receive feedback from subspecialist experts, who helped to make sure I didn't miss any developments and that my understanding of the latest updates in their fields were correct, precise, and practical. I extend my utmost gratitude to Dr. Jong Woo Lee (Epilepsy, Brigham and Women's Hospital), Dr. Tracey Milligan (Epilepsy, New York Medical College), Dr. Justin Sattin (Vascular Neurology, University of Wisconsin), Dr. Eli Zimmerman (Vascular Neurology, Vanderbilt University), Dr. Casey Albin (Neuro-Critical Care, Emory), Dr. Arun Venkatesan (Neuro-Infectious Disease, Johns Hopkins), Dr. Pria Anand (Neuro-Infectious Disease, Boston University), Dr. Shamik Bhattacharyya (Multiple Sclerosis and Autoimmune Neurology, BWH), Dr. Emmanuelle Waubant (Multiple Sclerosis, UCSF), Dr. Andrew Stern (Cognitive/Behavioral Neurology, BWH), Dr. Emily Ferenczi (Movement Disorders, BWH), Dr. Joshua Budhu (Neuro-Oncology, BWH/MGH), Dr. Maya Graham (Neuro-Oncology, Memorial Sloan-Kettering), Dr. Rebecca Burch (Headache, BWH), Dr. Christopher Doughty (Neuromuscular, BWH), Dr. Tabby Kennedy (Neuroradiology, University of Wisconsin).

Acknowledgments

I am very fortunate to have trained in neurology under two of the field's great luminaries, Dr. Allan H. Ropper and Dr. Martin A. Samuels. They are not only two virtuosic neurologists, they are extraordinary teachers, inspiring and dedicated mentors, and serve as role models of the Complete Physician toward which to strive.

Dr. Steve Feske has also been an extremely important guru in my development as a neurologist. I have learned so much from discussing cases with him, and admire his balance of clinical wisdom and rigorous analysis of the evidence (or lack thereof) when approaching the most complex cases with extreme clarity. I often find myself "trying to ask my inner Feske" when faced with vexing clinical dilemmas.

I would also like to thank the faculty of the Partners Neurology Residency Program who trained me, with special gratitude to Dr. Tracey Milligan, Dr. Nagagopal Venna, Dr. Steve M. Greenberg, Dr. Albert Hung, Dr. Sashank Prasad, Dr. Anthony Amato, Dr. Tracey Cho, Dr. Joshua Klein, and Dr. Sherry Chou for their clinical teaching and mentorship.

I have learned so much from the residents and students with whom I have been privileged to work in Boston, in Haiti, and in Malawi. Their questions and their pursuit of answers to questions I could not answer have enriched my own knowledge, and in turn, have helped me to develop as a teacher of neurology and neuroanatomy.

In Haiti, where there is one neurologist for 10 million citizens, I have had the honor of teaching neurology to family practitioners and internists for the last several years. Dr. Patrick Jouissance, my long-time colleague in Haiti, once said to me after a week of neurology training for his family medicine residents, "We need a clear and concise neurology textbook- please write one for us!" I hope he and his residents will find that this book fulfills their request.

In writing the first edition of this book, I was fortunate that my expert subspecialty colleagues from Brigham and Women's Hospital (BWH) and Massachusetts General Hospital (MGH) took time out of their busy schedules to review individual chapters in their areas of expertise, and this book has benefited greatly from their thoughtful reviews and insightful suggestions. I extend enormous thanks to Dr. Anthony Amato (Neuromuscular Diseases, BWH), Dr. Shamik Bhattacharyya (Multiple Sclerosis and Autoimmune Neurology, BWH), Dr. Tracey Cho (Neuro-infectious Diseases, MGH), Dr. Thomas Cochrane (Neuromuscular Diseases, BWH), Dr. Barbara Dworetzky (Epilepsy, BWH), Dr. Claudio DeGusmao (Pediatric and Transitional Neurology, BWH), Dr. Steven Feske (Vascular neurology and Neurocritical care, BWH), Dr. Steven M. Greenberg (Vascular neurology, MGH), Dr. Albert Hung (Movement Disorders, BWH/MGH), Dr. Tamara Kaplan (Fellow in Multiple Sclerosis and Demyelinating Diseases, BWH), Dr. Joshua Klein (Neuroradiology and Neurology, BWH), Dr. Jong Woo Lee (Epilepsy, BWH), Dr. Jennifer Lyons (Neuro-infectious Diseases, BWH), Dr. Scott McGinnis (Behavioral and Cognitive Neurology, BWH), Dr. William Mullally (Headache, BWH), Dr. Lakshmi Nayak (Neuro-oncology, BWH), Dr. Page Pennell (Epilepsy, BWH), Dr. Sashank Prasad (Neuro-ophthalmology, BWH), and Dr. James Stankiewicz (Multiple Sclerosis and Demyelinating Diseases, BWH).

I am also grateful to the residents and medical students who took the book for a "test drive" and provided thoughtful feedback: Dr. Emer McGrath, Dr. Pooja Raibagkar, Dr. Francois Roosevelt, Dr. Michael Erkkinen, and Cathy Hao.

The first edition of this book would not have been possible without the phenomenal stewardship of Andrew Moyer and the efforts of his team at McGraw Hill. Andrew guided this book from idea to production and he and his team developed creative ways to enhance the pedagogy of the text and figures through their layout and presentation. I am grateful to Tim Hiscock, Peter Boyle, and their team at McGraw Hill for shepherding this book through its second edition. Tasneem Kauser and her team at KnowledgeWorks Global Ltd. effectively and efficiently transformed the countless text and image files with which I provided them into the book you are holding and were a pleasure to work with.

Finally, to the patients who have taught me all of the neurology I know, I hope that this book will honor your courage in facing neurologic disease and your generosity in allowing us to learn from you.

Diagnostic Reasoning in Neurology & the Neurologic History & Examination

Differential diagnosis in neurology is based on two main components determined from the clinical history and physical examination:

- The **localization** of the neuroanatomic origin(s) of the patient's symptoms and signs
- The **time course** over which these symptoms and signs have arisen and evolved

These give rise to what I call the "fundamental equation" of differential diagnosis in neurology:

Differential Diagnosis = Localization × Time course

Localization relies on the clinical history and neurologic examination to determine *where* in the nervous system the problem is. To some extent, knowing *where* the problem is already begins to circumscribe *what* the problem is, since each level of the nervous system has a particular differential diagnosis for the types of disease processes that can affect it. The time course over which neurologic symptoms arise and evolve provides crucial information in determining *what* the problem is, since different disease processes emerge and evolve over different time frames.

LOCALIZATION IN NEUROLOGIC DIAGNOSIS: DETERMINING *WHERE* THE PROBLEM IS

Localization is the process of determining *where* in the nervous system the patient's disease process is occurring: Is the problem in the central nervous system (CNS), the peripheral nervous system (PNS), or both? Within the CNS, is there a lesion in the brain, brainstem, cerebellum, or spinal cord? More precisely, *where* is the lesion within those structures? For example, which *level* of the brainstem or spinal cord? Which hemisphere(s), lobe(s), and gyrus/gyri of the brain? Within the PNS, is the lesion at the level of the spinal roots, dorsal root ganglia, peripheral nerves, neuromuscular junction, or muscles? If there is a root, nerve, or muscle problem, which root(s), nerve(s), and/or muscle(s) is/are involved?

Nervous system diseases may affect particular **structures** (e.g., the basal ganglia, the cerebellum, the peripheral nerves), a particular **tissue type** (e.g., white matter vs gray matter of the brain; myelin of peripheral nerves vs their axons), or one or more particular **systems** (e.g., the motor system, the limbic system).

Localization requires a detailed understanding of neuroanatomy. Part 1 of this book presents clinical neuroanatomy alongside the clinical approach to symptoms and signs related to the anatomy under discussion. Diseases that are mentioned in Part 1 of this book are discussed in more detail with respect to their clinical features, diagnosis, and treatment in Part 2.

Localization begins with the clinical history, which should elucidate the nature of the patient's presenting symptom(s) and allow for an initial idea of potential localization(s). For example, is a chief concern of "difficulty walking" due to weakness, impaired coordination, altered sensation, pain, decreased vision, higher-order motor dysfunction, or a non-neurologic (e.g., orthopedic) condition? The neurologic examination provides further clues as to the neuroanatomic localization of the patient's symptoms (see "Introduction to the Neurologic Examination").

TIME COURSE IN NEUROLOGIC DIAGNOSIS: DETERMINING *WHAT* THE PROBLEM IS (FIG. 1–1)

The time course of symptom onset and evolution may be described as **sudden/hyperacute** (seconds to minutes), **acute** (hours to days), **subacute** (weeks to months), or **chronic** (months to years). The following is a general "first pass" in neurologic differential diagnosis based on the timing of symptom onset and pace of symptom evolution (with a few exceptions noted below):

- **Hyperacute (seconds to minutes):**
  - **Vascular** (e.g., ischemic stroke, intracerebral hemorrhage, subarachnoid hemorrhage)
  - **Seizure**
  - **Migraine**
  - **Metabolic** (e.g., hyperglycemia or hypoglycemia)
  - **Medications/Toxins**
  - **Trauma**

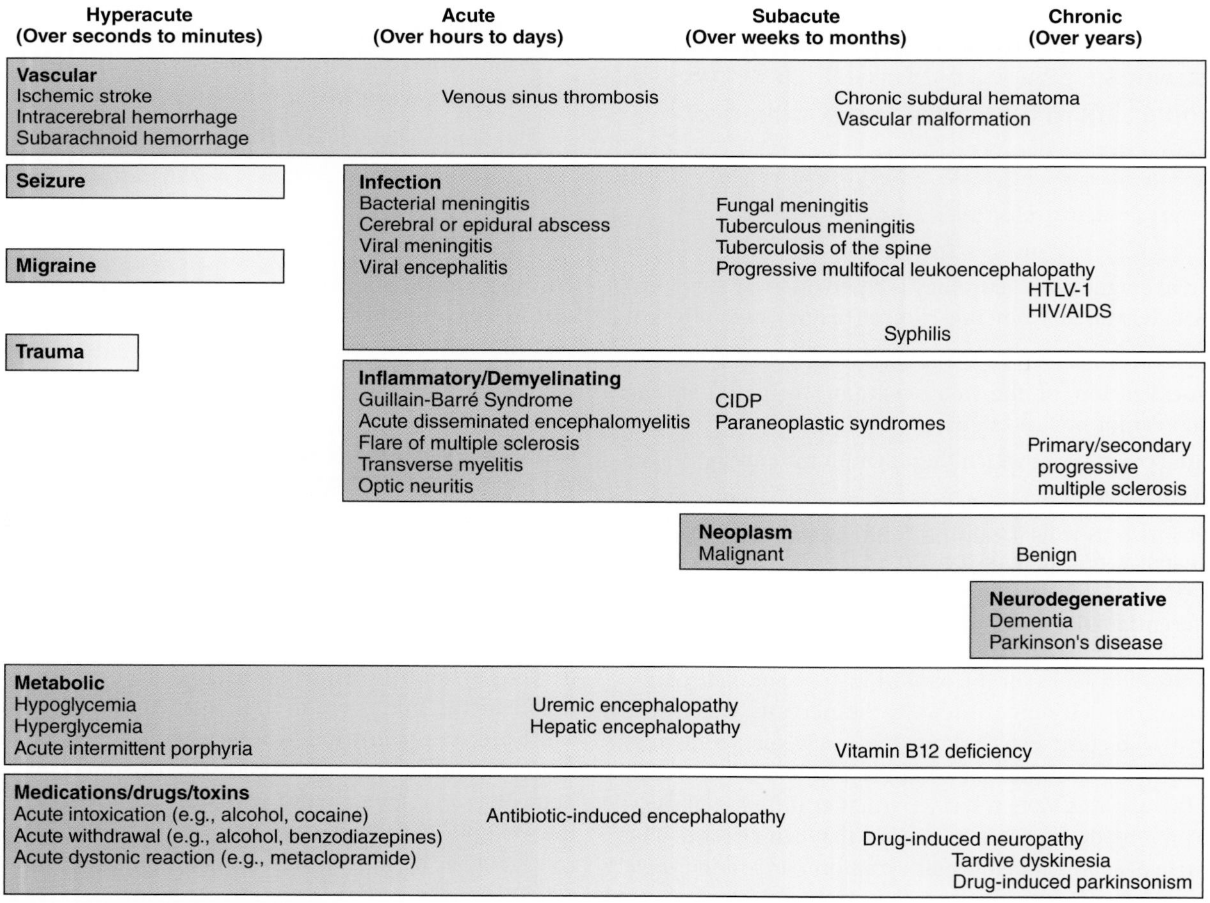

Hyperacute (Over seconds to minutes)	Acute (Over hours to days)	Subacute (Over weeks to months)	Chronic (Over years)
Vascular Ischemic stroke Intracerebral hemorrhage Subarachnoid hemorrhage	Venous sinus thrombosis	Chronic subdural hematoma Vascular malformation	
Seizure			
	Infection Bacterial meningitis Cerebral or epidural abscess Viral meningitis Viral encephalitis	Fungal meningitis Tuberculous meningitis Tuberculosis of the spine Progressive multifocal leukoencephalopathy	HTLV-1 HIV/AIDS
Migraine			
		Syphilis	
Trauma			
	Inflammatory/Demyelinating Guillain-Barré Syndrome Acute disseminated encephalomyelitis Flare of multiple sclerosis Transverse myelitis Optic neuritis	CIDP Paraneoplastic syndromes	Primary/secondary progressive multiple sclerosis
		Neoplasm Malignant	Benign
			Neurodegenerative Dementia Parkinson's disease
Metabolic Hypoglycemia Hyperglycemia Acute intermittent porphyria	Uremic encephalopathy Hepatic encephalopathy	Vitamin B12 deficiency	
Medications/drugs/toxins Acute intoxication (e.g., alcohol, cocaine) Acute withdrawal (e.g., alcohol, benzodiazepines) Acute dystonic reaction (e.g., metaclopramide)	Antibiotic-induced encephalopathy	Drug-induced neuropathy Tardive dyskinesia Drug-induced parkinsonism	

FIGURE 1–1 Schematic showing differential diagnosis of neurologic disease by time course.

- **Acute (hours to days):**
  - **Infectious** (bacterial and viral infections of the nervous system; e.g., meningitis, encephalitis, abscess)
  - **Immune-mediated** (e.g., Guillain-Barré syndrome, flare of multiple sclerosis)
  - **Metabolic** (e.g., uremia, hepatic encephalopathy, hyponatremia or hypernatremia)
  - **Medications/Toxins**
- **Subacute (weeks to months)**
  - **Neoplastic**
  - **Immune-mediated** (e.g., paraneoplastic/antibody-mediated syndromes)
  - **Infectious** (fungal, tuberculous, and parasitic infections, neurologic complications of HIV)
  - **Metabolic** (e.g., vitamin B12 deficiency)
  - **Medications/Toxins**
- **Chronic (months to years)**
  - **Degenerative diseases** (e.g., Alzheimer's disease, Parkinson's disease)
  - **Genetic** (e.g., Charcot-Marie-Tooth, hereditary spastic paraplegia, Huntington disease)
  - **Metabolic**
  - **Medications/Toxins**

Note that if one keeps in mind that metabolic abnormalities, medications, and toxins can cause neurologic dysfunction over nearly any time course (depending on the metabolic abnormality, medication, or toxin), the rest of this schema distills to:

- **Hyperacute**: vascular, seizure, migraine, trauma
- **Acute to subacute**: infectious, immune-mediated
- **Subacute to chronic**: neoplastic, immune-mediated, infectious
- **Chronic**: degenerative, genetic

There are a few important exceptions to this general schema:

- Nonacute disease processes may present acutely. For example, although focal deficits from tumors usually emerge and evolve subacutely, a brain tumor may be asymptomatic until it causes a seizure. Another example is relapsing-remitting multiple sclerosis, a chronic disease characterized by acute flares.
- Although most vascular problems present hyperacutely, chronic subdural hematoma is an example of a vascular condition that presents subacutely/chronically (see Ch. 19).
- Fungal infections, tuberculosis, and neurologic complications of HIV can present subacutely compared to bacterial and viral infections, which present more acutely (see Ch. 20).

With the exception of seizure and migraine, which are exclusively cerebral phenomena, the other categories apply across most levels of the neuraxis. For example, sudden-onset findings localizing to a particular part of the brain suggest a vascular cause, and this is also true of the spinal cord (e.g.,

spinal infarct, spinal epidural hemorrhage) and even of a sudden-onset peripheral nerve palsy (e.g., nerve infarction as can be seen in vasculitis). Acute inflammatory disease of the brain (e.g., acute flare of multiple sclerosis), spine (e.g., transverse myelitis), or peripheral nerves (e.g., Guillain-Barré syndrome) all emerge and evolve over hours to days.

ASSOCIATED SYMPTOMS & SIGNS IN NEUROLOGIC DIAGNOSIS

In addition to the time course of symptom onset and evolution, the history must elicit associated concurrent or preceding symptoms to contextualize the patient's primary symptom. For example, if the presenting symptom is weakness, is this weakness accompanied by sensory changes and/or pain? Is the presenting symptom restricted to the limb most prominently noted by the patient or is it also present elsewhere? If the symptom is headache, is there associated nausea/vomiting or are there visual changes? Such questions establish the full range of the patient's symptoms beyond the "chief concern" most salient to the patient, aiding in localization of the cause of the patient's symptoms.

Of course, as in all areas of medicine, each symptom must also be fully characterized with respect to its quality, severity, exacerbating and alleviating factors, and any accompanying symptoms. The patient's presenting symptom(s) must also be contextualized with respect to the past medical history, family history, social history, and medications.

The clinical history should allow for an initial hypothesis to be generated about *where* in the nervous system the problem may be as well as *what* it may be, and the neurologic examination provides further information to support or refute this hypothesis.

INTRODUCTION TO THE NEUROLOGIC EXAMINATION

The neurologic examination is a critical tool in localization, confirming or refuting hypotheses generated during the history, or sometimes giving rise to new ones entirely. For example, is the patient's presenting problem of "difficulty moving one hand" due to weakness, slowed movement, numbness, pain, incoordination, or inability to execute a complex movement plan? Each of these possibilities can be tested in the course of the neurologic examination.

With each element of the neurologic examination, it is important to consider which systems and structures within the nervous system are being evaluated and how their dysfunction could manifest. When working toward mastery of the neurologic examination and its interpretation, it is helpful to try to imagine the pathways involved while examining them. For example, when testing the pupillary light reflex, think: "afferent via optic nerve to pretectal nuclei of the midbrain, efferent via Edinger-Westphal nuclei to the oculomotor nerves" (see Ch. 10). When testing a muscle, think about the name of the muscle and its nerve and nerve root supply (see Chs. 16–17).

The neurologic examination is divided into seven components:

1. **Mental status**
2. **Cranial nerves**
3. **Motor**
4. **Sensory**
5. **Reflexes**
6. **Coordination**
7. **Gait**

Each of these components of the neurologic examination has countless individual examination maneuvers, and only the basic elements are briefly introduced here. Many more detailed aspects of the examination of each system are described in Chapters 3–17 alongside a more in-depth discussion of the neuroanatomic localization and clinical significance of abnormal examination findings.

Examination of Mental Status

The examination of the patient's mental status evaluates two aspects of the mental state:

- The **level of consciousness**
- The integrity of individual **cognitive functions** (e.g., attention, memory, language, calculation, abstract reasoning, praxis)

Examination of the Level of Consciousness: Assessment of the Reticular Activating System, Thalami, & Cerebral Hemispheres

The neuroanatomic substrates of consciousness include the reticular activating system and other ascending projections from the brainstem, which project to the bilateral thalami and to the bilateral cerebral hemispheres.

The level of consciousness refers to the patient's state of arousal: Is the patient awake? If the patient is awake, is she or he alert? If the patient is alert, is she or he attentive? If the patient is not awake, can she or he be awakened by voice or is vigorous stimulation required to awaken the patient? Once awakened, is wakefulness maintained or does the patient fall back to sleep? These types of descriptions are more precise for clinical communication than stating that a patient is **delirious** (fluctuating acute confusion), **lethargic** or **somnolent** (falls asleep without repeated stimulation), **stuporous** (requires vigorous and/or painful physical stimulation to be awakened), **obtunded** (somewhere between somnolent and stuporous), or **comatose** (not able to be aroused by any stimulus of any sort and no response to the environment). These terms may mean different things to different clinicians, and so the precise descriptions noted above are generally preferable when describing a patient's mental state.

Examination of the Integrity of Cognitive Functions: Assessment of the Cerebral Hemispheres

The neuroanatomic substrates of cognition reside in the cerebral hemispheres. Individual cortical regions, networks of these regions and subcortical structures, and their interconnections are specialized for different cognitive functions (see Ch. 7).

Generally, the examiner develops a good sense of the patient's mental status during the history: Is the patient's flow of ideas logical and clear? Is the patient's speech fluent? Does the recounting of recent and past events demonstrate that the patient's memory is intact? Does the patient respond appropriately to questions? Difficulties with any of these may give initial inklings of cognitive deficits that can be further evaluated on the mental status examination.

If the patient is not awake, or not arousable for long enough to engage in the examination, cognition cannot be tested. If the patient is awake and alert, the first cognitive modality to test is **attention**. If the patient's attention is impaired, the other cognitive domains cannot be effectively evaluated. For example, if you are sending or reading a text message during a lecture, despite hearing what the lecturer says, you may not remember it later: without paying attention, you cannot store the information in memory. Similarly, if you are not paying attention to what someone is saying to you, you may not understand what is said, and your response may not make sense, so your language comprehension in that moment may be suboptimal. Therefore, cognitive modalities beyond attention can only be reliably tested if attention is intact.

Examination of Attention: A Function of the Frontal and Parietal Lobes—Attention cannot occur without perception. For example, if a patient is blind, the patient cannot pay attention to a visual stimulus. The ability to select what to pay attention to and the ability to maintain attention are subserved by the frontal and parietal lobes. Attention can be tested by assessing the patient's ability to recite a string of numbers forward and backward (digit span), asking the patient to recite the days of the week (or the months of the year) backward, asking the patient to spell the word "world" backward (or another word of similar length), or asking the patient to subtract seven serially from 100 (100, 93, 86, and so on). These tasks require maintaining attention and concentration on the task at hand, and any lapse in attention will cause the patient to get lost, or make other errors (e.g., start going forward rather than backward). Note that the spelling task requires language ability and the subtraction task requires calculation, so forward and backward repetition of a string of numbers of increasing length provided by the examiner or recitation of the days of the week (or months of the year) backward may be simpler and less confounded ways of testing attention.

Inattention is a core feature of the altered mental state in delirium (see Ch. 22), and inattention to one-half of the world (**neglect**) can be seen with parietal lesions (most commonly right parietal lesions producing left-sided neglect; see Ch. 7).

Examination of Memory: A Function of the Temporal Lobes—Short-term memory can be tested by asking patients about the recent past (e.g., what they had for breakfast that morning, current events), and long-term memory can be tested by asking about the remote past (e.g., where they were born, went to school), although accuracy of the responses may be hard for the examiner to verify if the patient is being examined alone. Note that even patients with the most profound deficits in memory due to neurologic conditions should never forget their own names. Forgetting one's own name is almost always an indication of a psychiatric condition.

Short-term memory can also be tested by asking the patient to remember three or more words and then asking the patient to recall these words 5 minutes later after the rest of the examination. The words used should be in different categories so they cannot be easily "joined" by the patient (e.g., "blue" and "shirt" could be stored and recalled as one element "blue shirt"); the words "red," "window," and "honesty" are commonly used for this test. If the patient cannot recall one or more of the words spontaneously after 5 minutes, category clues can be given (for "red," "window," and "honesty": a color, a part of a building, and a character trait). If these cues do not elicit a memory of the words, the patient can then be given a list of choices to see if the patient can recognize the words from a list.

Memory loss is called **amnesia**. **Retrograde amnesia** refers to the inability to recall events from the past, and **anterograde amnesia** refers to the inability to form new memories. Amnesia generally occurs due to dysfunction of one or both temporal lobes, particularly medial temporal lobe structures such as the hippocampus. Deficits in memory are a core feature of Alzheimer's disease and transient global amnesia (see Ch. 22).

Examination of Language: A Function of the Frontal and Temporal Lobes (Most Commonly in the Left Hemisphere)— Language has several components: production (spoken and written), comprehension (hearing and reading), and repetition. The various combinations of deficits in aspects of spoken language are called **aphasias**, and are described in Chapter 7. In right-handed patients (and in most left-handed patients), language is predominantly a function of the left hemisphere: Broca's area for language production is in the left inferior frontal gyrus, and Wernicke's area for language comprehension is in the left posterior superior temporal gyrus (see Ch. 7). Language can be affected by any lesion in one or both of these regions including stroke (see Ch. 19), tumor (see Ch. 24), or neurodegenerative diseases such as primary progressive aphasia (see Ch. 22). Aphasia should be distinguished from **dysarthria**, which refers to a difficulty articulating speech but with preserved language content and structure.

Many other aspects of cognitive function can be tested depending on the clinical context, including visuospatial ability, abstract reasoning, calculation, and ability to perform complex learned motor tasks (**praxis**), some of which are discussed in more detail in later chapters.

The Mini-Mental State Examination (MMSE) and the Montreal Cognitive Assessment (MoCA) are examples of bedside tests that evaluate a number of cognitive functions in different domains. These tests are useful in characterizing a patient's cognitive deficits as well as in making comparisons over time. More extensive neuropsychological testing batteries can also be performed.

Examination of the Cranial Nerves

The cranial nerve examination evaluates the neurologic functions of the structures of the head and neck. Although this portion of the examination is called the "cranial nerve" examination, it also tests the brainstem (the site of the cranial nerve nuclei), and, in many cases, the cerebral hemispheres (which are the ultimate recipients of incoming sensory information from the cranial nerves [e.g., vision, hearing, taste, smell, facial sensation], and which provide descending control of the motor functions of the motor cranial nerves to the muscles of the head and neck). The brainstem and cranial nerves, their functions and pathways, and the conditions that affect them are discussed in Chapters 9–14.

Cranial Nerve 1: Olfactory Nerve
Cranial nerve 1 (CN 1) is the olfactory nerve, which conveys the sense of smell from the nose to the olfactory cortex (inferior frontal and medial temporal lobes). This is the only sensory modality that sends information directly to the cortex without a stop in the thalamus en route (although the olfactory cortex does send projections to the thalamus). Thus, testing smell is a test not only of CN 1, but also its corresponding sensory cortex (see Ch. 14).

Cranial Nerve 2: Optic Nerve
Cranial nerve 2 (CN 2) is the optic nerve, which transmits visual information from the retinae to the occipital cortex (see Ch. 6). CN 2 also transmits light information to the midbrain as the afferent limb of the pupillary light reflex. The pupillary light reflex tests CN 2 (afferent), CN 3 (efferent), and the midbrain nuclei and pathways that connect them (see Ch. 10). Examining visual acuity and visual fields tests the eyes, optic nerves, the visual cortex in the occipital lobes, and the pathways that connect them (see Ch. 6). CN 2 is the only cranial nerve—and the only nerve for that matter—that can be directly visualized on the physical examination: The optic nerve head can be seen by fundoscopy. CN 2 is also the only cranial nerve that is part of the CNS; all others are peripheral nerves.

Cranial Nerve 3 (Oculomotor Nerve), Cranial Nerve 4 (Trochlear Nerve), & Cranial Nerve 6 (Abducens Nerve)
Cranial nerves 3 (the oculomotor nerve), 4 (the trochlear nerve), and 6 (the abducens nerve) control the movements of the eyes. CN 3 also controls elevation of the eyelid and constriction of the pupil. Therefore, tests of eye movements examine these three nerves and their interconnections in the brainstem. Examining the ability to follow instructions to look in a specific direction

(**saccades**) and to follow the examiner's finger (**smooth pursuit**) tests not only cranial nerves 3, 4, and 6 and their brainstem pathways, but also the cerebellum and cortical eye fields (see Ch. 11).

Cranial Nerve 5: Trigeminal Nerve

Cranial nerve 5 is the trigeminal nerve, which transmits facial sensation to the sensory cortex by way of the brainstem and ventral posterior medial nucleus of the thalamus, and also controls the muscles of mastication (chewing). Testing facial sensation (i.e., light touch, temperature, and pain) and evaluation of the strength of jaw opening and closure are tests of the trigeminal nerve, its brainstem nuclei, and the sensory and motor centers with which they communicate in the cerebral hemispheres (VPM of the thalamus and postcentral gyrus for facial sensation; precentral gyrus for motor supply to the jaw musculature). The trigeminal nerve carries the afferent limb of the corneal reflex (eye closure with stimulation of the cornea); the efferent limb travels in CN 7. CN 5 provides both the afferent and efferent limbs of the jaw jerk reflex (see Ch. 13).

Cranial Nerve 7: Facial Nerve

Cranial nerve 7 is the facial nerve, the main function of which is to control the movements of facial musculature (it has a number of other functions discussed in Ch. 13). Asking the patient to raise the eyebrows and close the eyes tightly tests the upper facial muscles, and asking the patient to smile tests the lower facial muscles. Differences in patterns of facial weakness with respect to the upper and lower face can help localize the site of dysfunction to the facial nerve itself or the motor cortex and descending pathways that control it (see Ch. 13).

Cranial Nerve 8: Vestibulocochlear Nerve

Cranial nerve 8 is the vestibulocochlear nerve, responsible for transmitting auditory and vestibular information to the brain. The auditory portion is tested by assessing patients' hearing in both ears (which tests the integrity of the pathway from the inner ear, through the nerve, through the brainstem and thalamus up to the auditory cortex in the superior temporal lobe). The vestibular portion and its brainstem connections with the eye movement nuclei (CNs 3, 4, and 6) can be assessed by various maneuvers that examine the interaction of head movements and eye movements (see Ch. 12).

Cranial Nerve 9 (Glossopharyngeal Nerve) & Cranial Nerve 10 (Vagus Nerve)

Cranial nerve 9 (the glossopharyngeal nerve) and cranial nerve 10 (the vagus nerve) have a number of roles including innervation of the muscles of the larynx and pharynx, and afferent and efferent visceral autonomic functions (see Ch. 14). Dysfunction may cause difficulty with articulation of speech (**dysarthria**), decreased speech volume (**hypophonia**), and/or difficulty swallowing (**dysphagia**). Aside from assessing for dysarthria and hypophonia, CNs 9 and 10 can only be evaluated on examination by assessing palate elevation (primarily a function of CN 10) and the gag reflex (afferent limb is supplied primarily by CN 9; efferent limb primarily by CN 10; see Ch. 14).

Cranial Nerve 11: Spinal Accessory Nerve

Cranial nerve 11 is the spinal accessory nerve, which controls the trapezius (shoulder elevation) and the sternocleidomastoid (turning the head) (see Ch. 14). CNs 1 and 11 are the only cranial nerves that do not make any contact with the brainstem. CN 11 is comprised of spinal roots, but exits the skull with other cranial nerves through the jugular foramen.

Cranial Nerve 12: Hypoglossal Nerve

Cranial nerve 12 is the hypoglossal nerve, which controls the muscles of the tongue. It is assessed by asking the patient to protrude and move the tongue. Like CN 7 and the motor component of CN 5, its motor control comes from the motor cortex (precentral gyrus), so weakness of the tongue on one side can localize anywhere along the pathway from the contralateral motor cortex to its connections with the CN 12 nucleus in the medulla to the hypoglossal nerve itself (see Ch. 14).

Examination of the Motor System

The motor system spans the entire nervous system: brain, brainstem, spinal cord, (ventral) nerve roots, peripheral nerves, neuromuscular junction, and muscle (see Ch. 4). In addition to testing the strength of all muscles during the motor examination and looking for weakness or differences between the left and right sides, the motor examination assesses for muscle bulk (**atrophy** refers to loss of muscle bulk), muscle **tone** (increased tone refers to resistance when passively moving a joint; decreased tone or flaccidity refers to decreased resistance), speed of movements (**bradykinesia** refers to a slowing of movements), or any abnormal movements (e.g., fasciculations of muscle, tremor). The ways in which these features of the examination can aid in localizing motor problems along the neuraxis are discussed in Chapter 4.

Strength is graded on a 0–5 scale:

- 5: Full strength
- 4: Able to apply force against resistance but less than full strength
- 3: Able to move against gravity but not against resistance
- 2: Able to move from side to side but not against gravity
- 1: Most minimal detectable movement (a "flicker" of movement)
- 0: Unable to move at all

+ and – may be added to these designations. For example, 5– suggests strength that is nearly but not quite full.

Weakness is referred to as **paresis**, and complete paralysis is called **plegia**. For example, weakness of both legs is called

paraparesis, paralysis of both legs is called **paraplegia**, weakness on one side of the body is referred to as **hemiparesis**, and paralysis of one limb is called **monoplegia**.

Examination of the Sensory System

The sensory system begins in the skin (for pain, temperature, light touch, and vibration sensation), and tendons/muscles (for **proprioception**—perception of where the body is in space). Peripheral nerves transmit this information to the spinal cord via dorsal root ganglia and dorsal roots. Sensory information then travels in various pathways to and through the brainstem, the thalamus, and ultimately the somatosensory cortex in the anterior parietal lobe (postcentral gyrus). The distribution of sensory loss on the body and the affected sensory modalities are the key points that help localize lesions of the sensory pathways (see Ch. 4). Pain sensation is generally assessed with a pin (to assess the spinothalamic tracts; see Ch. 4). Vibration sensation is assessed by holding a 128 Hz tuning fork to a joint (e.g., interphalangeal joint of big toe) and assessing if the patient can feel it and, if so, for how long (to assess the dorsal columns; see Ch. 4). Proprioception can be assessed by moving a joint up or down and asking the patient to identify the direction of movement with their eyes closed (this also assesses the dorsal columns, but is considered less sensitive than testing vibration [see Ch. 4]). Proprioception can also be assessed by having the patient stand with the feet together and eyes closed: If proprioception is impaired, without vision to compensate when the eyes are closed, the patient will be unable to maintain balance (**Romberg sign**).

Examination of the Reflexes (Fig. 1–2)

Reflexes test the nerves and roots that provide sensory input to the spinal cord and receive motor output from the spinal cord, as well as the interconnections between the motor and sensory pathways in the spinal cord. Reflexes can be diminished (**hyporeflexia**) or absent (**areflexia**) with lesions in the PNS (roots, nerves) and increased (**hyperreflexia**) with lesions in the CNS (brain, brainstem, spinal cord), discussed further in Chapter 4. The most commonly tested reflexes are the biceps (C5-C6, musculocutaneous nerve), brachioradialis (C6, radial nerve), and triceps (C7-C8, radial nerve) in the upper extremities; and the patella (L3-L4, femoral nerve) and ankle/Achilles (S1-S2, tibial nerve) in the lower extremities. The associated nerve roots can be remembered by the mnemonic 1-2 – 3-4 – 5-6 – 7-8, counting from the ankle (S1,2), upward to the patella (L3,4), to the biceps (C5,6) and brachioradialis (C6), and, finally, to the triceps (C7,8).

If a patient's reflexes are not able to be elicited in the usual manner, reinforcement maneuvers may be attempted. For the upper extremities, the patient can be asked to bite down while the reflexes are being tested. For the lower extremities, the patient can be asked to curl the fingers of one hand into the fingers of the other and pull at the moment the reflex hammer strikes (**Jendrassik maneuver**). Elicitation of reflexes only by reinforcement is a sign of hyporeflexia.

Reflexes are described as normal, increased (hyperreflexia), decreased (hyporeflexia), or absent (areflexia). 0 is used to designate areflexia, 1+ signifies hyporeflexia (diminished or requiring reinforcement), 2+ signifies normal reflexes, 3+ denotes hyperreflexia, and 4+ denotes hyperreflexia with

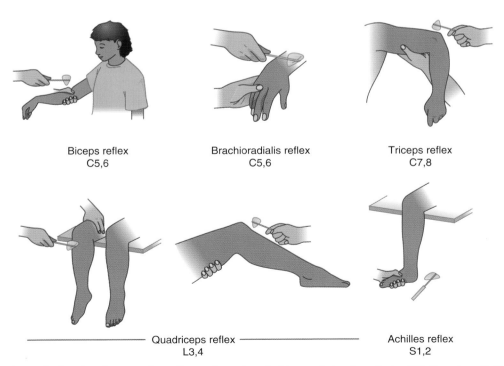

Biceps reflex C5,6 — Brachioradialis reflex C5,6 — Triceps reflex C7,8 — Quadriceps reflex L3,4 — Achilles reflex S1,2

FIGURE 1–2 Schematic showing deep tendon reflexes. Reproduced with permission from Aminoff M, Greenberg D, Simon R: *Clinical Neurology*, 9th ed. New York, NY: McGraw Hill; 2015.

TABLE 1–1 Neuroanatomic Structures & Pathways Evaluated in the Neurologic Examination.

	Structures/Pathways Evaluated	Chapter(s) Where Discussed
MENTAL STATUS		
Arousal	Reticular activating system, bilateral thalami, and cerebral hemispheres	Chapter 7
Attention	Frontal and parietal lobes	Chapter 7
Memory	Temporal lobes	Chapter 7
Language	Frontal and temporal lobes (usually left)	Chapter 7
Praxis	Frontal and parietal lobes	Chapter 7
Abstract reasoning	Frontal lobes	Chapter 7
Visuospatial processing	Occipital and parietal lobes	Chapter 6
CRANIAL NERVES		
Smell	CN 1 and olfactory cortex	Chapter 14
Pupillary light reflex	CNs 2 and 3; midbrain nuclei and pathways	Chapter 10
Visual acuity and fields	Eyes, CN 2, thalamus (lateral geniculate nucleus [LGN]), optic radiations, occipital cortex	Chapter 6
Eye movements	CNs 3, 4, and 6, brainstem pathways, frontal and parietal eye fields, cerebellum for saccades and smooth pursuit	Chapter 11
Facial sensation	CN 5, brainstem pathways, thalamus (ventral posterior medial nucleus [VPM]), somatosensory cortex	Chapter 13
Facial movements	CN 7, motor pathway from precentral gyrus to CN 7 nucleus in pons	Chapter 13
Hearing	Inner ear, CN 8, brainstem auditory pathways, thalamus (medial geniculate nucleus [MGN]), auditory cortex in superior temporal gyrus	Chapter 12
Vestibular system	Inner ear, CN 8, brainstem pathways and their connections with nuclei of CNs 3, 4, 6, and cerebellum	Chapter 12
Palate elevation and gag reflex	CNs 9 and 10, their pathways in the medulla, and motor control from the precentral gyrus	Chapter 14
Sternoclediomastoid and trapezius strength	CN 11 and motor control from the precentral gyrus	Chapter 14
Tongue movements	CN 12 and motor control from the precentral gyrus	Chapter 14
MOTOR		
Strength	Corticospinal tract (precentral gyrus through subcortical white matter, brainstem, and spinal cord), ventral roots, peripheral nerves, neuromuscular junction, and muscle	Chapters 4, 15–17, 29, 30
Higher-order motor control	Basal ganglia	Chapter 7
SENSORY	Peripheral nerves, dorsal root ganglia, dorsal roots, spinal cord and brainstem pathways, thalamus (ventral posterior lateral nucleus [VPL]), postcentral gyrus	Chapter 4
REFLEXES	Peripheral nerves, nerve roots, and spinal cord	Chapter 4
COORDINATION	Cerebellum and its sensory input	Chapter 8
GAIT	Motor, sensation, coordination pathways	Chapter 1

CN: Cranial nerve

clonus. Clonus is rhythmic oscillating movement at a joint, most commonly elicited by briskly dorsiflexing the ankle and holding the foot dorsiflexed. Clonus should be described in terms of the number of beats of clonus, and it should be noted whether clonus stops spontaneously or is sustained. Clonus is discussed further in Chapter 4.

Another sign of hyperreflexia that may be observed is **spread** of reflexes: eliciting one reflex leads to simultaneous activation of adjacent reflexes. For example, eliciting the biceps reflex causes simultaneous finger flexion or eliciting the patellar reflex leads to simultaneous ankle plantarflexion.

Pathologic Reflexes

The pathologic reflex tested for most commonly is the **Babinski sign**. To elicit this sign, the examiner strokes the sole of the foot slowly from the heel along the lateral aspect of the sole, and then continues medially along the base of the toes: The normal (non-pathologic) response is flexion of the toes. In contrast, the Babinski sign is characterized by an extensor response: extension of the big toe (a "thumbs-up" of the big toe; this may be accompanied by fanning of all toes and/or the triple flexion response of dorsiflexion, knee flexion, and hip flexion). The Babinski sign is associated with a lesion of the CNS (brain, brainstem, or spinal cord), specifically the corticospinal tract (see Ch. 4). The Babinski sign occurs normally in infants but is always abnormal in childhood and adulthood.

Other signs that can demonstrate a pathologic extensor response in the big toe like the Babinski sign include: **Chaddock sign** (stroke lateral aspect of dorsum of foot from lateral malleolus toward fifth toe), **Oppenheim sign** (stroke the tibia downward from the knee toward the foot), **Gordon sign** (squeeze the calf), and **Bing sign** (pinching one of the toes; pricking the dorsum of the fourth or fifth toe with pin in original description). If any of these maneuvers causes an extensor response of the big toe (which may be accompanied by the triple flexion response), this signifies corticospinal tract dysfunction.

Hoffman's sign is an upper-extremity analogue to Babinski's sign, elicited by flicking the middle finger and observing for flexion of the fingers and thumb (see Ch. 4).

A number of reflexes called **frontal release signs** can be seen in patients with dementia, but may also be seen in normal elderly adults (and like Babinski's sign, are normal in infants) (see Ch. 22).

Examination of Coordination

Coordination is usually tested by having the patient move the index finger back and forth between the examiner's finger and the patient's nose, sliding the heel down the shin, and performing rhythmic rapid alternating movements. When the patient is performing the finger–nose task, it is important that the target (i.e., the examiner's finger) be sufficiently far from the patient so that the patient must extend the arm fully to reach it, otherwise subtle ataxia at the extremes of motion may be missed. Note that coordination testing may be confounded if the patient has weakness, as actions attempted by weak muscles can appear uncoordinated.

Ataxia refers to uncoordinated movements, **dysmetria** refers to inaccuracy of movements (overshooting or undershooting a target), and **dysdiadochokinesia** refers to uncoordinated rapid alternating movements. All of these abnormalities in coordination are associated most commonly with disorders of the cerebellum, but note that the cerebellum needs proprioceptive input to perform its coordinating function. Therefore, ataxia can also be caused by impaired proprioception (e.g., due to nerve, dorsal root, dorsal root ganglia, or spinal cord disease), which is called **sensory ataxia** (see Ch. 8).

Examination of Gait

Gait relies on optimal function of all levels of the nervous system. The pattern of gait can suggest various types of lesions in the central or peripheral nervous system, and in some instances, particular diseases. Examples include:

- **Steppage gait:** The foot is lifted high off the ground and is slapped down. This occurs when there is dorsiflexion weakness causing foot drop (see Ch. 17).
- **Trendelenburg gait:** The pelvis drops toward the opposite side when the weight is balanced on the leg on the affected side during walking. This occurs when there is gluteal muscle weakness.
- **Parkinsonian gait:** Stooped, small-stepped, shuffling gait, with difficulty turning (see Ch. 23).
- **Magnetic gait:** The feet are lifted only briefly off the ground before being returned briskly to the ground (as if a magnet were pulling them down). This can be seen in normal pressure hydrocephalus (see Ch. 22) and with proprioceptive dysfunction (see Ch. 4).
- **Ataxic gait:** A wide-based and unsteady gait. This is seen in cerebellar dysfunction (as can be seen in alcohol intoxication) and severe proprioceptive dysfunction.
- **Spastic gait:** The leg is extended, the foot plantarflexed, and the entire leg **circumducted** (swung out to the side) with each step. If both legs are spastic, this pattern can lead to a **scissor** gait. This is a pattern seen with CNS dysfunction of the motor system (brain, brainstem, and/or spinal cord).

A summary of the localizing value of the various components of the examination is presented in Table 1–1 with references to chapters where these individual components are discussed further.

The General Examination in Neurologic Diagnosis

The general physical examination is also of great importance in patients with neurologic symptoms and signs to evaluate for any signs of systemic disease that may be producing neurologic manifestations. The following are a few of many possible examples. In patients with stroke, a detailed cardiovascular examination should evaluate for carotid bruit (a sign of possible carotid stenosis), cardiac arrhythmia, and cardiac murmur (which could suggest valvular disease including endocarditis). Orthostatic vital signs may be abnormal in patients with autonomic neuropathies (see Ch. 27) and multiple systems atrophy (see Ch. 23). Pallor could suggest anemia, which may be due to vitamin B12 deficiency, a cause of myelopathy and neuropathy. Signs of chronic illness could suggest underlying malignancy, inflammatory disease, or chronic infection (e.g., HIV), all of which can have neurologic manifestations. Characteristic skin findings may be seen in dermatomyositis (see Ch. 30) and in neurocutaneous syndromes such as tuberous sclerosis and neurofibromatosis (see Ch. 24).

Introduction to Neuroimaging & Cerebrospinal Fluid Analysis

Neurodiagnostic tests aid in determining both localization and diagnosis. The main neurodiagnostic tests are: neuroimaging, cerebrospinal fluid (CSF) analysis, electroencephalography (EEG), and electromyography/nerve conduction studies (EMG/NCS). EEG is discussed in the context of the diagnosis of seizures and epilepsy (see Ch. 18) and EMG/NCS in the context of the diagnosis of neuromuscular disease (see Ch. 15 for the principles; Chs. 16, 17 and 27–30 for clinical use). Neuroimaging and CSF analysis are discussed throughout this book, but an introduction to their use and interpretation is provided here.

NEUROIMAGING IN CLINICAL PRACTICE

Neuroimaging allows for visualization of the structures of the neuraxis, and is used as an extension of the neurologic examination. If a patient's symptoms and signs localize to a particular part of the neuraxis, neuroimaging of that region can provide additional information about the underlying pathologic process. The disease-based chapters of Part 2 of this book discuss when neuroimaging should be obtained with regard to particular symptoms and diseases, and how it can aid in diagnosis of various neurologic conditions.

In clinical practice, many patients have undergone neuroimaging studies before a neurologist has evaluated them, and some patients may be referred for neurologic evaluation because of neuroimaging findings rather than clinical findings. In such scenarios, part of the clinical reasoning process is interpreting the neuroimaging in the context of the clinical findings: Do the neuroimaging findings correlate with the patient's clinical presentation? Are there aspects of the patient's clinical presentation that do not have a neuroimaging correlate? Are there incidental findings that have no relationship to the patient's current presentation but require further evaluation or longitudinal clinical and radiologic surveillance? Whether neuroimaging is obtained and reviewed before evaluation of a patient or in the process of a patient's evaluation, neuroimaging must always be interpreted in the context of the patient's history and physical examination in order to prevent misinterpretation/overinterpretation/underinterpretation of radiologic findings.

The cornerstones of neuroimaging of the nervous system are computed tomography (CT) and magnetic resonance imaging (MRI), both of which can be performed with or without intravenous contrast, and both of which can be used to evaluate the cerebral vessels (CT angiography [CTA] and venography [CTV]; MR angiography [MRA] and venography [MRV]). More specialized radiographic techniques used in the evaluation of neurologic diseases include CT and MR perfusion studies, MR spectroscopy, nuclear imaging (positive emission tomography [PET] and single photon emission computed tomography [SPECT]), and transcranial Doppler ultrasound.

What follows is a primer on neuroimaging. It is not intended to be of sufficient scope and detail for radiologists and radiology trainees, but is meant to provide the clinician with an approach to interpreting neuroimaging studies of the brain and spinal cord (bone and extracranial soft tissues are not discussed).

OVERVIEW OF NEUROIMAGING INTERPRETATION

Whether using CT or MRI, and whether evaluating the brain or spine, the two main goals are as follows:

1. Identification of *normal* structures and any disturbance or distortion of these structures: **Is everything there that is supposed to be there, and does it look as it is supposed to look?**

    - Are tissue structures of normal size or is there atrophy or expansion of one or more regions of the brain or spinal cord?

    - Are the fluid compartments of normal size and configuration (i.e., ventricles, cisterns, sulci of the brain; central canal of spinal cord)?

    - Are structures where they are supposed to be or is there herniation (displacement of structures beyond their normal compartments)?

2. Identification and characterization of *abnormal* lesions: **Is there anything there that should not be there, and if so, how can it be characterized?**

    - CT: Are there regions of **hypodensity** (darker than normal tissue density) or **hyperdensity** (brighter than normal tissue density)?

    - MRI: Are there regions of **hypointensity** (darker than normal tissue intensity) or **hyperintensity** (brighter than normal tissue intensity)?

When interpreting neuroimaging studies, it is helpful to begin by scrolling once from top to bottom and then from bottom to top through all obtained sequences, first taking inventory of normal structures and abnormal findings, and then characterizing them in radiographic terms before interpreting them (e.g., "There is a hypodensity spanning the left frontal and temporal lobes with sharply demarcated borders and no other apparent abnormalities."). This will allow for an initial radiologic differential diagnosis that can be aligned with the clinical presentation and will avoid potentially premature conclusions (e.g., focusing on an obvious abnormality at the expense of not noting other more subtle abnormalities or global abnormalities).

The easiest neuroimaging abnormalities to see are asymmetries (e.g., a lesion on one side that contrasts with the normal contralateral side). It can be more challenging to note symmetric abnormalities (e.g., diffuse cerebral edema, symmetric ventriculomegaly, symmetric atrophy), especially when first learning to interpret neuroimaging. This skill emerges over time after reviewing a large number of normal and abnormal studies (just as appreciating what the range of normal is for a physical examination finding such as reflexes requires examining a large number of patients).

The main neuroimaging modalities used to examine the brain and spine are CT and MRI. Noncontrast CT has the advantages of being able to be completed rapidly and being better at analyzing abnormalities of bone. It may be more sensitive than MRI for detecting acute intracranial hemorrhage but is less sensitive for identifying subtle pathologic changes and is particularly insensitive in the posterior fossa (due to beam hardening artifact). MRI has several advantages: greater resolution than CT, increased ability to detect small and/or subtle abnormalities that may not be visible on CT, ability to use different MRI sequences (discussed below) to allow for abnormalities to be viewed in different ways (which aids in characterizing them), and no radiation exposure. Compared to CT, MRI takes longer to perform, is more expensive, and cannot be performed in patients with cardiac pacemakers, other implanted ferromagnetic medical devices, or exposure to shrapnel.

INTERPRETATION OF BRAIN CT

CT can be viewed using different windows that highlight different aspects of the image (e.g., brain vs bone) (Fig. 2–1). CT relies on differences in density of tissues to generate an image. Denser tissues (and some pathologic findings) are brighter (**hyperdense**), whereas less dense tissues (and some pathologic findings) are darker (**hypodense**). At the extremes, bone is the most dense structure on a head CT and appears the brightest, while air (e.g., in the sinuses) is the least dense and is therefore the darkest. CSF is denser than air but not as dense as brain. Brain is denser than CSF. Within the brain, the gray matter is denser than the white matter, so the cortex and deep gray matter structures (basal ganglia and thalamus) are slightly brighter than white matter. The most common CT window used by neurologists is the brain window, which allows for these various structures to be identified and differentiated, but is less sensitive for noting bony abnormalities (e.g., fractures), which are best visualized using the bone window.

Abnormal brain CT findings (e.g., beyond changes in the shape or size of normal structures such as atrophy, ventricular enlargement) can be classified as hyperdensities or hypodensities.

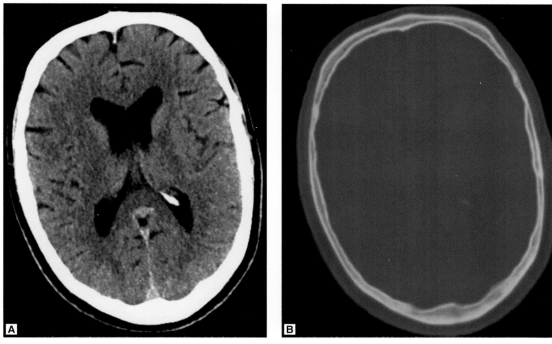

FIGURE 2-1 **Brain and bone windows on head CT. A:** Normal CT of the head, brain window. **B:** Normal CT of the head, bone window.

Causes of Hyperdensity on Brain CT (Fig. 2-2)

The most common causes of hyperdensity in the brain on CT are **hemorrhage** and **calcification**. Contrast enhancement is also hyperdense (see "Contrast-Enhanced Neuroimaging"). The distinction between hemorrhage and calcification as a cause of a CT hyperdensity can generally be made in the context of the clinical history (e.g., acute-onset focal deficits with a corresponding hyperdense lesion suggests hemorrhage), but if there is doubt, Hounsfield units can be determined (60–100 for blood, 100–200 for calcification; for reference, bone is typically greater than 1000). Calcifications may represent normal findings (e.g., in the choroid plexus, in the falx cerebri, in the pineal gland, and in some older individuals in the basal ganglia). Pathologic **hyperdensities** on brain CT can be caused by:

- Acute intracranial hemorrhage (intraparenchymal, intraventricular, subarachnoid, subdural, epidural; see Ch. 19)
- Calcification (tumors or infectious lesions may have calcified components; e.g., neurocysticercosis)
- Hypercellular tumor (e.g., lymphoma)
- Thrombosed blood vessel (e.g., hyperdense vessel sign in acute ischemic stroke and cord sign in venous sinus thrombosis; see Ch. 19)
- Atherosclerotic plaques within arteries
- Contrast-enhancing lesions such as tumor, abscess, acute demyelination, subacute stroke (see "Contrast-Enhanced Neuroimaging")

Causes of Hypodensity on Brain CT (Fig. 2-3)

Pathologic **hypodensities** on brain CT can be caused by:

- Any type of pathology that causes edema: tumor, inflammation, infection, trauma, ischemic stroke (although CT may be normal in the acute phase of ischemic stroke; see Ch. 19)
- Sequelae of prior injury (trauma, infarct, demyelinating lesion)

The differential diagnosis for a discrete region of hypodensity on brain CT includes stroke, tumor, inflammatory lesion, and infectious lesion. Since strokes respect a vascular territory, the hypodensities that they cause generally have clear, distinct borders. In contrast, edema around a tumor, infectious lesion, or an acute demyelinating lesion typically has less distinct boundaries. Additionally, if the hypodensity in question is near the cortical surface, an infarct will most often *include* the cortex since a cortical vessel will supply both the cortex and the underlying white matter. In contrast, most neoplastic, infectious, and demyelinating lesions involve the subcortical white matter and, therefore, the hypodensity caused by such lesions will usually respect the gray–white boundary, sparing the overlying cortex (Fig. 2-3).

INTERPRETATION OF BRAIN MRI

The main clinically important MRI sequences for evaluating the brain are T1, T2, FLAIR, DWI and ADC, and SWI (or GRE) (Fig. 2-4). These sequences differ in the way they are acquired in order to allow for visualization of different types of pathology.

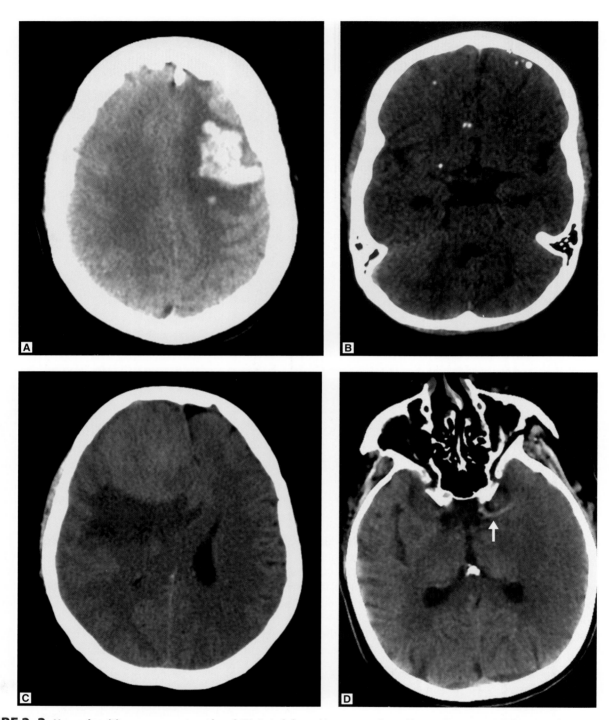

FIGURE 2–2 **Hyperdensities on noncontrast head CT. A:** Left frontal intraparenchymal hemorrhage. **B:** Multifocal calcifications caused by neurocysticercosis. **C:** Hyperdense mass in right frontal lobe (meningioma). **D:** Hyperdense left middle cerebral artery (MCA) in acute ischemic stroke.

T1-weighted, T2-weighted, & FLAIR MRI Sequences

On T1-weighted images, the gray matter appears darker than the white matter, and the CSF is dark. T2-weighted images appear like a "negative" of the T1-weighted images: white

matter is darker than gray matter, and CSF is bright. Most types of pathology in the brain show up as bright (hyperintense) on T2-weighted images and dark (hypointense) on T1-weighted images (e.g., stroke, tumor, infection, edema, demyelination).

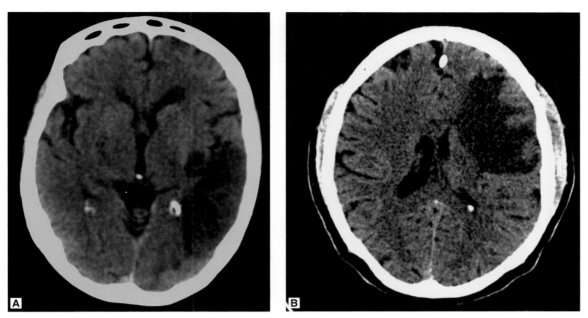

FIGURE 2–3 **Hypodensities on head CT. A:** Left temporo-occipital hypodensity caused by ischemic infarct in the middle cerebral artery territory causing hypodensity that extends to the inner table of the skull. **B:** Left frontal hypodensity due to toxoplasmosis. Note that the lesion respects the gray–white junction, sparing the overlying cortex (see text for explanation).

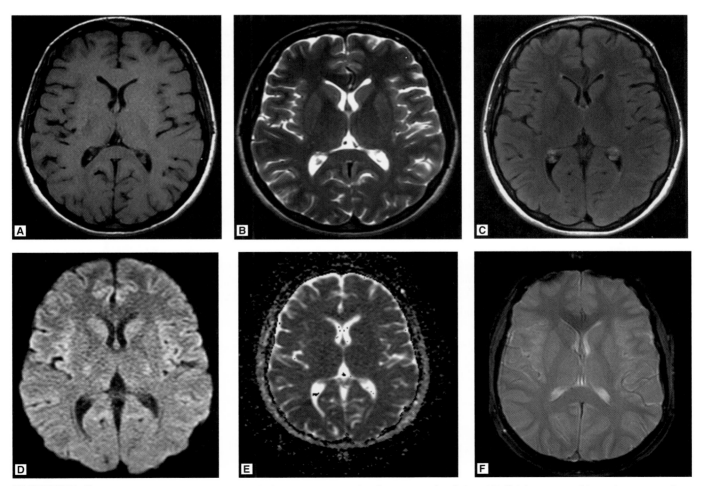

FIGURE 2–4 **MRI sequences (normal MRI of the brain). A:** T1-weighted. **B:** T2-weighted. **C:** FLAIR (fluid-attenuated inversion recovery). **D:** DWI (diffusion-weighted imaging) **E:** ADC (apparent diffusion coefficient) **F:** GRE (gradient echo).

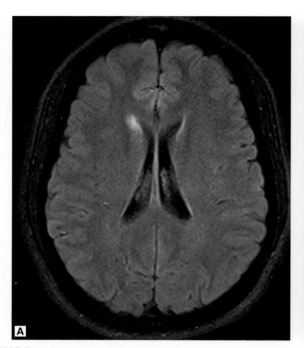
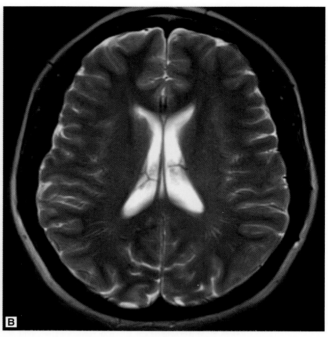

FIGURE 2–5 **FLAIR and T2-weighted MRI sequences demonstrating a periventricular lesion. A:** FLAIR sequence demonstrating hyperintensity adjacent to the frontal horn of the right lateral ventricle that is not well visualized on the corresponding T2 sequence in **B**.

The FLAIR (fluid-attenuated inversion recovery) sequence is a T2-weighted sequence with suppression of the bright CSF signal. By suppressing the bright CSF, the FLAIR sequence makes T2-hyperintense pathology in the brain more easily visible. For example, hyperintensity immediately adjacent to the ventricles may be difficult to visualize on T2-weighted images since the CSF is bright and may make it difficult to distinguish periventricular hyperintensities. FLAIR images resolve this problem by suppressing the CSF signal in the ventricles to make periventricular signal abnormalities more easily visible (Fig. 2–5). T2 hyperintensities in the brainstem may be more effectively visualized on T2-weighted images than on FLAIR images.

In general, T1 images are used to examine brain structure, and T2/FLAIR images are used to look for hyperintensities suggestive of pathology. When contrast is administered, postcontrast T1-weighted images are compared to precontrast T1-weighted images to look for abnormal regions of enhancement (see "Contrast-Enhanced Neuroimaging").

As described above, acute blood on CT is bright (hyperdense). On MRI, blood has different appearances on T1 and T2 sequences depending on the age of the blood, which can therefore help to determine the age of an intracranial hemorrhage (Table 2–1).

Diffusion-Weighted Imaging & Apparent Diffusion Coefficient MRI Sequences (Fig. 2–6)

Diffusion-weighted imaging (DWI) and apparent diffusion coefficient (ADC) sequences evaluate the ease with which

water can diffuse through tissue. The appearance of DWI and ADC sequences can be distinguished from T1 and T2 sequences by the fact that the brain anatomy is much less well defined on DWI/ADC and the scalp and subcutaneous soft tissues are not visible on DWI/ADC. Areas where water diffuses less easily are said to demonstrate **diffusion restriction.** Regions of diffusion restriction appear bright on DWI and dark on ADC. Foci that are bright on DWI but *not* dark on ADC do *not* represent true restricted diffusion (referred to as T2 shine-through if also bright on T2/FLAIR, but may also represent artifact).

DWI and ADC sequences are most commonly used in the evaluation of acute ischemic stroke (see Ch. 19), since acute ischemia may be visible within minutes on DWI and ADC, significantly earlier than any other MRI sequence (the cause of diffusion restriction in acute ischemic stroke is cytotoxic edema). In addition to stroke, diffusion restriction can be seen in Creutzfeldt-Jakob disease (in the cortical ribbon and

TABLE 2–1 **Signal Characteristics of Blood on MRI T1 & T2 Sequences.**

	T1	T2
Hyperacute blood	Isointense	Hyperintense
Acute blood	Isointense	Hypointense
Early subacute blood	Hyperintense	Hypointense
Late subacute blood	Hyperintense	Hyperintense
Chronic blood	Hypointense	Hypointense

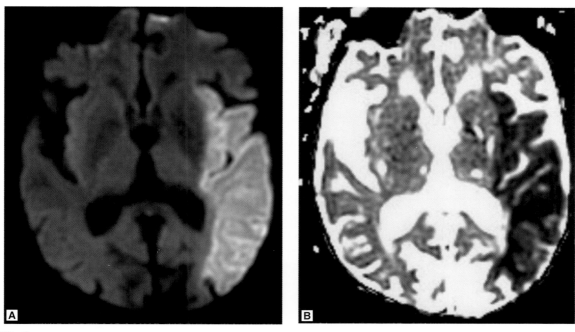

FIGURE 2–6 **DWI and ADC MRI sequences. A:** DWI sequence demonstrating bright region that corresponds to dark region on ADC (**B**) due to ischemic stroke in the left middle cerebral artery (MCA) territory.

basal ganglia [see Ch. 22]), hypercellular lesions (e.g., abscess [see Ch. 20], primary central nervous system lymphoma [see Ch. 24]), and in the setting of seizures (see Ch. 18).

Susceptibility-Weighted Imaging & Gradient Echo MRI Sequences (Fig. 2–7)

Susceptibility-weighted imaging (SWI) and gradient echo (GRE) sequences are mostly used to evaluate for blood, which is dark on these sequences. Calcification is also dark on SWI/GRE sequences. These sequences are particularly sensitive for detecting microhemorrhages (e.g., in the evaluation for cerebral amyloid angiopathy [see Ch. 19]) and may also reveal a thrombosed blood vessel in the setting of acute ischemic stroke or cortical vein or venous sinus thrombosis (see Ch. 19).

MR Spectroscopy (Fig. 2–8)

MR spectroscopy (MRS) quantitatively evaluates brain metabolites. The most common clinically relevant metabolites examined are *N*-acetyl aspartate (NAA) and choline. NAA can be thought of as a measure of neuronal health (higher NAA = healthier neurons; lower NAA = diseased neurons), and choline as a marker of membrane turnover. Decrease in the NAA peak is nonspecific, but the combination of decreased NAA peak and increased choline peak is suggestive of glial neoplasm (although this pattern can also be seen in acute demyelination). Normally, the NAA peak towers over the choline peak, and the angle of a line drawn between them

(Hunter's angle) is about 45 degrees. With glial neoplasms, the choline peak becomes equal to or rises above the NAA peak. Other MRS findings that may be useful in neurologic diagnosis are increased lactate (which can occur with tumor, ischemic stroke, mitochondrial disease) and increased NAA (which can occur in Canavan's disease [see Ch. 31]).

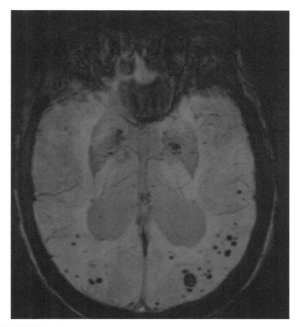

FIGURE 2–7 **GRE MRI sequence.** Multiple microhemorrhages are demonstrated, predominantly in the occipital lobes, in a patient with cerebral amyloid angiopathy (see Ch. 19).

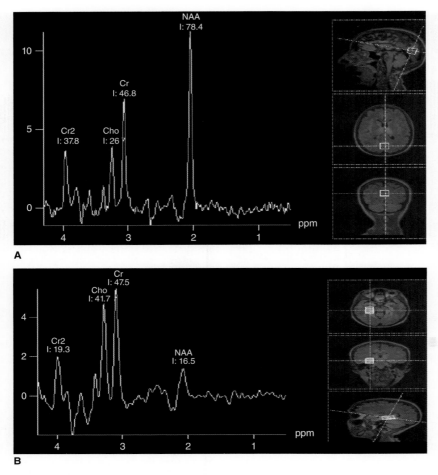

FIGURE 2–8 **MR spectroscopy. A:** MR spectroscopy in a normal region of the brain showing NAA peak towering over choline peak (labeled Cho). **B:** MR spectroscopy in glial neoplasm, showing elevated choline peak (labeled Cho) and reduced NAA peak in a glial neoplasm.

CONTRAST-ENHANCED NEUROIMAGING (FIG. 2–9)

Contrast administration can further improve the sensitivity of neuroimaging in detecting abnormalities, and can also improve the specificity with which the etiology of such abnormalities can be determined. CT uses iodinated contrast, and MRI uses gadolinium contrast. Blood vessels normally enhance with contrast administration, but if the meninges or brain parenchyma enhance, this suggests breakdown of the blood–brain barrier, allowing contrast to leak into these tissues. Contrast enhancement can occur in the setting of tumor, infection, inflammation, and in the subacute period after infarction. Contrast-enhanced images should always be compared to analogous images without contrast: CT with contrast should be compared to noncontrast CT; T1-weighted postcontrast MRI sequences should be compared with T1-weighted precontrast sequences. This is important so that a region that is hyperintense on T1 (or hyperdense on CT) *without* contrast is not mistakenly presumed to enhance with contrast if the region's intrinsic hyperintensity/hyperdensity is not noted on the precontrast image.

Many tumors and infectious lesions show a complete rim of enhancement, whereas demyelinating lesions may show open-rim or C-shaped regions of enhancement (see Ch. 21).

Contrast enhancement in the meninges can be characterized as **leptomeningeal** (affecting the pia and arachnoid) or **pachymeningeal** (affecting the dura) (Fig. 2–10). Leptomeningeal enhancement follows the contour of the surface of the brain, extending into the cerebral sulci and cerebellar folia. Pachymeningeal enhancement appears as a rim around the outer surface of the brain *without* invaginating into the sulci; it often involves other dural structures such as the falx and the tentorium (see Ch. 3). In general, leptomeningeal enhancement is most commonly due to infectious meningitis or malignant disease (leptomeningeal metastases), and pachymeningeal enhancement is most commonly due to inflammatory disease, tumor, or intracranial hypotension. However, some infections may cause pachymeningeal enhancement (e.g., tuberculosis, fungal infections, syphilis), and some inflammatory conditions may cause leptomeningeal enhancement (e.g., sarcoidosis). Pachymeningeal enhancement can also be caused by intracranial hypotension,

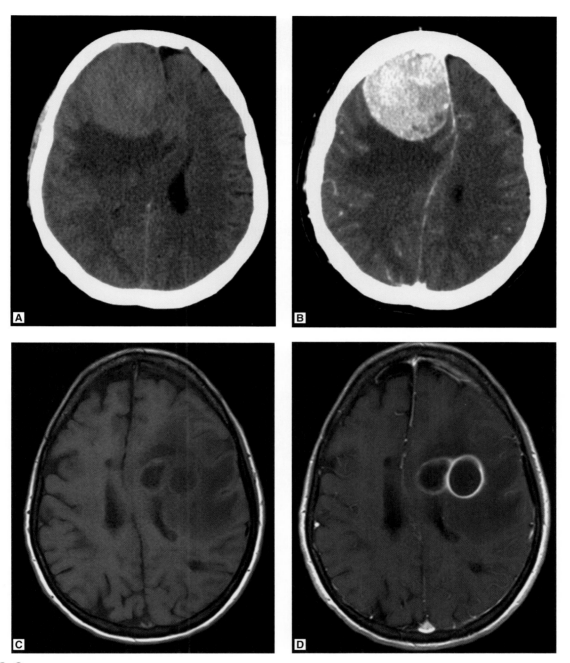

FIGURE 2–9 **Contrast-enhanced neuroimaging. A–B**: Noncontrast (**A**) and postcontrast (**B**) CT showing homogenous enhancement of a right frontal meningioma. **C–D**: T1 precontrast (**C**) and T1 postcontrast (**D**) sequences showing left frontal ring enhancing lesion caused by a cerebral abscess.

in which case the enhancement is typically smooth and uniform (see Ch. 25).

Potential complications of contrast agents include allergic reactions, contrast-induced nephropathy (with iodinated contrast used with CT), and nephrogenic systemic fibrosis (with gadolinium contrast used with MRI). The latter two complications occur in patients with underlying renal disease, so the risks and benefits of contrast in such patients must be carefully weighed, and contrast is generally contraindicated in patients with renal failure.

VASCULAR IMAGING (FIG. 2–11)

CT angiography (CTA) and **MR angiography (MRA)** allow for visualization of the vasculature. In the neck, brain, and spine, these studies can be used to look for aneurysms and other vascular malformations, arterial stenosis, occlusion, or dissection, and vascular irregularities that may suggest vasculopathy (see Ch. 19). MRA can be performed with contrast or without (time of flight imaging). Since time of flight MRA is dependent on flow velocity, the

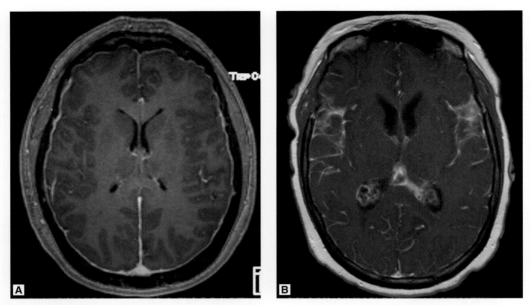

FIGURE 2-10 Meningeal enhancement. A: Pachymeningeal enhancement caused by inflammatory meningitis in a patient with rheumatoid arthritis (note that the enhancement surrounds the brain but does not enter the sulci). **B:** Leptomeningeal enhancement in a patient with bacterial meningitis (note that the enhancement enters the sulci).

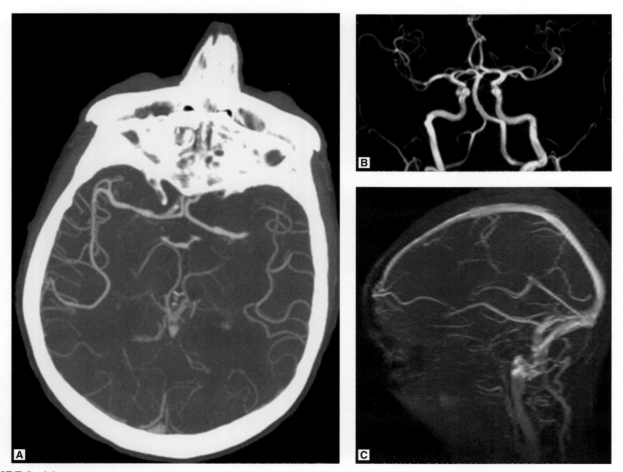

FIGURE 2-11 Vascular imaging. A: CT angiogram (showing left middle cerebral artery cutoff). **B:** MR angiogram (normal). **C:** MR venogram (normal).

degree of vascular stenosis may be overestimated with this technique. CTA (which can only be performed using contrast) allows for more accurate measurement of the degree of arterial stenosis than MRA.

CT venography (CTV) and **MR venography (MRV)** allow for the visualization of the veins and venous sinuses, and are used primarily in the evaluation for venous sinus thrombosis (see Ch. 19).

For patients who cannot undergo CTA (e.g., contrast allergy, renal failure) or MRA (e.g., pacemaker), the carotid arteries can be visualized by **Doppler ultrasound** to assess for carotid artery stenosis (see Ch. 19).

Transcranial Doppler (TCD) ultrasound is used to evaluate the proximal intracranial arteries. It is most commonly used as a screening tool for arterial vasospasm after aneurysmal subarachnoid hemorrhage (see Ch. 19). It can also detect high-intensity transient signals (HITS) that represent emboli passing through the intracranial arteries.

The gold standard for vascular imaging is catheter-based **digital subtraction angiography**. This technique is used most commonly for the evaluation of aneurysms and other vascular malformations, and in the setting of catheter-based interventions for acute stroke and vascular lesions (see Ch. 19).

CT perfusion and **MR perfusion** are used to study cerebral blood volume (CBV), cerebral blood flow (CBF), and mean transit time (MTT). CBV is the amount of blood in a region of the brain, CBF is the volume of blood moving through a region per unit time, and MTT is the average time for blood to traverse a given region. Perfusion imaging can be used to define the boundaries of tissue that is ischemic but not yet infarcted (**ischemic penumbra**), which will have decreased CBF and elevated MTT. Sometimes the CBV can actually be normal or increased in such at-risk regions (**luxury perfusion**).

NUCLEAR MEDICINE STUDIES: POSITRON EMISSION TOMOGRAPHY & SINGLE PHOTON EMISSION COMPUTED TOMOGRAPHY

Positron emission tomography (PET) and single photon emission computed tomography (SPECT) use injections of radioactive substances to evaluate brain metabolism (PET) and brain blood flow (SPECT). Particular patterns of reduced metabolism/blood flow are associated with particular neurodegenerative diseases (e.g., temporoparietal hypometabolism/decreased perfusion in Alzheimer's disease; temporo-parieto-occipital hypometabolism/decreased perfusion in dementia with Lewy bodies; frontotemporal hypometabolism/decreased perfusion in frontotemporal lobar degeneration, see Ch. 22). PET and SPECT are also used to aid in localization of an epileptic focus in patients undergoing evaluation for epilepsy surgery. Ictal SPECT is used to assess for a focal region of increased blood flow during seizures, and interictal PET evaluates for a focal region of hypometabolism between seizures (see Ch. 18).

NEUROIMAGING OF THE SPINE (FIG. 2–12)

X-ray, CT, and MRI can all be used to evaluate the spine. MRI is the most sensitive technique for evaluating the spinal cord and nerve roots, but x-ray and CT provide excellent visualization of bony structures. Like brain imaging, interpretation of spine imaging requires identifying normal structures and any abnormalities within them. Vertebrae should be assessed for alignment and fracture, and intervertebral disc spaces should be evaluated for appropriate height or displacement of the intervertebral discs. The spinal cord should be completely surrounded by CSF (bright on T2-weighted images). Loss of this CSF space suggests either compression from outside of the spinal cord (e.g., spondylosis, disc prolapse, epidural hematoma or abscess) or expansion of the cord itself (e.g., due to intramedullary tumor, infection, or inflammation). As with brain MRI, T2-weighted sequences are ideal for evaluating for pathologic hyperintensity in the cord, which could represent tumor, demyelination, infarction, or infection. Contrast administration can aid in identification of abnormalities. The nerve roots should be evaluated for compression (e.g., due to spondylosis or disc prolapse) and enhancement. Nerve root enhancement can occur in inflammatory conditions (e.g., Guillain-Barré syndrome, chronic inflammatory demyelinating polyradiculoneuropathy, and sarcoidosis) and due to leptomeningeal metastases.

On a midsagittal view of the cervical spine, C2 can be identified as the triangular shape at the top of the vertebral column anterior to the spinal cord, and subsequent cervical vertebrae can be numbered downward from there (Fig. 2–12A). On a midsagittal view of the lumbar spine, S1 can be identified as the first trapezoid-shaped vertebra, and the lumbar vertebrae can be numbered upward from there (Fig. 2–12C).

CEREBROSPINAL FLUID ANALYSIS (TABLE 2–2)

Lumbar puncture allows for the evaluation of the following parameters in the CSF:

- CSF pressure
- CSF chemistry: glucose and protein
- CSF cell counts and types: red and white blood cells, cytology, flow cytometry
- CSF microbiology: cultures, polymerase chain reaction (PCR), and antibodies
- Special studies:
  - Oligoclonal bands (see Ch. 21)
  - Paraneoplastic antibody panels (see Ch. 24)
  - Biomarkers for neurodegenerative diseases (e.g., Aβ-42, tau, 14-3-3, RT-QUIC) (see Ch. 22)

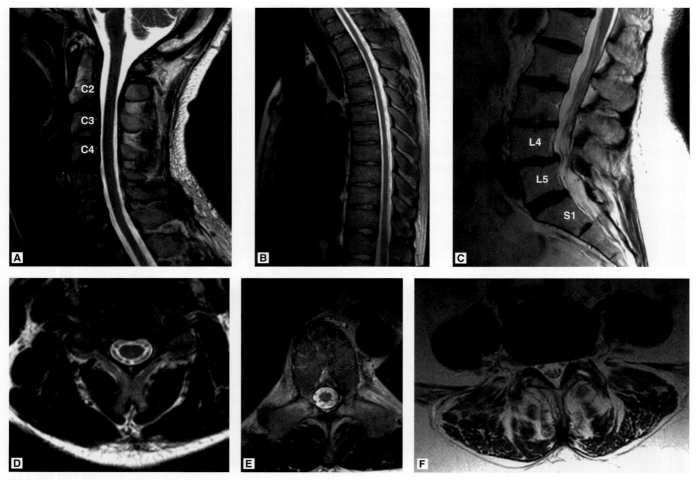

FIGURE 2–12   MRI of the spine. T2-weighted images of the cervical (**A, D**), thoracic (**B, E**), and lumbosacral (**C, F**) spine. **A:** Midsagittal view of the cervical spine, with C2, C3, and C4 vertebrae labeled. **B:** Midsagittal view of the thoracic spine. **C:** Midsagittal view of the lumbosacral spine with L4, L5, and S1 vertebrae labeled (note disc bulge at L4–L5). **D:** Axial view of the cervical spine. **E:** Axial view of the thoracic spine. **F:** Axial view of the lumbosacral spine (roots of the cauda equina are visible in the spinal canal).

CSF Pressure

CSF pressure is ascertained by attaching a manometer to the spinal needle. Measurement of CSF pressure should be made with the patient in the lateral decubitus position with the legs extended. Normal pressure is below 20 cm H_2O (200 mm H_2O). CSF pressure can be elevated due to any process raising intracranial pressure (intracranial hypertension), and can be decreased in any condition decreasing intracranial pressure (intracranial hypotension) (see Ch. 25).

CSF Chemistry: Glucose & Protein
CSF Glucose

CSF glucose should be approximately 60% of serum glucose. CSF glucose can be decreased in bacterial, fungal, and tubercular CNS infections (but not viral infections; see Table 20–2), as well as with leptomeningeal metastases (see Ch. 24). **Hypoglycorrhachia** is the technical term for decreased CSF glucose. Although the reason for decreased CSF glucose in CNS

infections is sometimes taught as the "infectious pathogens consuming the glucose," decreased CSF glucose in infection may be due to a combination of factors including impaired transport into the CSF in infectious states involving the meninges, CNS hypermetabolism in infectious states, and consumption of glucose by white blood cells.

A rare cause of decreased CSF glucose is GLUT1 deficiency, a rare genetic cause of infantile epilepsy due to a defect in a transporter of glucose (GLUT1) across the blood–brain barrier.

Increased CSF glucose can be seen when there is serum hyperglycemia.

CSF Protein

CSF protein should normally be less than 50 mg/dL. CSF protein can be elevated in any inflammatory or infectious state. CSF protein may also be elevated when there is obstructed circulation of CSF due to spinal lesions (spinal block); when extreme, this may cause the CSF to coagulate in the test tube (**Froin's syndrome**).

TABLE 2–2 Causes of Cerebrospinal Fluid Abnormalities.

	Increased	Decreased
Pressure	Intracranial hypertension	Intracranial hypotension
Glucose	Hyperglycemia	Bacterial, fungal, tuberculous CNS infection
		Leptomeningeal carcinomatosis
		GLUT1 Deficiency
Protein	Inflammation	(Normal <50 mg/dL)
	Infection	
	Spinal block	
	Leptomeningeal carcinomatosis	
WBC	Inflammation	(Normal is 0–5/mm^3)
	Infection	
	CNS hematologic malignancy	
RBC	Subarachnoid hemorrhage	(Normal is 0–5/mm^3)
	Traumatic lumbar puncture	
	Hemorrhagic encephalitis	

CSF Cell Counts & Cell Types

White Blood Cells in the CSF

The normal range of white blood cells (WBCs) in the CSF is 0–5 WBCs/mm^3. Increases in CSF WBC count can occur due to CNS infection, inflammation, and CNS hematologic malignancy (e.g., CNS lymphoma).

Polymorphonuclear cells (neutrophils) predominate in bacterial meningitis but may also be seen early in viral meningitis/encephalitis, whereas lymphocytes are generally predominant in viral, fungal, and tubercular CNS infections, CNS inflammation, and lymphoma. Flow cytometry can be used to characterize WBC populations in the CSF to evaluate for hematologic malignancy. Cytology can examine cells to look for malignant cells as can be seen in CNS lymphoma and leptomeningeal metastases from systemic cancer (see Ch. 24).

Red Blood Cells in the CSF

The normal range of RBCs in the CSF is 0–5 RBCs/mm^3. Elevated RBC can be seen in subarachnoid hemorrhage (see Ch. 19) or if a lumbar puncture is traumatic, causing bleeding into the CSF (see "Traumatic Lumbar Puncture"). If blood is present from subarachnoid hemorrhage, it will have been present in the CSF for some time and RBCs will have begun to break down. In contrast, a traumatic lumbar puncture will yield fresh RBCs that have not yet had the time to

break down. **Xanthochromia,** a yellow tinge to the CSF (more sensitively detected by spectrophotometry) is an indication of broken-down red blood cells in the CSF, suggesting that they were there prior to the lumbar puncture (i.e., suggestive of subarachnoid hemorrhage rather than traumatic lumbar puncture).

CSF Microbiology: Cultures, PCR, & Antibodies

Examination of CSF for a pathogen causing CNS infection can include Gram stain, culture, PCR, and evaluation for CSF production of IgM or IgG against a particular pathogen (see Ch. 20).

Patterns of CSF Abnormalities

Several patterns of CSF abnormalities are important to recognize.

Elevated Protein With No or Few Cells (Albuminocytologic Dissociation)

Albuminocytologic dissociation is suggestive of an inflammatory process. While this pattern is generally learned by most medical students as the classic finding in Guillain-Barré syndrome, it is a nonspecific indicator of inflammation and can be seen in chronic inflammatory demyelinating polyradiculoneuropathy (CIDP; see Ch. 27), CNS paraneoplastic conditions (see Ch. 24), acute disseminated encephalomyelitis (see Ch. 21), transverse myelitis (see Ch. 21), and primary CNS vasculitis (see Ch. 19). (Why does the CSF demonstrate an inflammatory pattern in peripheral nervous system disorders such as Guillain-Barré syndrome and CIDP? These disorders involve the nerve roots which pass through the CSF space.)

Elevated WBCs & Protein With Normal Glucose

This is suggestive of a viral process.

Elevated WBCs & Protein With Low Glucose

This pattern generally indicates a nonviral CNS infection (bacterial, fungal, or tubercular). The most extreme values for low glucose, elevated WBCs, and elevated protein are seen with CNS bacterial infections.

In CNS bacterial infections, the WBCs are predominantly neutrophils, whereas they are predominantly lymphocytes in other types of CNS infections (see Table 20–2 in Ch. 20).

Traumatic Lumbar Puncture

Elevations of protein and WBCs can occur in a traumatic lumbar puncture since there is contamination of the CSF with peripheral blood. Protein elevation and WBC elevation are both approximately 1 per 1000 RBCs (1 mg/dL of protein per 1000 RBCs/mm^3, and 1 WBC/mm^3 per 700–1000 RBCs/mm^3).

Additional Tests of CSF

Oligoclonal bands are a nonspecific marker of CNS inflammation, denoting intrathecal synthesis of IgG. Although they are most commonly assessed in the evaluation for multiple sclerosis (see Ch. 21), they can be seen in any CNS infectious or inflammatory condition.

CSF evaluation for antibodies causing CNS paraneoplastic syndromes (e.g., paraneoplastic limbic encephalitis, paraneoplastic cerebellar degeneration; see Ch. 24) is often more sensitive than serum evaluation.

14-3-3 protein is a nonspecific marker of neuronal degeneration. Although it can be present in Creuzfeldt-Jakob disease, the test is neither sensitive nor specific, and has largely been replaced by RT-QUIC for the diagnosis of this condition (see Ch. 22).

The ratio of amyloid-beta 42 ($A\beta$-42) to tau is a biomarker for Alzheimer's disease, discussed further in Chapter 22.

Overview of the Anatomy of the Nervous System

The nervous system serves three main functions: **perception, cognition**, and **action**. **Perception** is the translation of the outer world into electrochemical signals that can be interpreted by the brain. For example, light information is converted by the retina and then sent to the brain by the optic nerves (cranial nerve 2); sound is transformed by the inner ear apparatus and transmitted to the brain via the auditory nerves (cranial nerve 8). **Action** is the brain's way of allowing the organism to interact with the environment by moving the body (and in the case of humans and some other animals, by using movements of the vocal apparatus to communicate). **Cognition** includes all of the operations that interpret perceptual input to understand the external environment, and plan the interaction with the environment through action.

In neuroanatomic terms, perception is carried out by the input to the nervous system (**afferent** pathways), action is the output (**efferent** pathways), and cognition arises from interconnections within and between perceptual modalities, as well as between perception and action. Perception begins with the sense organs (skin, eyes, ears, nose, tongue) and travels in peripheral nerves (including cranial nerves for the structures of the head), ultimately transmitting information to the sensory cortices of the cerebral hemispheres (e.g., somatosensory cortex, visual cortex, auditory cortex). Motor output is controlled by the motor cortex, whose signals travel by way of the motor pathways to ultimately reach the peripheral nerves that will command muscles to move (see Ch. 4). The motor cortex collaborates with adjacent structures (premotor and supplementary motor cortices) and participates in circuits involving the basal ganglia (see Ch. 7) and cerebellum (see Ch. 8), all of which work to coordinate and execute movements.

CENTRAL NERVOUS SYSTEM (CNS) & PERIPHERAL NERVOUS SYSTEM (PNS) (FIG. 3–1)

The central nervous system (CNS) consists of the brain, brainstem, cerebellum, and spinal cord. The peripheral nervous system (PNS) includes the nerve roots that enter (dorsal roots) and exit (ventral roots) the spinal cord and continue into the peripheral nerves. Before devoting the rest of this chapter to the internal and external structures of the brain, a brief orientation to the brainstem, spinal cord, and cerebellum is provided here. The brainstem is divided into three levels from superior to inferior: **midbrain**, **pons**, and **medulla** (see Ch. 9). The medulla transitions inferiorly into the spinal cord, which itself is divided into four levels: cervical, thoracic, lumbar, and sacral (see Ch. 5). The cerebellum lies posterior to the brainstem and inferior to the posterior aspect of the cerebral hemispheres, and is connected to the brainstem by way of the three cerebellar peduncles (see Ch. 8).

HEMISPHERES & LOBES OF THE BRAIN (FIG. 3–2)

The brain is divided into two **hemispheres** (left and right), each of which is divided into four **lobes** (frontal, temporal, parietal, and occipital). In order to maximize surface to volume ratio of the brain in the skull, the cortical surface folds during development. The folds are called **gyri**, and the spaces between them are called **sulci.** Large divisions between the hemispheres or lobes are referred to as **fissures**.

The left and right hemispheres are separated by the **longitudinal (interhemispheric) fissure**. The frontal lobe is in

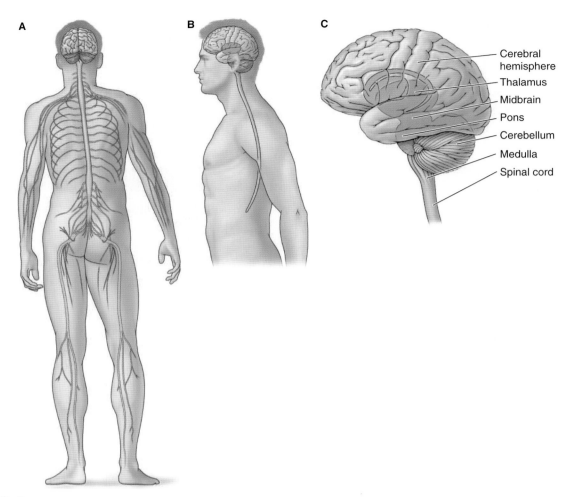

FIGURE 3–1 **The neuraxis. A:** Schematic of posterior view of the neuraxis. **B:** Schematic of lateral view of the central nervous system. **C:** Schematic of lateral view of the brain and brainstem. The central nervous system includes the brain, brainstem, cerebellum, and spinal cord. The peripheral nervous system includes the nerve roots and nerves (shown in yellow in [**A**]). The brainstem is composed of the midbrain, pons, and medulla (**C**). Reproduced with permission from Martin J: *Neuroanatomy Text and Atlas*, 4th ed. New York, NY: McGraw Hill; 2012.

the front, the occipital lobe is at the back (at the occiput), and the parietal lobe is between the occipital and frontal lobes. The temporal lobe is inferior to these three lobes. The frontal lobe is separated from the parietal lobe by the **central sulcus**. The frontal lobe is separated from the temporal lobe by the **Sylvian fissure**. The parietal lobe and occipital lobe have no clear boundary on the lateral surface of the brain, but are separated by the **parieto-occipital sulcus** on the medial surface of the brain.

GRAY MATTER & WHITE MATTER OF THE BRAIN & SPINAL CORD (FIG. 3–3)

The nervous system is composed of **neurons** and supporting cells (**glia**). The cell bodies of neurons comprise the **gray matter**, and their myelinated axons form the **white matter**. In the brain, cell bodies are found in the **cortex** on the outer surface of the brain, and the axons from those cell bodies travel in the subcortical white matter. There are also "islands" of subcortical gray matter structures within the subcortical white matter such as the basal ganglia and thalamus, which form nodes in a variety of networks, most of which begin and/ or end in the cortex (see Ch. 7).

In the spinal cord, the gray matter is on the inside, and the white matter is on the outside.

THE MENINGES: COVERINGS OF THE BRAIN & SPINAL CORD (FIG. 3–4)

The brain and spinal cord are covered by several protective layers called the **meninges**. The meninges have three layers. From external to internal these are the **dura mater**, **arachnoid**, and **pia mater**. The dura mater (literally "tough mother") is a tough outer "skin" that covers the entire brain,

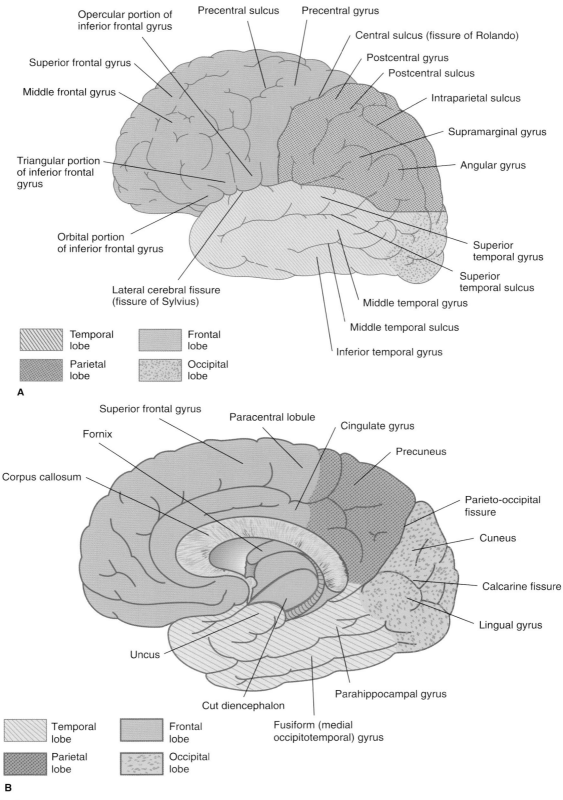

FIGURE 3–2 **The cerebral hemispheres. A:** Schematic of left lateral view. **B:** Schematic of midsagittal view. Reproduced with permission from Waxman S: *Clinical Neuroanatomy*, 27th ed. New York, NY: McGraw Hill; 2013.

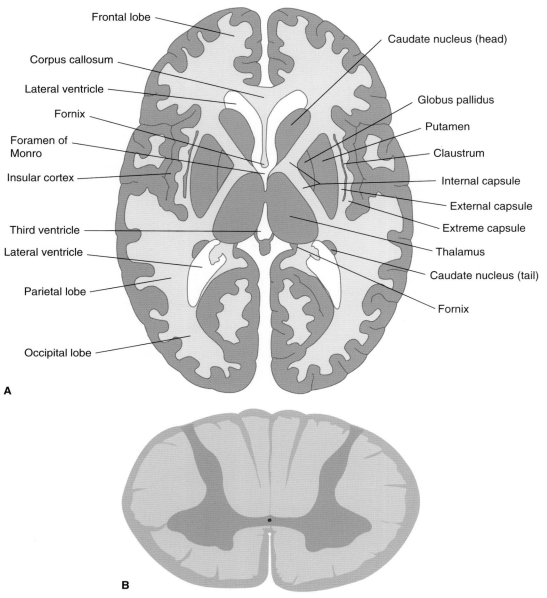

FIGURE 3–3 **Gray matter and white matter of the cerebral hemispheres and spinal cord. A:** Schematic of axial section of the cerebral hemispheres. **B:** Schematic of axial section of the spinal cord. Reproduced with permission from Waxman S: *Clinical Neuroanatomy*, 27th ed. New York, NY: McGraw Hill; 2013.

with folds that extend between the hemispheres (**falx cerebri**) and between the cerebral hemispheres and cerebellum (**tentorium cerebelli**). The dura surrounds the brain but does not invaginate into the sulci. The outer surface of the dura mater is tightly affixed to the skull.

The arachnoid is a thin membrane beneath the dura mater. Like the dura mater, the arachnoid also does not invaginate into the sulci. The dura mater can be thought of as being similar to the thick peel of an orange, and the arachnoid can be thought of as similar to the thin skin below the peel of an orange that can also be peeled off.

The pia mater is the only one of the three meningeal layers that invaginates into the sulci and therefore contacts the entire surface area of the brain.

The pia and arachnoid are collectively referred to as the **leptomeninges**, and the dura mater is referred to as the **pachymeninges** (*pachy* means thick, as used in the term *pachy*derm meaning elephant). In general, infectious meningitis predominantly affects the leptomeninges and inflammatory meningitis predominantly affects the pachymeninges, although there are exceptions (e.g., neurosarcoidosis can affect the leptomeninges, and tuberculosis and fungal infections can affect the

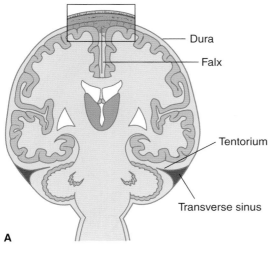

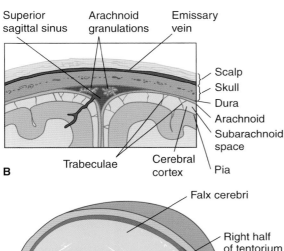

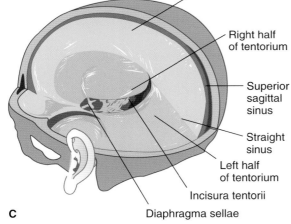

FIGURE 3–4 The meninges. A: Schematic of coronal section of the cerebral hemispheres showing surrounding dura mater. **B:** Schematic of detailed view of meninges. **C:** Schematic of relationship of dural folds and cerebral venous sinuses. Reproduced with permission from Waxman S: *Clinical Neuroanatomy*, 27th ed. New York, NY: McGraw Hill; 2013.

pachymeninges). Metastatic cancer can affect the leptomeninges or the pachymeninges.

The space between the bone and dura is the **epidural space**, the space between the dura and arachnoid is the **subdural space**, and the space between the arachnoid and pia is the **subarachnoid space**. Pathologic processes can lead to blood or infection in any of these spaces: epidural hematoma, subdural hematoma, and subarachnoid hemorrhage (see Ch. 19); epidural abscess, subdural empyema, and meningitis (infectious meningitis predominantly involves the leptomeninges and subarachnoid space; see Ch. 20).

THE CEREBRAL VENOUS SINUSES (FIG. 3–5)

Although arterial blood supply to the CNS will be discussed in more detail in relation to specific brain and brainstem regions (see Ch. 7), the venous drainage of the brain is discussed here since it is anatomically related to the meninges. The venous drainage from the brain ultimately ends up in the internal jugular veins that travel to the superior vena cava by way of the subclavian veins. To arrive in the jugular veins, the blood travels in venous sinuses formed by folds of dura.

The **superior sagittal sinus** travels along the superior surface of the brain at the midline and descends posteriorly to empty into the bilateral **transverse sinuses**. The transverse sinuses travel laterally through folds in the tentorium cerebelli and pass into the **sigmoid sinuses**, which empty into the **jugular veins**. The deep structures of the brain are drained by the **internal cerebral veins** and the **basal veins of Rosenthal**. These empty into the **great vein of Galen**, which empties into the **straight sinus**. The straight sinus joins the transverse sinuses and superior sagittal sinus at the **confluence of sinuses** (also called the **torcula**).

The lateral hemispheres are drained by superficial cortical veins. The largest of these are the veins of Trolard and Labbé. Mnemonic: **T**rolard is on **t**op and **L**abbé is **l**ower and more **l**ateral.

When venous drainage is impaired (e.g., due to venous sinus thrombosis), intracranial pressure rises, which can cause headache, visual disturbances, and ultimately coma. If pressure in the venous system rises to a sufficient level, intracerebral or subarachnoid hemorrhage can occur, causing focal deficits (see "Cerebral Venous Sinus Thrombosis and Cortical Vein Thrombosis" in Ch. 19).

THE VENTRICULAR SYSTEM & CEREBROSPINAL FLUID FLOW (FIGS. 3–6 AND 3–7)

The brain and spinal cord are bathed in cerebrospinal fluid (CSF) in order to provide buoyancy so as to create a shock absorber in the case of trauma. The CSF is produced in the **choroid plexus**, which lines the ventricles. The two **lateral ventricles** drain into the **third ventricle** via the **foramina of**

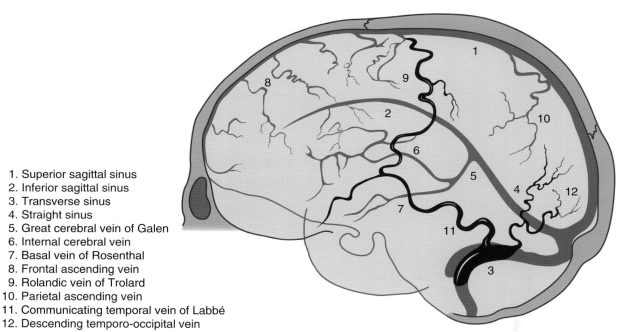

1. Superior sagittal sinus
2. Inferior sagittal sinus
3. Transverse sinus
4. Straight sinus
5. Great cerebral vein of Galen
6. Internal cerebral vein
7. Basal vein of Rosenthal
8. Frontal ascending vein
9. Rolandic vein of Trolard
10. Parietal ascending vein
11. Communicating temporal vein of Labbé
12. Descending temporo-occipital vein

A

B   **Sagittal view**   **C**   **Posterior view**

FIGURE 3–5 **Cerebral venous sinuses. A:** Schematic lateral view of cerebral venous sinuses. **B–C:** Magnetic resonance venogram (MRV) in lateral view (**B**) and posterior coronal view (**C**). A, Reproduced with permission from List CF, Burge CH, Hodges FJ: *Intracranial angiography, Radiology* 1945;45(1):1-14.

Monro (one for each lateral ventricle). The CSF then flows from the third ventricle to the **fourth ventricle** (between the brainstem and cerebellum) by way of the **cerebral aqueduct** in the midbrain. The fourth ventricle is continuous with the central canal of the spinal cord. From the fourth ventricle, CSF can exit the ventricular system into the subarachnoid space via the foramen of **M**agendie (**m**idline) and the foramina of **L**uschka (**l**ateral) to bathe the outer surface of the

brain and spinal cord. CSF is then reabsorbed via the arachnoid granulations into the venous sinuses. CSF is produced at a rate of approximately half a liter per day (approximately 20 mL per hour).

Disruption of CSF flow due to obstruction anywhere along this pathway can lead to **hydrocephalus**. Hydrocephalus can be classified as **communicating** or **noncommunicating**. The "communication" in question refers to the ability of the

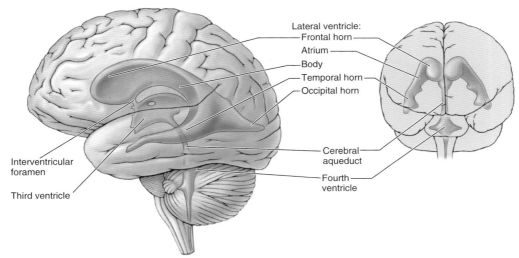

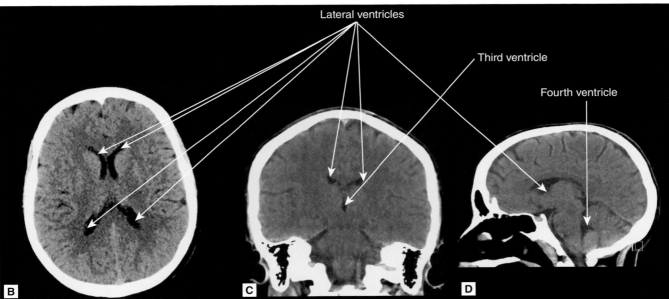

FIGURE 3-6 **The ventricular system and cerebrospinal fluid flow. A:** Schematic of the ventricular system in relation to the brain. **B–D:** CT images with ventricles labeled (**B.** Axial image, **C.** Coronal image, **D.** Sagittal image). A, Reproduced with permission from Waxman S: *Clinical Neuroanatomy*, 27th ed. New York, NY: McGraw Hill; 2013.

ventricles to communicate with one another. **Noncommunicating hydrocephalus** signifies a blockage in the ventricular system itself (e.g., by a tumor, mass effect from a large stroke with edema, intraventricular hemorrhage) such that the ventricles proximal to the obstruction dilate. **Communicating hydrocephalus** occurs when there is failure of CSF reabsorption in the arachnoid granulations such that the ventricles can still communicate with one another but hydrocephalus develops since CSF cannot be absorbed. In communicating hydrocephalus, all of the ventricles dilate.

The distinction between communicating and noncommunicating hydrocephalus is important because in chronic **communicating hydrocephalus**, lumbar puncture can relieve pressure from the ventricular system (e.g., in cryptococcal meningitis [see Ch. 20] and normal pressure hydrocephalus [see Ch. 22]), whereas in **noncommunicating hydrocephalus**, the elevated intracranial pressure proximal to the obstruction can lead to herniation if fluid is removed from below by lumbar puncture (see Ch. 25).

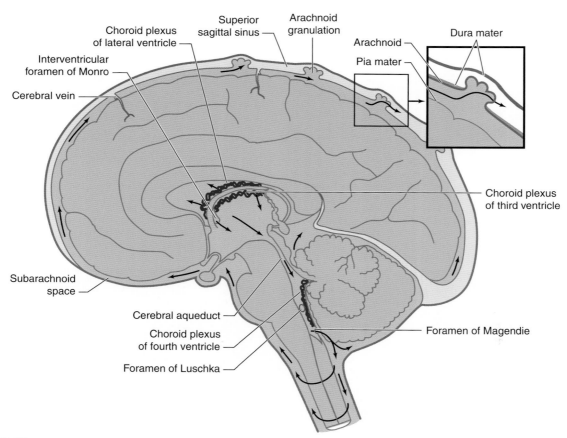

FIGURE 3–7   Schematic of CSF flow. Reproduced with permission from Aminoff M, Greenberg D, Simon R: *Clinical Neurology*, 9th ed. New York, NY: McGraw Hill; 2015.

The Motor and Somatosensory Pathways & Approach to Weakness and Sensory Loss

The cerebral hemispheres are where the motor pathways originate, and where the somatosensory pathways terminate. The left cerebral hemisphere controls the motor functions of the right side of the body, and the right cerebral hemisphere controls the motor functions of the left side of the body. This crossed system is maintained in other modalities including the somatosensory and visual pathways: If the left hemisphere controls the right side of the body, it makes sense that it would need somatosensory information about the right side of the body and visual information about the right side of the world.

There are three main clinically relevant tracts for motor and somatosensory function for the body—one motor and two sensory—that span the brain, brainstem, and spinal cord:

- Motor: The **corticospinal tracts** send motor information from the cortex to the spinal cord as the name suggests.
- Sensory: The **anterolateral (or spinothalamic) tracts** and **dorsal (or posterior) column pathways** bring sensory input from the spinal cord to the brain by way of the brainstem. The names of these pathways refer to their anatomic positions within the spinal cord.

In this chapter, the anatomy of these pathways will be described, providing a foundation for localizing symptoms of weakness and sensory changes, and also laying out anatomic landmarks in the brain, brainstem, and spinal cord that

will serve as points of orientation as additional pathways are described in subsequent chapters.

THE CORTICOSPINAL TRACTS (FIG. 4–1)

The corticospinal tracts convey the motor plan from the cerebral cortex to the spinal cord—specifically to the alpha motor neurons of the anterior (ventral) horns of the spinal cord. These alpha motor neurons exit the spinal cord as ventral roots that then travel through plexuses and peripheral nerves to relay impulses to the muscles. The corticospinal tracts are sometimes referred to as the **pyramidal system** (since they travel for part of their course in the medullary pyramids). The **extrapyramidal system** includes the basal ganglia and cerebellum, which participate in circuits with the motor cortex and are involved in action initiation and coordination (see Chs. 7 and 8).

Each corticospinal tract begins in the motor cortex, which is located in the precentral gyrus (immediately anterior to the central sulcus). The motor cortex is organized by the region of the body it controls: face lateral, hand and arm superior to this, and leg and foot most medial (with arm and leg representations connected at the shoulder/hip such that the hand is most lateral and the foot most medial with the arm

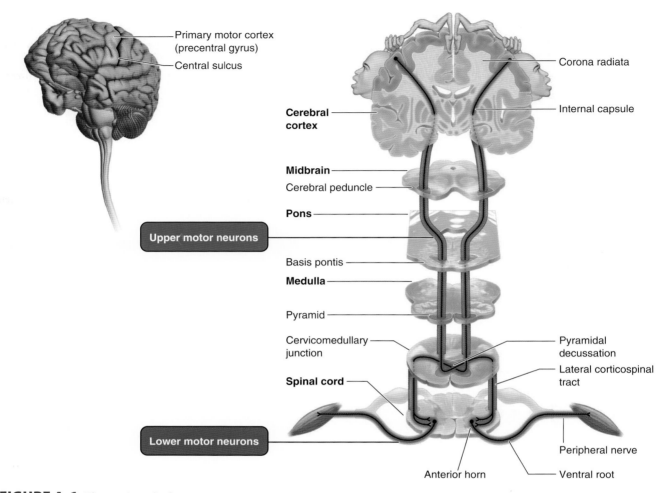

FIGURE 4–1 **The corticospinal tract.**

and leg between). This cortical map of the regions of the body is referred to as the **homunculus**.

The cell bodies from layer 5 of the motor cortex give rise to axons that travel in the subcortical white matter (specifically in the posterior limb of the internal capsule), then in the ventral/anterior brainstem (cerebral peduncles of the midbrain, basis pontis of the pons, and medullary pyramids of the medulla). At the junction of the medulla and the cervical spinal cord (cervicomedually junction), the corticospinal tracts cross (decussate), such that the corticospinal tract that began in the left hemisphere descends on the right side of the spinal cord and the corticospinal tract that began in the right hemisphere descends on the left side of the spinal cord.

Once in the spinal cord, the main clinically relevant corticospinal tracts are situated posterolaterally. In the spinal cord, the axons that have traveled all the way from the contralateral motor cortex synapse on alpha motor neurons in the anterior horns of the spinal cord gray matter. Axons of the alpha motor neurons leave the ventral/anterior spinal cord via ventral roots and enter peripheral nerves to travel to muscles.

For clinical purposes, the pyramidal motor system can be considered as a two-neuron system. First-order neurons have their cell bodies in the motor cortex (precentral gyrus), and their axons travel through the internal capsule, brainstem, and spinal cord (the corticospinal tract). Second-order neurons have their cell bodies in the anterior horn of the spinal cord, and their axons travel through nerve roots and peripheral nerves. The neurons of the central nervous system (CNS) component in the brain/brainstem/spinal cord (i.e., the corticospinal tract) are referred to as **upper motor neurons**, and the neurons of the peripheral nervous system (PNS) component (anterior horn of the spinal cord through the ventral roots into peripheral nerves) are referred to as **lower motor neurons**.

Two key anatomical points for clinical localization of weakness are:

• The corticospinal tracts *cross at the cervicomedullary junction*.

• The system is *divided into upper motor neurons (CNS) and lower motor neurons (PNS)*.

Because of the crossing (decussation) of the corticospinal tracts at the cervicomedullary junction, unilateral corticospinal tract lesions in the brain or brainstem cause *contralateral* weakness (i.e., on the *opposite* side of the body from the

TABLE 4–1 Upper & Lower Motor Neuron Signs.

	Upper Motor Neuron (CNS: Brain, Brainstem, Spinal Cord)	Lower Motor Neuron (PNS: Root, Plexus, Nerve)
Tone	Increased ("Up")	Decreased ("Lower")
Reflexes	Increased ("Up")	Decreased or absent ("Lower")
Babinski's sign	Present (Toe Goes "Up")	Absent (Toe Goes "Lower")
Muscle bulk	(Generally preserved except with prolonged disuse)	Atrophy ("Lower" bulk)
Fasciculations	Absent	May be present

lesion), whereas unilateral spinal cord lesions cause *ipsilateral* weakness (i.e., on the *same* side of the body as the lesion). Lesions in individual roots and nerves cause weakness in the particular muscle(s) they supply.

Upper Motor Neuron Lesions Versus Lower Motor Neuron Lesions (Table 4–1)

Understanding the differences in the clinical signs caused by upper motor neuron lesions (CNS) versus lower motor neuron lesions (PNS) is an essential component of the assessment of weakness. With upper motor neuron lesions, all of the signs go up: reflexes are "up" (increased: **hyperreflexia**), tone is "up" (increased: **spasticity**), and the big toe may go up when stroking the bottom of the foot (**Babinski sign**; for discussion of other related signs, see Ch. 1).

With lower motor neuron lesions, nearly all of the signs are *lowered*: diminished or absent reflexes (**hyporeflexia** or **areflexia**), decreased (**flaccid**) tone, decreased muscle bulk (**atrophy**), toes downgoing (no Babinski sign). Abnormal muscle twitches called **fasciculations** can occur with diseases affecting lower motor neurons. Fasciculations are an example of a sign of *increased* activity due to lower motor neuron dysfunction, and are therefore an exception to the "up" and "low" mnemonic for signs associated with pathology of upper and lower motor neurons (Table 4–1).

Another upper motor neuron sign is the **Hoffmann sign**, which can be thought of as a Babinski sign for the upper extremity. To see if a Hoffmann sign is present, the examiner holds the patient's hand by the middle finger with one hand, and uses the other hand to quickly flick the tip of the middle finger (as if snapping one's fingers, but with the patient's finger between). If a Hoffmann sign is present, the fingers and thumb will flex. As with the Babinski sign, this sign is indicative of upper motor neuron (CNS) dysfunction.

Another upper motor neuron sign that can be seen in the lower extremities is **triple flexion:** If the big toe is pinched, this stimulates simultaneous dorsiflexion, knee flexion, and hip flexion. The triple flexion response may also be observed as part of the Babinski sign.

A very important clinical point is that some of the classic upper motor neuron findings such as increased tone and hyperreflexia are often *not* present acutely after a CNS insult and take time to emerge. For example, with weakness caused by acute stroke or acute spinal cord trauma, the affected limb(s) will usually be flaccid and areflexic in the acute setting. Upper motor neuron signs emerge over time. Therefore, it may be more challenging to distinguish between upper and lower motor neuron causes of weakness in the acute setting. An upgoing toe (Babinski sign) may be present acutely (although not always), and when it is, can help point toward a CNS etiology of weakness.

Pronator drift is another indication of upper motor neuron pattern weakness: when the arms are held outstretched with the palms up and fingers spread (as if holding a tray), the hand may begin to close and the arm may begin to pronate and drift downward if upper extremity weakness is due to CNS/upper motor neuron pathology. (With parietal lesions, the affected arm may drift upward due to impaired proprioception.) Unlike the upper motor neuron signs described above that may not be present acutely, pronator drift can indeed be present acutely (since it is a reflection of the pattern of weakness).

When an upper motor neuron lesion causes weakness without causing complete paralysis, a distinct pattern of weakness may be seen in which the upper extremity extensors are weaker than the flexors, and the lower extremity flexors are weaker than the extensors. In other words, the arm is stronger when flexing the elbow compared to extending the elbow, and the leg is stronger when extending the knee compared to flexing the knee. This pattern can be remembered by recalling the posture of a patient with long-standing upper motor neuron injury (e.g., prior stroke): the arm, wrist, and fingers are flexed and pronated close to the body, whereas the lower extremity is extended at the knee with the foot plantarflexed and needs to be circumducted when the patient walks. This posture demonstrates that the stronger flexors of the arm have overcome the weaker extensors, and the stronger extensors of the leg have overcome the weaker flexors. As with pronator drift, this upper motor neuron pattern of weakness can be present acutely (as opposed to hyperreflexia and increased tone, which generally take time to emerge, as described above). Note that a radial nerve palsy will affect the triceps, wrist/finger extensors, and supinator, and can thus mimic an upper motor neuron lesion and vice versa (see Ch. 16).

THE CORTICOBULBAR TRACTS

The muscles of the face, tongue, larynx, and pharynx also have upper motor neurons and lower motor neurons. The upper motor neurons arise from the motor cortex and travel with the corticospinal tracts as the **corticobulbar tracts**. Instead of continuing to the spinal cord like the corticospinal tracts do, the corticobulbar fibers terminate in their respective cranial nerve nuclei in the brainstem. The lower motor neurons arise in the cranial nerve nuclei and travel in the cranial nerves. For example, corticobulbar fibers (upper motor neurons) synapse on the cranial nerve 7 nucleus in the pons for movements of the face, and the cranial nerve 12 nucleus for movements of the tongue. These pathways are discussed further in Chapters 13 and 14.

SOMATOSENSORY PATHWAYS FOR THE BODY

Overview of the Somatosensory Pathways for the Body (Fig. 4–2)

In contrast to the motor pathways that begin in the brain and end in the periphery, the sensory pathways begin in the periphery and end in the brain. Sensory information from the skin (light touch, pressure, pain, temperature, vibration) and from the muscle spindles and the Golgi tendon organs (proprioception) travels from the periphery via the peripheral nerves to arrive in the dorsal root ganglia. The dorsal root ganglia are cell bodies of pseudounipolar neurons, each of which has one process in a peripheral nerve and the other traveling in the dorsal roots to the spinal cord.

At the entrance to the spinal cord, somatosensory information is "sorted" into two pathways: pain and temperature information enters the **anterolateral tracts** (also known as the **spinothalamic tracts**), whereas proprioception and vibration information enters the **dorsal columns**. Light touch information travels to some extent in both pathways and, therefore, has less localizing value. Both sensory pathways ascend through the spinal cord and brainstem to arrive at the **ventral posterior lateral (VPL)** nucleus of the thalamus, and the thalamus transmits this somatosensory information to the somatosensory cortex in the postcentral gyrus, just posterior to the motor strip. Further details of these pathways are described below.

The anterolateral and dorsal column systems both cross to transmit sensory information from one side of the body to the contralateral cerebral hemisphere, but the sites of crossing differ. The crossing of the dorsal column system occurs in the medulla, just superior to the crossing of the corticospinal tracts (which cross at the cervicomedullary junction). Therefore, unilateral lesions of the dorsal column pathway from the upper medulla and superiorly (i.e., pons, midbrain, thalamus, subcortical white matter, somatosensory cortex) affect *contralateral* sensation, whereas unilateral lesions from the lower medulla through the spinal cord affect *ipsilateral* sensation. This pattern essentially mimics that of the corticospinal tracts.

Unlike the corticospinal tracts and dorsal column pathways, the anterolateral tracts cross just after entering the

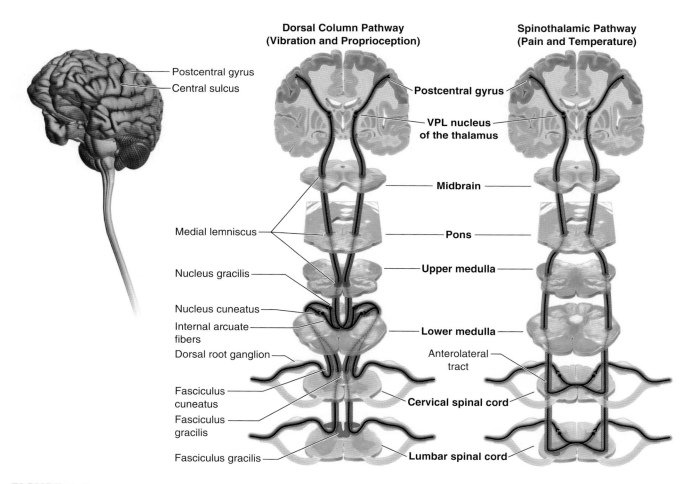

FIGURE 4-2 The somatosensory pathways for the body: Dorsal column pathway and spinothalamic pathway.

spinal cord (they actually cross over the course of a few spinal levels). Therefore, unilateral lesions anywhere in this pathway (spinal cord, brainstem, thalamus, brain) affect **contralateral** sensation, since it crosses almost immediately after entering the CNS. (Since the pathway crosses over the course of a few spinal levels, a small patch of ipsilateral pain/temperature loss involving the spinal levels over which the tract crosses may also be observed.)

The Dorsal Column–Medial Lemniscus Pathways

The dorsal columns travel dorsally (posteriorly) in the spinal cord. They are divided into the **fasciculus cuneatus** and **fasciculus gracilis** (one of each on each side). The fasiculi cuneatus run laterally in the dorsal columns and carry upper extremity sensory information, whereas the fasciculi gracilis run medially in the dorsal columns and carry lower extremity sensory information. The columns rise all the way to the lower medulla where they synapse in the nucleus cuneatus and nucleus gracilis on each side. The axons exiting the nuclei cuneatus and gracilis on each side (second-order neurons in the system) cross by way of the **internal arcuate fibers** to become the contralateral **medial lemniscus**. Each medial lemniscus ascends through the brainstem to synapse in the ipsilateral VPL nucleus of the thalamus, which provides the third-order neurons in the system that synapse in the somatosensory cortex in the postcentral gyrus (just posterior to the central sulcus).

Dysfunction in the dorsal column pathway leads to deficits in vibration sense and proprioception (joint position sense). Isolated dorsal column pathway dysfunction is most commonly due to large fiber peripheral neuropathy (see Ch. 27), dorsal root ganglionopathy (see Ch. 15), or spinal cord disease (see Ch. 5). Vibration sense is tested by placing a vibrating 128-Hz tuning fork on a joint, and comparing the length of time the patient feels the vibration with the time the examiner can feel it. Proprioception is tested by moving a particular joint up or down and asking the patient to determine if the joint has been moved up or down without looking. Evaluation of vibration sense is a more sensitive test for dorsal column pathway dysfunction than evaluation of proprioception.

Assessing for the **Romberg sign** is another test of dorsal column pathway dysfunction. Patients are asked to stand with their feet together, and once balance is achieved, they are asked to close their eyes. Patients with a deficit in proprioception can stand with their feet together when using vision to compensate, but closing their eyes removes this cue and requires them to rely exclusively on proprioception. If the dorsal column pathway is not working properly due to large fiber peripheral neuropathy, ganglionopathy, or spinal cord disease, patients will sway and take a step to maintain balance, which is Romberg's sign. If patients do not take a step when testing for Romberg's sign, but exhibit involuntary piano playing–like movements of the toes (**pseudoathetosis**), this is a sign of proprioceptive dysfunction (a sort of pre–Romberg sign).

The Anterolateral (Spinothalamic) Tracts

The dorsal root neurons carrying pain and temperature sensation enter the posterior spinal cord and go directly into the posterior gray matter via Lissauer's tract. In the dorsal gray matter, these fibers synapse, and the second-order neurons travel anteriorly and cross in the anterior commissure of the spinal cord to arrive in the anterior lateral spinal cord. The axons of these second-order neurons then ascend through the spinal cord as the anterolateral (spinothalamic) tracts to the brainstem, where they eventually join the medial lemniscus in the pons to travel together to the VPL nucleus of the thalamus. After synapsing in the thalamus, the third-order neurons of the pathway travel to the somatosensory cortex just like in the dorsal column pathways.

Pain sensation is generally assessed by determining if the patient can feel a pin as sharp, and if the pin feels of equal sharpness in different locations. Isolated diminished pain sensation can be due to peripheral neuropathy (affecting small fibers), radiculopathy, or dysfunction in the anterolateral system in the spinal cord. When sensory loss is due to spinal cord pathology, a distinct **spinal level** may be detected when pin prick is tested along the spine: Patients will note a discrete level above which the pin is felt as sharp and below which it is felt as dull (or not felt). Temperature can be assessed by using the side of a metal tuning fork to see if it feels equally cold in different locations.

Two key anatomical points for localization of sensory loss are:

- The dorsal column pathways and spinothalamic tracts *cross in different locations* (dorsal column pathways in inferior medulla and spinothalamic tracts in the spinal cord).
- The dorsal column pathways and spinothalamic tracts *travel in different locations in the spinal cord* (dorsal columns dorsally, spinothalamic tracts anterolaterally).

These points are particularly important in localizing lesions of the spinal cord, discussed further in Chapter 5.

Facial sensation is carried in the trigeminal nerve (cranial nerve 5) to the brainstem, from which facial sensory information is transmitted to the contralateral ventral posterior medial (VPM) nucleus of the thalamus and then to the somatosensory cortex. This pathway is discussed in further detail in Chapter 13.

LOCALIZATION OF MOTOR & SENSORY DEFICITS

Weakness can occur due to lesions anywhere in the motor pathways: brain, brainstem, spinal cord, ventral roots, peripheral nerves, neuromuscular junction, and/or muscles. Sensory changes (loss of sensation, paresthesias, proprioceptive deficits) can occur due to lesions anywhere along the sensory pathways: peripheral nerves, dorsal root ganglia, dorsal roots, spinal cord, brainstem, or brain.

The clinical evaluation of weakness or sensory disturbances requires determining the **distribution** of the patient's symptoms (i.e., unilateral, bilateral, proximal, distal) and the **time course** of the onset and evolution of the patient's symptoms (i.e., sudden, acute, subacute, chronic, and whether there has been progression and/or fluctuation).

For weakness, the examination must also determine whether the weakness is consistent with localization to the CNS (brain, brainstem, or spinal cord; i.e., upper motor neuron signs on examination), PNS (roots, peripheral nerves; i.e., lower motor neuron signs on examination), neuromuscular junction (i.e., fatigability on examination; see Ch. 29), or muscles (often proximal and symmetric, although not always; see Ch. 30).

For sensory disturbances, the affected sensory modalities must be determined (i.e., pain/temperature and/or vibration/proprioception). Light touch has less localizing value than vibration, proprioception, pain, and temperature.

Understanding the localization of particular distributions of motor and/or sensory symptoms rests on the foundation of the pathways discussed in this chapter.

Involvement of the Motor & Sensory Pathways in the Brain

The motor and sensory cortices are adjacent to one another, and their white matter tracts in the brain (descending from the motor cortex; ascending from the thalamus to the sensory cortex) are also close to one another. Isolated weakness or isolated sensory loss caused by a lesion of the brain can occur if there is a small lesion affecting just one of these pathways (e.g., small embolic stroke affecting just one gyrus, or a small deep [**lacunar**] infarct in either the posterior limb of the internal capsule [motor] or the thalamus [sensory]). Lesions in the brain will cause contralateral motor and/or sensory deficits. Since the anterolateral and dorsal column pathways are adjacent from the level of the pons until the thalamus (where both synapse in the VPL nucleus), lesions above the level of the medulla usually cause sensory loss affecting all modalities (although very small brainstem lesions affecting just one of these pathways can sometimes occur). Isolated proprioception/vibration or isolated pain/temperature deficit generally suggests a lesion in the lower medulla, spinal cord, dorsal roots/ganglia, or peripheral nerves.

Since the face and arm are adjacent on the cortical surface and share the vascular supply of the middle cerebral artery (the leg region is supplied by the anterior cerebral artery; see Ch. 7), a common pattern of motor and/or sensory changes due to a lesion in the brain is deficits in the face and hand on one side. Since the hand and the the mouth are among the most sensitive and dexterous, they have substantial cortical representation. Therefore, the symptom of sensory changes and/or weakness in the hand and ipsilateral perioral region (**cheiro-oral** pattern) is highly suggestive of a lesion in the contralateral cerebral hemisphere.

Isolated lesions of the somatosensory cortex may not lead to sensory loss but may lead to higher-level sensory deficits.

For example, the patient may be unable to recognize a number or letter drawn on the hand (**agraphesthesia**). If the patient's left and right sides of the body are touched simultaneously, the patient may not note the sensation in the limb contralateral to the lesion, despite being able to detect sensation when this limb is touched in isolation (**extinction to double simultaneous stimulation**). This occurs most commonly with nondominant (usually right) parietal lesions (see Ch. 7).

Involvement of the Motor and/or Sensory Pathways in the Brainstem

In the brainstem, the corticospinal tracts travel in the anterior (ventral) portion, whereas the sensory pathways are predominantly dorsolateral (the medial lemniscus beginning in the anterior medial medulla is an exception to this generalization). Therefore, anterior brainstem lesions can affect the motor pathways, whereas dorsolateral lesions can affect the sensory pathways. Since all of the cranial nerve nuclei are also in the brainstem, isolated motor or sensory symptoms limited to the extremities from a brainstem lesion are rare, although they can occur with small anterior lesions affecting only the corticospinal tracts, or small dorsal lesions affecting only the sensory tracts.

As will be discussed in Chapter 9, unilateral brainstem lesions can cause **crossed signs**: weakness and/or sensory changes in the ipsilateral face, but in the contralateral body. This is because nearly all cranial nerves control *ipsilateral* functions in the head, whereas the not-yet-crossed corticospinal tracts and the already-crossed ascending sensory tracts at the level of the brainstem control contralateral functions in the body.

Lesions at the level of the foramen magnum affecting the cervicomedullary junction can produce a pattern of weakness evolving in an **around the clock** progression, for example, from one arm to the ipsilateral leg to the contralateral leg to the arm contralateral to the original weak arm. This is thought to be due to the arm fibers of the corticospinal tracts decussating superiorly to the leg fibers, and thus susceptible to sequential compression by a growing mass in this region (e.g., meningioma). Lesions in this region can also lead to bilateral arm weakness (if the more superior arm fibers are affected in isolation; **cruciate paralysis of Bell**) or crossed paralysis with weakness of one arm and the contralateral leg (if the crossed arm fibers and not-yet-crossed leg fibers on one side are affected).

Involvement of the Motor and/or Sensory Pathways in the Spinal Cord

The anatomic arrangement of the long tracts in the spinal cord gives rise to several possible clinical syndromes, which are discussed in detail in Chapter 5. Since the spinal cord is relatively small, it is common for disease processes affecting it to cause bilateral symptoms and signs, although small lesions within the spinal cord (**intramedullary lesions**) or unilateral external compression of the spinal cord (**extramedullary lesions**) can lead to unilateral symptoms.

Involvement of the Motor and/or Sensory Pathways in the Peripheral Nervous System

As discussed in Chapter 27, peripheral neuropathies can be motor, sensory, or mixed, and can affect an individual nerve (**mononeuropathy**), multiple nerves (**mononeuropathy multiplex**), or all nerves (**polyneuropathy**), leading to varying patterns of weakness and/or sensory changes. When an individual limb is weak and/or has changes in sensation such as numbness or pain, the problem may be referable to an individual root or nerve, multiple roots or nerves, or to a nerve plexus (see Chs. 16 and 17).

In summary (Fig. 4–3):

- If there are sensory and/or motor changes in the face (with or without deficits in the extremities), this requires a lesion at the level of the brainstem or in the cerebral hemisphere. (Evaluation of facial weakness and sensory changes is discussed in further detail in Ch. 13.)
- If the arm and leg are affected on one side without the face being involved, the lesion is most likely in the medulla or cervical spinal cord.
- If one limb is affected in isolation, a lesion at nearly any level of the nervous system is possible: a small cortical or subcortical lesion, a spinal cord lesion, or a lesion at the level of the nerve roots, plexus, or one or more peripheral nerves. A brainstem lesion causing unilateral involvement of one limb is unlikely since the fibers of the motor and sensory pathways are packed so closely in the brainstem.
- Isolated bilateral weakness suggests a process affecting the spinal cord, peripheral nerves, neuromuscular junction, or

muscles. To have bilateral weakness from a brain or brainstem lesion would require bilateral lesions, which will usually cause symptoms/signs beyond just motor problems (e.g., changes in mental state if there are bilateral cerebral lesions or cranial nerve deficits if there are bilateral brainstem lesions). An exception is a very medial lesion affecting the bilateral leg areas of the motor cortices, which can lead to paraplegia mimicking a spinal cord lesion. This can be caused by a parasagittal meningioma or bilateral anterior cerebral artery strokes (which can occur when both anterior cerebral arteries arise from a common trunk, called azygous anterior cerebral arteries; see Ch. 7). In the case of bilateral anterior cerebral artery strokes, there are usually cognitive deficits in addition to the motor findings. Isolated bilateral sensory changes generally suggest a process affecting the spinal cord, dorsal roots, dorsal root ganglia, or peripheral nerves.

With respect to time course of symptom onset and evolution:

- **Hyperacute (sudden-onset) weakness and/or sensory changes.** Common causes of sudden-onset weakness and/or sensory changes localizing to the brain include stroke, seizure, or migraine. The most common cause of sudden-onset weakness and/or sensory changes localizing to the brainstem is stroke. Common causes of sudden-onset weakness and/or sensory changes localizing to the spinal cord include acute disc prolapse or vertebral collapse (e.g., due to trauma or metastatic malignancy to the vertebrae), which are typically painful. Spinal cord infarct occurs rarely (see Ch. 19). Sudden-onset weakness and/or sensory changes localizing to a particular nerve may be caused by a nerve infarct (as can be seen in vasculitic neuropathies; see Ch. 15)
- **Acute (onset over hours to days) weakness and/or sensory changes.** Acute-onset weakness and/or sensory changes at any level of the nervous system can be due to inflammatory conditions (e.g., Guillain-Barré syndrome [see Ch. 27],

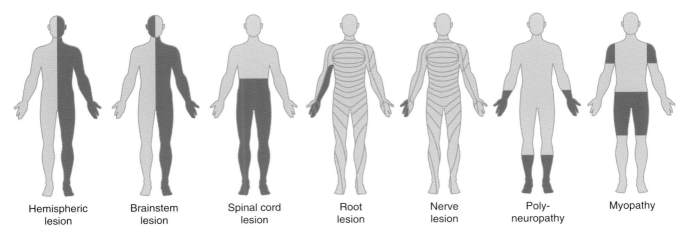

| Hemispheric lesion | Brainstem lesion | Spinal cord lesion | Root lesion | Nerve lesion | Poly-neuropathy | Myopathy |

FIGURE 4–3 **Schematic showing patterns of weakness and/or sensory disturbances caused by lesions at different levels of the nervous system.** Note that a myopathy will not cause sensory deficits. Adapted with permission from Aminoff M, Greenberg D, Simon R: *Clinical Neurology*, 9th ed. New York, NY: McGraw Hill; 2015.

transverse myelitis, or an acute demyelinating lesion in multiple sclerosis; see Ch. 21) or infectious processes (e.g., cerebral or epidural abscess; see Ch. 20).

- **Subacute- to chronic-onset (over weeks to months to years) weakness and/or sensory changes**. Subacute- to chronic-onset weakness and/or sensory changes can be caused by neoplasm, immune-mediated disease (e.g., chronic inflammatory demyelinating polyneuropathy [CIDP]; see Ch. 27), metabolic conditions (vitamin B12 or copper deficiency), or degenerative disease (e.g., spondylosis of the spine [see Chs. 16 and 17], or in the case of isolated weakness, motor neuron disease; see Ch. 28).

The Spinal Cord & Approach to Myelopathy

OVERVIEW OF SPINAL CORD ANATOMY

The spinal cord begins where the medulla ends, running from the foramen magnum at the base of the skull to about the level of the first lumbar vertebrae (L1-L2) (Fig. 5–1). The spinal cord is divided into cervical, thoracic, lumbar, and sacral regions. The cervical and thoracic regions of the spinal cord correspond to the cervical and thoracic regions of the spinal column. However, the spinal cord is shorter than the spinal column, and so the lumbar region of the spinal cord actually corresponds to the lower thoracic spine, and the sacral region of the cord is housed in a short region called the **conus medullaris** at about the level of the L1-L2 vertebrae. Throughout the spine, dorsal roots enter and ventral roots exit through the neural foramina of the vertebrae that correspond to their spinal cord level of origin/exit. At cervical and thoracic levels, the corresponding foramina are essentially adjacent to the spinal cord levels with which they are associated. Since the spinal cord ends at L1-L2, below this level, the lumbosacral nerve roots (**cauda equina**) must descend to reach their corresponding exiting foramina (discussed further in Chs. 15 and 17).

The lateral corticospinal tracts, dorsal column pathways, and anterolateral (spinothalamic) tracts are the three most clinically relevant pathways for clinical localization within the spinal cord. Sympathetic and parasympathetic pathways also traverse the spinal cord, and there are a number of other tracts (e.g., tectospinal, rubrospinal, vestibulospinal) that play roles in posture and motor control but are not generally assessed in clinical neurology. The spinocerebellar pathways that bring proprioceptive information to the cerebellum will be discussed in the context of the cerebellum in Chapter 8.

The lateral corticospinal tracts are lateral and posterior in the spinal cord, the dorsal columns are posterior and medial, and the anterolateral (spinothalamic) tracts are anterior and lateral (as their name suggests) (Figs. 5–2 and 5–3).

LAMINATION OF THE LONG TRACTS IN THE SPINAL CORD (FIGS. 5–3 AND 5–4)

Lamination refers to the arrangement of fibers within a pathway. For the corticospinal, anterolateral, and dorsal column pathways, this refers to where the arm, leg, and torso fibers run (there are no fibers for the head in the spinal cord since these are carried to/from the brainstem by the cranial nerves) (see Fig. 5–3).

As the corticospinal tracts descend from the brainstem, arm fibers synapse on lower motor neurons in the cervical cord, but leg fibers must wait until the lumbar cord to do so. Therefore, arm fibers must be most medial to have first access to the alpha motor neurons, and leg fibers are more lateral, gaining exposure to the anterior horn cells only after the arm fibers have done so and departed as the tracts descend. The corticospinal tracts are thus laminated with the arm fibers medial and the leg fibers lateral (see Fig. 5–4A).

The dorsal column fibers from the feet and legs enter the spinal cord at the lumbar and sacral levels, and are pushed medially by the addition of trunk and arm fibers as the tracts ascend. The dorsal columns are thus laminated with the legs medial and the arms lateral (see Fig. 5–4B).

The spinothalamic tracts' feet and leg fibers cross to the contralateral side and are pushed laterally as subsequent crossing fibers for the trunk and arms push them aside and layer more medially. The spinothalamic tracts are thus laminated

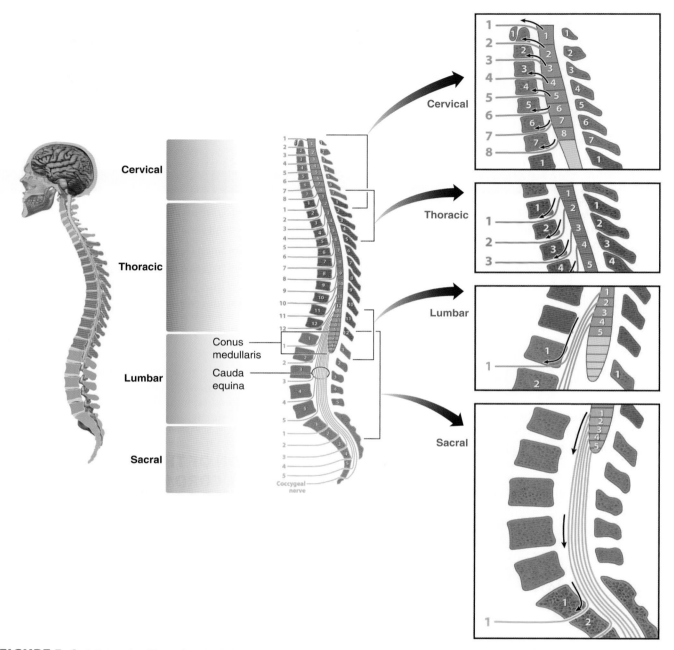

FIGURE 5–1 Schematic of lateral view of the spinal cord and nerve roots in relation to the spinal column.

with the arms medial and the legs lateral like the corticospinal tracts (see Fig. 5–4C).

In summary, in the corticospinal and anterolateral tracts, the arm fibers are medial and the leg fibers are lateral, and the pattern is reversed for the dorsal columns. As a mnemonic, imagine two people laying feet to feet on top of the spinal cord (dorsal columns: lower extremities medial, upper extremities lateral) and four people (two on each side) diving into the central canal (anterolateral and corticospinal tracts: upper extremities medial, lower extremities lateral) (see Fig. 5–3B). This lamination pattern is particularly important

for the understanding of **central cord syndrome** (e.g., as can be caused by a **syrinx**) (See "Central Cord Syndrome").

SPINAL CORD SYNDROMES

Spinal cord pathology is broadly referred to as **myelopathy** (which should not be confused with myopathy, which refers to pathology of the muscles; see Ch. 30). There are several important clinical patterns to recognize that signify localization to particular parts of the spinal cord, each

A. Corticospinal Pathway   **B.** Dorsal Column Pathway   **C.** Spinothalamic Pathway

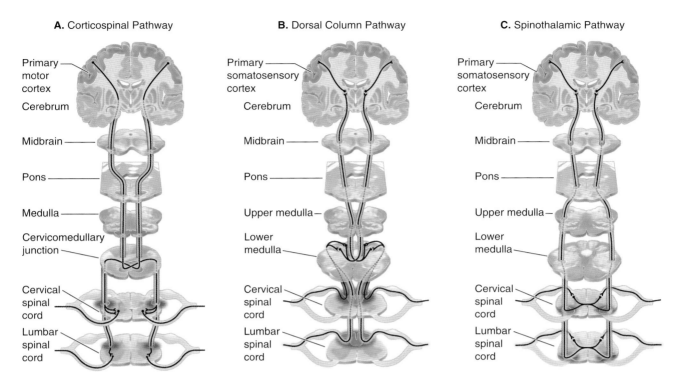

FIGURE 5–2 Schematic of the three long tracts. Anatomical location of the pathways in axial section of the spinal cord are highlighted in red.

with a particular differential diagnosis (Fig. 5–4A and Table 1–1).

Complete Transection of the Spinal Cord

Complete transection of the spinal cord will cause loss of all spinal cord functions below the level of the lesion, leading to weakness, sensory loss in all modalities, and bowel/bladder dysfunction (other features of dysautonomia can also occur). Upper motor neuron signs will be seen below the level of the lesion, though may be absent in the acute setting of spinal shock. Lower motor neuron signs may be seen at the level(s) of the lesion if anterior horn cells or ventral roots are affected. Lesions at or above the T1 level will affect both the upper and

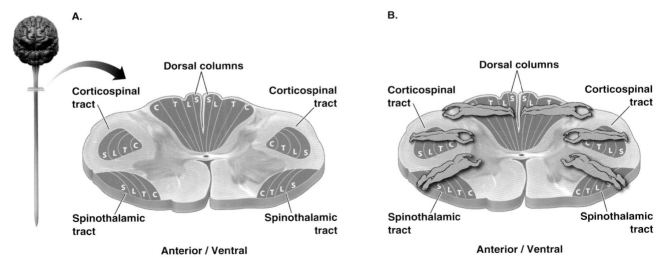

FIGURE 5–3 Schematic of axial section of the spinal cord. A. This schematic demonstrates the locations of the three main clinically relevant pathways and their lamination: corticospinal tracts, dorsal columns, and anterolateral (spinothalamic) tracts. **B.** This schematic shows mnemonically how the upper extremity, trunk, and lower extremity fibers are laminated; see text for explanation.

lower extremities, whereas lesions below the T1 level will affect only the lower extremities. A **spinal level** may be observed below which there is no sensation and above which sensation is preserved; the lesion is generally a few levels above the clinically determined spinal level. Complete transection can be caused by spinal injury or transverse myelitis, though it should be noted that not all transverse lesions are inflammatory, and not all inflammatory disorders of the spinal cord cause fully transverse lesions (see "Transverse Myelitis" in Ch. 21).

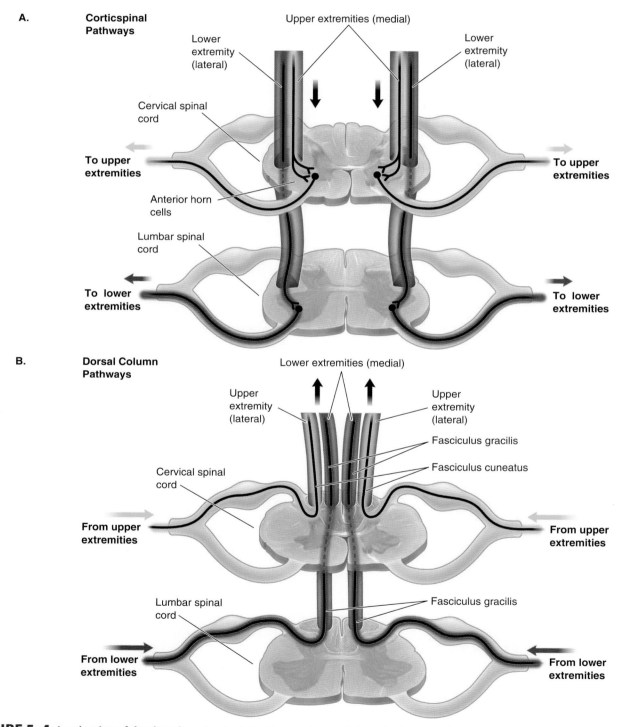

FIGURE 5–4 **Lamination of the three long tracts. A.** Corticospinal tracts. **B.** Dorsal columns. **C.** Spinothalamic (anterolateral) tracts.

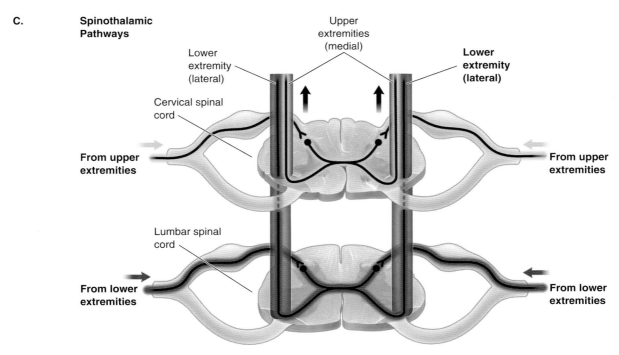

FIGURE 5-4 (*Continued*)

Brown-Séquard (Hemicord) Syndrome (Fig. 5–5A)

Hemicord syndrome affects all pathways on one side of the spinal cord. The corticospinal tracts cross in the medulla, which is just above their entry into the cervical spinal cord. Therefore, motor deficits caused by a unilateral spinal cord lesion will cause *ipsilateral* weakness below the level of the lesion. The dorsal column pathways remain ipsilateral until they cross in the medulla, so unilateral spinal cord lesions will cause *ipsilateral* deficits of proprioception and vibration sensation below the level of the lesion. Since the anterolateral (spinothalamic) tracts cross soon after they enter the spinal cord, lesions of one side of the spinal cord will affect already-crossed spinothalamic fibers, causing *contralateral* deficits in pain and temperature sensation below the level of the lesion (a small region of ipsilateral pain and temperature

sensation loss may also be seen at the levels over which the pathway is crossing).

In summary, a lesion affecting one lateral half of the spinal cord will cause:

- *Ipsilateral* weakness below the level of the lesion
- *Ipsilateral* loss of vibration sense and proprioception below the level of the lesion
- *Contralateral* loss of pain and temperature sensation below the level of the lesion

For example, in a lower thoracic Brown-Séquard syndrome affecting the *right* hemicord, there will be *right-sided* (ipsilateral) weakness and vibration sense/proprioception loss with spared pain/temperature sensation, and the opposite pattern on the *left* (contralateral) side: preserved strength and vibration sense/proprioception but impaired pain/temperature sensation.

TABLE 5-1 Spinal Cord Syndromes.

	Brown-Séquard Syndrome		Anterior Cord Syndrome	Central Cord Syndrome	Subacute Combined Degeneration
	Ipsilateral	**Contralateral**			
Motor	Affected	Spared	Affected bilaterally	Spared bilaterally (until very advanced)	Affected bilaterally
Vibration/ proprioception	Affected	Spared	Spared bilaterally	Spared bilaterally	Affected bilaterally
Pain/temperature	Spared	Affected	Affected bilaterally	Affected bilaterally (in hands/ upper extremities first)	Spared bilaterally

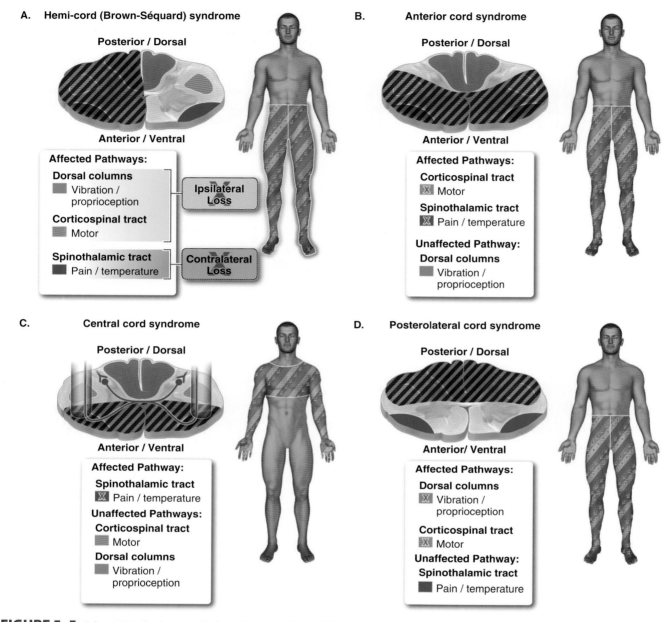

FIGURE 5–5 **Schematic of spinal cord lesions. A:** Brown-Séquard (hemicord) syndrome. **B:** Anterior cord syndrome. **C:** Central cord syndrome. **D:** Subacute combined degeneration.

Hemicord syndrome is most commonly caused by penetrating trauma (e.g., stab or gunshot wound), but can also be caused by a neoplasm compressing the cord from one side (e.g., meningioma) or a unilateral demyelinating lesion (e.g., transverse myelitis).

Anterior Cord Syndrome (Fig. 5–5B)

Anterior cord syndrome involves nearly the entire cross sectional area of the spinal cord with the exception of the dorsal columns. Therefore, motor function and pain and temperature sensation are impaired below the level of the lesion but

proprioception and vibration are spared. Both upper and lower motor neuron signs may be seen: upper motor neuron signs due to interruption of the descending corticospinal tracts and lower motor neuron signs due to involvement of the gray matter at the affected level(s) of the spinal cord. Anterior cord syndrome occurs most commonly due to infarction in the territory of the anterior spinal artery of the spinal cord, which is most often caused by aortic aneurysm rupture, or in the setting of surgery to repair an aortic aneurysm. The reasons why the anterior spinal cord is more vulnerable to ischemia than the posterior cord are discussed in Chapter 19, though it should be noted that anterior cord syndrome is not the only pattern of spinal cord involvement seen in spinal cord ischemia (see "Ischemic stroke of the Spinal Cord" in Ch. 19).

Central Cord Syndrome (Fig. 5–5C)

Central cord syndrome occurs most commonly due to **syrinx**, a dilatation of the central canal of the spinal cord. When the central canal enlarges in a syrinx, this usually occurs in the cervical spinal cord. The closest structure to the central canal is the anterior commissure where the anterolateral tracts cross. Since the upper extremity spinothalamic fibers enter and cross in the cervical spinal cord, these are affected first. This leads to bilateral loss of pain and temperature sensation in the upper extremities, which can cause a "cape-like" distribution of sensory deficits **(suspended sensory level)**. As a syrinx continues to expand, spinothalamic (and, in some cases, corticospinal) tracts may be compressed from medially to laterally. Since upper extremity fibers are medial in both pathways, these are affected first leading to involvement of the upper extremities before affecting the lower extremities if the syrinx progresses.

Syrinx can occur in the setting of a Chiari malformation (see "Chiari Malformation" in Ch. 26), or any lesion of the spinal cord leading to obstruction of the central canal (e.g., tumor, prior trauma (particularly with cervical hyperextension), demyelination, hemorrhage).

Subacute Combined Degeneration (Fig. 5–5D)

Selective involvement of the dorsal columns and corticospinal tracts together occurs in subacute combined degeneration. Subacute combined degeneration is most commonly caused by vitamin B12 deficiency, but can also be caused by copper deficiency. Vitamin B12 deficiency can be caused by malabsorption (e.g., pernicious anemia, small intestine pathology or surgery, gastric bypass) or a vegetarian or vegan diet. Copper deficiency can occur in the setting of excess zinc ingestion (which can be caused by zinc-containing denture creams), after gastric bypass surgery, or due to malabsorption. Both vitamin B12 deficiency and copper deficiency can result in concurrent myelopathy and neuropathy **(myeloneuropathy)**, which can cause mixed upper and lower motor neuron features on examination (e.g., absent ankle reflexes and brisk knee reflexes, or areflexia with Babinski signs).

The dorsal columns and corticospinal tracts are also selectively affected in the vacuolar myelopathy of AIDS (see "HIV-associated vacuolar myelopathy" in Ch. 20).

Involvement of the dorsal columns and dorsal roots together is seen in tabes dorsalis in syphilis (see Ch. 20).

SPINAL CORD PATHWAYS FOR BOWEL & BLADDER CONTROL (TABLE 5–2)

The pathways for bowel and bladder control also pass through the spinal cord. Recall that with upper motor neuron lesions affecting control of the limbs, the affected extremities are generally flaccid acutely, and upper motor neuron signs (e.g., hyperreflexia, spasticity) develop over time (see "Upper Motor Neuron Lesions vs Lower Motor Neuron Lesions" in Ch. 4). Similarly, acute spinal cord pathology causes flaccidity of the bowel and bladder, and spasticity develops over time.

For the bladder, this means that in the acute setting of spinal cord injury, the bladder is flaccid and does not contract, leading to urinary retention with overflow incontinence. Over time, an upper motor neuron pattern emerges whereby the bladder is spastic/hyperreflexic: it contracts too much, leading to urgency and incontinence.

For the bowel, acute spinal cord lesions lead to bowel and rectal flaccidity, causing constipation due to decreased bowel motility and incontinence due to decreased rectal tone. Chronic spinal cord lesions lead to increased bowel and rectal tone, which results in constipation (generally requiring physical stimulation of the rectum for a bowel movement to occur).

Lower motor neuron lesions for both bowel and bladder (sacral roots 2–4 of the cauda equina) lead to flaccidity, leading to retention of both stool and urine, with overflow incontinence of urine and bowel incontinence due to flaccid sphincter tone. (See "Cauda Equina and Conus Medullaris Syndromes" in Ch. 17.)

CAUSES OF MYELOPATHY

Common causes of myelopathy are classified here by time course of onset and evolution. Details of individual disorders are discussed in Part 2 of the book.

TABLE 5–2   Effects of Spinal Lesions on Bowel & Bladder Function.

	Acute Spinal Cord Injury	Chronic Spinal Cord Injury	Cauda Equina/Conus Medullaris Lesion
Bowel	Constipation	Constipation	Constipation
	Decreased rectal tone	Increased rectal tone	Decreased rectal tone
	Incontinence		Incontinence
Bladder	Retention	Spastic bladder	Retention
	Overflow incontinence	Frequency and incontinence	Overflow incontinence

Hyperacute-onset (minutes to hours) myelopathy can be caused by:

- Trauma
- Structural disease of the spine: acute central disc prolapse, acute vertebral collapse
- Vascular causes (see Ch. 19): stroke, epidural hemorrhage, or spinal cord hemorrhage (hematomyelia)

Acute-onset (hours to days) myelopathy can be caused by:

- Infections (see Ch. 20): viral myelitis, epidural abscess, schistosomiasis
- Immune-mediated (see Ch. 21): transverse myelitis, flare of multiple sclerosis, flare of neuromyelitis optica

Subacute-onset (weeks to months) myelopathy can be caused by:

- Structural disease of the spine (see Ch. 16): cervical stenosis
- Tumor (see Ch 24): primary or metastatic
- Infections (see Ch. 20): tuberculosis of the spine
- Vascular causes (see Ch. 19): spinal dural arteriovenous fistula
- Immune-mediated: sarcoidosis, paraneoplastic (anti-CRMP5, anti-Hu; see Ch. 24)
- Metabolic causes: vitamin B12 deficiency or copper deficiency

Chronic-onset (years) myelopathy can be caused by:

- Infections (see Ch. 20): human T-cell lymphocytic virus 1 (HTLV-1) associated myelopathy and HIV-associated vacuolar myelopathy
- Neurodegenerative myelopathies: hereditary spastic paraplegia (see below), spinocerebellar ataxia (see Ch. 8), adrenomyeloneuropathy (see Ch. 31)
- Radiation-induced myelopathy (see Ch. 24)

These conditions are discussed in Part 2, except hereditary spastic paraplegia, which is therefore discussed here.

Hereditary Spastic Paraplegia

Hereditary spastic paraplegia (HSP) is an inherited degenerative disorder that predominantly affects the corticospinal tracts in the spinal cord leading to progressive bilateral lower extremity weakness and spasticity. More than 50 subtypes of HSP have been identified with variable age of onset and inheritance pattern (autosomal dominant, autosomal recessive, and X-linked). Subtypes also vary in terms of whether the condition is limited to spastic paraplegia (pure or uncomplicated HSP) or accompanied by additional features (complicated HSP), which can include dementia, neuropathy, parkinsonism, epilepsy, ataxia, visual loss, and/or hearing loss. Treatment is supportive with agents to reduce spasticity (e.g., baclofen, tizanidine), use of assistive devices, and genetic counseling.

The Visual Pathway & Approach to Visual Loss

ANATOMY OF THE VISUAL PATHWAY (FIGS. 6–1 AND 6–2)

The optic nerve is the output of the retina. Therefore, each optic nerve carries all of the visual information from the eye from which it emerges. Since the left hemisphere moves the right side of the body and the right hemisphere moves the left side of the body, it makes sense that the left hemisphere should receive the visual information from the right half of the world and the right hemisphere should receive the visual information from the left half of the world. Therefore, some of the information in each optic nerve must cross so that the brain can work with the left and right **visual fields** rather than merely what is seen by the left and right eyes: The left hemisphere must receive right visual field information from both the left eye and the right eye; the right hemisphere must receive left visual field information from both the left eye and the right eye. The crossing of visual field information to convert the visual world from left eye–right eye organization to left field–right field organization occurs at the **optic chiasm**. Posterior to the optic chiasm, visual information is organized into fields: The left visual field is processed in the right hemisphere, and the right visual field in the left hemisphere.

Imagine viewing a simple rectangle that is half orange and half blue (Fig. 6–1). The right visual field (orange) projects onto the medial (nasal) retina in the right eye and the lateral (temporal) retina in the left eye. The left visual field (blue) projects to the medial (nasal) retina in the left eye and the lateral (temporal) retina in the right eye. The *medial* (nasal) retinas are, therefore, receiving the *lateral* (temporal) visual fields, and the *lateral* (temporal) retinas are receiving the *medial* (nasal) visual fields.

All visual information from the right visual field must end up in the left hemisphere, and all visual information from the left visual field must end up in the right hemisphere. Which visual information from each eye needs to cross to convert the organization of visual information from eyes to visual fields? The right visual field information in the left optic nerve (from the lateral retina of the left eye) is already on the correct (left) side of the brain, but the right visual field information in the right optic nerve (from the medial retina of the right eye) must cross from the right optic nerve to the left side of the brain to join it. The left visual field information in the right optic nerve (from the lateral retina of the right eye) is already on the correct side of the brain, but the left visual field information in the left optic nerve (from the medial retina of the left eye) must cross from the left optic nerve to the right side to join it.

In summary, the information seen by the lateral (temporal) retina of each eye is from the contralateral visual field, and so it is already on the correct side of the brain in the optic nerve and does not need to cross. The information in the medial (nasal) retina in each eye is from the ipsilateral visual field, so that information needs to cross at the chiasm. Therefore, at the chiasm, the information from the medial (nasal) retinas (representing the lateral [temporal] visual fields) crosses, and the information from the lateral (temporal) retinas (representing the medial [nasal] visual fields) remains ipsilateral.

Posterior to the optic chiasm, the visual world is separated into left and right visual fields, with the left visual field represented in the right hemisphere, and the right visual field represented in the left hemisphere. This information travels in the left and right optic tracts from the chiasm to the left and right **lateral geniculate nucleus** (LGN) of the thalamus. From each LGN, information travels to the visual cortex of the occipital lobes in a superior radiation and an inferior radiation on each side. Just as the left visual field goes to the opposite (i.e., right) side of the brain and the right visual field goes to the opposite (i.e., left) side of the brain, the *inferior* visual

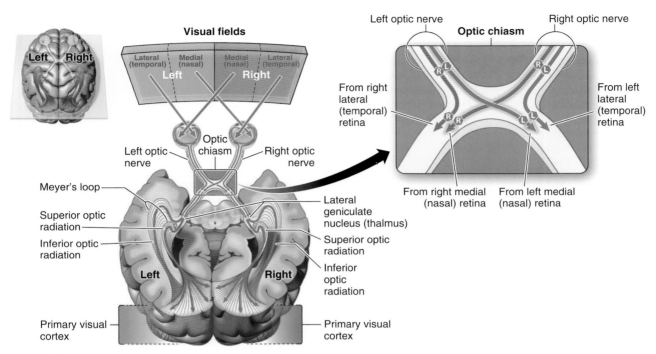

FIGURE 6-1 Anatomy of the visual pathways. The left visual field (blue) and right visual field (orange) are traced through the pathways, and the pop-out zooms in on the optic chiasm to demonstrate which visual field information crosses in the chiasm.

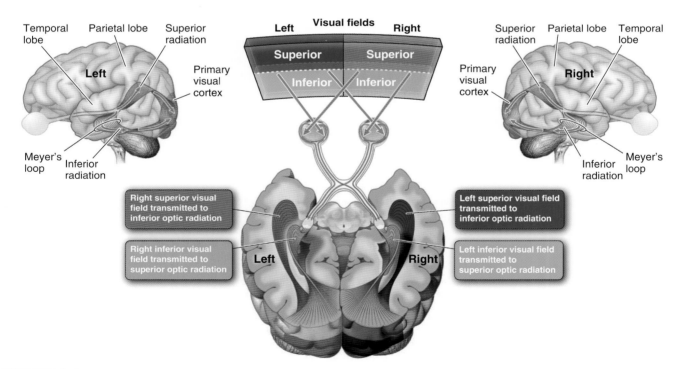

FIGURE 6-2 Anatomy of the visual pathways. The left visual field (blue) and right visual field (orange) are traced through the pathways with the superior visual fields darker and the inferior visual fields lighter as they are traced through the optic radiations to the primary visual cortex.

fields travel in the *superior* radiations to the *superior* bank of the calcarine cortex in the posterior occipital lobe, and the *superior* visual fields travel in the *inferior* radiations to the *inferior* bank of the calcarine cortex. The superior radiations travel through the parietal lobes to the occipital lobes, and the inferior radiations travel through the temporal lobes to the occipital lobes. The inferior radiations loop anteriorly before proceeding posteriorly, and this anterior loop is called **Meyer's loop**.

APPROACH TO VISUAL LOSS

Understanding the flow of visual information allows for the localization of visual deficits to particular regions of the visual pathway (Fig. 6–3).

A visual deficit limited to just one eye (i.e., the other eye sees the whole world normally when the problematic eye is closed) must be due to either ocular pathology (e.g., lens, anterior chamber, retina) or pathology of the optic nerve (Fig. 6–3A).

A visual deficit limited to a particular visual *field* in *both* eyes (i.e., the same deficit in each eye—a **homonymous** deficit) localizes posterior to the optic chiasm: optic tract, LGN, optic radiation(s), or occipital lobe (on the side *contralateral* to the homonymous deficit (Fig. 6–3C-H)).

- A lesion of the optic tract or LGN will cause contralateral **homonymous hemianopia** (Fig. 6–3C, D). Lesions of the optic tract may cause incongruous visual field deficits that are on the same side in each eye (homonymous) but of different shapes in each eye. Isolated lesions in the optic tract or LGN are rare in practice.
- A lesion affecting an individual optic radiation or individual bank of the calcarine cortex will cause a contralateral visual deficit in one quadrant in both eyes (**quadrantanopia**) (Fig. 6–3E-H):
  - A superior quadrantanopia localizes to the contralateral inferior radiation and/or inferior bank of the calcarine cortex (Fig. 6–3E, F).
  - An inferior quadrantanopia localizes to the contralateral superior radiation and/or superior bank of the calcarine cortex (Fig. 6–3G, H).
- A lesion of one occipital lobe that affects both the superior and inferior portions of the calcarine cortex will lead to a contralateral homonymous hemianopia, similar to a lesion of the optic tract or LGN on that side (Fig. 6–3C,D). Infarction of one occipital lobe (due to stroke in the posterior cerebral artery territory) may produce a homonymous hemianopia with **macular sparing** (preserved central vision). This may be due to the macula receiving some blood supply from the middle cerebral artery and/or the macula being bilaterally represented since it is at the center of vision and, therefore, does not fall into one "field."

A lesion at the optic chiasm creates a more complex visual deficit. As described previously, the chiasm is where information from the medial retina from each eye/optic nerve (representing the lateral visual field in each eye/optic nerve) crosses. Therefore, a lesion affecting this crossing information causes loss of vision in the bilateral lateral (temporal) visual fields, with sparing of the bilateral medial (nasal) visual fields. This pattern of visual loss is referred to as **bitemporal hemianopia**, and causes loss of peripheral vision on both sides (Fig. 6–3B).

It is important to note that to elicit bitemporal hemianopia at the bedside requires visual field testing of each eye *individually*. Take the example of an object in the left visual field: It is seen by the left nasal retina (information from here crosses in the chiasm) and the right temporal retina (information from here does *not* cross in the chiasm). Therefore, if there is a bitemporal hemianopia due to a chiasmal lesion, the visual information in this example (an object on the left) projected on to the medial (nasal) retina of the *left* eye will *not* "get through," and so will not be seen. However, the same left visual field information projected onto the temporal retina of the *right eye will* "get through," since this information does *not* cross at the chiasm. So if the visual fields are tested with both eyes open (i.e., rather than by having the patient cover one eye to test each eye separately) in a patient with a bitemporal hemianopia, an object in the left visual field will still be seen by the right eye/optic nerve and right hemisphere. If the right eye is covered so the left eye is tested in isolation, then the temporal field deficit in the left eye will be revealed (since the right eye information that does not traverse the chiasm is not available to the brain when the right eye is covered). Therefore, a bitemporal hemianopia may be missed if visual fields are tested with both eyes open, but should be evident if each eye is tested separately with one eye covered.

A **junctional scotoma** occurs when the optic nerve is affected at its junction with the chiasm. This produces an ipsilateral central scotoma (from optic neuropathy) and contralateral superior temporal quadrantanopia because the inferior nasal fibers (representing the superior temporal quadrant) loop anteriorly into the most distal portion of the contralateral optic nerve after crossing before proceeding posteriorly. The portion of the pathway that loops anteriorly is called **Wilbrand's knee**.

Another bilateral syndrome of the optic nerves is **Foster Kennedy syndrome**. In this syndrome, an enlarging mass lesion compresses the optic nerve on one side leading to optic neuropathy (with optic nerve pallor on examination due to chronicity), and the elevated intracranial pressure caused by the mass results in papilledema on the contralateral side.

Monocular Visual Loss

The causes of **monocular** visual loss include problems of the lens (e.g., cataract), anterior chamber (e.g., uveitis), retina (e.g., retinal ischemia, diabetic retinopathy), and optic nerve (i.e., optic neuropathy [see below for differential diagnosis]). In general, monocular vision loss is classified as acute or nonacute, and painful or painless. Sudden monocular visual loss is generally vascular in etiology (e.g., central retinal artery occlusion, central retinal vein occlusion, ischemic optic neuropathy), and all other causes are generally subacute to chronic in presentation. Vascular causes of monocular visual loss such as retinal ischemia and ischemic optic neuropathy are generally painless. (Patients with visual loss due to giant cell arteritis often have headache, although they do not typically have eye pain.) Painful monocular visual loss occurs with acute angle closure glaucoma and optic neuritis.

Optic neuropathy generally causes blurred vision centrally (**central scotoma** or **cecocentral scotoma** if it extends to the blind spot), decreased color vision, decreased visual acuity, and an afferent pupillary defect (see Ch. 10 for explanation of afferent pupillary defect). If optic neuropathy is due to an inflammatory cause (**optic neuritis**), optic nerve swelling may be visible on fundoscopy (unless the inflammation is more posterior in the optic nerve [**retrobulbar**], in which case the optic nerve may appear normal). Chronic optic neuropathies cause optic nerve pallor.

Hyperacute causes of optic neuropathy include:

- Ischemic:
  - Anterior ischemic optic neuropathy (AION):
    - Arteritic AION: giant cell arteritis or systemic vasculitis
    - Nonarteritic AION: small "crowded" optic disc increases risk; caused by hypotension and/or vascular risk factors
  - Posterior ischemic optic neuropathy (PION): usually caused by hypotension (e.g., postsurgical, especially with prone positioning during surgery)
- Traumatic: severe head trauma can cause shearing of optic nerves

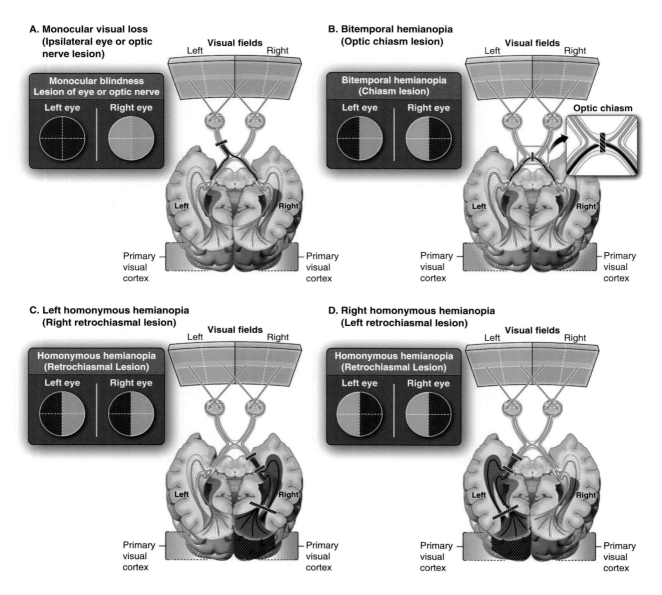

FIGURE 6–3 Patterns of visual loss and associated lesion locations. **A.** Monocular visual loss in the left eye due to a left eye ophthalmologic condition or left optic neuropathy. **B.** Bitemporal hemianopia due to a lesion of the optic chiasm. **C.** Left homonymous hemianopia due to a right retrochiasmal lesion affecting the right LGN, right optic radiations, or right occipital cortex. **D.** Right homonymous hemianopia due to a left retrochiasmal lesion affecting the left LGN, left optic radiations, or left occipital cortex.

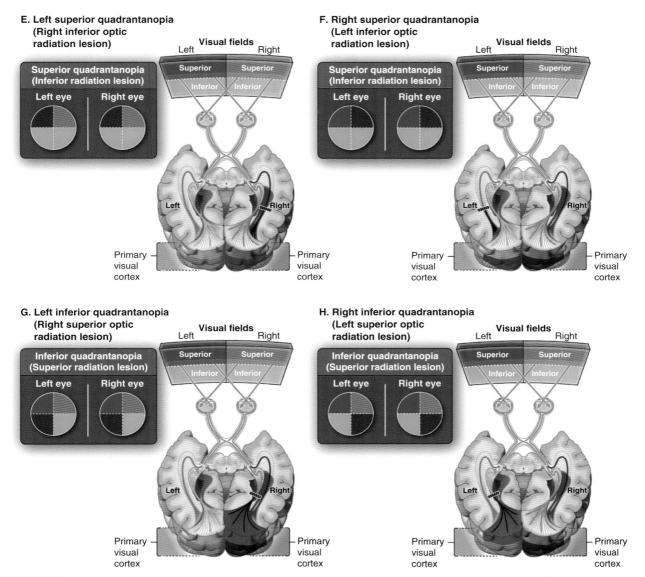

FIGURE 6–3 **E.** Left superior quadrantanopia due to a lesion of the right inferior optic radiation or inferior aspect of the right visual cortex. **F.** Right superior quadrantanopia due to a lesion of the left inferior optic radiation or inferior aspect of the left visual cortex. **G.** Left inferior quadrantanopia due to a lesion of the right superior optic radiation or superior aspect of the right visual cortex. **H.** Right inferior quadrantanopia due to a lesion of the left superior optic radiation or superior aspect of the left visual cortex.

Acute causes of optic neuropathy include:

- Elevated intracranial pressure with papilledema
- Immune-mediated (optic neuritis; see Ch. 21):
  - Demyelinating disease: multiple sclerosis, neuromyelitis optica, anti-MOG
  - Systemic inflammatory disease: sarcoidosis, vasculitis, paraneoplastic (anti-CRMP-5 antibodies)
- Infectious: syphilis, *Bartonella* (cat-scratch disease)

Subacute to chronic causes of optic neuropathy include:

- Neoplasm or treatment of neoplasm:
  - Intrinsic: optic nerve glioma
  - Extrinsic: compression from optic nerve sheath meningioma, skull base meningioma, pituitary tumor, leptomeningeal metastases
- Radiation-induced optic neuropathy
- Toxic:
  - Medications: ethambutol, linezolid
  - Toxins: methanol, tobacco-alcohol amblyopia
- Metabolic: vitamin B12 deficiency
- Hereditary: For example, Leber's hereditary optic neuropathy (a mitochondrial condition)

In general, ischemic, neoplastic, and inflammatory causes of optic neuropathy present unilaterally. In demyelinating disease, multiple sclerosis often causes unilateral optic neuritis, whereas

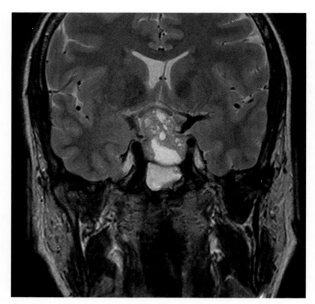

FIGURE 6–4 **Coronal T2-weighted MRI demonstrating pituitary macroadenoma compressing the optic chiasm.** This patient presented with bitemporal hemianopia.

neuromyelitis optic and anti-MOG disease can cause bilateral (or rapidly sequential) optic neuritis. Infectious causes of optic neuropathy can present unilaterally or bilaterally. Toxic, metabolic, and hereditary causes generally present bilaterally. Optic neuritis is typically painful (with worsening ocular pain with eye movement), whereas other etiologies of optic neuropathy are typically painless. Optic neuritis is discussed in Chapter 21.

Bitemporal Hemianopia

The most common cause of chiasmal lesions is pituitary pathology, but sellar menigiomas, craniopharyngiomas, and aneurysms (e.g., of the distal carotid) can also occur in this region. Figure 6–4 shows an MRI from a patient who presented with bitemporal hemianopia and was found to have a pituitary macroadenoma compressing the optic chiasm.

Homonymous Visual Field Deficits

The causes of lesions of the lateral geniculate nucleus (LGN), optic radiations, and occipital lobes include any diseases that can affect the cerebral hemispheres: for example, vascular, neoplastic, infectious, inflammatory. The LGN is in the territory of the anterior choroidal artery (a branch of the internal carotid artery), the superior radiation is in the territory of the middle cerebral artery, the inferior radiation is in the territory of the middle and posterior cerebral arteries, and the occipital cortex is in the territory of the posterior cerebral artery (see Ch. 7).

DISORDERS OF VISUAL COGNITION

Visual information from the primary visual cortex (at the occipital pole) is transmitted superiorly to the parietal lobe for spatial processing (the "where" pathway) and transmitted inferiorly to the temporal lobe for object identification/recognition (the "what" pathway). The left "what" pathway is specialized for processing of visual word forms, so lesions in the left inferior temporo-occipital region can lead to inability to read (**alexia**), sometimes with preserved ability to write (**alexia without agraphia**). The right "what" pathway is specialized for processing of faces, so lesions in the right inferior temporo-occipital region (in the fusiform gyrus) can lead to inability to recognize faces (**prosopagnosia**).

Balint Syndrome

Balint syndrome occurs with lesions of the bilateral parieto-occipital junctions (e.g., due to middle cerebral artery–posterior cerebral artery [MCA-PCA] watershed/borderzone infarcts; see Ch. 7). This syndrome is characterized by a triad of signs that are manifestations of deficits in visual attention: **optic ataxia, ocular apraxia**, and **simultanagnosia**.

Optic ataxia is an "ataxia" due to difficulty using visual attention to guide extremity movements. This can be demonstrated on the finger–nose test. Rather than the oscillatory movements seen in cerebellar ataxia, the patient's movements appear to be misdirected, as if the patient cannot determine how to direct the finger to the target.

Ocular apraxia is an inability to use visual attention to guide eye movements. The patient will not be able to track the examiner's finger, but may be able to move the eyes appropriately in response to commands such as "look left" and "look right."

Simultanagnosia is an inability to visually "survey" a scene and see the "forest for the trees." For example, if a patient is shown a drawing of one large letter or number composed of smaller versions of a different letter or number, the patient may see only the small letters or numbers but not the larger letter or number they create.

Cortical Blindness & Anton Syndrome

If enough of the occipital cortex is damaged bilaterally (e.g., bilateral posterior cerebral artery [PCA] strokes), this can lead to **cortical blindness**: The eyes and optic nerves still work (as can be proven by normal pupillary light reflexes), but the brain cannot decode visual information. Some patients with cortical blindness are unaware that they are blind and may deny being unable to see, a condition called **Anton syndrome**.

Charles Bonnet Syndrome

In patients with bilateral visual loss of any cause (most commonly ocular in older adults), patients may develop "release" hallucinations (**Charles Bonnet syndrome**). These hallucinations are generally of small people, are not threatening to the patient, and the patient usually knows they are not real.

The Cerebral Hemispheres & Vascular Syndromes

CHAPTER CONTENTS

Chapters 4 and 6 mapped the primary motor cortex (precentral gyrus of the frontal lobe), primary somatosensory cortex (postcentral gyrus of the parietal lobe), and the primary visual cortex (calcarine cortex of the posterior occipital lobe) onto the cerebral hemispheres. The primary auditory cortex is housed in the superior temporal gyrus of the temporal lobe. Knowing the locations of the motor cortex and these three primary sensory cortices allows for a logical deduction of the functions of the rest of the cortical surface as is discussed in the following text.

The hemisphere contralateral to the side of handedness is considered the **dominant hemisphere** (e.g., the left hemisphere in a right-handed patient), and the hemisphere ipsilateral to the side of handedness is considered the **nondominant hemisphere** (e.g., the right hemisphere in a right-handed patient). Most patients are right-handed, so their left hemisphere is the dominant hemisphere. Language dysfunction is most commonly due to lesions in the dominant (usually left) hemisphere, whereas neglect (see "Attention" below) is most commonly due to lesions in the nondominant (usually right) hemisphere (causing left-sided neglect).

CORTICAL REGIONS (FIG. 7–1)

Parietal Lobes: Spatial Attention & Praxis
Attention
The parietal lobe regions bounded by the somatosensory cortex anteriorly and the visual cortex posteriorly are ideally situated to combine visual and spatial information, playing roles in awareness of the body in space, spatial reasoning, and mathematical processing. The projection from the occipital lobe superiorly to the parietal lobe (the dorsal stream) is referred to as the "where" pathway: Visual information is processed here to determine where things are in space with respect to the body. Lesions here can cause **neglect:** The patient is unaware of one half of the world. Neglect is more common with lesions in the nondominant parietal lobe, which is most commonly the right parietal lobe causing left-sided neglect. Examination findings in patients with neglect may include extinction to double simultaneous stimulation (see Ch. 4), lack of awareness of deficits (**anosognosia**; e.g., not being aware that a paretic limb is weak despite inability to move it), and in severe cases, inability to recognize the neglected body parts as one's own.

Lesions in the angular gyrus of the dominant (usually left) parietal lobe can cause **Gerstmann's syndrome:** left-right confusion, inability to count (**acalculia**), inability to name the fingers (**finger agnosia**), and inability to write (**agraphia**).

Praxis
Parietal lesions can also cause difficulty performing a complex learned action (**apraxia**) despite intact strength, sensation, and coordination. This can be demonstrated by asking a patient to mime an action (e.g., "pretend you are taking out a

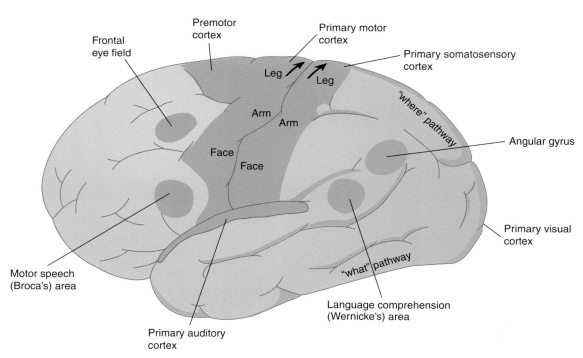

FIGURE 7–1 **Schematic of the left lateral surface of the brain showing selected clinically important cortical regions.** Reproduced with permission from Waxman S: *Clinical Neuroanatomy*, 27th ed. New York, NY: McGraw Hill; 2013.

pack of matches and lighting one," or "pretend you are brushing your teeth"). There are several types of apraxia, including:

- **Limb-kinetic apraxia** refers to a loss of dexterity in performing actions.
- **Ideomotor apraxia** refers to inability to correctly perform actions in response to verbal cues or by imitation, with errors in both spatial positioning and timing. A commonly made movement error in this condition is substituting the body part for the tool being pantomimed (e.g., instead of pantomiming brushing one's teeth by gripping an imaginary toothbrush, the patient pantomimes the hand itself as the toothbrush).
- **Ideational apraxia** refers to inability to perform an action sequence in the appropriate order. For example, if asked to perform a multistep movement sequence (e.g., fold a letter, put it in an envelope, and seal the envelope), despite preserved ability to perform individual component movements.

Apraxia is generally caused by lesions of the parietal lobe in the dominant (usually left) hemisphere, but can also be caused by lesions of the supplementary motor cortex or white matter tracts connecting parietal regions with frontal motor regions.

Temporal Lobes: Recognition Memory

The temporal lobes are ideally located to combine sensory input from olfactory, auditory, visual, and somatosensory cortices. The temporal lobes are thus ideally suited to play a role in **recognition memory**, since this type of memory relies on internal representations of sensory experiences. Lesions of the medial temporal lobes (including the hippocampus) can cause **amnesia**. The flow of visual information inferiorly to the temporal lobe (the ventral stream) is referred to as the "what pathway:" visual information is processed here to determine what things are (recognition memory). The dominant (usually left) inferior temporal lobe houses the visual word form area necessary for reading, and the nondominant (usually right) inferior temporal lobe houses the face recognition area. Inability to read is called **alexia** and inability to recognize faces is referred to as **prosopagnosia**.

Frontal & Temporal Lobes: Language

The inferior frontal gyrus lies in proximity to the auditory and motor cortices and is adjacent to the premotor cortex for the face. It is therefore ideally positioned to combine auditory and motor functions for speech production. The inferior frontal gyrus houses **Broca's area** for speech production. **Wernicke's area** for speech recognition lies at the junction of the auditory cortex (superior temporal gyrus) and the parietal cortex, where auditory regions are adjacent to parietal regions involved in awareness of one's surroundings. In most right-handed patients, language is localized to the left hemisphere, and this is true in many left-handed patients as well. However, in some patients (more commonly left-handed patients), language may localize to the right hemisphere. Lesions in and around Broca's and Wernicke's areas lead to speech disturbances (**aphasia**).

The aphasias can be categorized based on the patient's ability to produce speech, comprehend speech, and repeat

TABLE 7–1 Aphasias.

	Speech Production	Speech Comprehension	Repetition	Lesion Location (Most Commonly in Left Hemipshere)
Broca's aphasia	Impaired	Preserved	Impaired	Inferior frontal gyrus (Broca's area)
Transcortical motor aphasia	Impaired	Preserved	Preserved	Anterior/superior to Broca's area
Wernicke's aphasia	Preserved	Impaired	Impaired	Posterior superior temporal gyrus (Wernicke's area)
Transcortical sensory aphasia	Preserved	Impaired	Preserved	Parietal, posterior to Wernicke's area
Global aphasia	Impaired	Impaired	Impaired	Broca's and Wernicke's areas
Mixed transcortical aphasia	Impaired	Impaired	Preserved	Extensive lesions often involving middle cerebral artery–anterior cerebral artey (MCA-ACA) watershed region
Conduction aphasia	Preserved	Preserved	Impaired	Arcuate fasciculus

words and phrases (Table 7–1). In pure **Broca's aphasia**, the primary deficit is in production of speech (called **nonfluent** or **expressive aphasia**), but the patient can generally still comprehend. However, patients with Broca's aphasia may have difficulty with comprehension of grammatically complex phrases (e.g., "The tiger was eaten by the lion. Who survived?"). In the most severe Broca's aphasias, the patient is mute. When less severe, the patient may have effortful speech with frequent errors. Since comprehension is generally largely preserved in Broca's aphasia, the patient is aware of and frustrated by the inability to speak. In a pure Broca's aphasia, the patient cannot repeat phrases stated by the examiner but can comprehend (i.e., can follow commands). If a patient has an expressive aphasia with preserved repetition, this is called a **transcortical motor aphasia**.

In pure **Wernicke's aphasia**, comprehension is impaired (**receptive aphasia**), and although the prosody (melody and rhythm) of speech is preserved (**fluent aphasia**), the content is nonsensical. The patient cannot understand his or her own nonsensical speech, and so may not appear concerned by the deficit. In pure Wernicke's aphasia, a patient cannot repeat phrases. If repetition is preserved in a receptive aphasia, this is called a **transcortical sensory aphasia**.

If both production and comprehension are impaired, this is called **global aphasia**. Rarely, patients with both productive and receptive aphasia are still able to repeat what they hear, a scenario called **mixed transcortical aphasia**.

Note that all of the transcortical aphasias are characterized by preserved repetition, and named for the primary language *deficit*: Transcortical *motor* aphasia is characterized by a deficit in speech *production* (motor output), transcortical *sensory* aphasia is characterized by a deficit in speech *comprehension* ("sensation" of speech), and mixed transcortical aphasia is characterized by a mix of both expressive and receptive aphasia.

If a patient's only language deficit is repetition with preserved comprehension and production, this is called a **conduction aphasia**, since conduction between Wernicke's area and Broca's area (via the **arcuate fasciculus**) is disrupted.

Sudden-onset aphasia is most commonly due to stroke in the left middle cerebral artery territory, but can also be due to a seizure or postictal state if the seizure activity originates in or

spreads to language regions. More subacute development of aphasia can be seen with a left-sided chronic subdural hematoma or a tumor affecting language regions. Aphasia can also develop even more insidiously due to neurodegenerative diseases such as primary progressive aphasia (see Ch. 22).

In addition to regions involved in language and motor control, the frontal lobes support executive functions including working memory, decision making, abstract reasoning, and emotional processing. Frontal lobe lesions can cause **abulia** (decreased initiative, motivation, speech, and emotional response), behavioral disinhibition, and/or impairments in any of the above executive functions.

The higher order functions of the occipital lobes are discussed in Chapter 6.

SUBCORTICAL STRUCTURES: THALAMUS & BASAL GANGLIA

The thalamus and basal ganglia are "islands" of gray matter in the subcortical white matter. Both are nodes in a variety of circuits that begin and/or end in the cortex, brainstem, and/or cerebellum.

The Thalamus

The left and right thalamus are positioned on either side of the third ventricle, just superior to the midbrain. The thalamus is a collection of nuclei, most of which project to one or more cortical regions (only the reticular nuclei do not project to the cortex, but rather to other thalamic nuclei) (Table 7–2). Four basic types of circuitry pass through thalamic nuclei en route to the cortex:

1. **Sensory pathways**. All sensory pathways synapse in the thalamus, which transmits sensory information to the respective sensory cortices. Smell is the only sensory modality that reaches the cortex before the thalamus (transmitted directly to the olfactory cortex, which then transmits smell information to the thalamus [dorsomedial nucleus]).

2. **Motor control pathways**. The ventral anterior (VA) and ventral lateral (VL) nuclei of the thalamus participate in

TABLE 7–2 Thalamic Nuclei.

	Function	Input	Output
Sensory nuclei			
Ventral posterior lateral (VPL)	Somatosensory for body	Dorsal column pathway Anterolateral (spinothalamic) tracts	Postcentral gyrus (superior-medial)
Ventral posterior medial (VPM)	Somatosensory for face	Trigeminal pathways	Postcentral gyrus (lateral)
Lateral geniculate nucleus (LGN)	Visual pathway	Optic tracts	Occipital lobes
Medial geniculate nucleus (MGN)	Auditory pathway	Inferior colliculus	Superior temporal gyrus
Pulvinar	Visual attention	Superior colliculus	Occipital and parietal cortex
Motor nuclei			
Ventral anterior (VA)	Motor circuits	Basal ganglia	Motor/premotor/supplementary motor cortex
Ventral lateral (VL)	Motor circuits	Basal ganglia Cerebellum (via superior cerebellar peduncle)	Motor/premotor/supplementary motor cortex
Cognition, consciousness, and arousal nuclei			
Anterior	Memory and emotion (Papez circuit)	Mamillothalamic tracts (Papez circuit originates in hippocampus)	Anterior cingulate (Papez's circuit ultimately projects back to hippocampus)
Mediodorsal	Cognition	Cortex	Cortex (except reticular nuclei, which project to other thalamic nuclei)
Centromedian	Arousal	Basal ganglia	
Reticular	Consciousness	Reticular activating system	
Intralaminar		Other thalamic nuclei	

cortical–basal ganglia–cortical loops and cerebellar–cortical pathways.

3. **Consciousness/arousal pathways.** These pathways begin in the brainstem reticular activating system and project to both thalami, which in turn project diffusely throughout the cortex.

4. **Cognition/emotion pathways.** Corticocortical loops pass through the thalamus, playing roles in diverse cognitive functions. One such loop is the **circuit of Papez** which participates in memory and emotion: hippocampus → fornix → mamillary bodies → anterior nucleus of the thalamus → anterior cingulate → entorhinal cortex → hippocampus.

Individual thalamic nuclei can be affected by small strokes (e.g., lacunar stroke in ventral posterior medial/ventral posterior lateral [VPM/VPL] thalamic nuclei causing contralateral sensory loss). Larger lesions of the thalamus can cause decreased level of consciousness. The thalamus is commonly affected by intracerebral hemorrhage (e.g., due to hypertension, or bilateral due to internal cerebral vein thrombosis), which also often affects the adjacent posterior limb of the internal capsule, leading to contralateral hemiparesis/hemiplegia (in addition to contralateral hemisensory loss and depressed level of consciousness due to thalamic involvement). Given its diffuse connections with diverse cortical regions, lesions of the thalamus are said to be able to "do anything" (i.e., cause any type of deficit), including causing "cortical" signs (e.g., aphasia, neglect, cognitive deficits) and eye movement abnormalities (in part due to effects on nearby midbrain pathways for eye movements).

The Basal Ganglia

The basal ganglia include the caudate, putamen, globus pallidus, and subthalamic nucleus (Figs. 7–2, 7–3, and 7–4). The caudate and putamen together are referred to as the **striatum**, and the putamen and globus pallidus together are referred to as the **lenticular nuclei**. The basal ganglia are part of circuits that initiate and control movements, and dysfunction in the basal ganglia leads to movement disorders (e.g., Parkinson's disease; see Ch. 23). When the basal ganglia are affected by cerebrovascular disease, the surrounding internal capsule is also often affected, causing the predominant manifestation to be contralateral weakness, with movement disorders being relatively uncommon in this scenario. One exception is stroke of the subthalamic nucleus, which can produce contralateral hemiballismus (unilateral ballistic movements). Slower growing lesions involving the basal ganglia (e.g., tumors, toxoplasmosis) can cause contralateral movement disorders.

One model of basal ganglia circuitry provides an explanation for some aspects of certain movement disorders (Fig. 7–5). The model includes a loop circuit that goes from cortical motor regions to the basal ganglia to the thalamus (VL/VA nuclei) back to cortical motor regions. The cortical motor regions excite the basal ganglia and the thalamus

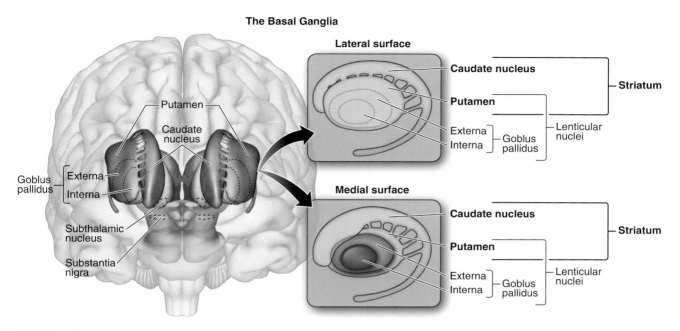

FIGURE 7–2 The basal ganglia. Hologram frontal view of brain to show internal aspects of basal ganglia, with lateral and medial views projected to the right.

excites cortical motor regions. Basal ganglia output to the thalamus is inhibitory, so the degree of thalamic excitation of cortical motor regions depends on whether this inhibitory basal ganglia output is excited (increased inhibition leading to decreased cortical motor activity) or inhibited

(decreased inhibition leading to increased cortical motor activity).

The basal ganglia have two overlapping pathways within them: the direct pathway and the indirect pathway. The direct pathway leads to decreased inhibitory output to the thalamus

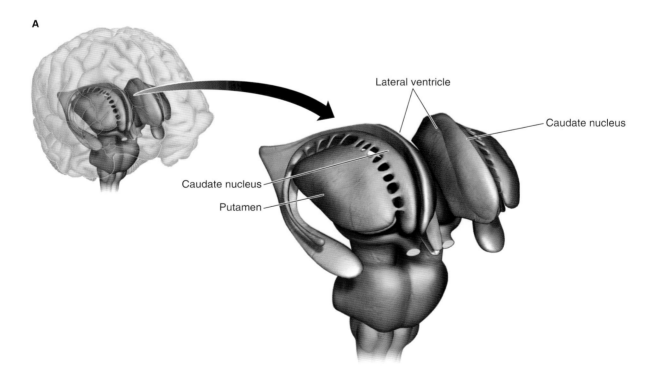

FIGURE 7–3 The basal ganglia. Basal ganglia "removed" from brain to show three-dimensional relationships. **A.** In relation to lateral ventricles (gray). **B.** Caudate and putamen translucent to view globus pallidus and thalamus (the latter not considered part of the basal ganglia).

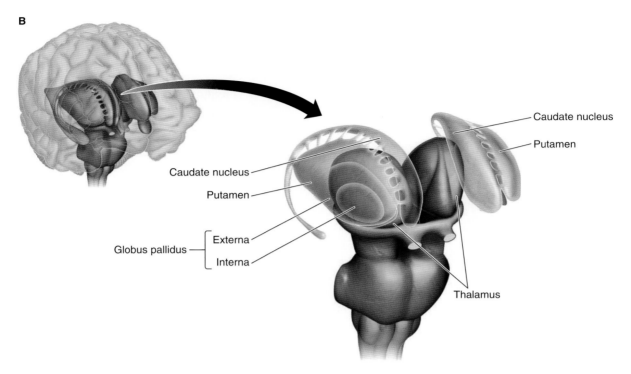

FIGURE 7-3 (*Continued*)

and therefore increased excitation of cortical motor regions; the indirect pathway leads to increased inhibitory output to the thalamus and therefore decreased excitation of the cortical motor regions.

Both the direct and indirect pathways begin in the striatum and end in the globus pallidus interna (GPi), which is the output of the basal ganglia to the thalamus in this circuit. The direct pathway proceeds from the striatum to the GPi to

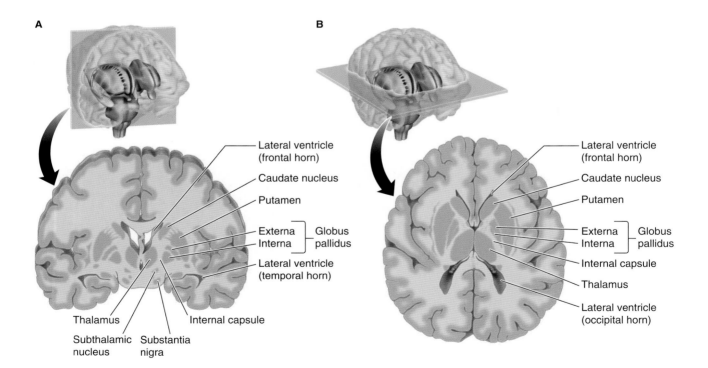

FIGURE 7-4 **The basal ganglia. A.** Coronal view. **B.** Axial view.

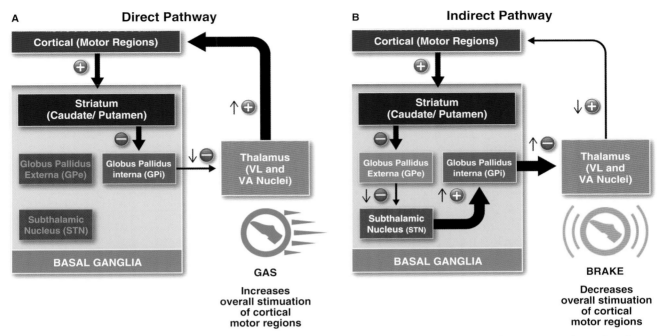

FIGURE 7–5 **Schematic of the direct and indirect pathway model. A.** Direct pathway. **B.** Indirect pathway. See text for explanation.

the thalamus. The indirect pathway proceeds from the striatum to the globus pallidus externa (GPe) to the subthalamic nucleus (STN) to the GPi to the thalamus. All synapses within the direct and indirect pathways are inhibitory (GABA) *except* for from the STN to the GPi, which is excitatory (glutamate). In the direct pathway, the striatum inhibits the GPi from inhibiting the thalamus, therefore disinhibiting the thalamus and leading to overall increased activity of cortical motor regions (mnemonic: *di*rect pathway *di*sinhibits). In the *in*direct pathway, the striatum *in*hibits the GPe from inhibiting the STN,

therefore disinhibiting the STN, which increases its excitation of the GPi, which in turn inhibits the thalamus, leading to overall decreased cortical motor activity (mnemonic: *in*direct pathway *in*hibits). Thus, the direct pathway serves as a "gas pedal," and the indirect pathway as a "brake" in this model.

Dopaminergic projections from the substantia nigra to the striatum lead to increased direct pathway activity (through stimulation of D1 receptors) and decreased indirect pathway activity (through stimulation of D2 receptors) (Fig. 7–6). Therefore, dopamine leads to increased excitation and decreased

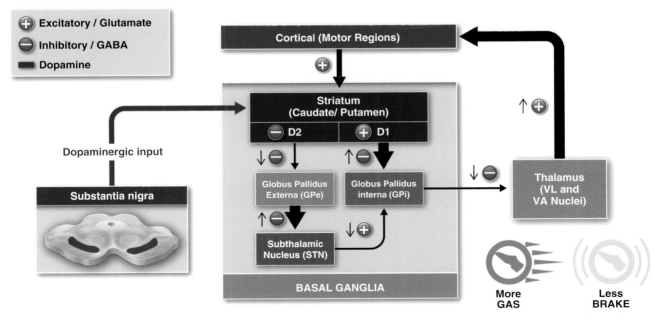

FIGURE 7–6 **Relationship of substantia nigra dopaminergic input with direct and indirect pathway model.** See text for explanation.

inhibition, resulting in overall increased motor activity. In Parkinson's disease (see Ch. 23), substantia nigra degeneration leads to decreased dopaminergic input to the striatum (Fig. 7–7A). This leads to decreased direct pathway activity and increased indirect pathway activity, which may explain the bradykinesia of Parkinson's disease (but does not explain the tremor).

In Huntington's disease (see Ch. 23), there is thought to be selective degeneration of indirect pathway neurons in the striatum. This leads to decreased indirect pathway (inhibitory)

activity, resulting in excess stimulation of cortical regions, which may explain the hyperkinetic nature of this movement disorder that causes chorea (Fig. 7–7B).

If the STN is affected unilaterally (most commonly by stroke or hemorrhage), this decreases excitation of the GPi, leading to decreased indirect pathway (inhibitory) activity, resulting in excess stimulation of cortical regions (Fig. 7–7C). This causes contralateral increased motor activity, most commonly hemiballismus.

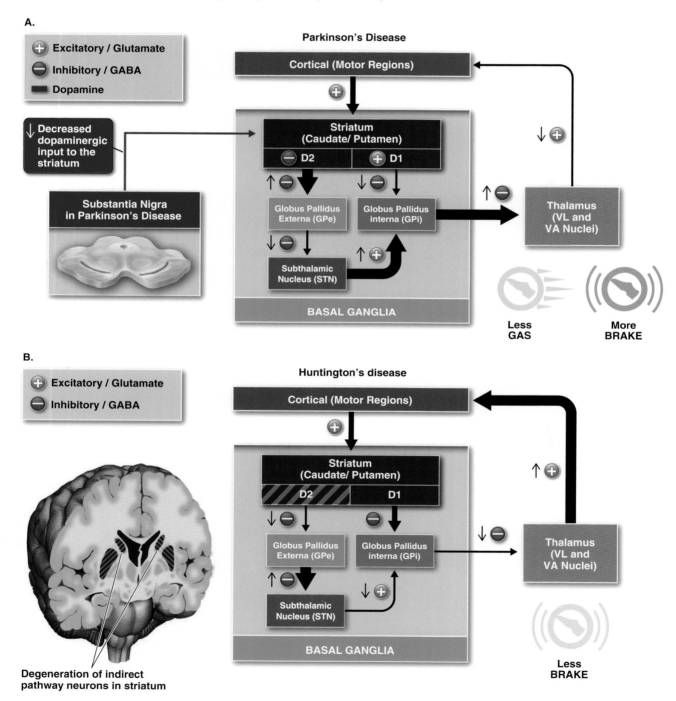

FIGURE 7–7 **Direct and indirect pathway model in neurologic disease. A.** Parkinson's disease. **B.** Huntington's disease. **C.** Hemiballismus. See text for explanation.

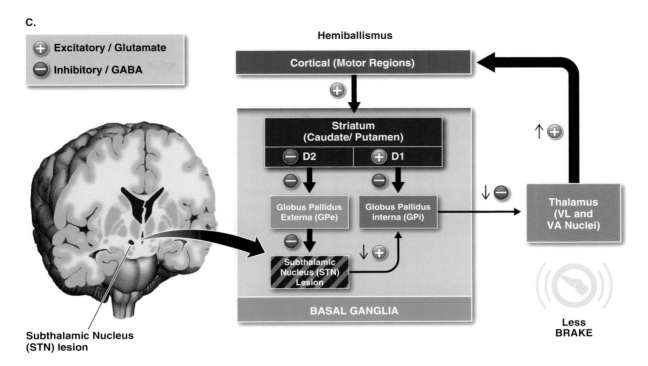

C.

Hemiballismus

- Excitatory / Glutamate
- Inhibitory / GABA

Cortical (Motor Regions)

Striatum
(Caudate/ Putamen)

⊖ D2   ⊕ D1

Globus Pallidus
Externa (GPe)

Globus Pallidus
interna (GPi)

Subthalamic
Nucleus (STN)
Lesion

BASAL GANGLIA

Thalamus
(VL and
VA Nuclei)

Less
BRAKE

Subthalamic Nucleus
(STN) lesion

FIGURE 7–7 *(Continued)*

ARTERIAL SUPPLY OF THE CEREBRAL HEMISPHERES (FIGS. 7–8 AND 7–9)

The brain, brainstem, and cerebellum are supplied by arteries arising from the paired internal carotid arteries (the **anterior circulation**) and the paired vertebral arteries (the **posterior circulation**). The internal carotid arteries arise from the common carotid arteries, which themselves arise from the aortic arch (from the brachiocephalic trunk on the right and directly from the aortic arch on the left). Each carotid artery ultimately gives rise to a **middle cerebral artery** (MCA) and an **anterior cerebral artery** (ACA), and these arteries together supply the majority of the cerebral hemispheres including the frontal lobes, parietal lobes, and superior and lateral temporal lobes.

Each internal carotid artery also gives rise to an ophthalmic artery (which supplies the retina) and an anterior choroidal artery (which supplies the posterior thalamus and internal capsule).

The vertebral arteries arise from the subclavian arteries, join to form the **basilar artery** at around the level of the pontomedullary junction, and end by giving off the **posterior cerebral arteries** (PCAs) at the level of the upper midbrain. The PCAs supply the regions of the cerebral hemispheres not supplied by the MCAs and ACAs: the occipital lobes and inferior and medial temporal lobes.

Before giving rise to the PCAs, the vertebrobasilar system gives off three paired circumferential arteries that supply the lateral brainstem and cerebellum (superior cerebellar arteries [SCAs], anterior inferior cerebellar arteries [AICAs],

and posterior inferior cerebellar arteries [PICAs]), which are discussed in relation to the cerebellum and brainstem in Chapters 8 and 9.

The anterior circulation and posterior circulation are linked by the **posterior communicating arteries**, and the ACAs are linked by the **anterior communicating artery**. These connections form the circle of Willis on the inferior surface of the brain, which provides routes for collateral flow. Not all patients have a complete circle of Willis, and some patients have anatomic variants, the most common of which are introduced here. The clinical implications of some of these variants are discussed later in this chapter.

- **Hypoplastic vertebral artery.** Many patients have one dominant vertebral artery and a smaller hypoplastic nondominant vertebral artery. When this occurs, the basilar artery appears to swing to the side of the nondominant vertebral artery, and the vertebral canal is smaller on the side of the congenitally smaller vertebral artery. These features help to distinguish a congenitally smaller vertebral artery from a pathologically smaller one (e.g., due to dissection or atherosclerosis). In Figure 7–9A, the left vertebral artery (on the right of the image) is dominant, the right vertebral artery (on the left of the image) is nondominant, and the basilar artery swings toward the nondominant right vertebral artery (toward the left of the image). Note that although it is common for the vertebral arteries to be different in caliber, the carotid arteries should *always* be symmetric. Any asymmetry of the internal carotid arteries is therefore abnormal.

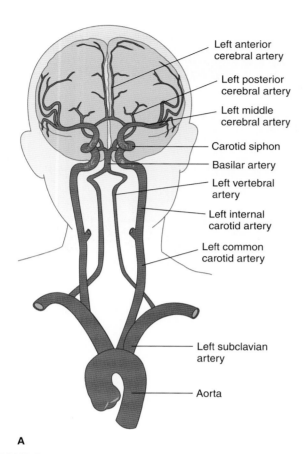

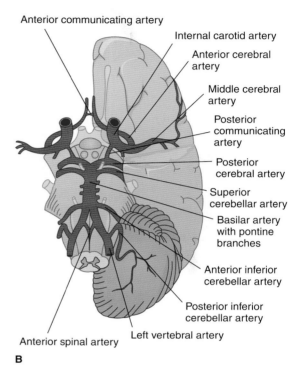

A

B

FIGURE 7–8 **Schematic of the blood supply to the brain. A:** Frontal view of the cerebral circulation (as if looking at the patient; note that the circumferential branches of the vertebrobasilar system are not shown in this diagram). **B:** View of the inferior surface of the brain (and anterior surface of the brainstem) showing the arterial supply to the cerebral hemispheres, brainstem, and cerebellum. Reproduced with permission from Waxman S: *Clinical Neuroanatomy*, 27th ed. New York, NY: McGraw Hill; 2013.

- **Azygous ACA**. In this variant, both ACAs emerge from a common trunk.
- **Fetal PCA**. In this variant, the PCA arises from the internal carotid artery rather than the top of the basilar. This variant may occur unilaterally or bilaterally (Fig. 7–10).
- **Artery of Percheron**. In this variant, a single artery from one of the PCAs supplies both thalami (rather than an individual supply on each side).

The Vascular Territories of the ACA, MCA, & PCA (Fig. 7–11)

Most generally, the ACAs and MCAs supply the anterior, medial, and lateral aspects of the hemispheres, and the PCAs supply the posterior and inferior aspects. On the cortical surface, the MCAs supply the lateral surface of the frontal, temporal, and parietal lobes, the ACAs supply the medial surface of the frontal and parietal lobes, and the PCAs supply the occipital lobes and the inferior temporal lobes. Subcortically, the MCAs supply the majority of the hemispheres, creating a trapezoidal territory in the axial plane—anteriorly

and medially to this trapezoid are supplied by the ACAs, and posteriorly and inferiorly are supplied by the PCAs (including the thalamus, which is supplied by penetrating vessels arising from the PCAs and posterior communicating arteries).

Watershed (Borderzone) Territories (Fig. 7–12)

The watershed (borderzone) territories are the regions at the border of two arterial territories. The MCA-ACA and MCA-PCA borderzones are the most commonly discussed borderzones, but there is also a borderzone between AICA and PICA, as well as a deep borderzone territory between the lenticulostriate branches of the MCA (penetrating from below) and the leptomeningeal branches of the MCA (penetrating from above). Although the common teaching is that borderzone infarction is due to hypoperfusion, borderzone strokes can also be caused by emboli: If the smallest possible emboli travel as distally as possible before causing an occlusion, they will arrive at the end-arterial territories, which are the borderzones. So although borderzone infarction can certainly be due

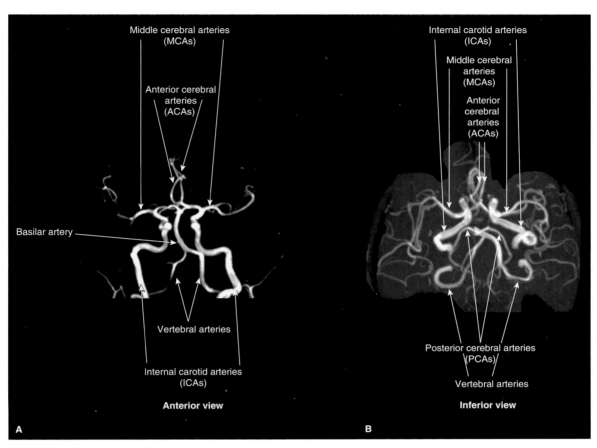

Middle cerebral arteries
(MCAs)

Anterior cerebral
arteries
(ACAs)

Basilar artery

Vertebral arteries

Internal carotid arteries
(ICAs)

Anterior view

A

Internal carotid arteries
(ICAs)

Middle cerebral
arteries
(MCAs)

Anterior
cerebral
arteries
(ACAs)

Posterior cerebral arteries
(PCAs)

Vertebral arteries

Inferior view

B

FIGURE 7–9 **MR angiogram (MRA) of the intracranial arterial circulation. A:** Frontal view (as if looking at the patient). **B:** Inferior view (as if looking up at the base of the brain from below).

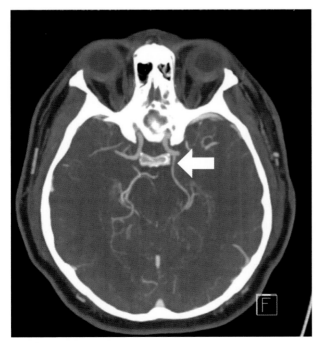

FIGURE 7–10 **Fetal PCA.** Axial CT angiogram (CTA) demonstrating left PCA emerging from the left internal carotid artery (arrow).

to hypoperfusion, this is not always the cause, and an embolic etiology should also be considered as the etiology of border-zone infarction (for an interesting discussion of this topic, see Caplan and Hennerici, 1998).

CLINICAL SYNDROMES ASSOCIATED WITH CEREBRAL VASCULAR TERRITORIES

Any artery or arterial branch may be affected in ischemic stroke, with corresponding symptoms related to the location and size of the infarct. The diagnosis and management of stroke are discussed in Chapter 19.

MCA Territory Infarction (Fig. 7–13)

The MCA territory includes the majority of the cerebral hemisphere, including portions of the frontal, temporal, and parietal lobes with the exception of the anterior, medial, and superior frontal lobes and the medial and superior parietal lobes (supplied by the ACA), and the occipital and inferior temporal lobes (PCA territory). The functional regions supplied by the MCA therefore include the motor and premotor

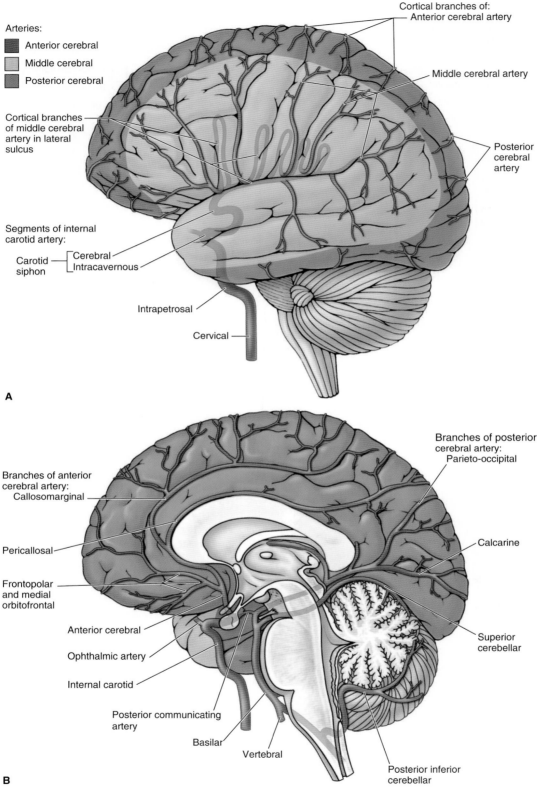

FIGURE 7–11 Schematic of vascular territories of the cerebral hemispheres. A: Lateral surface of the cerebral hemisphere. **B:** Medial surface of the cerebral hemisphere. **C:** Axial section of the cerebral hemispheres. **D:** Coronal section of the cerebral hemisphere. A-C, Reproduced with permission from Martin J: *Neuroanatomy Text and Atlas*, 4th ed. New York, NY: McGraw Hill; 2012. D, Reproduced with permission from Ropper A, Samuels M, Klein J: Adams and Victor's *Principles of Neurology*, 10th ed. New York, NY: McGraw Hill; 2014.

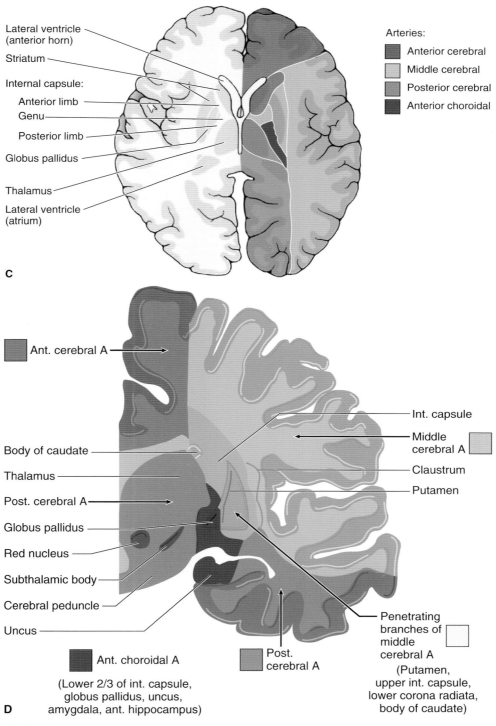

C

Arteries:
- Anterior cerebral
- Middle cerebral
- Posterior cerebral
- Anterior choroidal

Lateral ventricle (anterior horn)
Striatum
Internal capsule:
Anterior limb
Genu
Posterior limb
Globus pallidus
Thalamus
Lateral ventricle (atrium)

Ant. cerebral A
Body of caudate
Thalamus
Post. cerebral A
Globus pallidus
Red nucleus
Subthalamic body
Cerebral peduncle
Uncus

Int. capsule
Middle cerebral A
Claustrum
Putamen
Penetrating branches of middle cerebral A (Putamen, upper int. capsule, lower corona radiata, body of caudate)

Ant. choroidal A
(Lower 2/3 of int. capsule, globus pallidus, uncus, amygdala, ant. hippocampus)

Post. cerebral A

D

FIGURE 7–11 (Continued)

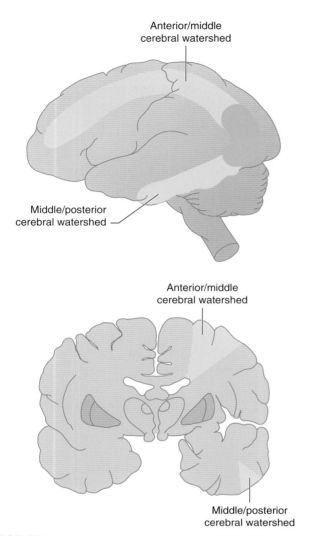

FIGURE 7–12 **Schematic of ACA/MCA and MCA/PCA watershed (borderzone) territories**. Reproduced with permission from Aminoff M, Greenberg D, Simon R: *Clinical Neurology*, 9th ed. New York, NY: McGraw Hill; 2015.

regions, somatosensory cortex, the frontal eye fields, the language areas (found on the left in the majority of patients), parietal regions responsible for spatial attention (right parietal lesions may cause left-sided neglect), and the superior and inferior radiations of the visual pathways as they pass through the parietal and temporal lobes, respectively. Therefore, a full left MCA syndrome causes right hemiplegia and hemisensory loss, aphasia, gaze deviation toward the left, and right homonymous hemianopia. A full right MCA syndrome causes left hemiplegia and hemisensory loss, left-sided neglect, gaze deviation to the right, and left-sided homonymous hemianopia. Gaze deviation is discussed in Chapter 11 and visual field deficits in Chapter 6.

The MCA stem is called the M1 segment of the MCA. The MCA stem gives off the lenticulostriate penetrating branches that supply the basal ganglia and internal capsule before dividing into superior and inferior branches known as

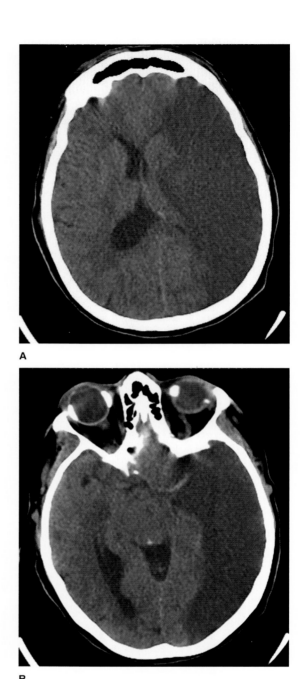

FIGURE 7–13 **MCA infarct.** Axial CT scan demonstrating full-territory left MCA infarct. Note *spared* areas including: **A:** caudate (supplied by recurrent artery of Huebner), thalamus (supplied by PCA), ACA and PCA territories, as well as the medial temporal lobe (**B**). Note also hyperdense left MCA in **B** (see Ch. 19 for explanation of this sign).

the M2 segments. The superior M2 branch of the MCA supplies Broca's area (most commonly on the left), the motor cortex, and the superior visual radiation, whereas the inferior M2 branch supplies Wernicke's area (most commonly on the left) and the inferior optic radiation. The M2 segments divide into further branches—the smaller and more

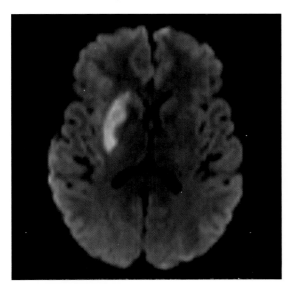

FIGURE 7–14 MCA stem infarct. Axial diffusion-weighted MRI (DWI) demonstrating ischemic infarct in the territory of the MCA stem on the right.

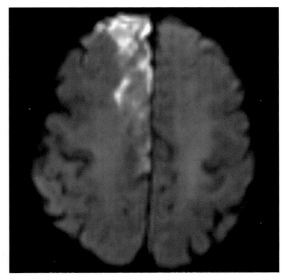

FIGURE 7–15 ACA infarct. Axial diffusion-weighted MRI (DWI) demonstrating ischemic infarct in the territory of the right ACA.

distal the vessel occluded in ischemic stroke, the smaller the corresponding deficit. However, if a small penetrating (lenticulostriate) branch of the MCA stem is affected, this can affect the convergence of descending motor fibers and lead to a complete contralateral hemiparesis despite a small infarct (pure motor lacunar syndrome; see "Lacunar Strokes").

The MCA stem is quite poorly collateralized, and MCA stem occlusion (proximal to the origin of the lenticulostriate branches) can lead to a large subcortical infarct with sparing of more distal regions if there is good collateral flow distally (Fig. 7–14).

ACA Territory Infarction (Fig. 7–15)

The ACAs supply the anterior, superior, and medial frontal lobes and the superior and medial parietal lobes—essentially all of the frontal and parietal lobes not supplied by the MCAs. Due to the position of the leg area in the motor homunculus (medial; see Ch. 4), ACA strokes cause contralateral leg weakness and sensory loss more so than face and arm weakness and sensory loss. ACA strokes can also cause cognitive changes such as abulia. The ACAs are connected by the anterior communicating artery. Proximal to the anterior communicating artery, the ACAs are labeled A1 segments; distal to the anterior communicating artery, they are labeled A2 segments.

In some patients, both ACAs arise from a common trunk (**azygous ACA**). Occlusion of both ACAs simultaneously can cause acute paraplegia, mimicking acute spinal pathology. The presence of cognitive symptoms usually distinguishes bilateral ACA infarction from acute spinal cord pathology.

The ACAs can also be compromised by subfalcine herniation (see Ch. 25).

One typically learns that the MCA supplies the face and arm areas on the lateral surface of the homunculus and the ACA supplies the leg area, so that MCA strokes cause contralateral face and arm weakness much more so than leg weakness, and ACA strokes cause contralateral leg weakness much more so than face and arm weakness. This is true for strokes affecting the cortical surface. However, the motor fibers from the face, arm, and leg travel together subcortically in the internal capsule, so an MCA stroke that affects the subcortical white matter pathways can cause contralateral hemiparesis or hemiplegia affecting the face, arm, and leg (e.g., a full MCA territory infarct affecting the cortex and subcortical white matter).

Recurrent Artery of Huebner Territory Infarction

The recurrent artery of Huebner is a branch of the ACA that supplies the head of the caudate and the adjacent internal capsule. Infarction can cause contralateral hemiparesis and/or movement disorder, which may be accompanied by cognitive deficits.

Anterior Choroidal Artery Territory Infarction

The anterior choroidal artery branches directly from the internal carotid artery and supplies the posterior thalamus (including the lateral geniculate nucleus) and the internal capsule (including descending motor and ascending thalamocortical pathways). Infarction in the territory of the anterior choroidal artery can cause contralateral visual field defects, contralateral hemiparesis, and/or contralateral hemisensory loss, and can also cause cortical signs (e.g., neglect if the right hemisphere is affected) due to interruption of thalamocortical pathways.

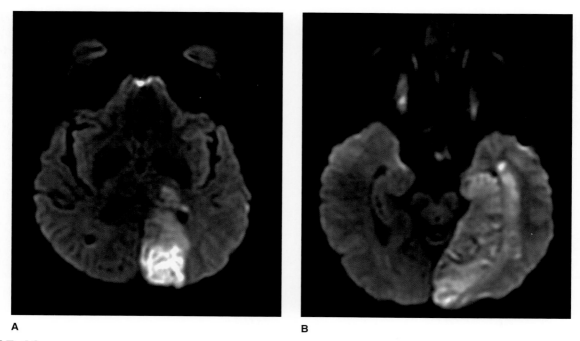

A   **B**

FIGURE 7–16 **PCA infarct.** Axial diffusion-weighted MRI (DWI) demonstrating ischemic infarct in the territory of the left PCA. Note that this territory involves not only the posterior occipital lobe but also the thalamus (**A**) and medial temporal lobe (**B**).

PCA Territory Infarction (Fig. 7–16)

The PCAs supply the occipital lobes, inferior medial temporal lobes, and the thalami. Depending on the extent of infarction in the PCA territory, deficits can include contralateral homonymous hemianopia or quadrantanopia (see Ch. 6), impaired short-term memory (if there is medial temporal/hippocampal involvement), inability to read with spared ability to write (**alexia without agraphia**) (if there is involvement of the left visual cortex and splenium of the corpus callosum, or involvement of the visual word form area in the left inferior temporal lobe), decreased ability to recognize faces (**prosopagnosia**) (if there is right inferior temporal involvement), and/or changes in cognition and/or level of arousal (if there is thalamic involvement).

The PCAs are connected to the anterior circulation by the posterior communicating arteries. Proximal to each posterior communicating artery, the PCA is called the P1 segment, and distal to the posterior communicating artery, it is called the P2 segment. In some patients, one or both PCAs arise from the internal carotids rather than the top of the basilar artery, a variant referred to as a **fetal PCA** (see Fig. 7–10). Although strokes in the PCA territory are generally considered posterior circulation strokes, if a patient has a PCA stroke in the setting of a fetal PCA, the stroke would be considered to have arisen from the anterior circulation. This is important to recognize in patients with PCA stroke and ipsilateral carotid stenosis: A fetal PCA on the side of a PCA stroke and carotid stenosis suggests that the stenotic carotid may be symptomatic (see Ch. 19).

In some patients, the left and right thalami are both supplied by a single artery that arises from the PCA, referred to as the **artery of Percheron**. Occlusion of this artery can lead to bithalamic infarction causing acutely altered mental status, a rare global, rather than focal, stroke syndrome (Fig. 7–17).

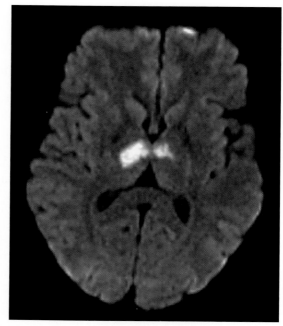

FIGURE 7–17 **Artery of Percheron infarct.** Axial diffusion-weighted MRI (DWI) demonstrating ischemic infarct in the bilateral thalami due to occlusion of the artery of Percheron.

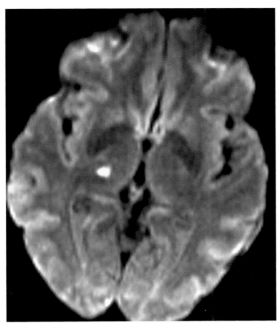

FIGURE 7–18 **Lacunar infarct.** Axial diffusion-weighted MRI (DWI) demonstrating lacunar infarction in the right thalamus.

Lacunar Strokes

Lacunar strokes are caused by occlusion of small penetrating arteries affecting the subcortical white matter (internal capsule), subcortical gray matter (basal ganglia, thalamus [Fig. 7–18]), or anterior pons. Lacunar stroke syndromes include:

- **Pure motor stroke:** unilateral hemiparesis due to involvement of the posterior limb of the internal capsule or the anterior pons.

- **Pure sensory stroke:** unilateral hemisensory loss due to involvement of the VPL/VPM nuclei of the thalamus.
- **Ataxia-hemiparesis:** unilateral hemiparesis (due to involvement of the corticospinal tract) with ataxia in the weak limb(s) (due to interruption of the corticopontocerebellar fibers destined for the middle cerebellar peduncles [see Ch. 8]). This can occur due to lacunar stroke in either the internal capsule or the anterior pons, both of which are places where the corticospinal tract and corticopontocerebellar fibers run together.
- **Dysarthria–clumsy hand:** dysarthria and unilateral upper limb ataxia; localization is the same as for ataxia-hemiparesis (internal capsule or anterior pons).

Infarction in the Watershed (Borderzone) Territories (Fig. 7–19)

The MCA-ACA watershed regions span the "stripes" at the border of the two territories. Recalling the homunculus (see Fig. 4–1), the part of the motor homunculus supplied by the MCA-ACA watershed region includes the proximal arm and leg, which are joined at the shoulder and hip in the homunculus. Therefore, infarction in the MCA-ACA borderzone can cause proximal arm and leg weakness with preserved strength distally in the hands and feet. When this occurs bilaterally, it causes what is called the "person in a barrel" syndrome since the distal arms and legs have preserved strength while the proximal limbs are weak (simulating a person in a barrel with the hands and feet sticking out).

The MCA-PCA watershed region is at the parieto-occipital junction. When the MCA-PCA watershed region is affected bilaterally, the patient will often have deficits in visual attention that can include some or all of the elements

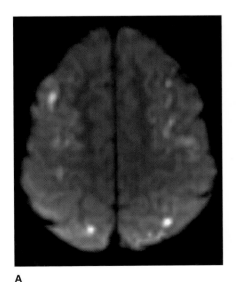

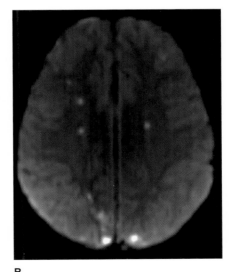

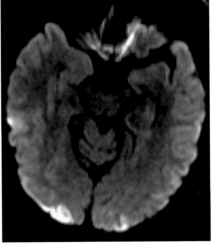

A   **B**   **C**

FIGURE 7–19 **Watershed (borderzone) infarcts.** Axial diffusion-weighted MRI (DWI) demonstrating ischemic infarction in the borderzones. **A:** Bilateral MCA-ACA borderzone infarctions. **B:** Bilateral deep borderzone infarctions. **C:** Bilateral MCA-PCA borderzone infarctions.

of **Balint's syndrome**: optic ataxia, ocular apraxia, and simultanagnosia (see Ch. 6).

The evaluation and management of patients with cerebral infarction is discussed in detail in Chapter 19.

REFERENCE

Caplan LR, Hennerici M. Impaired clearance of emboli (washout) is an important link between hypoperfusion, embolism, and ischemic stroke. *Arch Neurol* 1998;55:1475-1482.

The Cerebellum & Approach to Ataxia

The output of the motor cortex (and the adjacent premotor and supplementary cortices) is shaped by input from the basal ganglia and cerebellum. The basal ganglia and cerebellum participate in corticocortical loops that begin and end in cortical motor regions. The basal ganglia are involved in the initiation and control of movements (see Ch. 7), and the cerebellum is involved in the coordination of movements. Both structures are also involved in cognition and eye movements. Lesions of the cerebellum can lead to incoordination of movements (**ataxia**), imprecision of movements (**dysmetria**), difficulty with rapid alternating movements (**dysdiadochokinesia**), truncal and gait instability, and difficulty with articulation of speech (**dysarthria**). Due to cerebellar involvement in oculomotor and vestibular function, cerebellar lesions can also cause nystagmus, vertigo, nausea, and vomiting.

ANATOMY & FUNCTION OF THE CEREBELLUM

Overall Structure of the Cerebellum (Fig. 8–1)

Like the brain, the cerebellum has two hemispheres consisting of a cortex, deep white matter, and deep gray matter (the bilateral dentate, emboliform, globose, and fastigial nuclei). At the midline, a cerebellar structure called the **vermis** lies between the hemispheres. The midline vermis controls coordination of the middle of the body, so pathology of the vermis leads to truncal and gait instability. The laterally placed cerebellar hemispheres control the lateral parts of the body: the limbs. Therefore, lesions of one or both cerebellar hemispheres can cause limb ataxia. Lesions in the cerebellar hemispheres cause deficits in the arm and/or leg ipsilateral to the affected hemisphere (in contrast to lesions of the cerebral hemispheres which cause deficits in the arm and/or leg contralateral to the affected hemisphere).

The left and right **flocculi** and the midline **nodulus** (together referred to as the **flocculonodular lobe**) are anterior cerebellar structures involved in vestibular function and eye movements.

The Cerebellar Peduncles (Figs. 8–2, 8–3, and 8–4)

In order to coordinate movements, the cerebellum must have access to two types of information:

- What the brain wants the body to do
- Where the body is in space

After determining what needs to be done to get the body from where it is to where the brain wants it to go, the cerebellum computes a plan and sends it back to the motor regions to carry out the appropriate adjustments to coordinate ongoing movements.

To accomplish these goals, the cerebellum needs two inputs (one with information about what the brain wants the body to do, one with information about where the body is in space) and one output (to tell the brain how to guide further movements). This information travels in the three paired **cerebellar peduncles** (superior, middle, and inferior cerebellar peduncles on each side), which are the conduits of information into and out of the cerebellum. The cerebellar peduncles should not be confused with the *cerebral* peduncles (the name given to the anterior portions of the midbrain that house the corticospinal tracts and substantia nigra).

Inferior Cerebellar Peduncles: Input From Below

The **inferior cerebellar peduncles** mostly carry in*put in* from *in*feriorly: The vestibulocerebellar tracts (vestibular information about where the head is in space), spinocerebellar tracts (proprioceptive information about where the body is in

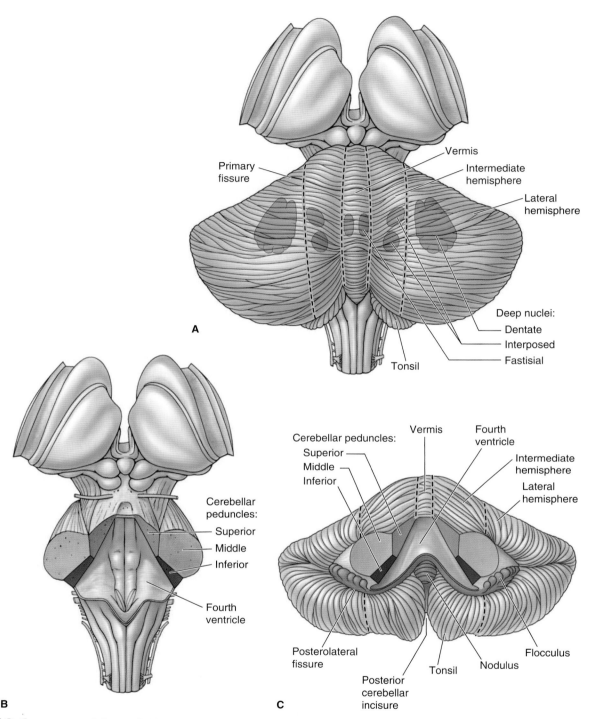

FIGURE 8–1 **Anatomy of the cerebellum. A:** Schematic posterior view of the cerebellum. **B:** Schematic posterior view of the brainstem with the cerebellum removed, demonstrating the three cerebellar peduncles. **C:** Schematic anterior view of the cerebellum with the brainstem removed. **D:** Schematic midsagittal view of the cerebellum. **E:** T1-weighted MRI, sagittal view. **F:** Schematic axial section of the cerebellum at the level of the pons and middle cerebellar peduncle demonstrating the deep cerebellar nuclei. Reproduced with permission from Martin J: *Neuroanatomy Text and Atlas*, 4th ed. New York, NY: McGraw Hill; 2012.

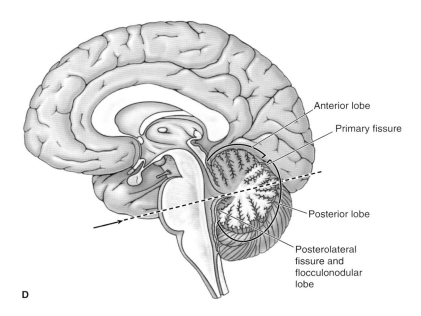

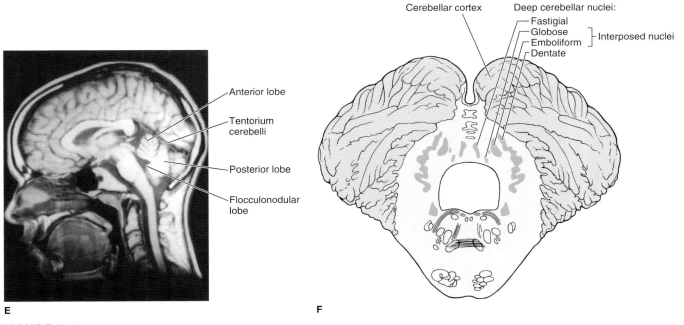

FIGURE 8-1 (*Continued*)

space), and olivocerebellar tracts (involved in motor learning) all travel through the inferior cerebellar peduncles to the cerebellum. The inferior cerebellar peduncles enter the cerebellum at the most *inferior* level of the brainstem: the medulla. All pathways traveling through the inferior cerebellar peduncles project to the ipsilateral cerebellar hemisphere except the olivocerebellar tracts, which cross. There is one minor exception to the inferior cerebellar peduncles being input pathways: The cerebellum sends output back to the vestibular system and this passes through the inferior cerebellar peduncles.

Middle Cerebellar Peduncles: Input From The Cerebral Hemispheres

The **middle cerebellar peduncles** carry input from the cerebral hemispheres to the cerebellum about what the brain wants the body to do. The corticopontocebellar fibers arise from cortical motor regions, descend with the corticospinal tracts, and cross in the anterior pons to enter the contralateral cerebellum via the middle cerebellar peduncles. The majority of fibers in the "bulge" of the anterior pons are these crossing

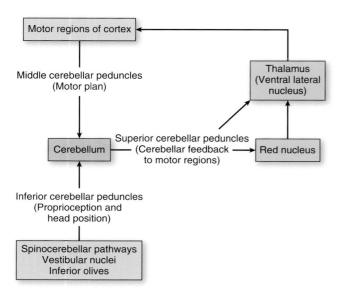

FIGURE 8–2 Schematic of the flow of information through the cerebellar peduncles.

corticopontocerebellar fibers en route to the middle cerebellar peduncles.

Superior Cerebellar Peduncles: Output Back to the Brain

The **superior cerebellar peduncles** predominantly send information *superiorly*, communicating the cerebellum's plan back to the brain. The superior cerebellar peduncles exit the cerebellum by way of the upper pons, and cross at the junction of the upper pons/lower midbrain. Some crossed fibers synapse with the red nucleus (contralateral to the cerebellar hemisphere of origin), while others continue to the ventral lateral (VL) nucleus of the thalamus (contralateral to the cerebellar hemisphere of origin), which projects to cortical motor regions. There is one minor exception to the superior cerebellar peduncles being output pathways: One component of the spinocerebellar tracts (the ventral spinocerebellar tracts) enters the cerebellum through the superior cerebellar peduncles.

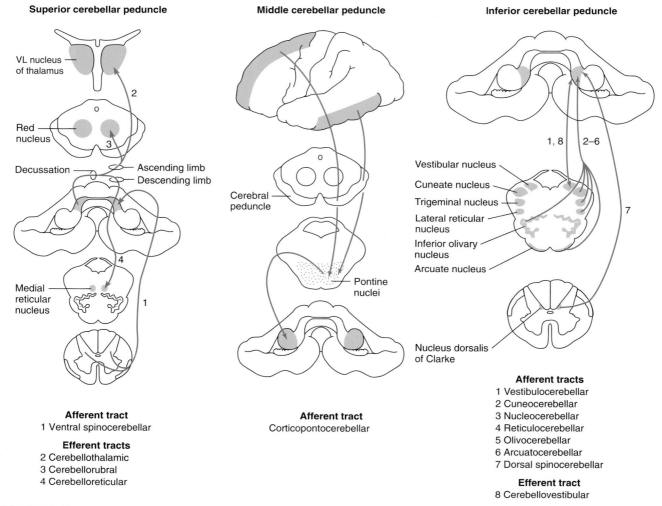

FIGURE 8–3 Schematic of the pathways that traverse the cerebellar peduncles demonstrating projections to and from the cerebellum.
Reproduced with permission from Aminoff M, Greenberg D, Simon R: *Clinical Neurology*, 9th ed. New York, NY: McGraw Hill; 2015.

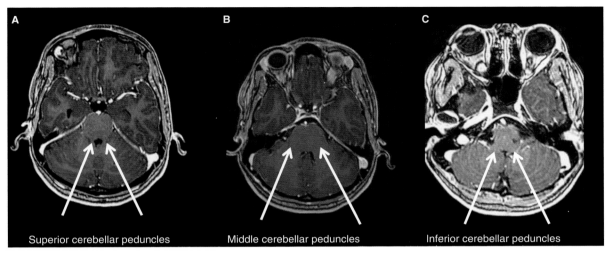

FIGURE 8–4 **Axial T1-weighted postcontrast MRI demonstrating the cerebellar peduncles. A:** At the level of the upper pons showing the superior cerebellar peduncles. **B:** At the level of the midpons showing the middle cerebellar peduncles. **C:** At the level of the medulla showing the inferior cerebellar peduncles.

The middle cerebellar peduncles and superior cerebellar peduncles both cross, creating a loop between each cerebral hemisphere and the contralateral cerebellar hemisphere. For example, motor regions in the left cerebral hemisphere project to the right cerebellar hemisphere via the crossing middle cerebellar peduncle, and the right cerebellar hemisphere projects back to the motor regions of the left hemisphere by way of the crossing superior cerebellar peduncle. This double crossing means that the relationship between cerebellar deficits and the body is ipsilateral: Lesions of the left cerebellar hemisphere (connected with the right cerebral hemisphere) cause left-sided deficits and lesions of the right cerebellar hemisphere (connected with the left cerebral hemisphere) cause right-sided deficits.

All three cerebellar peduncles pass through the brainstem. It would have been simple if each peduncle corresponded to one level of the brainstem, but it does not quite work out this way: The inferior cerebellar peduncles connect the cerebellum and the brainstem at the level of the medulla, and the middle and superior cerebellar peduncles both connect the cerebellum and the brainstem at the level of the pons (mid-pons for the middle cerebellar peduncle, and upper pons for the superior cerebellar peduncle).

ARTERIAL SUPPLY OF THE CEREBELLUM

The vascular supply of the cerebellum comes from three pairs of circumferential arteries that arise from the vertebrobasilar system: the superior cerebellar arteries (SCAs), the anterior inferior cerebellar arteries (AICAs), and the posterior inferior cerebellar arteries (PICAs). The SCAs and AICAs arise from the basilar artery, and the PICAs usually arise from the vertebral arteries. Since these blood vessels also supply the brainstem, they are discussed in more detail with the vascular supply of the brainstem in Chapter 9.

APPROACH TO ATAXIA

Ataxia may be present in the limbs if there is pathology of the cerebellar hemispheres. This can be demonstrated on finger–nose and heel–shin testing, and by testing the patient's ability to rapidly mirror the examiner's movements (see "Examination of coordination" in Ch. 1). Gait instability/ataxia may be present if there is midline cerebellar (vermis) pathology.

When a patient presents with clumsiness, incoordination, and/or difficulty walking, the history and evaluation must determine whether such symptoms are due to sensory disturbances, weakness, or ataxia. If the problem is indeed ataxia, it is important to note that the lesion is not necessarily cerebellar. The cerebellum is only as good as its inputs and outputs. For example, a lesion affecting any of the cerebellar peduncles can lead to cerebellar ataxia by depriving the cerebellum of the inputs and outputs necessary to perform its functions. Ataxia can also be seen with disruption of the corticopontocerebellar fibers in their descent in the internal capsule or anterior pons, as demonstrated by the ataxia-hemiparesis and dysarthria-clumsy hand lacunar syndromes (see Ch. 7). If the cerebellum does not receive adequate proprioceptive information (from the inferior cerebellar peduncles), it cannot adequately coordinate movements. Therefore, problems anywhere along the dorsal column pathways (large fiber neuropathy, sensory ganglionopathy, pathology of the dorsal columns in the spinal cord) can lead to a type of ataxia known as **sensory ataxia**.

Distinguishing Cerebellar Ataxia From Sensory Ataxia (Table 8–1)

Ataxia due to cerebellar causes may be accompanied by additional cerebellar signs such as nystagmus (see Ch. 12), titubation (oscillation of the head and/or trunk at rest), and/or

TABLE 8-1 Distinguishing Cerebellar Ataxia From Sensory Ataxia.

	Cerebellar Ataxia	Sensory Ataxia
Finger–nose testing	Intention tremor	"Searching/meandering" movements
		Worsens with eyes closed
Accompanying features	Nystagmus	Decreased proprioception
	Dysarthria	Romberg's sign
		Pseudoathetosis
		(Hyporeflexia or areflexia if due to neuropathy or ganglionopathy)
Gait	Wide based	Wide based

dysarthria. Such findings should not be present if ataxia is caused by sensory dysfunction due to neuropathy, gangli-onopathy, or dorsal column dysfunction (unless there is also concurrent cerebellar pathology). If there is a sensory etiology of ataxia, other sensory signs may be present such as diminished proprioception and vibration sense and Romberg's sign. If sensory dysfunction is due to peripheral nervous system pathology (i.e., nerves, dorsal root ganglia, or dorsal roots), diminished or absent reflexes may be present.

Romberg's sign is commonly mistakenly attributed to cerebellar pathology, but it is actually indicative of impaired proprioception or vestibular dysfunction. Patients with severe cerebellar dysfunction are often unable to stand with their feet together even with their eyes open, let alone closed. Patients with a deficit in proprioception can stand with their feet together when using vision to compensate, but closing the eyes removes this cue and requires the patient to rely on proprioception, so the patient may lose her/his balance (**Romberg's sign**).

On finger–nose testing, cerebellar and sensory ataxia have different appearances. Cerebellar ataxia appears as an oscillatory movement perpendicular to the plane of movement (i.e., side-to-side when the patient approaches the target in the finger–nose task) and worsens as the patient approaches the target. Sensory ataxia causes what resembles a "searching" movement in which the affected limb looks as if it is approaching the target with meandering, circular movements. With slow movements under visual guidance, a patient with sensory ataxia may be able to gain reasonable accuracy with finger–nose testing. However, if the examiner leaves the target finger in the same place and asks the patient to continue going back and forth from nose to finger with the eyes closed, the patient will become increasingly inaccurate. This is because removing the patient's visual compensation requires complete reliance on proprioception, which is impaired in sensory ataxia.

An additional subtle sign of diminished proprioception that may be seen is **pseudoathetosis**. (Not to be confused with athetosis, a movement disorder characterized by writhing

movements [see Ch. 23]). In a patient with diminished proprioception, when the patient's arms and hands are stretched out in front of her/him with the eyes closed (as in testing pronator drift), subtle writhing piano playing–like movements of the fingers may be noted. Similar movements of the toes may be noted when testing for Romberg's sign. These movements may be the digits trying to "find themselves in space" without adequate proprioception to serve that function, and are referred to as pseudoathetosis.

Differential Diagnosis of Cerebellar Ataxia

As with any neurologic problem, once localized, the differential diagnosis arises from an understanding of the time course of symptom onset and evolution.

Hyperacute-onset (over seconds to hours) of cerebellar pathology can be caused by:

- Vascular causes: ischemic stroke, cerebellar hemorrhage (see Ch. 19)
- Toxic: alcohol, cytarabine (see Ch. 24)

Acute-onset (over hours to days) of cerebellar pathology can be caused by:

- Immune-mediated:
  - Postinfectious cerebellitis (most commonly seen in children after a viral illness, most commonly varicella infection)
  - Flare of multiple sclerosis (see Ch. 21)

Subacute-onset (over weeks to months) of cerebellar pathology can be caused by:

- Infection: progressive multifocal leukoencephalopathy (see Ch. 20)
- Paraneoplastic cerebellar degeneration, which can be associated with anti-Yo (ovarian and breast cancer), anti-Hu (small cell lung cancer), anti-Tr (Hodgkin's lymphoma), anti-Ma2 (testicular cancer), and anti-GAD (often not associated with a malignancy) antibodies (see Ch. 24)
- Tumor: medulloblastoma (in children), metastatic tumor (in adults)
- Metabolic causes: vitamin E deficiency (acquired or inherited)

Chronic-onset (over years) of cerebellar pathology can be caused by:

- Chronic medication/toxin exposure: phenytoin, alcohol
- Degenerative etiologies
  - Acquired: multiple systems atrophy cerebellar type (MSA-C) (see Ch. 22)
  - Inherited:
    - Friedreich's ataxia (autosomal recessive)
    - Spinocerebellar ataxias (autosomal dominant)
    - Fragile X–associated tremor ataxia syndrome (X-linked)

Vascular, infectious, multiple sclerosis lesion–related, and malignant etiologies of cerebellar disease usually lead to *unilateral* cerebellar dysfunction, whereas drug-related, metabolic, degenerative, and non-multiple sclerosis inflammatory etiologies (e.g., paraneoplastic or postinfectious) more commonly lead to *bilateral* cerebellar dysfunction.

Most of these etiologies of cerebellar dysfunction are discussed in Part 2 of this book except the inherited ataxias, which are therefore discussed here.

Inherited Causes of Cerebellar Ataxia

Friedreich's ataxia—This autosomal recessively inherited ataxia affects the spinocerebellar tracts as well as the dorsal columns, corticospinal tracts, and peripheral nerves. In addition to ataxia and sensory loss developing in young adulthood, most patients develop cardiomyopathy. The causative mutation is in the ***frataxin*** gene (caused by GAA repeat).

Spinocerebellar ataxia—This term is applied to a growing number (more than 30) of autosomal dominantly inherited ataxias that are all characterized by adult-onset ataxia, but which can have a variety of additional features such as pyramidal, extrapyramidal, or cognitive dysfunction, and/or neuropathy. The most common spinocerebellar ataxia (SCA) is SCA3 (**Machado-Joseph disease**), which causes cerebellar dysfunction, cognitive impairment, neuropathy, and, in some cases, extrapyramidal features (e.g., parkinsonism; see Ch. 23). The highest prevalence of SCA3 is in the Azores, and the causative mutation is in the ***ATXN3*** gene (caused by CAG repeat).

Fragile X–associated tremor/ataxia syndrome (FXTAS)—An adult-onset progressive ataxia called fragile X–associated tremor/ataxia syndrome (FXTAS) can be caused by mutations in the same gene (*FMR1*) that causes fragile X syndrome (a common cause of intellectual disability in boys, accompanied by dysmorphic facial features and large testicles). FXTAS occurs in patients with a lower number of trinucelotide

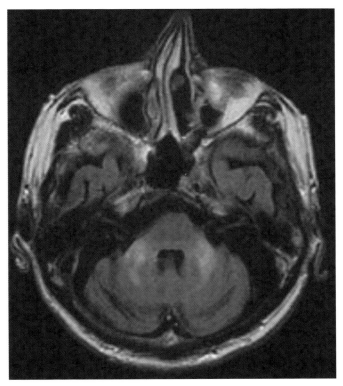

FIGURE 8–5 Axial FLAIR MRI in fragile X-associated tremor ataxia syndrome (FXTAS) demonstrating bilateral hyperintensities in the middle cerebellar peduncles.

(CGG) repeats than are necessary to produce fragile X syndrome (e.g., in the parent or grandparent of a child with fragile X syndrome), referred to as a **premutation**. As an X-linked condition, the disorder most commonly occurs in men, but can rarely occur in women in a milder form. Onset of cerebellar ataxia begins most commonly after age 50, and may be accompanied by parkinsonism and/or dementia. A characteristic MRI finding is T2/FLAIR hyperintensities in the bilateral middle cerebellar peduncles (Fig. 8–5).

The Brainstem & Cranial Nerves

OVERVIEW OF BRAINSTEM ANATOMY

The three levels of the brainstem from superior to inferior are the midbrain, pons, and medulla. The midbrain is just inferior to the bilateral thalami, and the medulla transitions inferiorly into the cervical spinal cord. Most simply, the brainstem can be thought of as a "spinal cord for the head and neck": Just as the spinal cord has sensory information coming in and motor information going out for the extremities and torso, the brainstem has sensory information coming in and motor information going out for the head and neck. In addition to somatic sensory information, however, the brainstem also receives vestibular, auditory, taste, and visceral sensory information. Motor functions of the brainstem include control of ocular, pupillary, facial, laryngeal, pharyngeal, and visceral musculature (Figs. 9–1 and 9–2).

   Understanding the brainstem requires a general framework for *what* is there and *where* it is. As far as *what* is in the brainstem, there are five general categories of structures:

1. The descending motor pathways for the extremities and torso (**corticospinal tracts;** see Ch. 4)

2. The ascending somatosensory pathways from the extremities and torso (**dorsal columns and spinothalamic tracts;** see Ch. 4)

3. The **cranial nerve nuclei** and associated structures. The **cranial nerve nuclei** are the collections of cell bodies whose axons give rise to the **cranial nerves.** Before the cranial nerves exit the brainstem, their fibers are referred to as **fascicles.**

4. Connections with the cerebellum (the **cerebellar peduncles;** see Ch. 8)

5. The reticular activating system and ascending neurotransmitter-specific projection pathways: **substantia nigra** (dopamine), **locus coeruleus** (norepinephrine), **median raphe nuclei** (serotonin), **pedunculopontine nuclei** (acetylcholine)

   As points of orientation for *where* structures are in the brainstem, the following principles apply at all three levels of the brainstem (see Fig. 9–1):

- The corticospinal tracts run in the *anterior (ventral)* aspect of the brainstem

- The somatosensory pathways for the extremities and torso move a bit over the course of their ascent, but are most often *posterior (dorsal)* within the brainstem (with the exception of the mid-medulla, where the medial lemnisci are medial and extend anteriorly; see Ch. 4)

- The cranial nerve nuclei are all *posterior (dorsal)*:

  - In general, the motor cranial nerve nuclei are closest to the midline, and their cranial nerves emerge medially/anteriorly (CN 4 is an exception in that it exits posteriorly)

    - The motor cranial nerve nuclei innervating *skeletal* muscle are at the midline: CNs 3, 4, and 6 (innervating extraocular muscles) and CN 12 (innervating tongue muscles)

    - The motor cranial nerve nuclei innervating *branchial* muscles are more lateral: CN 5 (jaw muscles), CN 7 (facial muscles), and CNs 9 and 10 (muscles of the larynx/pharynx)

  - The sensory and special sensory cranial nerve nuclei are all more lateral than the motor cranial nerve nuclei: sensory nuclei of CN 5, vestibular and cochlear nuclei (CN 8), and nucleus solitarius (for taste and visceral sensation)

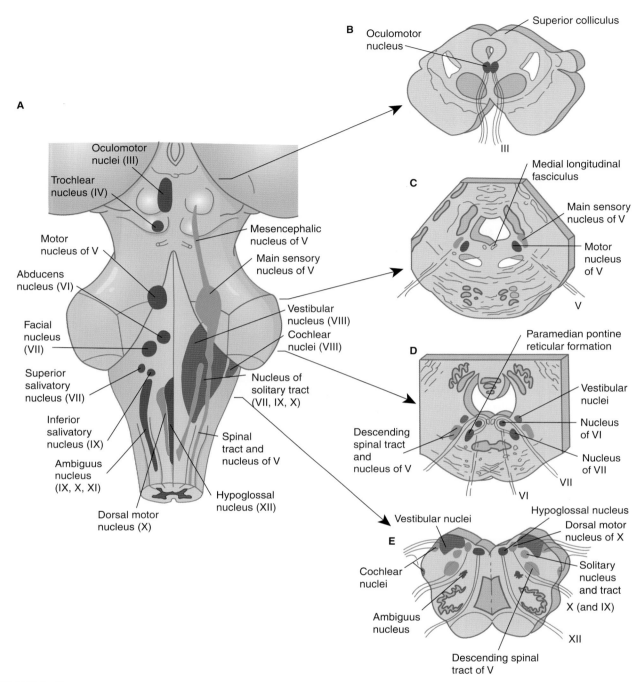

FIGURE 9–1 **Schematic of brainstem anatomy. A:** Posterior view of the brainstem with cerebellum removed revealing the locations of the cranial nerve nuclei. **B–E:** Axial sections demonstrating locations of cranial nerve nuclei and exiting cranial nerves in the midbrain (**B**), upper pons (**C**), midpons (**D**), and medulla (**E**). Reproduced with permission from Waxman S: *Clinical Neuroanatomy*, 27th ed. New York, NY: McGraw Hill; 2013.

- The cerebellar peduncles all arise from the posterior/dorsal brainstem (logically, since the cerebellum is posterior to the brainstem)
- The ascending neurotransmitter-specific projection pathways are found throughout the brainstem, but the reticular-activating system involved in maintaining arousal and consciousness resides in the upper pons and midbrain

The Cranial Nerve Nuclei

The 12 cranial nerves can be divided into three groups of four that mostly correspond to the three brainstem levels with a few exceptions denoted by asterisks:

- Midbrain: 1*-2-3-4
- Pons: 5*-6-7-8*
- Medulla: 9-10-11*-12

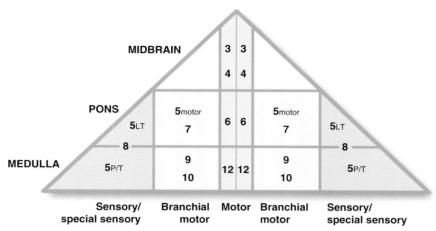

FIGURE 9–2 **Schematic for locations of cranial nerve nuclei.** Motor nuclei for CNs innervating skeletal muscle are medial (CNs 3, 4, 6, and 12). Motor nuclei for CNs innervating branchial muscle are more lateral (CN 5 [motor for muscles of mastication], CN 7, CN 9, CN 10). Somatic sensory and special sensory cranial nerve nuclei are most lateral (CNs 5 and 8). LT: Light touch. P/T: Pain/Temperature.

The exceptions are as follows:

- CN 1 and CN 11 do not connect with the brainstem
- CN 5 has nuclei at all three levels of the brainstem (although its fibers enter at the level of the pons as would be expected from the pons = 5*-6-7-8* schema; see Ch. 13)
- For CN 8, the vestibular nuclei are in the medulla and the cochlear nuclei are at the pontomedullary junction
- CN 2 can be considered a partial exception: Although CN 2's main projections are the visual pathways, which do not project to the brainstem (see Ch. 6), the afferent limb of the pupillary light reflex is communicated by CN 2 to the midbrain as would be expected by the midbrain = 1*-2-3-4 schema

The Cerebellar Peduncles

The three cerebellar peduncles nearly correspond to the three levels of the brainstem, with one exception (point 3 below; see also Fig. 8–3).

1. The inferior cerebellar peduncles connect the medulla to the cerebellum
2. The middle cerebellar peduncles connect the pons to the cerebellum
3. Although things would have been simpler if the superior cerebellar peduncles connected to the midbrain to give one pair of cerebellar peduncles per brainstem level, the superior cerebellar peduncles connect the cerebellum to the upper pons (en route to connections with the midbrain and thalamus)

The Arterial Supply of the Brainstem (Fig. 9–3)

The vascular supply of the brainstem corresponds to its three levels, with one pair of circumferential arteries per level of the brainstem:

1. Superior cerebellar arteries (SCAs) for the midbrain (though the superior midbrain is supplied by the PCAs)
2. Anterior inferior cerebellar arteries (AICAs) for the pons
3. Posterior inferior cerebellar arteries (PICAs) for the medulla

These arteries all have "cerebellar" in their names since they not only supply the brainstem, but also the cerebellum posterior to it. Most commonly, the SCAs and AICAs arise from the basilar artery and the PICAs from the vertebral arteries. The anterior spinal artery arises from the vertebral arteries and supplies the medial medulla and anterior spinal cord. At the level of the pons and midbrain, the midline basilar artery supplies the medial brainstem through penetrating branches.

Tables 9–1, 9–2, 9–3, and 9–4 summarize the structures of the brainstem (Table 9–1), the afferent and efferent limbs of the brainstem reflexes (Table 9–2), the cranial nerve functions, associated nuclei, and skull foramina of entry and exit (Table 9–3), and the cranial nerve nuclei (Table 9–4). Individual cranial nerves and their associated pathways are discussed in more detail in Chapters 10–14.

CLINICAL APPLICATIONS OF BRAINSTEM ANATOMY

Crossed Signs due to Brainstem Lesions

Recall that the corticospinal tracts do not cross until the cervicomedullary junction, the dorsal column pathways cross in the medulla, and the spinothalamic tracts cross in the spinal cord (see Ch. 4). Therefore, throughout most of the brainstem, lesions lead to *contralateral* weakness and/or sensory symptoms in the extremities. However, with the exception of CN 4, all cranial nerves project *ipsilaterally*. Therefore, unilateral lesions of the brainstem cause ipsilateral sensory and/or motor symptoms in the face, but *contralateral* symptoms in the body (**crossed signs**). For example, a lesion affecting the

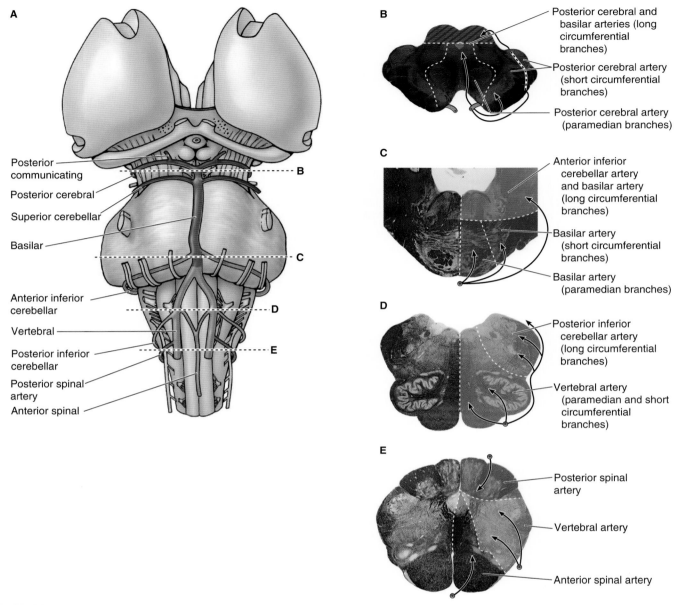

FIGURE 9–3 Schematic of the arterial supply of the brainstem. A: Anterior view of the brainstem demonstrating the vertebrobasilar system and circumferential vessels (SCA, AICA, PICA). **B–E**: Axial sections demonstrating blood supply of brainstem at the level of the midbrain (**B**), pons (**C**), upper medulla (**D**), and lower medulla (**E**). Reproduced with permission from Martin J: *Neuroanatomy Text and Atlas*, 4th ed. New York, NY: McGraw Hill; 2012.

left pons would cause *ipsilateral* (left-sided) facial weakness (CN 7) and *contralateral* (right-sided) arm/leg weakness (not-yet-crossed corticospinal tract).

Medial versus Lateral Brainstem Syndromes (Fig. 9–4)

As discussed previously, the descending corticospinal tracts are anterior and medial throughout the three levels of the brainstem, and the motor cranial nerve nuclei for skeletal muscle (CN 3, CN 4, CN 6, CN 12) are posterior and medial

and their associated cranial nerves exit anteriorly and medially (with the exception of CN 4, the only cranial nerve that exits posteriorly). The sensory and special sensory cranial nerve nuclei are *dorsolateral* in the brainstem. Therefore, lesions of the *medial* brainstem cause predominantly *motor* symptoms and signs, whereas lesions of the dorsolateral brainstem cause predominantly sensory and special sensory symptoms and signs. Since the cerebellar peduncles are positioned on the dorsal/dorsolateral aspects of the brainstem (and the cerebellum is just posterior to the brainstem and supplied by the same circumferential arteries), dorsolateral brainstem pathology

TABLE 9-1 Brainstem Structures.

	Blood Supply	Cerebellar Peduncles	Cranial Nerve Nuclei	Ascending Projections
Midbrain	PCA/SCA/Basilar		Pretectal nuclei (CN 2)	Reticular activating system
			Edinger-Westphal nuclei (CN 3)	Substantia nigra (dopamine)
			Oculomotor nuclei (CN 3)	Median raphe nuclei (serotonin)
			Trochlear nuclei (CN 4)	
			Mesencephalic nuclei of CN 5	
Pons	AICA/Basilar	Superior	Motor and principal sensory nuclei of CN 5	Reticular activating system
			Abducens nuclei (CN 6)	Locus coeruleus (norepinephrine)
		Middle	Facial nuclei (CN 7)	
			Superior salivatory nuclei (CN 7)	Pedunculopontine nuclei (acetylcholine)
			Cochlear nuclei at pontomedullary junction (CN 8)	Median raphe nuclei (serotonin)
Medulla	PICA/Vertebral arteries	Inferior	Spinal tract/nuclei of CN 5	Median raphe nuclei (serotonin)
			Vestibular nuclei (CN 8)	
			Nucleus solitarius (CNs 7, 9, and 10)	
			Inferior salivatory nuclei (CN 9)	
			Nucleus ambiguus (CNs 9 and 10)	
			Hypoglossal nuclei (CN 12)	

AICA: anterior inferior cerebellar artery; CN: cranial nerve; PICA: posterior inferior cerebellar artery; SCA: superior cerebellar artery.

may cause cerebellar symptoms (e.g., ataxia, nausea/vomiting; see Ch. 8).

For example, in the medulla, the schema to recall the relevant cranial nerve nuclei is "9-10-11*-12," but we must remove CN 11 (an exception), and add the spinal nucleus of CN 5 (pain and temperature sensation in the face; see Ch. 13) and the vestibular nuclei of CN 8. CN 12 innervates skeletal muscle, and so its nuclei are medial with the bilateral CN 12 exiting anteriorly and medially. The branchial motor nuclei associated with CN 9 and CN 10 are lateral to the CN 12 nuclei. The sensory nuclei (spinal nucleus of CN 5; see Ch. 13) and special sensory nuclei (vestibular nuclei [CN 8]) of the medulla are lateral to the nuclei of CN 9 and CN 10. Therefore, unilateral *medial medullary* infarction causes *ipsilateral*

tongue weakness (CN 12) and *contralateral* extremity weakness (due to involvement of the not-yet-crossed corticospinal tract). In contrast, *lateral medullary* infarction causes *ipsilateral* loss of facial pain/temperature sensation (spinal tract and nucleus of CN 5) and *contralateral* pain/temperature sensation loss in the extremities (due to involvement of the already-crossed anterolateral tract) as well as vertigo (vestibular nuclei), nausea/vomiting and ataxia (inferior cerebellar peduncle and cerebellum), dysarthria and dysphagia (nucleus ambiguus), and ipsilateral Horner's syndrome (descending oculosympathetic pathway; see Ch. 10). This constellation of findings in lateral medullary infarction is called **Wallenberg's syndrome**. Medial medullary infarction is caused by stroke in the territory of the anterior spinal artery, and lateral medullary infarction is caused by stroke in the territory of the PICA, often caused by disease of the vertebral artery.

When brainstem syndromes are caused by stroke, a *lateral syndrome* generally suggests occlusion of a circumferential artery (SCA, AICA, PICA), whereas a *medial syndrome* generally suggests occlusion of a penetrating branch of the vertebrobasilar system (or the anterior spinal artery at the level of the medulla). Pathophysiologically, a distal occlusion of a circumferential artery can suggest embolism as the mechanism, whereas a more medial stroke in the territory of a penetrating branch from one of the vertebral arteries or the basilar artery can suggest atherosclerosis (see Ch. 19).

TABLE 9-2 Brainstem Reflexes.

	Cranial Nerves	
	Afferent	**Efferent**
Pupillary	CN 2	CN 3
Jaw jerk	CN 5	CN 5
Corneal	CN 5	CN 7
Oculocephalic	CN 8	CNs 3, 4, and 6
Gag	CN 9	CN 10

CN: cranial nerve

TABLE 9–3 Cranial Nerve Functions, Brainstem Nuclei, and Associated Skull Foramina.

Cranial Nerve	Somatic Motor	Somatic Sensory	Special Sensory	Visceral Motor	Visceral Sensory	Brainstem Nuclei	Foramen of Exit
CN 1 (Olfactory)			Olfaction				Cribriform plate
CN 2 (Optic)			Vision			Pretectal nuclei (midbrain)	Optic canal
CN 3 (Oculomotor)	Superior rectus Inferior rectus Medial rectus Inferior oblique Levator palpebrae Pupilloconstrictors					Oculomotor nucleus Edinger-Westphal nucleus (midbrain)	Cavernous sinus→ superior orbital fissure
CN 4 (Trochlear)	Superior oblique					Trochlear nucleus (midbrain)	Cavernous sinus→ superior orbital fissure
CN 5 (Trigeminal)	Muscles of mastication (temporalis, masseter, pterygoids) Anterior belly of digastric Tensor veli palitini Tensor tympani Mylohoid	Face Anterior 2/3 of tongue Dura mater (shared with CN 10)				Mesencephalic nucleus of CN 5 (midbrain) Main sensory nucleus of CN 5 (pons) Motor nucleus of CN 5 (pons) Spinal nucleus of CN 5 (medulla)	Ophthalmic (V1): Cavernous sinus→ superior orbital fissure Maxillary (V2): Cavernous sinus→ foramen rotundum Mandibular (V3): foramen ovale
CN 6 (Abducens)	Lateral rectus					Abducens nucleus (pons)	Cavernous sinus→ superior orbital fissure
CN 7 (Facial)	Facial muscles Stapedius Stylohoid Posterior belly of digastric	External ear	Taste anterior 2/3 of tongue	Lacrimal glands Nasal glands Submandibular glands Sublingual glands (i.e., all glands of head **except** parotid)		Facial nucleus (pons) Superior salivatory nucleus (pons) Nucleus solitarius (medulla)	Internal auditory canal
CN 8 (Vestibulocochlear)			Hearing Balance			Cochlear (pontomdullary junction) Vestibular (medulla)	Internal auditory canal
CN 9 (Glossopharyngeal)	Stylopharyngeus	External and middle ear Posterior tongue	Taste posterior 1/3 of tongue	Parotid glands	Carotid body	Nucleus ambiguus (medulla) Inferior salivatory nucleus (medulla) Nucleus solitarius (medulla)	Jugular foramen

	Motor	Sensory	Taste	Visceral sensory	Parasympathetic	Nucleus	Foramen
CN 10 (Vagus)	All pharyngeal and laryngeal muscles **except** mylohyoid (CN 5), tensor veli palitini (CN 5), stylohyoid (CN 7), and stylopharyngeus (CN 9)	Pharynx External auditory meatus Dura of posterior fossa (**except** tentorium)	Taste epiglottis/pharynx	Thoracic and abdominal viscera (**except** distal 1/3 of colon and genitourinary system)	Aortic arch Thoracic and abdominal viscera (**except** distal 1/3 of colon and genitourinary system)	Nucleus ambiguus (medulla) Dorsal motor nucleus of vagus (medulla) Nucleus solitarius (medulla)	Jugular foramen
CN 11 (Spinal accessory)	Sternocleidomastoid Trapezius						Jugular foramen
CN 12 (Hypoglossal)	Muscles of the tongue					Hypoglossal nucleus	Hypoglossal canal

CN: cranial nerve.

TABLE 9–4   Cranial Nerve Nuclei (Aside From Those Named for Their Associated Cranial Nerves).

	Brainstem Level	Function(s)	Cranial Nerve(s) (CN(s))
Edinger-Westphal nucleus	Midbrain	Pupillary constriction	CN 3
Superior salivatory nucleus	Pons	Submandibular glands	CN 7
		Sublingual glands	
		Lacrimal glands	
		Nasal/palatal glands	
Inferior salivatory nucleus	Medulla	Parotid gland	CN 9
Nucleus ambiguus	Medulla	Laryngeal muscles	CNs 9 and 10
		Pharyngeal muscles	
Nucleus solitarius	Medulla	Taste	CNs 7, 9, and 10
		Visceral afferent	CNs 9 and 10

CN: cranial nerve.

Top of the Basilar Syndrome

Occlusion at the top of the basilar artery can affect the midbrain and/or the PCA territory of the cerebral hemispheres unilaterally or bilaterally. Midbrain involvement can lead to ocular abnormalities such as vertical gaze palsies (due to involvement of the vertical gaze centers and nuclei of CN 3 and CN 4 in the midbrain; see Ch. 11), convergence spasm, ptosis (due to involvement of CN 3 nucleus) or lid retraction (due to involvement of the dorsal midbrain; see Parinaud syndrome in Ch. 11); altered level of consciousness (due to involvement of the reticular activating system); and peduncular hallucinosis (often appearing to patient as embellished versions of existing visual scenes). PCA territory infarction can cause visual field deficits, visual cognitive syndromes (e.g., Balint syndrome, Anton syndrome; see Ch. 6), amnesia (due to involvement of the medial temporal lobe(s) or thalamus), and confusion or altered level of consciousness (due to involvement of the thalamus). For review, see Caplan, 1980.

Multiple Cranial Neuropathies

A patient presenting with multiple cranial neuropathies may have a process affecting the brainstem (cranial nerve nuclei or fascicles); the cranial nerves as they traverse the subarachnoid space (e.g., meningeal process), skull base, or face/neck; or a generalized process affecting the peripheral nerves (e.g., Guillain-Barré syndrome, see Ch. 27; all cranial nerves are peripheral nerves except CN 2). Processes that may also affect multiple cranial nerve-innervated muscles but are caused by lesions outside the brainstem/cranial nerves include neuromuscular junction disorders (myasthenia gravis, botulism) and myopathies (e.g., oculopharyngeal muscular dystrophy).

The first step in localizing the site of pathology in a patient with multiple cranial neuropathies is determining if the pattern of involved cranial nerves fits into a pattern associated with a particular location in the brainstem versus a particular location in a skull foramen. In the brainstem, common patterns include CN 6 and CN 7 affected together in the pons, and CNs 8, 9, 10 affected together in the lateral medulla. Cranial neuropathies due to brainstem lesions are commonly associated with contralateral motor or somatosensory deficits in the limbs/torso (motor if medial lesion; somatosensory if lateral lesion).

If the clinically affected cranial nerves have nuclei in more than one level of the brainstem and the patient has no deficits below the neck and a preserved level of consciousness, a brainstem localization is less likely.

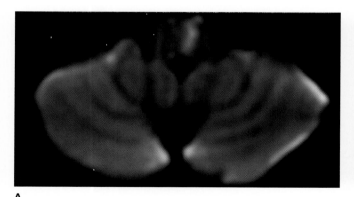
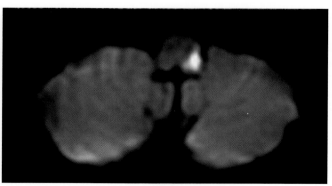

A   **B**

FIGURE 9–4   **Axial diffusion-weighted MRI of medial and lateral medullary infarction: A:** Left medial medullary infarction. **B:** Left lateral medullary infarction.

TABLE 9–5 Syndromes of Multiple Cranial Neuropathies.

	CN2	CN3	CN4	CN5	CN6	CN7	CN8	CN9	CN 10	CN 11	CN 12	Horner's
Orbital apex	✓	✓	✓	V1	✓							
Cavernous sinus		✓	✓	V1 and V2	✓							
Petrous apex (Gradenigo)				✓	✓							
Cerebellopontine angle				✓		✓	✓	(✓)	(✓)			
Internal auditory canal						✓	✓					
Jugular foramen (Vernet)								✓	✓	✓		
Jugular foramen/ Intercondylar space (Collet-Sicard)								✓	✓	✓	✓	
Retropharyngeal space (Villaret)								✓	✓	✓	✓	✓

Patterns of unilateral multiple cranial neuropathies referable to particular localization outside the brainstem include (Table 9–5):

- CNs 2, 3, 4, 6, and V1 branch of CN 5: orbital apex
- CNs 3, 4, 6, and V1 and V2 branches of CN 5: cavernous sinus (see Ch. 11)
- CN 5 and CN 6: petrous apex (Gradenigo syndrome if caused by suppurative otitis media)
- CNs 5, 7, 8 (+/− CN 9 and CN 10): cerebellopontine angle
- CN 7 and CN 8: internal auditory canal
- CN 9, CN 10, and CN 11: jugular foramen (Vernet syndrome; + CN 12 is Collet-Sicard syndrome; + Horner syndrome is Villaret syndrome)
- CN 9, CN 10, CN 11, CN 12, and/or Horner's syndrome: carotid dissection

When multiple cranial neuropathies do not correspond to a particular brainstem location or skull base location, the following localizations should be considered:

- **Meninges:**
  - Infectious meningitis (bacterial, tubercular, syphilitic, fungal)
  - Immune-mediated meningitis (e.g., sarcoidosis, IgG4-related disease)
  - Neoplasia: carcinomatous meningitis (leptomeningeal metastases), head/neck cancer, perineural spread,
  - Vascular: aneurysm/subarachnoid hemorrhage
- **Skull base:**
  - Primary disorders of bone (osteopetrosis, Paget's disease)
  - Skull base neoplasm: metastases, primary tumors of bone (e.g., chordoma affecting clivus)
- **Neck:**
  - Carotid dissection

- **Peripheral nervous system:**
  - Immune-mediated: Guillain-Barré syndrome
  - Infectious: diphtheric neuropathy, botulism (disorder of neuromuscular junction, not cranial nerves proper)

Neuromuscular junction disorders (e.g., myasthenia, botulism) and myopathies (e.g., oculopharyngeal muscular dystrophy) can also cause weakness in multiple cranial nerve innervated muscles that could mimic multiple cranial neuropathies.

Locked-in Syndrome

In **locked-in syndrome**, the patient is awake and conscious, but cannot move or communicate with the exception of blinking and vertical gaze. The portion of the reticular activating system responsible for maintaining consciousness and arousal is in the dorsal pons (pontine tegmentum) and midbrain. Ventral pontine lesions (e.g., basilar artery thrombosis, pontine hemorrhage, central pontine myelinolysis) cause loss of all motor function controlled by the pons (resulting in quadriplegia, bilateral facial weakness, horizontal gaze palsy), but the patient may still be awake and able to blink and look vertically if the dorsal pons, midbrain, and structures superior to it (i.e., thalami, cerebral hemispheres) are spared. (In basilar thrombosis, these regions can be perfused by collateral flow through the posterior communicating arteries to the posterior circulation distal to the occlusion). It is important to distinguish the locked-in state from coma, since a patient who is locked in is conscious (as compared to a patient in coma, who is not).

REFERENCE

Caplan LR. Top of the basilar syndrome. *Neurol* 1980;30:72-79.

Pupillary Control & Approach to Anisocoria

Cranial Nerves 2 & 3

C H A P T E R

10

CHAPTER CONTENTS

PUPILLARY CONSTRICTION: THE PARASYMPATHETIC PATHWAY

    Impaired Pupillary Constriction

PUPILLARY DILATION: THE SYMPATHETIC PATHWAY

    Impaired Pupillary Dilation

APPROACH TO ANISOCORIA & OTHER PUPILLARY ABNORMALITIES

    Anisocoria

    Bilateral Pupillary Abnormalities

Pupillary constriction is a parasympathetic function and pupillary dilation is a sympathetic function ("wide eyed with fear"). The pupils constrict in response to light and accommodation, and dilate in response to darkness and adrenergic states. Pupillary asymmetry is referred to as **anisocoria**, and can be caused by a variety of neurologic and ophthalmologic conditions. Changes in pupil size can also be caused by medications. **Miosis** refers to an abnormally constricted pupil, and **mydriasis** refers to an abnormally dilated pupil (mnemonic: mydriasis is a longer word than miosis, and mydriasis refers to the larger pupil size [i.e., dilated]).

PUPILLARY CONSTRICTION: THE PARASYMPATHETIC PATHWAY (FIG. 10–1)

Pupillary constriction in response to light requires transmission of light information from the retina to the brain (**afferent pathway**), and signals from the brain to constrict the pupils (**efferent pathway**). The afferent pupillary light reflex fibers travel through the optic nerves, optic chiasm, and optic tracts, and then separate from the optic tracts to proceed to the pretectal nuclei of the dorsal midbrain (note the separation of light reflex afferents from visual pathway fibers at this point—the visual pathway fibers in the optic tracts proceed to the lateral geniculate nuclei; Fig. 6–1). In the dorsal midbrain, the pretectal nuclei communicate with the Edinger-Westphal nuclei, which give rise to the efferent pupillary constrictor fibers that travel in the oculomotor nerves (CN 3). These parasympathetic pupillomotor fibers of CN 3 synapse in the ciliary ganglion in the orbit, and short ciliary neurons arising from the ciliary ganglion innervate the pupillary constrictor muscles of the iris. Each pretectal nucleus projects bilaterally to both

Edinger-Westphal nuclei so that both pupils constrict equally in response to light input from either side. For example, light shined in the left eye causes constriction of both the left pupil (direct response) and the right pupil (consensual response) and vice versa.

Impaired Pupillary Constriction

Impaired pupillary constriction to light can be caused by dysfunction in the afferent pathway (most commonly CN 2 dysfunction) or the efferent pathway (CN 3 dysfunction).

Impaired Pupillary Constriction due to a Lesion of the Afferent Pathway

If CN 2 is not functioning properly on one side (e.g., optic neuritis), no light will enter on that side, and so there will be neither a direct (ipsilateral) nor a consensual (contralateral) response to light shined on the affected pupil. However, since CN 2 is functioning on the unaffected side and both CN 3s are functioning, both pupils will constrict in response to light shined in the unaffected eye.

For example, if there is a lesion of CN 2 on the right (and the right CN 3, left CN 2, and left CN 3 are all intact), there will be no (or minimal) pupillary constriction in either eye when light is shined in the right eye, but both pupils will constrict when light is shined in the left eye (Fig. 10–2). In the **swinging flashlight test** in this situation, one would note bilateral pupillary constriction when light is shined in the left eye, but bilateral pupillary dilation (back to normal size) when light is shined in the right eye, since that light is not "seen" on the right due to right optic nerve dysfunction. The apparent dilation of the right eye after swinging the flashlight from the left pupil to the right pupil is due to the fact that the right pupil had constricted when light was shined in the

91

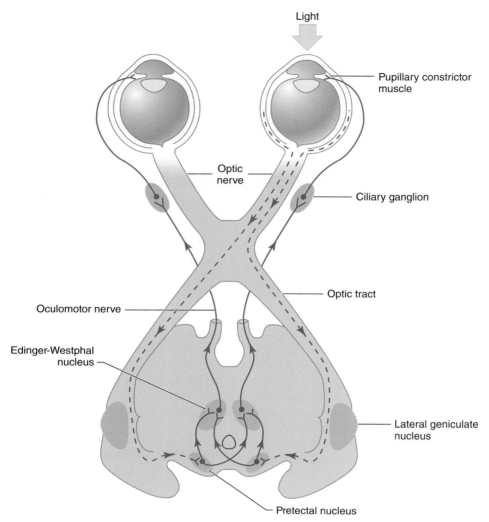

FIGURE 10-1 **The parasympathetic pathway for pupillary constriction.** Reproduced with permission from Aminoff M, Greenberg D, Simon R: *Clinical Neurology*, 9th ed. New York, NY: McGraw Hill; 2015.

left eye, and is returning to normal size since it does not "see" the light when the flashlight returns to the right eye. This is called a **relative afferent pupillary defect** (RAPD or Marcus Gunn pupil), which is most commonly caused by lesions of CN 2 (i.e., optic neuropathy; see "Monocular visual loss" in Ch. 6), but can also occur with severe unilateral or asymmetric retinal disease, or rarely with lesions in the optic chiasm, optic tract, or dorsal midbrain. An optic tract lesion as the cause of an RAPD results in contralateral hemianopia (see Ch. 6) and contralateral RAPD. A dorsal midbrain lesion as the cause of an RAPD will not cause any visual loss (since visual information proceeds to the lateral geniculate nucleus en route to the visual cortex, not the midbrain).

Impaired Pupillary Constriction due to a Lesion of the Efferent Pathway

If there is CN 3 dysfunction on one side and all else is working, the pupil on the side of the dysfunctional CN 3 will not respond to light in either eye since its pupillary constrictors

cannot be activated. However, since CN 2 on the side of CN 3 dysfunction is still intact, light shined in the pupil on the side of CN 3 dysfunction will be seen and will signal the constriction of the contralateral pupil. For example, if there is left CN 3 dysfunction, light shined in either eye will cause right-sided pupil constriction, but the left pupil will not constrict in response to light shined in either eye since CN 3 is not working on that side to "transmit the message" to the left pupil to constrict no matter which eye has light shined in it.

CN 3 also controls several extraocular movements and eyelid elevation in addition to pupillary constriction (see Ch. 11). Therefore, a complete CN 3 palsy will cause multiple eye movement abnormalities in addition to pupillary dilation/lack of response to light. However, since the pupillary constrictor fibers run on the medial exterior of the nerve, they can be compressed in isolation without causing eye muscle weakness (e.g., by posterior communicating artery aneurysm, tumor, or uncal herniation). See Chapter 11 for further discussion of CN 3 palsy.

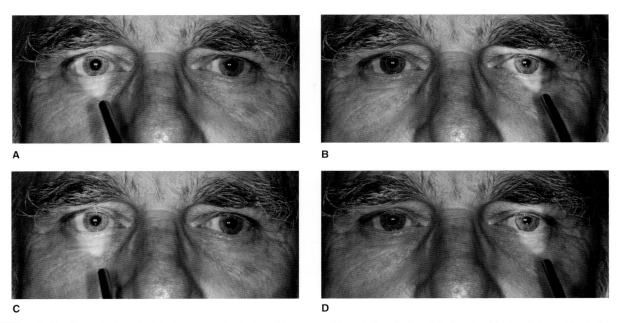

FIGURE 10–2 **The swinging flashlight test and relative afferent pupillary defect.** When light is shined in the right pupil (**A**), there is minimal reaction of the pupils on both sides. When light is shined in the left pupil (**B**), both pupils constrict. When the light is returned to the right pupil (**C**), the right pupil appears to dilate as compared to (**B**) when it returns to its normal size. When light is returned to the left pupil (**D**), both pupils constrict. This patient has a right optic neuropathy. Reproduced with permission from Martin T, Corbett J: *Practical Neuroophthalmology*. New York, NY: McGraw Hill; 2013.

PUPILLARY DILATION: THE SYMPATHETIC PATHWAY (FIG. 10–3)

The pathway for pupillary dilation begins in the hypothalamus, travels in the dorsolateral brainstem, and descends to the lower cervical/upper thoracic spinal cord before traveling over the lung apex, and then along the internal carotid through the neck and cavernous sinus en route to the orbit. This pathway has three components:

1. **First-order** neurons travel from the hypothalamus through the brainstem to the intermediolateral column (**ciliospinal center of Budge**).
2. **Second-order (preganglionic)** neurons travel from the spinal cord over the lung apex to the superior cervical ganglion.
3. **Third-order (postganglionic)** neurons travel from the superior cervical ganglion to the eye, traveling alongside the internal carotid artery in the neck and cavernous sinus.

Impaired Pupillary Dilation

Lesions along the oculosympathetic pathway can cause a triad of findings called **Horner's syndrome:**

- **Miosis:** pupillary constriction due to impaired dilation
- **Ptosis:** drooping of the upper eyelid (usually mild in Horner's syndrome). The sympathetic pathways innervate Müller's muscle (also known as the superior tarsal muscle), which raises the eyelid (helping the eyes look "wide-eyed with fear" when the sympathetic system is active). Decreased oculosympathetic activity in Horner's syndrome leads to weakness in Müller's muscle, causing ptosis. The ptosis in Horner's syndrome is generally more subtle than that seen in CN 3 palsy. There is often also slight elevation of the lower lid (again, the eye is less "wide-eyed" with loss of sympathetic input)
- **Anhidrosis:** decreased sweating on the face ipsilateral to the lesion

The fibers for facial sweating travel with the external carotid, whereas the fibers to the pupil and eyelid muscles travel with the internal carotid. Therefore, if Horner's syndrome is due to third-order neuron pathology (i.e., along the internal carotid artery or in the cavernous sinus), ptosis and miosis will be present, but facial sweating will *not* be affected (except for one small patch on the medial forehead and medial nose that may have impaired sweating because the sweating fibers that supply these regions travel with the internal carotid).

If Horner's syndrome occurs due to pathology in the first- or second-order components of the pathway (hypothalamus–brainstem–spinal cord–superior cervical ganglion), there will be ipsilateral facial anhidrosis along with ptosis and miosis, since the facial sweating fibers do not diverge until the third-order component of the pathway.

Horner's syndrome can be caused by pathology anywhere along the oculosympathetic pathway, with common causes including:

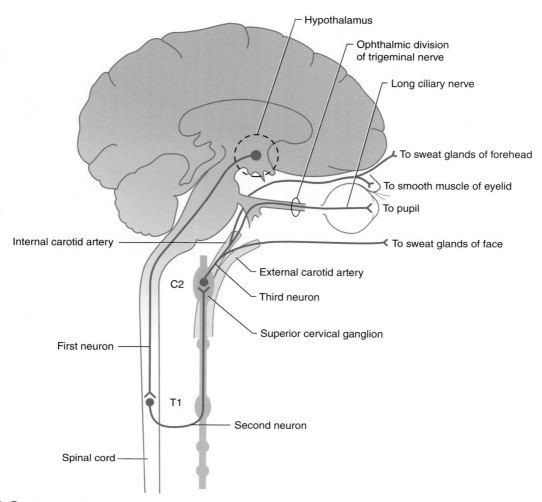

FIGURE 10–3 **The sympathetic pathway for pupillary dilation.** Reproduced with permission from Aminoff M, Greenberg D, Simon R: *Clinical Neurology*, 9th ed. New York, NY: McGraw Hill; 2015.

- **At the level of the first-order neuron:**
  - Lateral medullary infarct (Wallenberg's syndrome), accompanied by nausea, vomiting, ataxia, vertigo, dysarthria, dysphagia, ipsilateral diminished facial pain/temperature sensation and contralateral diminished bodily pain/temperature sensation (see Ch. 9)
- **At the level of the second-order neuron:**
  - Pathology of the brachial plexus, including trauma and malignant compression/infiltration (see Ch. 16)
  - Malignancy at the lung apex (Pancoast tumor) or in the head/neck
  - Thoracic surgery (or chest tube placement)
- **At the level of the third-order neuron:**
  - Internal carotid artery dissection (see Ch. 19)
  - Neck surgery
  - Cavernous sinus pathology, usually accompanied by multiple deficits in ocular movements and/or numbness in the upper face, since CNs 3, 4, and 6 and the V₁ and V₂ branches of CN 5 also travel through the cavernous sinus (see Ch. 11, Fig. 11–6)

Depending on the symptoms and signs associated with Horner's syndrome, radiologic tests are ordered to assess the brain, brainstem, spinal cord, lung apex, and/or neck (including vascular imaging to evaluate the internal carotid artery on the affected side). If the etiology remains unclear, a series of pharmacologic maneuvers with eye drops can aid in localization.

Pharmacologic Diagnosis of Horner's Syndrome

The neurotransmitter at the final synapse between the oculosympathetic fibers and the pupillary dilator muscle is norepinephrine. Cocaine eye drops, apraclonidine eye drops, and hydroxyamphetamine eye drops all have effects on norepinephrine transmission, and the responses of anisocoric pupils to these eye drops can help to determine localization of lesions along the oculosympathetic pathway (Table 10–1).

Cocaine eye drops decrease norepinephrine reuptake, allowing more norepinephrine to stay in the synapse. This dilates a normal pupil. However, in Horner's syndrome, no norepinephrine is being released at this synapse, so there is no norepinephrine reuptake to block, and the constricted pupil

TABLE 10–1 Pharmacologic Localization in Horner's Syndrome.

	Normal Pupil	Pupil With Sympathetic Dysfunction	Effect on Both Pupils in Patient With Horner's Syndrome	Localizing Value
Cocaine	Dilates	Does not dilate	Anisocoria worsens	Confirms Horner's syndrome
Apraclonidine	No effect or mild dilation	Dilates	Anisocoria reverses	Confirms Horner's syndrome
Hydroxyamphetamine	Dilates	Does **not** dilate if third-order lesion Dilates if first-order **or** second-order lesion	(Not tested in both eyes)	Distinguishes third-order lesion from first-order or second-order lesion

will not dilate in response to cocaine. Therefore, in Horner's syndrome, cocaine eye drops in both eyes make the anisocoria more prominent: The normal pupil dilates, but the pupil on the side of the Horner's syndrome does not dilate (Fig. 10–4A–C). This confirms that a Horner's syndrome is present but does not localize where along the pathway the problem is since either the third-order neuron is not releasing norepinephrine due to its own dysfunction, or it is not being stimulated to release norepinephrine if there is first-order or second-order neuron dysfunction.

Apraclonidine eye drops weakly stimulate the postsynaptic norepinephrine receptors. In Horner's syndrome due to pathology at any level, norepinephrine is not being released at the final synapse, and so the postsynaptic receptors become hypersensitive over time since they have been deprived of norepinephrine. In a normal pupil, there is no (or very little) change in pupil size when apraclonidine is administered, but in a chronically denervated Horner's pupil, the supersensitive receptors are easily excitable by stimulation, so apraclonidine causes the pupil to dilate. In Horner's syndrome, if apraclonidine drops are administered to both eyes, the Horner's pupil dilates *more* than the normal pupil, leading to reversal of the anisocoria (i.e., the formerly smaller pupil is now larger) (Fig. 10–4D–F). Note that since supersensitivity takes time to develop, there will be no pupillary dilation with apraclonidine in a recently developed Horner's syndrome. Like cocaine eye drops, apraclonidine confirms that there is a Horner's syndrome present but does not localize it.

Hydroxyamphetamine eye drops cause norepinephrine release from third-order oculosympathetic neurons. If the third-order neurons are the site of the lesion, there will be no norepinephrine released since the third-order neurons are not working. However, if the third-order neurons are intact but are not receiving stimulation due to a lesion at the level of the first-order or second-order neurons, the third-order neurons will have a large amount of norepinephrine waiting to be released, and hydroxyamphetamine will cause the pupil to dilate (Fig 10–4G–I). Therefore, hydroxyamphetamine eye drops can determine whether a Horner's syndrome is due to third-order pathology or not, but cannot distinguish between first-order and second-order lesions.

In sum, cocaine and apraclonidine eye drops can confirm the presence of Horner's syndrome but do not localize it. Hydroxyamphetamine distinguishes whether the cause of Horner's syndrome is third-order or not. No eye drop can distinguish between first-order and second-order causes of Horner's syndrome (Figs. 10–5 and 10–6).

APPROACH TO ANISOCORIA AND OTHER PUPILLARY ABNORMALITIES

Anisocoria (Table 10–2 and Fig. 10–7)

The first task in the diagnosis of anisocoria is to determine which pupil is abnormal: the smaller one or the larger one. If pupillary asymmetry is more pronounced in darkness, this suggests that the smaller pupil is the abnormal one: It has not dilated adequately in darkness as it should have and the normal pupil has dilated, exaggerating the difference between them. If pupillary asymmetry is more pronounced in the light, this suggests that the larger pupil is the abnormal one: It has not constricted adequately in response to light as it should have and the normal pupil has constricted, exaggerating the difference between them (Fig. 10–7)

If ptosis is present on the side of the small pupil, this suggests Horner's syndrome. If ptosis is present on the side of the large pupil, this suggests CN 3 pathology (Table 10–2).

Anisocoria can be due to:

- CN 3 lesion (larger pupil abnormal); for example, due to compression from posterior communicating artery aneurysm or uncal herniation (see Ch. 24)
- Lesion along the sympathetic pathway (smaller pupil abnormal; see "Impaired Pupillary Dilation")
- Pharmacologic effect: ipratropium nebulizer blowing into one eye and scopolamine patch (if patient touches patch then touches eye) are both common pharmacologic causes of pupillary dilation
- Local iris pathology (e.g., prior ophthalmologic surgery or trauma)
- Migraine
- Seizure and postictal state

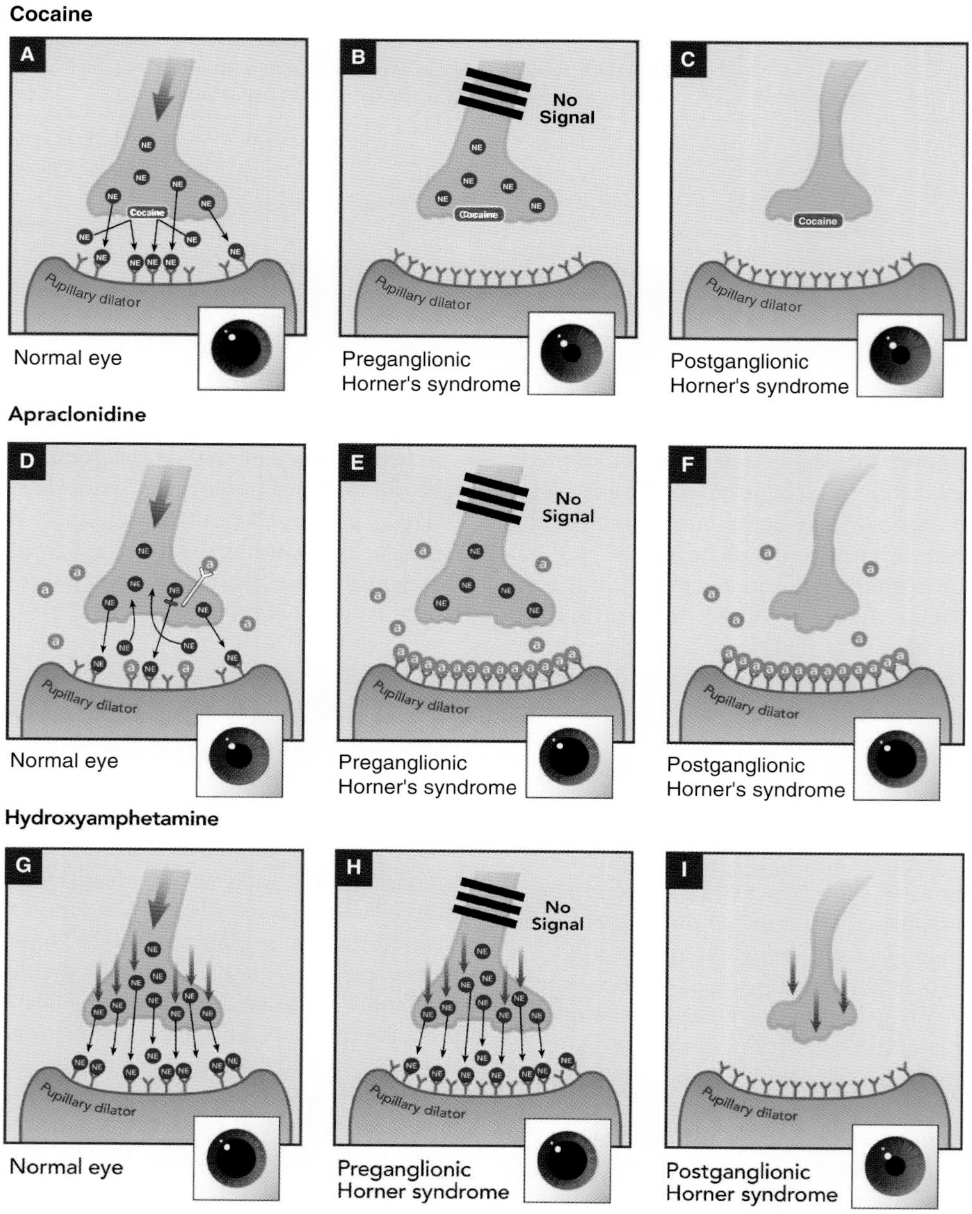

Cocaine

Apraclonidine

Hydroxyamphetamine

FIGURE 10–4 **The physiologic basis of pharmacologic localization in Horner's syndrome**. **A–C:** Cocaine eye drops in Horner's syndrome. **A:** A normal pupil dilates when cocaine eye drops are administered because norepinephrine reuptake is blocked. **B–C:** In Horner's syndrome, the abnormal pupil does not dilate when cocaine eye drops are administered, whether the lesion is preganglionic (first order or second order) (**B**) or postganglionic (third order) (**C**). **D–F:** Apraclonidine eye drops in Horner's syndrome. **D:** Apraclonidine has minimal effect on a normal pupil. **E–F:** In Horner's syndrome, supersensitivity to norepinephrine leads to dilation of the pupil in response to apraclonidine, whether the lesion is preganglionic (first order or second order) (**E**) or postganglionic (third order) (**F**). **G–I:** Hydroxyamphetamine eye drops in Horner's syndrome. **G:** Hydroxyamphetamine causes dilation of a normal pupil. **H:** In Horner's syndrome due to first-order or second-order lesions, hydroxyamphetamine leads to pupil dilation. **I:** In Horner's syndrome due to third-order lesions, hydroxyamphetamine has no effect. See text for explanations. Reproduced with permission from Martin T, Corbett J: *Practical Neuroophthalmology*. New York, NY: McGraw Hill; 2013.

- Physiologic anisocoria: a benign finding. In physiologic anisocoria, both pupils usually react symmetrically, and there is no difference in the appearance of the pupils in light versus in dark
- Tonic pupil: a dilated pupil that constricts with accommodation but not in response to light, which can be due to:

- Local ciliary ganglion pathology (e.g., orbital tumor, trauma, surgery, or inflammation)
- Idiopathic, known as Adie's pupil (mnemonic: **Adi**e's pupil is **a di**lated pupil). Adie's pupil is more common in young women and may be accompanied by hyporeflexia

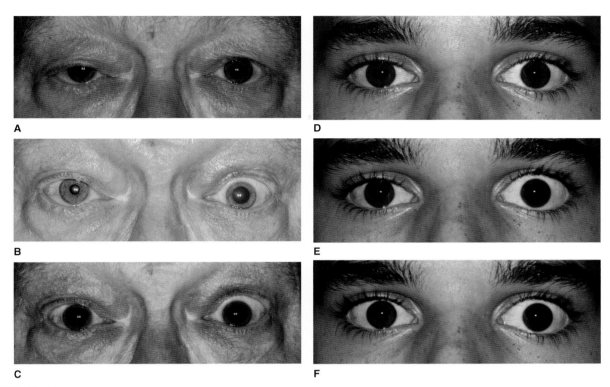

FIGURE 10–5 **Cocaine and hydroxyamphetamine testing in Horner's syndrome. A:** Right ptosis and miosis. **B:** After administration of cocaine eye drops, the left pupil dilates but the right pupil does not dilate, confirming Horner's syndrome on the right. **C:** After administration of hydroxyamphetamine eye drops, the right pupil dilates, confirming functioning third-order neurons, localizing the problem to the first-order *or* second-order neurons. **D:** Right ptosis and miosis. **E:** After administration of cocaine eye drops, the left pupil dilates but the right pupil does not dilate, confirming Horner's syndrome. **F:** After administration of hydroxyamphetamine eye drops, the right pupil does not dilate, localizing the problem to the third-order neurons. Reproduced with permission from Martin T, Corbett J: *Practical Neuroophthalmology*. New York, NY: McGraw Hill; 2013.

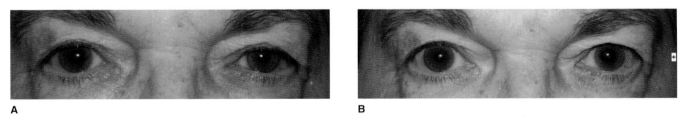

FIGURE 10–6 **Apraclonidine eye drops in Horner's syndrome. A:** Left ptosis and miosis. **B:** Apraclonidine administration leads to reversal of anisocoria (left pupil now larger) as well as resolution of left ptosis. Reproduced with permission from Martin T, Corbett J: *Practical Neuroophthalmology*. New York, NY: McGraw Hill; 2013.

TABLE 10–2 **Pattern of Anisocoria and Ptosis in Horner's Syndrome and Cranial Nerve (CN) 3 Palsy.**

	Anisocoria Worse in:	Ptosis (If Present) Will Be on Side of:
Horner's syndrome	Dark (Failure of abnormal pupil to dilate)	Small pupil (Ptosis due to weakness of Müller's muscle; lower lid elevation may also be present)
CN 3 palsy	Light (Failure of abnormal pupil to constrict)	Large pupil (Ptosis due to weakness of levator palpebrae)

With a tonic pupil, the pupillary constrictor muscle is deprived of cholinergic input from the ciliary ganglion and becomes supersensitive (just as with the pupillary dilator muscle in Horner's syndrome that is deprived of norepinephrine; see discussion of apraclonidine eyedrops in the previous section). **Pilocarpine** eyedrops stimulate the supersensitive tonic pupil, leading to constriction more so than would occur in a normal pupil. Therefore, pilocarpine administered to both pupils will cause the tonic pupil to constrict more than the normal pupil, reversing the anisocoria (i.e., the larger pupil becomes the smaller pupil). If the pupil is large due to pharmacologic effect as opposed to it being a tonic pupil, pilocarpine will not have this effect.

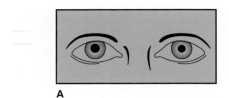

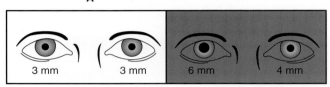

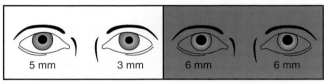

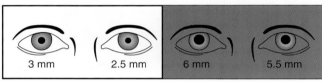

FIGURE 10–7 **Examining anisocoria in light and dark. A:** Anisocoria with the larger pupil on the patient's right. **B:** If the anisocoria is worse in darkness, this suggests that the smaller pupil (on the patient's left) has failed to dilate and is the abnormal pupil. **C:** If the anisocoria is worse in light, this suggests that the larger pupil (on the patient's right) has failed to constrict and is the abnormal pupil. **D:** In physiologic anisocoria, subtle anisocoria is generally present in both light and dark. Reproduced with permission from Martin T, Corbett J: *Practical Neuroophthalmology.* New York, NY: McGraw Hill; 2013.

Bilateral Pupillary Abnormalities

Bilateral pupillary dilation can be seen with:

- Bilateral CN 3 lesions
- Midbrain lesions
- Sympathomimetic medications (e.g., amphetamines, cocaine)

Bilateral pupillary constriction can be seen with:

- Pontine pathology
- Opiate medications
- Old age
- Syphilis. In syphilis, the pupils constrict to accommodation but not to light, which is called Argyll-Robertson pupils (mnemonic: **A**ccommodates—**yes**, **R**eacts—**no**: **A**rg**Y**ll-**R**obertso**N**). Light-near dissociation is not specific to syphilis and can be seen in any condition affecting parasympathetic input to the pupil (e.g., pathology of midbrain or CN 3, autonomic neuropathy, or local pathology [i.e., tonic pupil; see in the previous text]). This is because most CN 3 pupillomotor fibers support the near/accommodation response and fewer support the reaction to light, so in conditions that damage the parasympathetic pathway, regeneration favors the fibers responsible for accommodation.

Dilated or constricted pupils can also be seen bilaterally with widespread sympathetic and/or parasympathetic dysfunction as can be caused by autonomic neuropathy (see Ch. 27).

Extraocular Movements & Approach to Diplopia

Cranial Nerves 3, 4, & 6

Each eye is moved by six muscles: four rectus muscles and two oblique muscles. These muscles are controlled by three nerves: cranial nerves (CNs) 3, 4, and 6. These cranial nerves all originate from brainstem nuclei that communicate with one another through the **medial longitudinal fasciculus** (MLF) to coordinate movements between the left and right eyes. These nuclei are controlled by brainstem gaze centers that coordinate the eyes to move together horizontally or vertically, and these gaze centers are stimulated by cortical eye fields. From the top down, the cortical eye fields stimulate the gaze centers in the brainstem, the brainstem gaze centers communicate with the cranial nerve nuclei of CN 3, CN 4, and CN 6, and CN3, CN 4, and CN 6 activate the extraocular muscles.

The vestibular system also interacts with the eyes to coordinate eye movements with head movements. This pathway involves CN 8 and the cerebellum, and is discussed further in Chapter 12.

EXTRAOCULAR MOVEMENTS I: MUSCLES & THEIR INNERVATION (FIG. 11–1 & TABLE 11–1)

The six muscles that control each eye are the four rectus muscles (superior, inferior, medial, lateral) and the two oblique muscles (superior and inferior) (Fig. 11–1, Tables 11–1 and 11–2).

CN 4 controls the superior oblique, CN 6 controls the lateral rectus, and CN 3 controls the rest (superior, inferior, and medial recti and inferior oblique). The principal eye movements performed by the rectus muscles are easy to understand (Fig. 11–2):

- Lateral rectus (CN 6) moves the eye laterally (abducts)
- Medial rectus (CN 3) moves the eye medially (adducts)
- Superior rectus (CN 3) primarily moves the eye superiorly (elevates)
- Inferior rectus (CN 3) primarily moves the eye inferiorly (depresses)

The principal eye movements performed by the oblique muscles are slightly more complicated. In addition to moving up, down, left, and right, the eyes can also rotate when the head is tilted to either side. Rotation of the eye toward the nose/midline is called **intorsion** and rotation toward the ear is called **extorsion**. As the head is tilted to the left and the eyes attempt to maintain fixation straight ahead, the left eye must intort (turn toward the nose) and the right eye must extort (turn toward the ear). As the head is tilted to the right, the right eye intorts and the left eye extorts. In sum, when the head tilts to one side, the eye on the side to which the head is tilted (bottom eye) intorts and the other eye (top eye) extorts (Fig. 11–3). This is important in understanding the symptoms and signs of a CN 4 palsy, which is discussed further below.

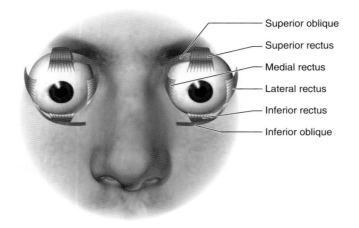

FIGURE 11–1 The six extraocular muscles.

Intorsion of the eye is the main role of the superior oblique muscle. However, when the eye is fully adducted, the superior oblique depresses the eye (Fig. 11–4). To understand the actions of the superior oblique, take your left hand and place it on the crown of your head with your elbow sticking out to the left. Look straight ahead. Your head now represents the right eye and your arm represents the right superior oblique muscle, bent at the elbow to represent the bend of the superior oblique muscle as it passes through the pulley (trochlea) for which CN 4 is named (i.e., trochlear nerve). If you pull with your hand, this will tilt the head inward—this is intorsion. If you turn your head all the way to the left so you are looking at your elbow crease (adducting the right eye), now pulling with your hand causes the head to look down (depressing the eye). The angle of the superior oblique allows for it to intort the eye when the eye is midline or abducted, and to depress the eye when the eye is adducted (Fig 11–1B). The inferior oblique performs an equal but opposite function: extorsion of the eye when the eye is midline or abducted, and elevation of the eye when the eye is adducted.

The primary actions of the superior rectus and inferior rectus are what would be expected based on their names: superior rectus elevates the eye, inferior depresses it. However, these two muscles also perform rotatory functions. Just as the superior oblique intorts the eye, the superior rectus also contributes to intorsion; just as the inferior oblique extorts the eye, the inferior rectus also contributes to extorsion (mnemonic to recall that inferior muscles extort and superior muscles intort: *Inf*EXions will leave you *Sup*INe). Just as the superior and inferior oblique perform their secondary actions (depression and elevation) in the adducted position, the superior and inferior recti also perform their secondary actions (intorsion and extorsion) in the adducted position.

EXTRAOCULAR MOVEMENTS II: CRANIAL NERVES 3, 4, & 6

All of the ocular motor nerves originate in brainstem nuclei (CN 3 and CN 4 in the midbrain; CN 6 in the pons), and travel in the subarachnoid space, through the cavernous sinus, and then into the orbit (Fig. 11–5). Lesions causing dysfunction of these cranial nerves can occur at one of four locations:

1. **Nucleus or fascicle of CNs 3, 4, or 6 in the brainstem.** The term **fascicle** refers to the portion of a cranial nerve that is still in the brainstem. Potential pathology in the brainstem includes stroke, tumor, and demyelination.

2. **CNs 3, 4, or 6.** Trauma and nerve infarct are the most common causes of isolated 3, 4, or 6 palsy. Trauma can affect CNs 3, 4, and 6 because their length and course render them susceptible to trauma. Nerve infarct of CNs 3, 4, or 6 is most commonly caused by diabetes. CNs 3, 4, and 6 can also be affected by skull base tumors, aneurysms, subarachnoid hemorrhage, meningitis, and Guillain-Barré syndrome (especially the Miller Fisher variant; see "Guillain-Barré syndrome" in Ch. 27).

TABLE 11–1   Innervation & Actions of the Extraocular Muscles.

	Cranial Nerve Innervation	Principal Action	Secondary Action	Effect of Weakness
Superior rectus	CN 3	Elevation	Intorsion in adducted position	Impaired upgaze
Inferior rectus	CN 3	Depression	Extorsion in adducted position	Impaired downgaze
Medial rectus	CN 3	Adduction	–	Impaired medial gaze
Lateral rectus	CN 6	Abduction	–	Impaired lateral gaze
Superior oblique	CN 4	Intorsion	Depression in adducted position	Impaired intorsion
				Impaired depression in adducted position
Inferior oblique	CN 3	Extorsion	Elevation in adducted position	Impaired extorsion
				Impaired elevation in adducted position

TABLE 11–2 Extraocular Muscles Controlled by Cranial Nerves 3, 4, & 6.

Nerve	Muscle
CN3 (oculomotor)	• Superior rectus
	• Inferior rectus
	• Medial rectus
	• Inferior oblique
CN4 (trochlear)	• Superior oblique
CN6 (abducens)	• Lateral rectus

3. **Cavernous sinus.** CNs 3, 4, and 6 pass through the cavernous sinus along with the V_1 and V_2 branches of the trigeminal nerve (Fig. 11–6). Potential pathology here includes cavernous sinus thrombosis, carotid-cavernous fistula, pituitary tumors or pituitary apoplexy, and Tolosa-Hunt syndrome (an idiopathic inflammatory condition of the cavernous sinus).

4. **Orbit.** When CNs 3, 4, and/or 6 are affected in the orbit, the optic nerve is also often affected (this is not the case with cavernous sinus pathology since the optic nerve does not pass through the cavernous sinus). Potential orbital pathology includes tumors, infections (orbital cellulitis), and orbital pseudotumor (an idiopathic inflammatory condition of the orbit).

Cranial Nerve 3: The Oculomotor Nerve

CN 3 originates in the medial dorsal midbrain and exits the midbrain anteriorly. It travels along the medial skull base, passing adjacent to the medial temporal lobe, through the cavernous sinus, and into the orbit. CN 3 innervates:

• Superior rectus, medial rectus, inferior rectus, and inferior oblique (all extraocular muscles except superior oblique [innervated by CN 4] and lateral rectus [innervated by CN 6])
• Levator palpebrae, which elevates the eyelid
• Parasympathetic fibers to the pupil, which constrict it (see Ch. 10)

A complete third nerve palsy (Fig. 11–7) causes:

• Weakness of the four supplied extraocular muscles, leaving the eye down and out: down due to the unopposed action of the superior oblique (CN 4) and out due to the unopposed action of the lateral rectus (CN 6)
• Weakness of the levator palpebrae, causing ptosis
• Decreased parasympathetic input to the pupil, leading to pupillary dilation (mydriasis)

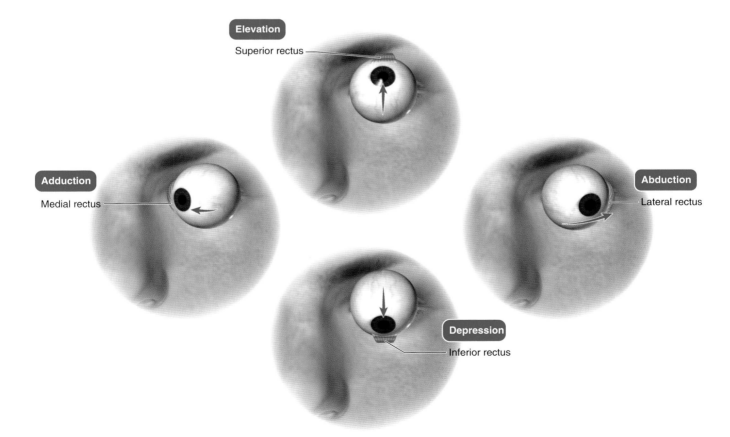

FIGURE 11–2 **The actions of the four rectus muscles.**

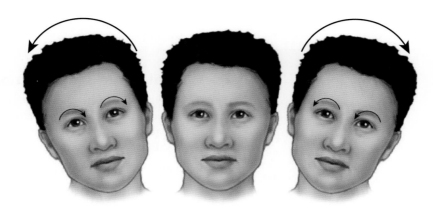

FIGURE 11–3 Schematic of intorsion and extorsion of the eyes with head tilting.

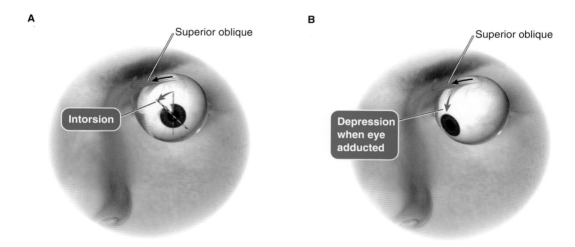

FIGURE 11–4 **Actions of the superior oblique muscle. A.** Intorsion. **B.** Depression in adduction.

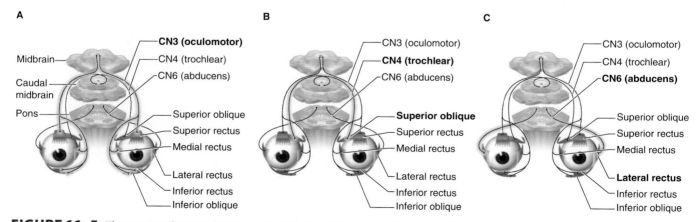

FIGURE 11–5 **The extraocular muscles innervated by Cranial Nerves 3, 4, and 6. A.** Cranial nerve 3 (oculomotor nerve) innervates the superior, inferior, and medial recti and inferior oblique (as well as supplying the levator palpebrae and parasympathetic fibers for pupillary constriction, not shown). **B.** Cranial nerve 4 (trochlear nerve) innervates the superior oblique. **C.** Cranial nerve 6 (abducens nerve) innervates the lateral rectus.

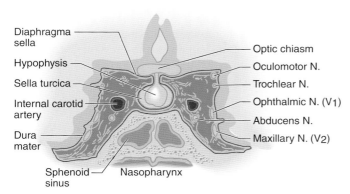

FIGURE 11-6 Schematic of a coronal view of the cavernous sinus. Reproduced with permission from Ropper A, Samuels M, Klein J: *Adams and Victor's Principles of Neurology*, 10th ed. New York, NY: McGraw Hill; 2014.

Due to the way the different fibers run in the third nerve, partial lesions of the third nerve can affect the pupillary fibers in isolation or the ocular motor fibers in isolation. The pupillary fibers run on the medial exterior part of the nerve, whereas the oculomotor fibers run in the interior of the nerve. A lesion compressing the third nerve affects the outermost fibers first, which can lead to impaired pupillary constriction with no extraocular muscle dysfunction (or preceding the development of extraocular muscle dysfunction). On the other hand, an ischemic insult to the nerve will affect the innermost fibers supplied by small penetrating vessels, and can cause extraocular dysfunction with sparing of pupillary reactivity. This is called a **pupil-sparing** third nerve palsy (Fig. 11-7).

Compressive lesions that can affect CN 3 causing isolated (or initially isolated) pupillary dilatation without eye movement abnormalities include posterior communicating artery aneurysms, skull base tumors, and uncal herniation. Pupil-sparing third nerve palsy is most commonly due to nerve infarct caused by diabetes, which usually resolves over months. Pupil-involving third nerve palsy requires urgent neuroimaging to evaluate for aneurysm or other intracranial mass lesion. When the pupil is not involved in an otherwise complete CN 3 palsy, neuroimaging can be deferred, although in practice it is often obtained in this scenario as well.

Each CN 3 nuclear complex in the dorsal midbrain has several subnuclei: one for each extraocular muscle (superior rectus, inferior rectus, medial rectus, inferior oblique). The **Edinger-Westphal nuclei** provide parasympathetic input for pupillary constriction. The levator palpebrae muscles (which elevate the eyelid) are supplied bilaterally by a single nucleus called the **central caudal nucleus**. The central caudal nucleus projects bilaterally to allow for symmetric eyelid elevation. The superior rectus subnucleus of each third nerve nucleus projects contralaterally, and the crossing fibers pass in close proximity to the contralateral CN 3 nucleus. Therefore, a very small focal lesion of the entire third nerve nuclear complex on one side will cause ipsilateral impairment of all third nerve functions and bilateral involvement of the superior rectus. Lesions of the third nerve nucleus cause *bilateral* superior rectus weakness because the affected superior rectus subnucleus projects contralaterally (causing contralateral impairment of upgaze), and the crossing fibers projecting from the unaffected contralateral superior rectus subnucleus pass in close proximity to the affected nucleus, causing involvement of the eye ipsilateral to the side of the nuclear lesion. If the adjacent

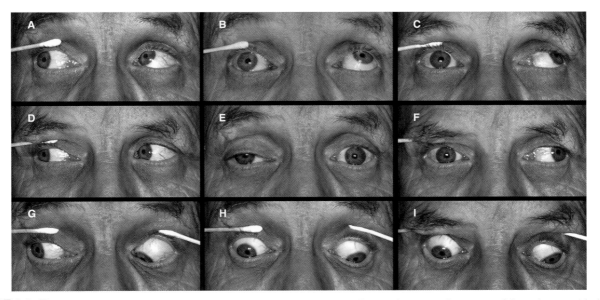

FIGURE 11-7 Right pupil-sparing third nerve palsy (due to diabetic CN 3 infarct). The patient has ptosis of the right eye with the eye "down and out" (**E**). There is impaired adduction (**C, F, I**), impaired elevation (**A, B, C**), and impaired depression (**G, H, I**) of the right eye. Abduction is spared (**A, D, G**). Sparing of superior oblique function is difficult to observe in the setting of impaired adduction. Reproduced with permission from Martin T, Corbett J: *Practical Neuroophthalmology*. New York, NY: McGraw Hill; 2013.

central caudal nucleus in the dorsal midbrain is also involved, this will cause bilateral ptosis.

The fascicle of each CN 3 travels anteriorly in the midbrain in proximity to the red nucleus, substantia nigra, and descending (not-yet-crossed) corticospinal tract before exiting as the third nerve itself. Fascicular lesions cause the same ocular findings as nerve lesions (without any contralateral/bilateral findings as can occur with lesions of the nucleus), and may be associated with contralateral weakness due to involvement of the not-yet-crossed corticospinal tract (**Weber's syndrome**), contralateral movement disorder due to involvement of the substantia nigra and/or red nucleus (**Benedikt's syndrome**), or contralateral ataxia due to involvement of the red nucleus and/or crossed superior cerebellar peduncle (coming from the contralateral cerebellar hemisphere; see Ch. 8) (**Claude's syndrome**).

Cranial Nerve 4: The Trochlear Nerve

CN 4 originates in the dorsal midbrain and is the only cranial nerve to exit posteriorly and the only cranial nerve that crosses to project contralaterally. It innervates one muscle, the superior oblique. Like CN 3 and CN 6, it is susceptible to trauma and diabetic nerve infarct (although diabetic nerve infarct occurs less commonly in CN 4 than in CN 3 or CN 6). CN 4 can also be compressed by dorsal midbrain pathology (e.g., pineal mass).

When the head is tilted to one side, the eye that intorts is the one on the side of the head to which the patient is tilting the head (e.g., if the patient tilts the head to the left, the left eye must intort, rotating equal and opposite to the direction that the head is tilting). When intorsion is impaired due to a CN 4 palsy, double vision (**diplopia**) occurs when the head is tilted *toward* the affected side since that eye cannot intort to maintain fixation. Therefore, the patient's preferred head position is to tilt the head *away* from the affected side to keep the eyes aligned. In a left CN 4 palsy, a patient's double vision will worsen when tilting the head to the left, and so the patient will prefer to keep the head tilted to the right. In a right CN 4 palsy, a patient's double vision will worsen when tilting the head to the right, and so the patient will prefer to keep the head tilted to the left.

Patients with CN 4 palsy have vertical double vision that is worst in downgaze when looking *away* from the side of the affected eye (e.g., looking left if the right eye is affected). This is because looking away from the side of the affected eye puts the affected eye in adduction, the position in which the superior oblique functions to depress the eye. When placed in the position that most needs the superior oblique (down and in), CN 4 dysfunction will be most evident, leading to double vision that is worst in this position (Fig. 11–8).

In summary for superior oblique palsies, the patient tilts the head *away* from the side of the palsy, and the diplopia worsens with downgaze *away* from the side of the affected eye (i.e., affected eye in adducted position). The trochlear nerve is

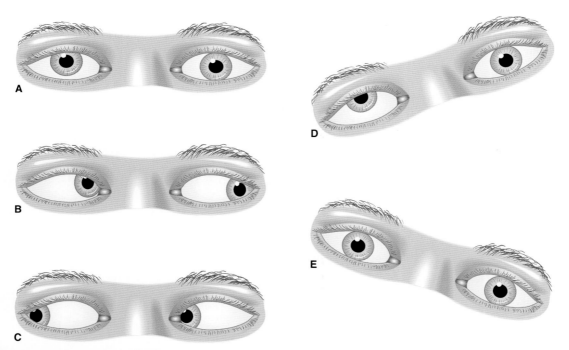

FIGURE 11–8 Schematic of right fourth nerve palsy. The right eye appears higher at baseline due to impaired depression (**A**). Depression of the eye is most impaired when looking away from the side of the affected eye, placing the affected eye in the adducted position (**B**), with less deficit when looking toward the affected side (affected eye abducted) (**C**). When the head is tilted toward the side of the affected eye, the affected eye cannot intort as it normally would, leading to increased dysconjugate gaze (**D**). When the head tilts away from the affected side, the eyes are aligned since extorsion is preserved (**E**). Reproduced with permission from Aminoff M, Greenberg D, Simon R: *Clinical Neurology*, 9th ed. New York, NY: McGraw Hill; 2015.

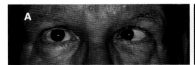
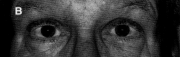
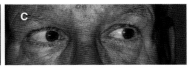

FIGURE 11–9 Right sixth nerve palsy (due to diabetic CN 6 infarct). The patient's right eye is slightly medially deviated at baseline (**B**) and the patient is unable to abduct the right eye (**A**). Leftward gaze is preserved (**C**). Reproduced with permission from Martin T, Corbett J: *Practical Neuroophthalmology*. New York, NY: McGraw Hill; 2013.

the only cranial nerve that crosses, and as a mnemonic, its deficits can also be thought of as "crossed": The head tilts *away* from the side of the superior oblique palsy, and diplopia worsens when looking *away* from the side of the superior oblique palsy (i.e., adducting the affected eye).

In **Brown's syndrome,** the superior oblique is restricted in the trochlea, causing inability to elevate the eye in adduction (i.e., the restricted superior oblique keeps the eye depressed, preventing elevation in adduction by the inferior oblique). Brown syndrome may be congenital or can occur secondary to ocular trauma, ophthalmologic, surgery, or inflammatory conditions (e.g., rheumatoid arthritis).

Cranial Nerve 6: The Abducens Nerve

The abducens nuclei reside in the dorsomedial pons, and the bilateral CN 6 run from their nuclei through the anterior pons, exit anteriorly, and then pass over the clivus, through the cavernous sinus, to the orbits.

An abducens palsy leads to failure to abduct the affected eye (Fig. 11–9). Abduction weakness causes horizontal diplopia that worsens when looking toward the side of the abduction deficit (e.g., a right-sided CN 6 palsy will cause diplopia when looking to the right, which requires right eye abduction). If there are no other cranial nerve or extraocular muscle deficits, looking *away* from the side of the deficit should lead to complete resolution of double vision, since adduction and contralateral eye abduction are spared. If a CN 6 palsy causes complete paralysis of the lateral rectus, the affected eye may be misaligned medially at rest with no lateral movement of the eye on attempted gaze toward the affected side. With partial weakness, the eye may be able to abduct only partially, allowing some of the lateral sclera to remain visible on attempted lateral gaze (called inability to "bury the sclera").

CN 6 has a long and tortuous intracranial course that takes it over the clivus. Like CNs 3 and 4, the length of CN 6 makes it susceptible to trauma. CN 6 infarct, most commonly due to diabetes, is another common cause of unilateral CN 6 palsy. Unilateral or bilateral CN 6 palsy can also occur when intracranial pressure is elevated since this pressure leads to stretching of the nerve(s) (see Ch. 25). This is sometimes referred to as a "false localizing" sign since it is a focal deficit that may not necessarily be caused by a focal lesion.

If CN 6 and CN 7 are affected on the same side, this suggests pontine localization since the CN 6 and CN 7 nuclei are adjacent in the pons. With a larger unilateral pontine lesion, contralateral hemiparesis may accompany CN 6 and CN 7

lesions (due to involvement of the not-yet-crossed corticospinal tract). If CN 6 is affected with CN 3 and/or CN 4 without involvement of CN 2, localization of the lesion in the cavernous sinus should be considered. Involvement of CNs 3, 4, and/or 6 *and* CN 2 suggests localization in the orbit.

EXTRAOCULAR MOVEMENTS III: SUPRANUCLEAR CONTROL OF HORIZONTAL & VERTICAL GAZE

The ocular motor nuclei of CNs 3, 4, and 6 for the two eyes must be coordinated for conjugate binocular movements such as horizontal gaze, vertical gaze, convergence, and divergence. These conjugate movements are under the control of gaze centers in the brainstem, which in turn are under the control of higher cortical centers.

Rapid conjugate eye movements to a target are called **saccades**, which are tested by having the patient look rapidly from one place to another (e.g., from the examiner's nose to the examiner's finger held out to one side or above or below the eyes). Conjugate eye movements that track an object are called **smooth pursuit** movements, which are tested by asking the patient to follow the examiner's finger. Saccades may occur voluntarily (a conscious decision to look at something), or can occur involuntarily (e.g., eyes move reflexively in the direction of a loud noise). The **frontal eye fields** initiate intentional saccades, and the **parietal eye fields** are involved in reflex saccades and smooth pursuit. This is logical if one recalls that intentional actions originate in the frontal lobes, whereas spatial attention is supported by the parietal lobes (see Ch. 7).

Optokinetic Reflex (Fig. 11–10)

The saccadic (frontal) and smooth pursuit (parietal) systems can be tested by evaluating the **optokinetic reflex**. An optokinetic nystagmus (OKN) strip typically has vertical alternating white and red stripes, and an OKN drum typically has vertical alternating white and black stripes. When an OKN strip is moved across the visual field in one direction (or an OKN drum is rotated in one direction), the eyes follow it in the direction it is moving. However, in order for the patient to continue following it, the patient must make saccades in the direction opposite the direction of movement of the strip/drum (like when watching trees pass by out of the window of a train). For example, when moving the OKN strip from left to

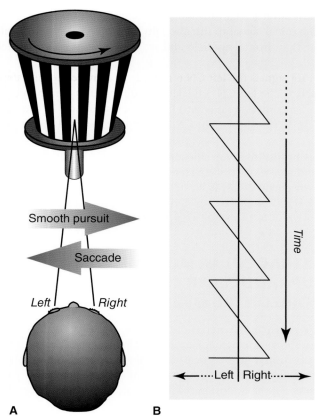

FIGURE 11–10 Schematic of optokinetic nystagmus induced by OKN drum. A: OKN drum rotated toward patient's right leads to right-ward smooth pursuits and left-ward saccades (**B**). Reproduced with permission from Martin T, Corbett J: *Practical Neuroophthalmology*. New York, NY: McGraw Hill; 2013.

right (or spinning the OKN drum from left to right), the eyes follow smoothly to the right with interrupting saccades back to the left. The pursuit in the direction that the OKN strip is moving/drum is turning is supported by the parietal lobe ipsilateral to the direction that the strip is moving/drum is turning (in this example, the right parietal lobe supports rightward smooth pursuit when the OKN strip is moving to the right). The saccades in the opposite direction from the direction of motion of the OKN strip/drum (left in this example) are supported by the frontal lobe ipsilateral to the direction of movement of the OKN strip/drum (in this example, the right frontal lobe generates leftward saccades when the OKN strip is moving to the right).

In addition to utilizing OKN to localize frontal versus parietal lesions, the optokinetic reflex is very hard to inhibit and so may be used to distinguish functional blindness from structural causes of visual loss.

Horizontal Gaze (Fig 11–11)

Horizontal gaze requires synchronizing the eyes for conjugate movements. For example, to look to the left, the left eye must abduct (left lateral rectus controlled by left CN 6) and the right eye must adduct (right medial rectus controlled by right CN 3). To achieve conjugate horizontal gaze, there must be a communication between the CN 6 nucleus on one side and the CN 3 nucleus on the other. This communication is the **medial longitudinal fasciculus** (MLF), a tract that connects each CN 6 nucleus with the contralateral CN 3 nucleus.

The MLF crosses from the CN 6 nucleus en route to the contralateral CN 3 nucleus almost immediately, spending most of its course contralateral to its point of origin. For this

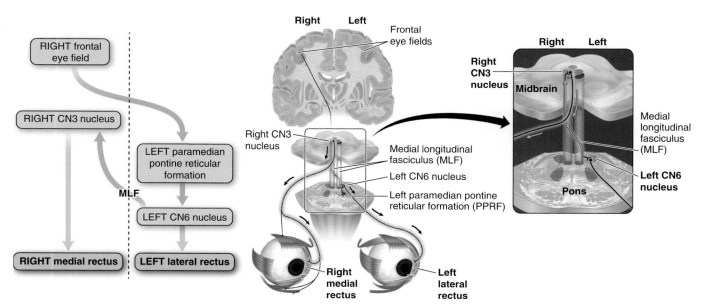

FIGURE 11–11 Schematic of pathway for conjugate horizontal gaze to the left. See text for explanation.

reason, the MLF is named for the side of the CN 3 nucleus with which it connects rather than the CN 6 nucleus from which it originates: The *left* MLF travels from the right CN 6 nucleus to the left CN 3 nucleus, and the *right* MLF travels from the left CN 6 nucleus to the right CN 3 nucleus.

The signal to voluntarily move the eyes comes from the frontal eye fields. Just as each hemisphere controls the contralateral side of the body and sees the contralateral visual field, the frontal eye fields send the eyes to the contralateral side: The left frontal eye field sends the eyes to the right, and the right frontal eye field sends the eyes to the left.

The frontal eye fields do not communicate directly with the cranial nerve nuclei but rather through horizontal and vertical gaze centers. These are the centers that communicate with the cranial nerve nuclei, which in turn communicate with each other to synchronize conjugate eye movements. The horizontal gaze center is the **paramedian pontine reticular formation** (PPRF). There is a left PPRF in the left pons for leftward gaze and a right PPRF in the right pons for rightward gaze. The flow of information for horizontal gaze is from frontal eye fields → contralateral PPRF → CN 6 nucleus → contralateral CN 3 nucleus (via MLF).

For example, to look to the left, the left eye must abduct (left lateral rectus controlled by left CN 6) and the right eye

must adduct (right medial rectus controlled by right CN 3). The initial signal to intentionally move the eyes comes from the right frontal eye field and crosses to connect with the left PPRF, which is adjacent to the left CN 6 nucleus. The left PPRF signals the left CN 6 nucleus to activate the left lateral rectus. The left CN 6 nucleus simultaneously communicates to the contralateral (right) CN 3 nucleus by way of the right MLF to signal the right CN 3 to activate the right medial rectus. A lesion of the right frontal eye field, the left PPRF, or the left CN 6 nucleus would, therefore, all lead to impaired left gaze in *both* eyes. Both eyes are affected because the problem is with *gaze in a particular direction* rather than a problem with an individual nerve or muscle. In contrast, a lesion of the abducens nerve (CN 6) itself would preclude lateral movement of that eye, but on attempted lateral gaze, the contralateral eye would still be able to adduct.

Conjugate Horizontal Gaze Abnormalities (Fig. 11–12 & Table 11–3)

A patient with a large middle cerebral artery (MCA) stroke that affects the frontal eye field will have gaze deviation toward the hemisphere of the stroke, which is away from the side of the hemiparesis. For example, a large right MCA stroke can cause left hemiparesis and right gaze deviation with inability

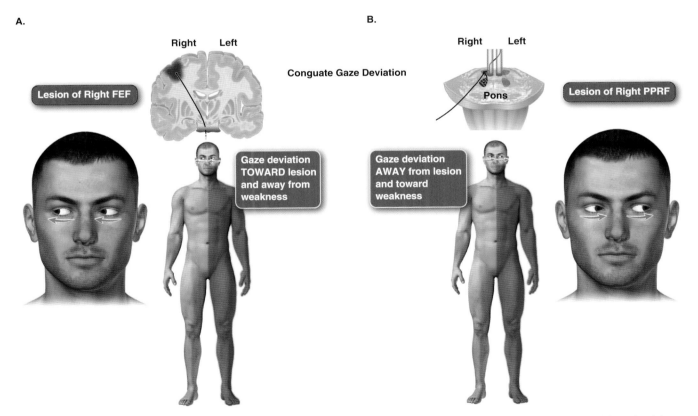

FIGURE 11–12 **Gaze deviation in cortical vs pontine stroke. A.** Lesions of FEF cause conjugate gaze deviation *toward* the side of the hemispheric lesion and *away* from the side of hemiparesis/plegia. In this instance, a lesion of the right FEF causes conjugate gaze deviation to the right with left hemiparesis/plegia. **B.** Lesions of PPRF cause conjugate gaze deviation *away* from the side of the pontine lesion and *toward* the side of hemiparesis/plegia. In this instance, a lesion of the right FEF causes conjugate gaze deviation to the left with left hemiparesis/plegia.

TABLE 11–3 Gaze Deviation in Stroke & Seizure.

	Hemispheric Stroke (Frontal Eye Field Affected)	Pontine Stroke (Lateral Gaze Center Affected)	Seizure (Frontal Eye Field Affected)
Direction of gaze deviation	Toward lesion	Away from lesion	Away from lesion (May be toward lesion in postictal state)
	Away from hemiparesis	Toward hemiparesis	Toward shaking limb(s) (May be away from Todd's paralysis in postictal state, mimicking stroke)

to look to the left. In contrast, patients with unilateral pontine stroke affecting the not-yet-crossed corticospinal tract and the lateral gaze center on one side will be unable to look toward the side of the lesion, which can produce gaze deviation toward the side of the hemiparesis, which is away from the side of the lesion. For example, a right pontine stroke can cause left hemiparesis with gaze deviation to the left and inability to look right. Gaze deviation may also be toward the side of the hemiparesis (and away from the lesion) in thalamic hemorrhage, a phenomenon called "wrong way eyes."

If seizure activity reaches a frontal eye field and activates it, this will cause the eyes to look contralaterally (i.e., deviate away from the seizure focus and toward the shaking limb if the seizure is focal). When the seizure is over and the seizure focus is in a refractory state, the eyes may deviate toward the focus in

the postictal period (which would be away from the side of a Todd's paralysis, if present).

Dysconjugate Horizontal Gaze

Dysconjugate horizontal gaze can be caused by pathology of the extraocular muscles (lateral or medial rectus), neuromuscular junction, lesions of cranial nerve 3 (affecting medial rectus) or 6 (affecting lateral rectus), or a lesion of the MLF (called internuclear ophthalmoplegia).

Internuclear ophthalmoplegia (Figs. 11–13 and 11–14)—
A lesion of the MLF impairs the coordination of CN 6 and contralateral CN 3. This leads to inability to adduct the eye on the side of the MLF lesion with gaze in the opposite direction. For example, a lesion of the left MLF causes impaired left eye adduction on rightward gaze. The phenomenon of impaired

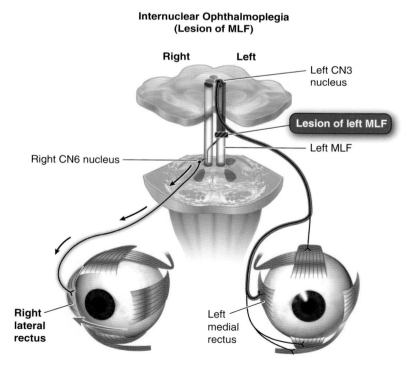

FIGURE 11–13 Schematic of left INO. A lesion of the left MLF prevents communication between the right CN 6 nucleus and left CN 3 nucleus such that there is failure of left eye adduction on right gaze.

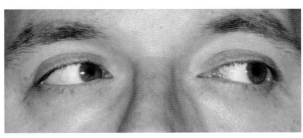

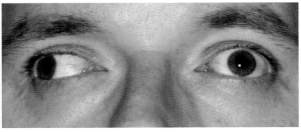

FIGURE 11–14 **Left internuclear ophthalmoplegia in a patient with multiple sclerosis. A:** Left gaze is normal. **B:** On attempted rightward gaze, the left eye does not adduct. Reproduced with permission from Hauser A, Josephson S: *Harrison's Neurology in Clinical Medicine*, 3rd ed. New York, NY: McGraw Hill; 2013.

adduction on horizontal gaze due to an MLF lesion is called **internuclear ophthalmoplegia** (INO)—*inter*nuclear because the lesion of the MLF is *between* the nuclei of CN 6 and CN 3. In INO, there is often nystagmus in the abducting eye, appearing as though it is "trying to tell the other (non-adducting) eye to come along."

Consider the example of a lesion of the left MLF. Recall that the MLF is named for the side of the CN 3 nucleus with which it communicates (i.e., *not* the contralateral CN 6 nucleus where the signal to the CN 3 nucleus originates for conjugate horizontal gaze). Therefore, a lesion of the left MLF is a lesion of the MLF that connects the right CN 6 nucleus with the left CN 3 nucleus. Leftward gaze will be normal since the left CN 6 nucleus, right MLF, and right CN 3 nucleus are not affected (Fig. 11–14A). On rightward gaze, the right eye can abduct, but the right CN 6 nucleus is unable to tell the left CN 3 nucleus to adduct the left eye (Fig. 11–14B). Therefore, the right eye abducts, but the left eye does not adduct. The patient will have double vision worst on right gaze since the eyes become dysconjugate with gaze in that direction when the left eye cannot adduct, and there will be right-beating nystagmus in the right eye on rightward gaze.

INO is seen commonly in multiple sclerosis (since the MLF is a highly myelinated tract and thus prone to the effects of demyelination), but can also be caused by pontine stroke or tumor. INO can also occur bilaterally (most commonly seen in multiple sclerosis). With bilateral INO, patients have no adduction on horizontal gaze to either side, but preserved abduction to both sides.

How can INO be distinguished from failure of adduction due to a partial CN 3 palsy or medial rectus muscle problem? In INO, CN 3 (and its nucleus) are functioning, but are cut off from their communication with the contralateral CN 6 nucleus. If convergence (bilateral adduction) is found to be preserved, this demonstrates normal function of the medial rectus, CN 3, and CN 3 nucleus by activating them through the convergence pathway that does not involve the MLF, confirming INO due to an MLF lesion. However, note that convergence is not always spared with MLF lesions: If the MLF is affected in the midbrain (as opposed to the pons), INO may be accompanied by impaired convergence (the convergence center is in the midbrain). Additionally, skew deviation (see next page) may accompany INO, causing vertical dysconjugate gaze in addition to INO, which can make it difficult for the patient to converge.

A condition called the posterior INO of Lutz occurs when there is a "reverse" INO: failure of abduction in one eye with adducting nystagmus in the contralateral eye; the distinction of this condition from a CN 6 palsy and its localization are debated.

One-and-a-half-syndrome (Fig. 11–15)—The PPRF, CN 6 nucleus, and MLF are all very close to each other in the dorsal pons. If the PPRF and/or CN 6 nucleus *and* the already-crossed MLF are affected together on one side, this has two consequences:

1. Ipsilateral conjugate gaze is impaired due to the lesion of the PPRF and/or CN 6 nucleus.

2. Adduction of the ipsilateral eye on contralateral gaze is impaired since the MLF that has crossed over from the contralateral CN 6 nucleus en route to the CN 3 nucleus on the side of the lesion is unable to signal CN 3 to adduct.

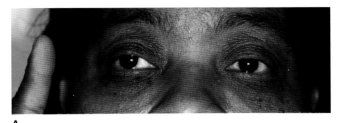

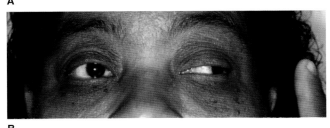

FIGURE 11–15 **One-and-a-half syndrome in a patient with multiple sclerosis. A:** On attempted right gaze, neither eye moves. **B.** On attempted left gaze, the left eye abducts, but the right eye does not adduct. This is consistent with a lesion in the right PPRF and/or CN 6 nucleus as well as the right MLF. Reproduced with permission from Martin T, Corbett J: *Practical Neuroophthalmology*. New York, NY: McGraw Hill; 2013.

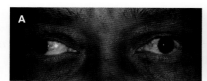
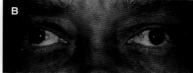
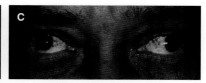

FIGURE 11–16 **Wall-eyed bilateral internuclear ophthalmoplegia (WEBINO) in a patient with pontine stroke.** At baseline (**B**), the patient's eyes appear bilaterally abducted ("wall-eyed"). On attempted right gaze (**A**), the right eye abducts, but the left eye does not adduct, consistent with left INO due to involvement of the left MLF. On attempted left gaze (**C**), the left eye abducts, but the right eye does not adduct, consistent with right INO due to involvement of the right MLF. Reproduced with permission from Martin T, Corbett J: *Practical Neuroophthalmology.* New York, NY: McGraw Hill; 2013.

For example, a lesion of the right PPRF and/or CN 6 nucleus and the right MLF (i.e., the MLF that crossed over from the left CN 6 nucleus en route to the right CN 3 nucleus) will cause:

- Loss of conjugate horizontal gaze to the right (due to the lesion of the right PPRF and/or right CN 6 nucleus)
- Loss of right eye adduction on left gaze (due to the lesion of the right MLF, which connects the left CN 6 nucleus to the right CN 3 nucleus)

This leaves only one horizontal movement: abduction of the eye contralateral to the lesion on contralateral gaze (because the contralateral PPRF and CN 6 nucleus are spared). In Figure 11–15, out of all of the horizontal eye movements, only left eye abduction is preserved. This syndrome is called **one-and-a-half syndrome** since three "half-movements" are impaired, where each "half" is one direction of horizontal gaze (left eye abduction + left eye adduction + right eye abduction + right eye adduction).

The CN 7 nucleus is adjacent to the CN 6 nucleus in the dorsal pons, so CN 6 and CN 7 nuclei may be affected simultaneously by a dorsal pontine lesion. If one-and-a-half syndrome is accompanied by CN 7 palsy, this condition is called eight-and-a-half syndrome (i.e., 1.5 + 7).

WEBINO (Fig. 11–16)—If a lesion affects *both* MLFs, there will be no adduction of either eye on horizontal gaze in either direction (bilateral INO). In some such cases, the eyes are abducted in primary gaze (exotropic), causing a "wall-eyed" appearance. This constellation of findings is called wall-eyed bilateral INO, or **WEBINO**. As with INO, multiple sclerosis and stroke are the most common causes.

A comparison of various horizontal gaze palsies is presented in Fig. 11–17 and Table 11–4.

Vertical Gaze

Vertical eye movements are controlled by two brainstem nuclei, the **rostral interstitial nucleus of the MLF** (vertical and torsional saccades) and the **interstitial nucleus of Cajal** (vertical gaze holding; eye-head coordination), both located in the dorsal midbrain close to the CN 3 and CN 4 nuclei, as would be expected (CN 6 does not participate in vertical gaze). Like the brainstem horizontal gaze centers, these nuclei are under the control of the cortical eye fields.

Impaired conjugate vertical gaze can be caused by lesions of the dorsal midbrain or in the region of the fourth ventricle (e.g., pineal pathology, tectal glioma, hydrocephalus with expansion of the fourth ventricle) and neurodegenerative diseases (e.g., progressive supranuclear palsy; see Ch. 23). Conjugate upgaze limitation may also be a normal finding in older individuals.

Pathology that compresses the dorsal midbrain can cause a constellation of ocular motor findings known as **Parinaud's syndrome:**

- Impaired upgaze with downgaze preference
- Light-near dissociation of pupillary reactions (constriction on accommodation but not in response to light)
- Eyelid retraction (called **Collier's sign**), causing a wide-eyed appearance to the eyes
- Convergence-retraction nystagmus, in which the eyes are pulled medially and retracted inward. This can be brought out in upward gaze

Skew Deviation

Skew deviation is a *supranuclear* dysconjugate vertical gaze palsy, meaning that it is due to a problem "above" (hierarchically speaking) the CN 3 or CN 4 nuclei. In skew deviation, the eyes are misaligned vertically (one higher than the other), and which eye is higher may change in different positions of gaze.

Skew deviation is caused by a unilateral lesion in the vestibular pathways (inner ear, CN 8, brainstem, or cerebellum; see Ch. 12). Central lesions (i.e., in the brainstem or cerebellum) are the cause of skew deviation more commonly than peripheral lesions (i.e., inner ear or CN 8).

In some patients with skew deviation, an **ocular tilt reaction** is also present: The asymmetric disruption in vestibular function leads the brain to think that the head is tilted when it is not, so the eyes assume positions as if the head were tilted to the side of the lesion (i.e., eye on the side of the lesion higher and intorted).

Skew deviation must be distinguished from a CN 4 palsy as a cause of vertical misalignment of the eyes, discussed further below. A unique finding in skew deviation is that it may improve (or even resolve entirely) when the patient goes from the seated to supine position (Wong et al., 2011).

There is no vertical gaze correlate to the INO, although a vertical-one-and-a-half syndrome has been rarely reported.

Dysconjugate Gaze

Right CN 3 Palsy	Right CN 4 Palsy	Right CN 6 Palsy	Right MLF Lesion

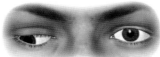

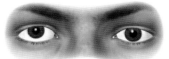

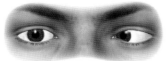

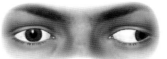

Right CN 3 Palsy

Affected eye
• Down
• Out
• Dilated pupil
• Ptosis

Right CN 4 Palsy

Right hypertropia

Right CN 6 Palsy

Failure to abduct in
ipsilateral gaze

Right MLF Lesion

Failure to adduct in
contralateral gaze

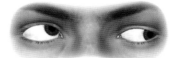

Failure to depress in adduction

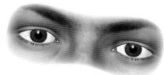

Contralateral head tilt

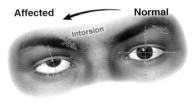

Affected   Normal

Intorsion

Worse with ipsilateral head tilt

FIGURE 11–17 Comparison of dysconjugate horizontal gaze palsies due to lesions of CN 3, CN 4, CN 6, or the MLF.

Supranuclear versus Nuclear/Infranuclear Lesions Affecting Eye Movements

Lesions in the frontal eye fields and brainstem gaze centers that control the cranial nerve nuclei are referred to as **supranuclear lesions**. Supranuclear lesions lead to problems with gaze in *both eyes* rather than in just one eye, because the gaze centers are responsible for bilateral conjugate gaze. Another system that interfaces with the brainstem horizontal and vertical gaze centers is the vestibular system. To maintain ocular fixation with head movement, the eyes have to move in the opposite direction of the head (the **vestibulo-ocular reflex [VOR]**). This is accomplished by transmitting information from the inner ear to the brainstem via CN 8, and then to the cranial nerve nuclei for CNs 3, 4, and 6 by way of the MLF. This pathway is discussed in Chapter 12. Here, the vestibulo-ocular

reflex is introduced because of its utility in localizing a gaze palsy as supranuclear or nuclear/infranuclear.

If a gaze palsy is *supranuclear*, the gaze palsy can often be *overcome by passive head movement* because the VOR pathway goes straight from the vestibular nuclei to the CNs 3, 4, and 6 nuclei, bypassing the supranuclear control systems (i.e., bypassing PPRF, rostral interstitial nucleus of the MLF, interstitial nucleus of Cajal). If a gaze palsy is caused by a lesion in CNs 3, 4, and/or 6 (or one or more of their nuclei), it *cannot* be overcome by passive head movement because the nerves/nuclei are not able to respond to the vestibular signals. Vertical gaze abnormalities in neurodegenerative disease are supranuclear and, therefore, can be overcome by the VOR. Supranuclear vertical gaze palsies may also be overcome by lifting the patient's eyelids while the patient attempts to close

TABLE 11–4 Summary of Findings in Conjugate & Dysconjugate Gaze Abnormalities.

	Effects of Lesion	Left-Sided Lesion	Right-Sided Lesion
Frontal eye field	Conjugate movements away from lesion impaired; deviation *toward* lesion	Left gaze deviation	Right gaze deviation
PPRF	Conjugate movements impaired toward side of lesion; deviation *away from* lesion	No left gaze; right gaze deviation	No right gaze; left gaze deviation
Abducens nucleus	Conjugate movements impaired toward side of lesion; deviation *away from* lesion	No left gaze; right gaze deviation	No right gaze; left gaze deviation
Abducens nerve	Dysconjugate with failure to abduct affected eye	On left gaze, right eye adducts, left eye does not abduct	On right gaze, left eye adducts, right eye does not abduct
MLF	Internuclear ophthalmoplegia: • Dysconjugate with failure to adduct one of the eyes on contralateral gaze; all other horizontal movements preserved • Convergence may be spared	On right gaze, right eye abducts, left eye does not adduct; right (abducting) eye often has right-beating nystagmus	On left gaze, left eye abducts, right eye does not adduct; left (abducting) eye often has right-beating nystagmus
PPRF or CN 6 nucleus *and* MLF	One-and-a-half syndrome: Contralateral abduction is the only functioning horizontal movement	No movement of either eye on attempted left gaze; on right gaze, right eye abducts, but left eye does not adduct	No movement of either eye on attempted right gaze; on left gaze, left eye abducts, but right eye does not adduct
Bilateral MLF	Bilateral INO: No adduction in contralateral gaze in either eye	On attempted gaze in either direction, abducting eye abducts, but contralateral eye does not adduct. In some cases eyes may appear abducted bilaterally at baseline (WEBINO).	

CN: cranial nerve; MLF: medial longitudinal fasciculus; PPRF: paramedian pontine reticular formation

the eyes tightly: The upgaze palsy in supranuclear vertical gaze palsies will be overcome by **Bell's phenomenon** (spontaneous conjugate elevation of the eyes upon eye closure).

APPROACH TO DIPLOPIA

Double vision (**diplopia**) is most commonly caused by misalignment of the two eyes (**strabismus**), leading to **binocular** double vision (i.e., double vision only with both eyes open). In binocular double vision, the double vision resolves if the patient covers either eye. If diplopia is **monocular** such that the patient sees double when looking out of just one eye, this suggests ocular pathology (usually pathology of the lens).

For diplopia due to ocular misalignment, the potential localizations of pathology from distal to proximal include:

• Neuromuscular junction (e.g., myasthenia gravis)
• Extraocular muscles (e.g., thyroid ophthalmopathy, intraorbital tumor or inflammation, myasthenia gravis)
• CNs 3, 4, and/or 6 (in the subarachnoid space, cavernous sinus, or orbit)
• Brainstem: nuclei of CN 3, 4, or 6; medial longitudinal fasciculus

Supranuclear lesions (e.g., PPRF, frontal eye fields) generally do not lead to diplopia since gaze is affected in one particular direction in both eyes symmetrically (skew deviation is an exception in that it is a supranuclear lesion that leads to ocular misalignment).

If diplopia is intermittent rather than constant, this may indicate fatigability of the extraocular muscles, and myasthenia gravis should be considered (see Ch. 29). Myasthenia can mimic cranial neuropathy of CN 3, 4, and/or 6, and even INO (called pseudo-INO in this context).

In patients with constant binocular diplopia, the clinician must determine which particular muscle(s) is/are affected. Extraocular muscles may be either weak or restricted. For example, inability of one eye to look laterally could be due to weakness of the lateral rectus or restriction of the medial rectus preventing lateral movement. A common cause of restriction of eye movements is thyroid eye disease, in which extraocular muscle inflammation leads to restriction of eye movement. In thyroid eye disease, the rectus muscles are most commonly affected, and among those the inferior rectus is most commonly affected (impeding elevation of the eye). In thyroid eye disease, the examiner will note restriction when attempting to passively move the patient's globe.

If weakness is the issue, once the weak muscle(s) is/are determined, the problem can be localized to one or more extraocular muscles, cranial nerves, or their pathways in the brainstem. *When there is only one muscle involved, diplopia will be worse when looking in the direction of the weak muscle.* For example, if the left lateral rectus is weak and the patient attempts to look right, up, or down, both eyes will move normally. However, when attempting to look left, the right eye will adduct but the left eye will not abduct, leading to increased misalignment of the eyes. Double vision will be worst when looking to the left in this example (i.e., in the direction of the weak muscle).

When the eyes are misaligned at rest or with testing of extraocular movements, the localization can generally be easily deduced by seeing which movements are impaired. This condition is called **strabismus** or **tropia**, and the type of tropia is named for the abnormal deviation (i.e., hypertropia for superior deviation, hypotropia for inferior deviation, esotropia for medial deviation, and exotropia for lateral deviation). However, some patients report diplopia but do not have obvious misalignment on initial evaluation of the extraocular movements. In such cases, subtle misalignment may be elicited on examination by using the **alternate cover test** and the **Maddox rod** (see below). Misalignment elicited with these tests is called **phoria** (i.e., hyperphoria for superior deviation, hypophoria for inferior deviation, esophoria for medial deviation, and exophoria for lateral deviation).

Horizontal Diplopia

Horizontal diplopia caused by extraocular muscle weakness (i.e., not by restriction as seen in thyroid eye disease) can be due to either lateral rectus weakness, medial rectus weakness, or INO.

If the patient has horizontal diplopia on left gaze, this could be due to left lateral rectus weakness, right medial rectus weakness, or right INO. If the patient has horizontal diplopia on right gaze, this could be due to right lateral rectus weakness, left medial rectus weakness, or left INO.

Vertical Diplopia

By convention, when the eyes are vertically misaligned, the condition is referred to as a hypertropia (or hyperphoria) of the eye that appears higher compared to the other, even if it is the downwardly deviated contralateral eye that is the abnormal one. For example, if the right eye appears higher than the left, it is called a right hypertropia whether it is due to pathologic elevation of the right eye (e.g., right inferior rectus or superior oblique palsy causing weakness in depression of the right eye) or pathologic depression of the left eye (e.g., left superior rectus palsy or left inferior oblique palsy causing weakness in elevation of the left eye).

With vertical misalignment, it can be challenging to determine which eye is abnormal and which muscle is abnormal since 4 muscles participate in vertical gaze in each eye (superior and inferior rectus and superior and inferior oblique). The Bielschowsky three-step test can be used to aid in localization:

1. Which eye is hypertropic?
2. In which direction of horizontal gaze does the hypertropia worsen?
3. In which direction of head tilt does the hypertropia worsen?

For example, consider the scenario of a patient with a left hypertropia. This could be due to left eye superior deviation or right eye inferior deviation. Is this a problem with left eye depression (left superior oblique muscle or inferior rectus muscle weakness), or a problem with right eye elevation (right inferior oblique muscle or superior rectus muscle weakness)?

Moving to step 2, if the left hypertropia worsens in right gaze, this suggests that there is a problem with either left eye depression in adduction (left superior oblique) or right eye elevation in abduction (right superior rectus); if the left hypertropia worsens in left gaze, this suggests that there is a problem with either left eye depression in abduction (left inferior rectus) or right eye elevation in adduction (right inferior oblique). So once it is determined in which direction the diplopia worsens, two muscles can be eliminated. For this example, let's say that the left hypertropia worsens on right gaze, leaving the possibilities of left superior oblique or right superior rectus weakness.

Moving to step 3, recall that the superior oblique intorts the eye (in addition to depressing the eye in the adducted position). If there is superior oblique weakness, the patient's diplopia may worsen when the head tilts *toward* the affected side and improve when the head is tilted away from the affected side (see "Cranial Nerve 4"). So, continuing the example of left hypertropia worsening on right gaze, if the diplopia worsens on left head tilt, this would suggest a left superior oblique palsy: the left eye is deviated superiorly compared to the right worsening in adduction and with ipsilateral head tilt.

Now consider the scenario of a right hypertropia. This could be due to left eye inferior deviation or right eye superior deviation. Is this a problem with left eye elevation (left inferior oblique muscle or superior rectus muscle weakness), or a problem with right eye depression (right superior oblique muscle or inferior rectus muscle weakness)?

Moving to step 2, if the right hypertropia worsens in left gaze, this suggests that there is a problem with either left eye elevation in abduction (left superior rectus) or right eye depression in adduction (right superior oblique); if the right hypertropia worsens in right gaze, this suggests that there is a problem with either left eye elevation in adduction (left inferior oblique) or right eye depression in abduction (right inferior rectus). So once it is determined in which direction the diplopia worsens, two muscles can be eliminated. For this example, let's say that the right hypertropia worsens on left gaze, leaving the possibilities of left superior rectus or right superior oblique weakness.

Moving to step 3, recall that the superior oblique intorts the eye (in addition to depressing the eye in the adducted position). If there is superior oblique weakness, the patient's diplopia may worsen when the head tilts *toward* the affected side and improve when the head is tilted away from the affected side (see "Cranial Nerve 4"). So, continuing the example of right hypertropia worsening on left gaze, if the diplopia worsens on right head tilt, this would suggest a right superior oblique palsy: the right eye is deviated superiorly, worsening in adduction and with ipsilateral head tilt.

The superior and inferior recti and the inferior oblique muscle are all controlled by CN 3, so if vertical diplopia is due to a third nerve palsy, it is common to see multiple eye movement abnormalities in the affected eye. If weakness can be isolated to the superior and/or inferior rectus in isolation, extraocular muscle pathology (e.g., thyroid eye disease) or myasthenia gravis should be considered.

Skew deviation can also cause vertical misalignment of the eyes (see "Skew Deviation"). How can skew deviation be distinguished from a CN 4 palsy? If skew deviation is accompanied by an ocular tilt reaction, the more elevated eye is intorted. This is in contrast to a CN 4 palsy, in which intorsion is *impaired* in the hypertropic eye (because CN 4 palsy leads to impaired intorsion and impaired depression). Skew deviation may improve in the supine position, whereas CN 4 palsy will not. Finally, skew deviation is usually comitant (i.e., same in all directions of gaze) although it can be incomitant, whereas CN 4 palsy will be incomitant (i.e., worse in when looking in direction of the weak muscle; in the case of CN 4 palsy when the eye is adducted).

Alternate Cover Test in the Diagnosis of Diplopia (Fig. 11–18)

In the alternate cover test, the examiner moves from covering one of the patient's eyes to covering the other, looking for subtle movements of each eye as it is uncovered. When the eye is covered, it assumes its most natural position, so if a muscle is weak, that muscle "gives up" all of the extra work it was trying to do to try to overcome its weakness and fixate when the eye was not covered. When uncovered, it must resume its hard work, so it moves once again in the direction of the weakness.

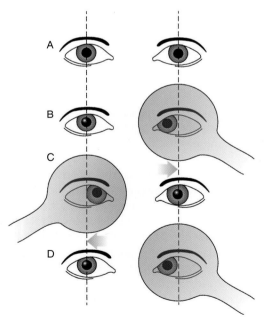

FIGURE 11–18 Schematic of alternate cover testing in bilateral esophoria. A: The eyes appear conjugate at baseline. **B:** When the left eye is covered, it moves inward. **C:** When the left eye is uncovered it moves outward, demonstrating esophoria. When the right eye is covered it moves inward. **D:** When the right eye is uncovered, it moves outward, demonstrating esophoria. Reproduced with permission from Martin T, Corbett J: *Practical Neuroophthalmology.* New York, NY: McGraw Hill; 2013.

For example, imagine that the right lateral rectus is slightly weak. To try to fixate, the right lateral rectus must work harder than normal because it is weaker. So when the right eye is covered and no longer fixating, the weak right lateral rectus can relax, and the eye moves inward. When uncovered, the weak right lateral rectus must get back to work, and so the eye moves outward. This is an **esophoria**—an inward deviation when covered (noted by seeing the eye move *outward* when uncovered). In this scenario, the *left* (normal) eye will also have an esophoria revealed when uncovered. This is because all of that neural "work" being used to try to maintain the right eye abducting in spite of its weak lateral rectus also gets applied to the left medial rectus for the left eye to look right (a phenomenon called **Hering's law**). Therefore, the left eye "overworks" in adduction. So when the left (normal) eye is covered and the right lateral rectus has to work extra hard, the left eye is also working extra hard by overadducting. When the left eye is uncovered and the right eye is covered, the left eye relaxes outward since the extra force applied to the right lateral rectus (and "shared" with the left medial rectus) is relaxed while the right eye is covered. So lateral rectus weakness on *either side* will cause *bilateral* esophoria on alternate cover testing.

To determine which eye/muscle is the problem, the alternate cover test is repeated in all of the cardinal positions of gaze. If the degree of phoria(s) is the same in all positions of gaze, this is called a **comitant** phoria. This generally suggests a congenital misalignment (congenital strabismus). In some patients, a latent congenital phoria becomes symptomatic as patients age (**decompensated phoria**). In such cases, phorias should be *comitant*.

If the degree of phoria differs in different positions of gaze, this is called an **incomitant** phoria and suggests focal weakness of a particular extraocular muscle. In an incomitant phoria, the degree of movement of each eye when it is uncovered *worsens* when the patient looks *in the direction of the weak muscle*. Resuming the example above, if there is isolated right lateral rectus weakness, the alternate cover test should reveal the greatest degree of movement of each eye when uncovered when the patient is looking to the right, and there should be less (or no) phoria seen on left gaze (since that movement does not involve the weak muscle).

The Maddox Rod in the Diagnosis of Diplopia (Fig. 11–19)

The Maddox rod is a red lens that is placed over the patient's right eye (by convention) when used in assessing diplopia. When the examiner shines a penlight in the patient's eyes at a distance, the uncovered (left) eye will see the dot of light, and the Maddox rod converts the light into a red line in the covered (right) eye. The line may be oriented vertically or horizontally depending on how the Maddox rod is held. If the eyes are perfectly aligned, the white dot and the red line should overlap perfectly. If there is misalignment, the patient will see separation between the white dot and the red line.

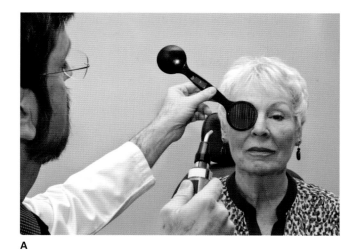

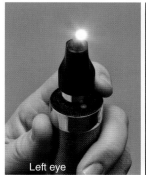
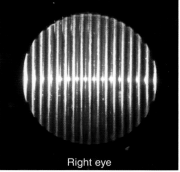

FIGURE 11–19 **Maddox rod testing demonstrating right hypertropia/left hypotropia. A:** The red lens is held over the right eye by convention. **B:** The patient's point of view (light on the left, red lens on the right). **C:** The patient sees the light (left eye image) as being higher than the horizontal line (right eye image). This means that light is hitting the left eye at a point inferior to that in the right eye (causing the left eye image to be seen superior to the right eye image), consistent with a right hypertropia. Reproduced with permission from Martin T, Corbett J: *Practical Neuroophthalmology.* New York, NY: McGraw Hill; 2013.

The separation of the dot and line worsen when the patient looks in the direction of the weak muscle (just as diplopia worsens when the patient looks in the direction of the weak muscle).

To interpret the pattern of separation of the white dot and red line in patients with ocular misalignment, recall that each part of the retina sees the opposite side of the world: The medial retina sees the lateral visual field, the lateral retina sees the medial visual field, the superior retina sees the inferior visual field, and the inferior retina sees the superior visual field (see Ch. 6). If an eye is deviated, light will hit a different part of the retina than it normally would have. For example, if the eye is medially deviated, light will end up hitting the retina more medially; if the eye is superiorly deviated, light will end up hitting the retina more superiorly. When light hits the retina in the "wrong place" compared to where it should normally land, the white dot (left eye) or red line (right eye) will be displaced in the direction *opposite* the deviation of the eye, since each part of the retina sees the opposite part of the visual field. For example, if light hits the left eye more medially, the white dot will be seen as being more lateral; if light hits the left eye more superiorly, this white dot will be seen as being more inferior.

For horizontal diplopia, the Maddox rod is used to create a vertical red line so the degree of horizontal separation between the white dot and red line can be determined. If there is esodeviation (medial deviation due to abduction weakness) in *either* eye, the white dot will be seen to the left of the red line. This is because if the left eye is medially deviated, light will hit the left eye more medially, projecting the white dot more laterally (i.e., further left); if the right eye is medially deviated, light will hit the right eye more medially projecting the red line more laterally (i.e., further right). So if the white dot is seen to the left of the red line there is either left or right esodeviation (abduction weakness). If the separation worsens when the patient looks to the left, there is left lateral rectus weakness; if the separation worsens when the patient looks to the right, there is right lateral rectus weakness.

For vertical diplopia, the Maddox rod is used to create a horizontal red line so that the degree of vertical separation between the red line and white light can be determined. If there is a left hypertropia this means either the left eye is pathologically higher or the right eye is pathologically lower (in either case, this is called a left hypertropia by convention, even if the right eye is the abnormal one). If there is left hypertropia due to the left eye being deviated upward (i.e., weakness of left eye depression), the light will hit a more superior part of the left retina than normally, projecting the white dot below the red line. If there is left hypertropia due to the right eye being deviated downward (i.e., weakness of right eye elevation), light will hit a more inferior part of the right retina than normal, projecting the red line above the white dot. So if the left eye is superior to the right eye due to vertical deviation in either eye (left hypertropia), the white dot will be seen below the red line.

If there is a right hypertropia this means either the right eye is pathologically higher or the left eye is pathologically lower (in either case, this is called a right hypertropia by convention, even if the left eye is the abnormal one). If there is right hypertropia due to the left eye being deviated downward (i.e., weakness of left eye elevation), the light will hit a more inferior part of the left retina than normally, projecting the white dot above the red line. If there is right hypertropia due to the right eye being deviated upward (i.e., weakness of right eye depression), light will hit a more superior part of the right retina than normal, projecting the red line below the white dot. So if the right eye is superior to the left eye due to vertical deviation in either eye (right hypertropia), the white dot will be seen above the red line.

Once the side of the hypertropia is determined, the Bielschowsky 3-step test can be utilized to localize the specific extraocular deficits (see "Vertical Diplopia").

REFERENCE

Wong AMF, Colpa L, Chandrakumar M. Ability of upright-supine test to differentiate skew deviation from other vertical strabismus causes. *Arch Ophthalmol* 2011;129:1570-1575.

The Auditory and Vestibular Pathways & Approach to Hearing Loss and Dizziness/Vertigo

Cranial Nerve 8

Cranial nerve 8 (CN 8) contains two components: auditory (cochlear) and vestibular. Both begin in the inner ear and travel to the brainstem: the auditory component projects to the cochlear nuclei (at the pontomedullary junction) and the vestibular component projects to the vestibular nuclei (in the medulla).

THE AUDITORY SYSTEM (FIG. 12–1)

Auditory information travels from the inner ear through the auditory (cochlear) portion of CN 8 to arrive at the cochlear nuclei at the pontomedullary junction. The cochlear nuclei project to the inferior colliculi of the lower midbrain via the lateral lemniscus, and also project to the superior olives. Each inferior colliculus projects to the ipsilateral medial geniculate nucleus (MGN) of the thalamus, and each MGN projects to the ipsilateral auditory cortex in the superior temporal gyrus (Heschel's gyrus).

APPROACH TO HEARING LOSS

Auditory information crosses to become bilateral early in its connections within the brainstem, so unilateral hearing loss can only occur due to pathology of the inner ear or CN 8 (or rarely the entry zone of CN 8 or cochlear nuclei at the pontomedullary junction). Central lesions (in the brainstem or temporal lobe) only rarely cause deafness, and must be extensive and bilateral

to do so. Therefore, central etiologies of deafness are usually associated with other signs due to involvement of neighboring structures. Left temporal lobe lesions can lead to deficits in word processing (**pure word deafness**) and right temporal lobe lesions can cause deficits in music processing (**amusia**).

Hearing loss due to a peripheral lesion is called **conductive hearing loss** if it is caused by problems in the outer or middle ear, and called **sensorineural hearing loss** if it is due to problems in the cochlea or auditory component of CN 8. Both conductive and sensorineural etiologies of hearing loss may be acquired or may have a congenital/genetic basis. Acquired causes of hearing loss are listed below.

Acquired causes of conductive hearing loss include:

- Outer ear: cerumen impaction
- Middle ear: infection (otitis media), otosclerosis

Acquired causes of sensorineural hearing loss include:

- Unilateral
  - Internal auditory artery infarct (the internal auditory artery [also called the labyrinthine artery] is usually a branch of the anterior inferior cerebellar artery [AICA])
  - Sudden sensorineural hearing loss (often idiopathic; may respond to steroids)
  - Ménière's disease (see "Ménière's Disease")
  - Vestibular schwannoma (also called acoustic neuroma; see "Vestibular Schwannoma" in Ch. 24)

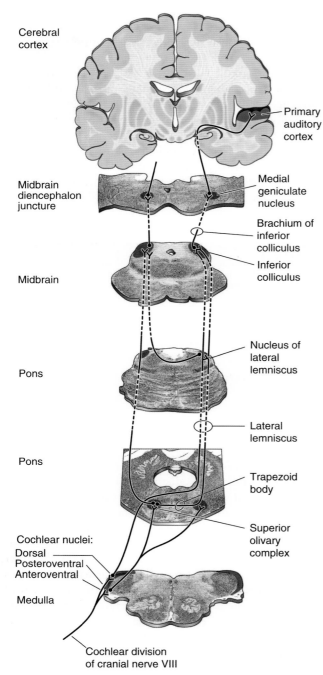

FIGURE 12–1   The auditory pathway. See text for explanation. Reproduced with permission from Martin J: *Neuroanatomy Text and Atlas*, 4th ed. New York, NY: McGraw Hill; 2012.

- Bilateral
  - Aging (**presbyacusis**)
  - Ototoxic medications (e.g., aminoglycosides)
  - Sequela of meningitis (especially in children)
  - Neurofibromatosis type II with bilateral vestibular schwannomas (see "Neurocutaneous Syndromes" in Ch. 24)

- Susac's syndrome (a syndrome causing branch retinal artery occlusion, sensorineural hearing loss, and encephalopathy; see "Susac Syndrome" in Ch. 19)
- Superficial siderosis (which causes hearing loss accompanied by cerebellar dysfunction and/or upper motor neuron signs; see "Superficial Siderosis" in Ch. 19)
- Mitochondrial disorders (see "Mitochondrial Diseases" in Ch. 31)

Sudden-onset unilateral hearing loss can be caused by infarction of the inner ear structures due to ischemia in the territory of the internal auditory artery (also called the labyrinthine artery), which is usually a branch of the AICA. This diagnosis should be strongly considered in patients whose acute-onset unilateral hearing loss is accompanied by vertigo or other brainstem or cerebellar symptoms/signs. If hearing loss is episodic with a sense of ear fullness and vertigo, Ménière's disease should be considered.

Distinguishing Conductive Hearing Loss From Sensorineural Hearing Loss

The function of the eardrum and middle ear bones is to amplify sound waves for transmission into neural impulses. In conductive hearing loss, CN 8 works properly, but sound is not able to be transmitted to it by the outer/middle ear. In sensorineural hearing loss, the pathway for auditory conduction is not functioning properly. The **Weber** and **Rinne** tests can help to distinguish between conductive and sensorineural hearing loss (Table 12–1).

Weber's Test

In Weber's test, a 512 Hz tuning fork is placed on the top of the patient's head. Normally, the pitch should be heard equally in both ears. If the pitch is louder on one side, this means that either the opposite (softer) side is affected by sensorineural hearing loss *or* the ipsilateral (louder) side is affected by conductive hearing loss (outer/middle ear blockage masks outside noise, making conduction by way of the skull louder in that ear).

TABLE 12–1   Conductive Versus Sensorineural Hearing Loss.

	Conductive	Sensorineural
Localization	Outer or middle ear	Inner ear or cranial nerve 8
Weber	Louder in affected ear	Louder in opposite ear
Rinne	Bone conduction louder than air conduction	Air conduction louder than bone conduction (but both diminished)
Frequencies affected	Low frequencies	High frequencies

Rinne's Test

In Rinne's test, a vibrating tuning fork is placed on the patient's mastoid and then next to the ear, and the patient is asked which is louder. Normally, the sound next to the ear should be louder because it takes advantage of the amplifier function of the middle ear bones. In conductive hearing loss, the middle ear bones are not working normally (e.g., otosclerosis, otitis media), or sound cannot adequately access the middle ear (e.g., cerumen impaction, otitis externa). Therefore, the tuning fork will sound softer next to the ear (since the amplifying mechanism of the middle ear is not functioning), but louder on the mastoid because it uses skull vibration to arrive directly at CN 8, taking a "detour" around the problem in the outer or middle ear. In sensorineural hearing loss, the tuning fork will be heard as diminished both on the mastoid and next to the ear since the final pathway (inner ear/CN 8) is not functioning. Air conduction is still usually louder than bone conduction in sensorineural hearing loss, as is the case normally.

THE VESTIBULAR SYSTEM (FIG. 12–2)

The inner ear vestibular structures (saccule, utricle, and semicircular canals) detect movements of the head. This information is transmitted by the vestibular portion of each CN 8 to the vestibular nuclei in the dorsolateral medulla, which then communicate with the cranial nerve nuclei for eye movements (CNs 3, 4, 6) via the medial longitudinal fasciculus (MLF). Vestibular information is also communicated to the vestibulocerebellum (the flocculus/nodulus of the cerebellum) via the inferior cerebellar peduncles (see Ch. 8). This coordination of eye movements with head movements allows for the **vestibulo-ocular reflex**.

The Vestibulo-Ocular Reflex (VOR) (Fig. 12–3)

When attempting to fixate gaze on a point while moving the head, the eyes must move in the opposite direction

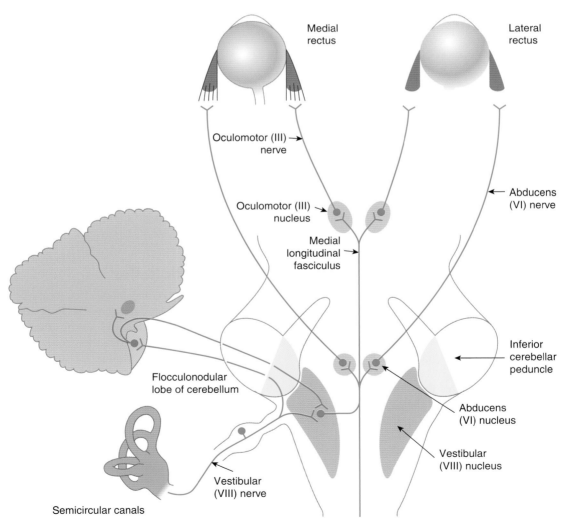

FIGURE 12–2 The vestibular pathway. See text for explanation. Reproduced with permission from Aminoff M, Greenberg D, Simon R: *Clinical Neurology*, 9th ed. New York, NY: McGraw Hill; 2015.

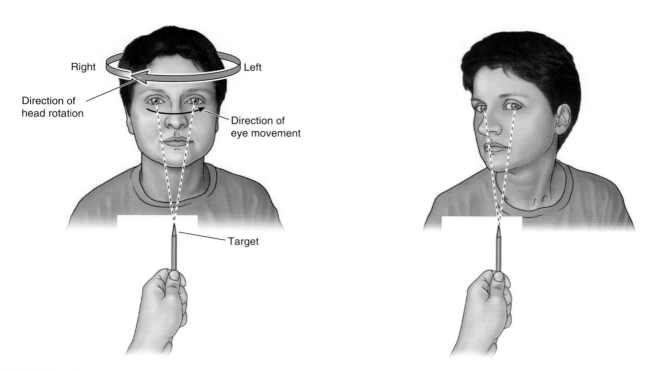

FIGURE 12–3 **The vestibulo-ocular reflex**. See text for explanation. Reproduced with permission from Martin J: *Neuroanatomy Text and Atlas*, 4th ed. New York, NY: McGraw Hill; 2012.

from the head. For example, if you ask a patient to continue looking at your nose while they turn their head to the right, the patient's eyes will have to move to the patient's left to maintain fixation. The horizontal **vestibulo-ocular reflex (VOR)** is accomplished by communication between the vestibular nuclei and the abducens nucleus on the left so as to coordinate left eye abduction (via CN 6) and right eye adduction (via MLF to CN 3; see Ch. 11).

The brain determines which way the head is turning by comparing information from the left and right vestibular systems. The side to which the head turns stimulates greater vestibular system excitation on that side, and this is communicated to the ocular motor nuclei by way of the MLF to turn the eyes to the opposite side. Turning the head toward the left causes the left vestibular system to become more activated than the right side, and this activation pattern is communicated through the MLF to the right abducens nucleus to send the eyes to the right (via the right CN 6 and left CN 3). Turning the head toward the right causes the right vestibular system to become more excited than the left side, and this excitement pattern is communicated through the MLF to the left abducens nucleus to send the eyes to the left (via the left CN 6 and right CN 3).

The VOR can be suppressed when needed. For example, if you want to turn both your head and your eyes to the left to look at something on the left side, you would not want your eyes being dragged to the right against your will as you try to look left. Although the decision to suppress the VOR likely comes from the hemispheres, suppression of the VOR is mediated by the vestibular portion of the

cerebellum (flocculus and nodulus). The ability to suppress the VOR can be tested by having the patient sit in a swivel chair with the thumb held out at arms' length, and then rotating the chair from side to side while the patient maintains fixation on the thumb. If the VOR cannot be suppressed, the eyes will move in the direction opposite chair/head turning rather than following the thumb. Failure to suppress the VOR can be seen in neurodegenerative disorders such as progressive supranuclear palsy (see "Progressive Supranuclear Palsy" in Ch. 23).

Oculocephalic Reflex

The **oculocephalic reflex** can be used to assess the VORs in a comatose patient to determine the integrity of brainstem pathways (although this should not be attempted if the cervical spine is injured). To test the oculocephalic reflex, the head is turned passively to look for the presence of conjugate eye movements in the opposite direction. Although the term "doll's eyes" is often used for this test, it can be unclear whether "having doll's eyes" means having an intact oculocephalic reflex or an abnormal one, so it is more precise to state whether the oculocephalic reflex is present or absent in each direction. Presence of oculocephalic reflexes in a comatose patient indicates that the brainstem pathways are intact, suggesting that the comatose state is due to pathology affecting the hemispheres. Oculocephalic reflexes may be impaired with brainstem pathology, but can also be diminished or absent with sedating medications, complicating assessment in comatose patients who are sedated.

Cold Caloric Testing

If a patient has neck trauma prohibiting oculocephalic reflexes from being safely tested by passive head turning, cold caloric testing can be pursued (as long as the tympanic membrane is intact). In this test, cold water is placed into one ear. Cold water "turns off" the vestibular apparatus. If one side is turned off, the other side's normal baseline activity is "greater than off," so the brain thinks the head is moving toward the not-cold side. This causes the eyes to move away from the not-cold side and toward the cold side.

For example, cold water in the left ear causes the left ear to be "off," so the brain detects more activity from the right vestibular system compared to the "off" left ear. This simulates the head turning toward the right, and so the eyes move to the left (if the VOR pathway is intact). If the frontal lobes are intact, there will be nystagmus with the fast phase in the direction opposite the slow phase (i.e., the fast phase of the nystagmus is away from the cold side).

Cold caloric testing assesses both brainstem and hemispheric function. If both the brainstem and hemispheres are functioning, there will be both a slow phase toward the cold water side and nystagmus with fast phase away from the cold water side. If the brainstem is functioning but there is hemispheric dysfunction, there will *only* be a slow phase (toward the cold water side) and no fast phase. If there is no slow phase at all, this suggests that there is either disruption of brainstem vestibulo-ocular pathways or that the patient has taken or received sedating medications.

Nystagmus

Nystagmus is involuntary rhythmic movement of the eyes. The type of nystagmus most commonly seen has a slow-phase in one direction and a fast phase in the opposite direction (**jerk nystagmus**). When nystagmus is present, the goal is to determine if the cause is peripheral (inner ear or CN 8) or central (brainstem/cerebellum).

Several types of nystagmus occur exclusively with *central* pathology (i.e., lesions of brainstem/cerebellum or medications affecting them):

- **Gaze-evoked, direction-changing nystagmus:** The fast phase is *in the direction of gaze* in all eye positions (i.e., fast phase is toward the left when the patient looks left and toward the right when the patient looks right). This is called direction-changing nystagmus because the direction of the fast phase changes depending on the direction of gaze (i.e., right-beating when looking right, left-beating when looking left; see "Direction-Changing Nystagmus Due to Central Lesions").
- **Pure vertical nystagmus** (i.e., downbeat or upbeat nystagmus with no torsional component). Downbeat nystagmus is commonly associated with lesions at the cervicomedullary junction (e.g., Chiari malformation, foramen magnum meningioma).

- **Pure torsional nystagmus** (i.e., with no horizontal or vertical component).
- **Pendular nystagmus:** In contrast to the more common jerk nystagmus, pendular nystagmus consists of symmetrically oscillating eye movements rather than movements with alternating slow and fast phases.
- **Periodic alternating nystagmus** is horizontal nystagmus that beats in one direction for a period of minutes, stops, and then beats in the other direction. This may be congenital or caused by an acquired disorder of the cerebellum (specifically the uvula and/or nodulus).
- **See-saw nystagmus** is elevation/intorsion nystagmus of one eye with simultaneous depression/extorsion nystagmus of the other. This is most commonly caused by a sellar mass (e.g., pituitary adenoma, craniopharyngioma).
- **Bruns nystagmus** is direction-changing horizontal nystagmus that is higher in frequency and lower in amplitude when looking away from the side of lesion. This is most commonly associated with a lesion at the cerebello-pontine angle (e.g., vestibular schwannoma, meningioma) that causes combined central (direction-changing, low frequency, large amplitude) and peripheral (direction-constant, high frequency, low amplitude accentuated when looking away from the side of the lesion) patterns of nystagmus.
- **Convergence-retraction nystagmus** is rhythmic convergence and retraction of the eyes (into the orbit) elicited on attempted upgaze: caused by dorsal midbrain lesions as part of Parinaud syndrome (see "Vertical Gaze" in Ch. 11).

Other useful localizing principles for nystagmus include:

- Nystagmus of peripheral origin can be suppressed by fixation, whereas nystagmus of central origin cannot. This is because when nystagmus is peripheral in origin, central mechanisms controlling fixation can overcome it.
- Nystagmus of central origin can be associated with additional brainstem and/or cerebellar signs. Nystagmus of peripheral origin may have accompanying hearing loss, but no other neurologic signs should be present. Both central and peripheral causes of nystagmus can be associated with nausea, dizziness, and imbalance.

Causes of nystagmus of central origin include:

- Stroke, demyelinating lesion, or tumor in the lower brainstem or cerebellum
- Medications (e.g., antiseizure medications and lithium)
- Toxins (e.g., alcohol)
- Paraneoplastic cerebellar degeneration (see "Paraneoplastic Syndromes of the Nervous System" in Ch. 24)
- Genetic cerebellar degenerative diseases (e.g., spinocerebellar ataxia; see "Inherited Causes of Ataxia" in Ch. 8)

Causes of nystagmus of peripheral origin include:

- Vestibular neuritis (usually postinfectious)
- Benign paroxysmal positional vertigo
- Ménière's disease

Direction-Changing Nystagmus Versus Nystagmus With the Fast Phase in the Same Direction in All Directions of Gaze

Direction-changing nystagmus due to central lesions— Eye movements are generated by a neural **pulse** that sends the eyes to a target and then a **step** of continued neural impulses maintaining them there. With central (brainstem/cerebellar) etiologies of nystagmus, there is a problem with the step causing difficulty *maintaining* gaze. Imagine the consequences of a lesion affecting the step: When the eyes look to the left, there is difficulty maintaining left-gaze, so the eyes drift away from the direction of gaze (slow phase to the right) and are sent back quickly in the direction of gaze (fast phase to the left) to try to maintain fixation—drift away (slow phase to the right), sent back (fast phase to the left), and so on. The same thing would happen when looking to the right: In attempting to maintain rightward gaze with a lesion affecting the step, the eyes would drift away (slow phase to the left) and be sent back quickly (fast phase to the right). So with a central lesion (affecting the step that maintains gaze), there would be nystagmus with the fast phase in the direction of gaze—left when looking left, right when looking right. Since the direction of the fast phase of the nystagmus changes depending on the direction of gaze, this is called **direction-changing nystagmus** or **gaze-holding nystagmus**, and is characteristic of a *central* cause of nystagmus.

In normal healthy patients, a few beats of nystagmus with the fast phase in the direction of gaze may be seen at the extremes of gaze when testing extraocular movements. This is called **end-gaze nystagmus** and is generally a benign finding if symmetric and not sustained.

Nystagmus with the fast phase in the same direction in all directions of gaze due to peripheral lesions— When peripheral lesions cause nystagmus, the problem is usually unilateral: either the left or right vestibular apparatus or CN 8 is not working normally.

Imagine what would happen if there is unilateral peripheral vestibular dysfunction (inner ear or CN 8). Recall that head turning to either side causes increased CN 8 activity on the side to which the head is turned compared to the other side, leading to movement of the eyes in the direction opposite the direction of head turning (see "The Vestibulo-Ocular Reflex" earlier). Consider the case of a left vestibular lesion (e.g., vestibular neuritis). If there is a lesion affecting the left vestibular apparatus or CN 8, activity in the left CN 8 will be decreased. This leads to an imbalance such that there is relatively more activity in the right CN 8 than in the malfunctioning left side. The brain perceives the greater degree of activity on the right (normal) side compared to the left (malfunctioning side) as the same pattern as when the head is turned toward the right side (right-sided CN 8 activity > left-sided activity), and so this sends the eyes to the left. (The lesion has the same effect as cold water in cold caloric testing; see "Cold Caloric Testing.") Since the patient is not trying to look left, the brain tries to correct the eye movements by sending them briskly back to the right. The eyes drift to the left (slow phase),

flick back to the right (fast phase), drift to the left, flick back to the right. No matter what position the eyes are in, they drift to the left, flick back to the right. The fast phase of the nystagmus is therefore *always in the same direction* no matter what position of gaze the eyes are in: slow phase toward the abnormal side, fast phase away from the abnormal side.

Continuing with the example of a left vestibular lesion, if the eyes do look all the way to the left, this is where the lesion is causing the brain to "want" them to be, so the nystagmus may diminish and even disappear. But when the eyes look furthest away from the lesion—to the right in this example—they are furthest from where the brain "wants" them to be, and so the nystagmus is intensified. This is called **Alexander's law**: Peripheral vestibular lesions cause nystagmus that is most pronounced when looking *away from the side of the lesion* (which is looking in the *direction of the fast phase*).

APPROACH TO DIZZINESS & VERTIGO

Dizziness can be caused by a problem in the nervous system or due to systemic causes. Within the nervous system, the problem can arise from the structures of the inner ear, the vestibulocochlear nerve, the brainstem, or the cerebellum. The inner ear and CN 8 are the peripheral components of this system, and the brainstem and cerebellum are the central components. Localizing the etiology of dizziness requires first determining whether the problem is neurologic or not, since dizziness can be caused by cardiovascular disease (e.g., arrhythmia, orthostatic hypotension), anemia, and endocrine dysfunction (e.g., hypoglycemia, thyroid disease) in addition to neurologic disorders. If dizziness is neurologic in etiology, one must determine whether the problem is peripheral (inner ear or CN 8) or central (brainstem/cerebellum). Medications can also cause dizziness through effects on the nervous system (e.g., antiseizure medications), the inner ear (e.g., aminoglycoside toxicity), or the cardiovascular system (e.g., antihypertensives causing orthostatic hypotension).

The classic teaching is that the history in a dizzy patient should aid in classifying the symptom of dizziness as one of the following four entities (Drachman and Hart, 1972):

1. **Vertigo**: a sensation of movement (spinning or tilting)—generally associated with a neurologic etiology
2. **Light-headedness/presyncope**: generally associated with a cardiovascular etiology
3. **Dysequilibrium/imbalance**: generally associated with a gait disorder (which may be neurologic or orthopedic, for example)
4. **Other/nonspecific**: generally associated with a psychogenic etiology

Although it is certainly important to elicit patients' descriptions of their symptoms, research suggests that patients are inconsistent and imprecise in their descriptions of whether their dizziness is true room-spinning vertigo or not (Newman-Toker et al., 2007), and that patient descriptions do not

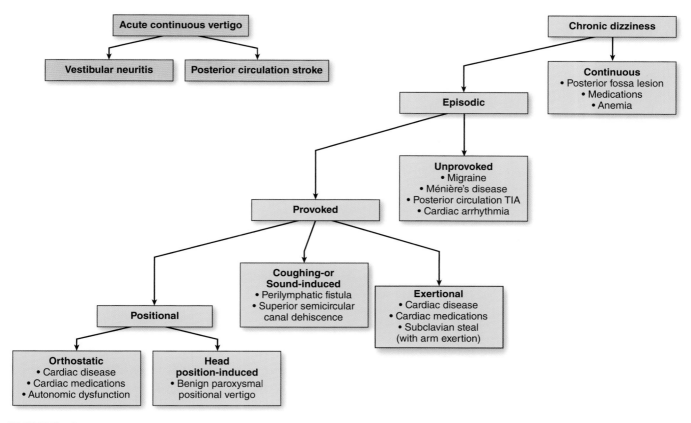

FIGURE 12–4 Approach to vertigo.

necessarily correlate well with underlying etiology. An approach centered around timing, triggers, and associated symptoms correlates more closely with pathophysiologic etiology, and these elements of the history are more consistently and accurately reported by patients (Newman-Toker, 2007; Newman-Toker et al., 2007). Within this framework, dizziness is classified as acute or chronic, and chronic dizziness is classified as continuous or episodic. Episodic dizziness is then categorized based on whether the episodes are triggered or spontaneous (Fig. 12–4). If episodes are triggered, the trigger(s) must be determined (discussed further below).

Evaluation of Acute-Onset Continuous Vertigo

Acute-onset continuous vertigo is referred to as the **acute vestibular syndrome**. If there is no history of head trauma or intoxication, the differential diagnosis is essentially between posterior circulation stroke and vestibular neuritis (a presumed viral or postviral inflammation of the vestibular portion of CN 8). This is a paradigmatic example of a scenario in which peripheral and central etiologies of vertigo must be distinguished to determine whether dizziness is caused by a benign self-limited condition (vestibular neuritis) or a life-threatening condition (posterior circulation infarct). When obvious localizing findings are present (e.g., ataxia, eye

movement abnormalities), the diagnosis of a central nervous system etiology is generally clear. However, many patients with posterior circulation infarct present with isolated vertigo, nausea, vomiting, and/or gait unsteadiness without obvious localizing findings on general neurologic examination. Moreover, MRI may be normal in the acute setting of posterior circulation infarction, so a normal MRI is not as reassuring as one would hope in an acutely vertiginous patient.

Fortunately, research has shown that a battery of three bedside tests is highly sensitive and specific for predicting posterior circulation stroke as the cause of acute continuous vertigo: the **head impulse test**, evaluation of the **pattern of nystagmus**, and the **cover-uncover test for vertical skew** deviation of the eyes (Kattah et al., 2009). This battery of tests was given the mnemonic HINTS (**h**ead **i**mpulse—**n**ystagmus—**t**est of **s**kew) by the authors of the study. A concerning finding on any of these three tests (normal head impulse test, direction-changing nystagmus, presence of skew deviation; see following text) should raise the index of suspicion for posterior circulation stroke as the cause of acute vertigo and warrants MRI, with repeat MRI after 24–48 hours if initial MRI is normal.

Head Impulse Test

The **head impulse test** is a test of vestibular function. The examiner asks the patient to fixate on the examiner's nose and maintain fixation while the examiner moves the head briskly to one side, observes the eyes, and then moves the head briskly to the other side. Normally, the VOR keeps the eyes fixated on the examiner's nose, so when the head is moved to the right, the eyes instantly conjugately go to the left to maintain fixation; when the head is moved to the left, the eyes instantly conjugately go to the right to maintain fixation. If there is unilateral peripheral dysfunction (e.g., vestibular neuritis), when the head is turned to the abnormal side, the signal that the head has been turned cannot be transmitted to the central nervous system. As a result, the VOR fails and the eyes go with the head, requiring a catch-up saccade to come back to the nose.

For example, with *left* peripheral vestibular dysfunction, when the head is turned briskly by the examiner to the right (normal side), the eyes move appropriately instantly back to the left (normal response). When the head is moved briskly by the examiner to the left (abnormal side) there is *no VOR*, so the eyes also go to the left with the head and then make a catch-up saccade to the right back to the target. A catch-up saccade on the head impulse test to one side only is suggestive of peripheral vestibular dysfunction (inner ear or CN 8), though can also be seen with lateral pontine stroke. In the setting of the acute vestibular syndrome, a *normal* head impulse test on both sides has been found to be predictive of stroke as the etiology. Note: The *normal* finding on this test is the concerning one in this context (i.e., concerning for stroke) since an abnormal head impulse test suggests a peripheral etiology in a patient with acute continuous vertigo. Note that a unilateral abnormal head impulse test may also be seen with lateral pontine stroke, so it is important to consider this finding in the context of the other two maneuvers in the HINTS examination.

Direction-Changing Nystagmus

With respect to nystagmus, the pattern concerning for a central etiology of the acute vestibular syndrome is **direction-changing nystagmus**. Direction-changing nystagmus refers to nystagmus in which the fast phase changes direction with changes in gaze direction: left-beating in left gaze and right-beating in right gaze. This suggests a problem with the gaze-holding mechanism, consistent with a central lesion (see "Direction-Changing Nystagmus Versus Nystagmus With the Fast Phase in the Same Direction in All Directions of Gaze").

Test of Skew

Skew deviation is discussed in Chapter 11. Although it can occur with peripheral lesions, it is more commonly seen with central lesions. When vertical skew deviation of the eyes is evident in the acutely dizzy patient, a central etiology should be considered. When subtle, it may not be apparent, but can be elicited by the cover-uncover test. In this test, the examiner asks the patient to fixate on the examiner's nose, and then the examiner moves one hand back and forth between the two eyes, looking for any vertical readjustment of each eye as it is uncovered. If vertical shifts of the eyes are seen with this test,

this is considered a concerning finding for posterior circulation infarct as the cause of acute continuous vertigo.

A mnemonic for remembering the concerning findings in HINTS testing is provided in the study in which it is described: INFARCT: **i**mpulse **n**ormal, **f**ast-phase (of nystagmus) **a**lternating, **r**efixation on **c**over-uncover **t**est (Kattah et al., 2009). The presence of any of these three findings in a patient with the acute vestibular syndrome is highly predictive of stroke as the etiology.

It should be noted that this interpretation of this three-test battery is not the same in patients who are *not* acutely dizzy at the time of examination. Patients often present following an episode of dizziness when they are no longer dizzy. A normal head impulse test will be a normal finding in normal patients, and some patients may have a few beats of end-gaze nystagmus (which is direction changing). Therefore, while the individual tests of the HINTS battery certainly have important utility in other contexts, the concerning findings in this battery suggest stroke only in a patient with acute-onset continuous vertigo.

Vertigo Accompanied by Acute Unilateral Hearing Loss

The presence of concurrent acute-onset vertigo and acute-onset unilateral hearing loss suggests a problem in the periphery (inner ear or CN 8) since hearing is represented bilaterally quite early in the brainstem auditory pathways and so is not easily disrupted by central lesions. Although most causes of peripheral vestibular lesions are benign, acute-onset unilateral hearing loss is a concerning finding: The inner ear can be infarcted by involvement of the internal auditory artery (also called the labyrinthine artery), which most commonly arises from the AICA. When the finding of acute hearing loss is added to HINTS ("HINTS plus"), the sensitivity for diagnosis of stroke as a cause of acute vertigo (and hearing loss) increases with slight decrease in specificity (Newman-Toker et al., 2013).

Vestibular Neuritis

Vestibular neuritis is diagnosed on clinical grounds when there is acute-onset vertigo following a viral illness and examination findings are consistent with a unilateral peripheral etiology (nystagmus with fast phase in the same direction irrespective of the direction of gaze, abnormal head impulse test). Vestibular neuritis may be treated with a short course of steroids, although data about their efficacy in vestibular neuritis are limited. If symptoms are severe and persistent, a vestibular suppressant (e.g., meclizine) may be considered, but it should be emphasized to the patient that only a short course should be utilized since prolonged use may impair central compensation for peripheral dysfunction.

Hearing loss should not be present in pure vestibular neuritis. If hearing loss is present, the diagnosis of labyrinthitis should be considered. Labyrinthitis may also be postviral, but can be bacterial (e.g., due to meningitis or otitis media). Bacterial labyrinthitis requires antibiotic treatment.

Evaluation of Chronic Dizziness

For patients in whom dizziness is not acute and sustained, the goal of the history is to determine whether dizziness is episodic or continuous, and if episodic, if episodes of dizziness are provoked or unprovoked/spontaneous.

Continuous chronic dizziness can be due to:

- Anemia
- Posterior fossa lesion (e.g., tumor, Chiari malformation)
- Medications (e.g., antiseizure, psychiatric, and cardiac medications)

In a patient who presents with episodic dizziness, one must first assess whether episodes of dizziness are unprovoked (i.e., spontaneous) or provoked. Spontaneous episodic dizziness may occur with:

- Cardiac arrhythmia
- Ménière's disease
- Vestibular migraine
- Posterior circulation transient ischemic attack (TIA)

When dizziness is provoked, specific triggers suggest particular underlying etiologies. Important triggers of episodic dizziness include:

- Moving from supine to seated or seated to standing (suggesting orthostatic hypotension)
- Changes in head position (suggesting benign paroxysmal positional vertigo; see below)
- Exertion (suggesting cardiac etiology)
- Sneezing/coughing/loud noises (suggesting perilymphatic fistula or superior canal dehiscence; see below)

Another feature of the clinical history that can be helpful is the length of episodes of vertigo:

- Seconds to minutes: benign paroxysmal positional vertigo (see "Benign Paroxysmal Positional Vertigo" below)
- Minutes to hours: Ménière's disease, transient ischemic attack (TIA), migraine

Episodic Dizziness Provoked by Positional Changes: Orthostasis and Benign Paroxysmal Positional Vertigo

Any patient who is already dizzy will likely feel that dizziness worsens with head position, as anyone who has been "sea sick" can confirm. The question here is whether the *onset* of dizziness is *provoked* by position change. Dizziness provoked by changes in body position (supine to seated or seated to standing) suggests orthostasis, and orthostatic vital signs should be obtained. Dizziness provoked by changes in head position (e.g., rolling over in bed) suggests **benign paroxysmal positional vertigo**.

Benign paroxysmal positional vertigo—Benign paroxysmal positional vertigo (BPPV) is caused by irritation of a particular semicircular canal by an otolith. The most commonly affected semicircular canal is the posterior canal, although anterior and horizontal canal BPPV occur rarely. BPPV is diagnosed by the **Dix-Hallpike test** in which the patient looks over one shoulder in the seated position and is then rapidly placed in the supine position with the head supported in the examiner's hands and tilted below the level of the examining table while still turned to the side. The test is repeated on each side. In classic BPPV of the posterior semicircular canal, when the head is turned toward the affected side, after a delay of several seconds, the patient will experience vertigo and a mixed upbeat rotatory nystagmus will emerge with the rotatory fast phase toward the ground and the up-beat component more prominent in the upper eye (Fig. 12–5).

If the Dix-Hallpike maneuver elicits downbeat nystagmus that appears without delay, a central etiology should be considered and neuroimaging should be obtained.

Posterior semicircular canal BPPV can be treated at the bedside through the **Epley maneuver** (Fig. 12–6). This begins like the Dix-Hallpike maneuver (head back and turned toward the affected side; Fig. 12–6A). After 1 minute, the patient's head is turned 90 degrees (now facing away from the affected side and still tilted below the level of the examining table; Fig. 12–6B) for 1 minute. Then the patient turns the body toward the head to lie on the side, which puts the head in the downward-facing position (Fig. 12–6C). After 1 minute, the patient returns to the seated position (now 90 degrees from the original seated position; Fig. 12–6D). It is common for the patient to feel a recurrence of vertigo when returning to the seated position, and nystagmus may reemerge in the direction opposite the direction observed during the Dix-Hallpike maneuver. If the symptoms are convincingly reproduced on one side only by the Dix-Hallpike maneuver but no nystagmus is observed, it is still reasonable to perform the Epley maneuver on that side since nystagmus may be quite subtle.

Anterior and horizontal canal BPPV are rare, and generally occur only as complications of the Epley maneuver for posterior canal BPPV such that the otolith that was originally in the posterior canal ends up in one of the other canals.

Anterior canal BPPV causes downbeat torsional nystagmus rotating toward the ceiling (away from the downward-facing ear) on Dix-Hallpike testing. However, as noted above, since downbeat nystagmus can be an indication of a central etiology of vertigo, and given the rarity of anterior canal BPPV, neuroimaging should be obtained if downbeat nystagmus is elicited. Since anterior canal BPPV is a rare condition, appropriate canal repositioning maneuvers for anterior canal BPPV are not well established.

Horizontal canal BPPV requires a different maneuver to be diagnosed: The patient is placed in the supine position and the head is rapidly rotated to one side and then the other, looking for pure horizontal nystagmus, which may be toward the ground (**geotropic**) or toward the ceiling (**ageotropic**), and typically changes direction when the head is turned to the opposite side. The affected side is generally considered the side toward which the nystagmus appears more prominent when the nystagmus is geotropic, and the side to which

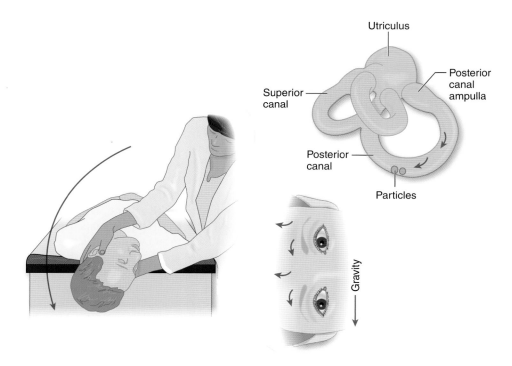

FIGURE 12–5 **Dix-Hallpike maneuver**. With BPPV of the right posterior semicircular canal, when the patient's head is turned over the right shoulder and the patient is brought into the supine position, upbeat-torsional nystagmus occurs with the rotatory component in the direction of the ground. Reproduced with permission from Ropper A, Samuels M, Klein J: *Adams and Victor's Principles of Neurology*, 10th ed. New York, NY: McGraw Hill; 2014.

it is less prominent with ageotropic nystagmus. Repositioning maneuvers to treat horizontal canal BPPV include the **360 roll maneuver** (also called the **Lempert maneuver**) and the **Gufoni maneuver**.

In the Lempert (360 roll) maneuver, the patient begins in the supine position with the head turned such that the affected ear is down, then begins a series of 90-degree turns of the head—to looking at the ceiling, to looking to the side opposite the original side, to lying prone and looking down, to laying on the side of the affected ear (affected ear down), to supine, to seated (360 degrees). In the Gufoni maneuver, the patient goes from the seated position to laying on the unaffected side, then looking down (head turned over shoulder) while in that position, followed by returning to the seated position with the head still turned over the shoulder.

Episodic Dizziness Provoked by Loud Noises (Tulio Phenomenon) or Coughing/Sneezing: Perilymphatic Fistula & Superior Semicircular Canal Dehiscence

The symptom of dizziness triggered by loud noises (called the **Tulio phenomenon**), coughing, and/or sneezing is suggestive of two rare conditions of the inner ear: **perilymphatic fistula** and **superior semicircular canal dehiscence**. Perilymphatic fistula is a fistula between the middle ear and the inner ear, usually secondary to trauma. In superior semicircular canal dehiscence there is thinning of the temporal bone superior to the superior semicircular canal. In addition to the symptoms

listed above, semicircular canal dehiscence can cause the symptom of **autophony**: patients report hearing their own heartbeat, chewing, and other internal sounds. Both conditions require imaging of the temporal bone and consultation with an otolaryngologist since surgical intervention may be indicated.

Unprovoked Episodic Dizziness

Ménière's disease—Ménière's disease is caused by idiopathic development of increased pressure in the inner ear (endolymphatic hydrops). The condition usually develops between early adulthood and late middle age (20s–50s). Episodes last hours and include vertigo, hearing loss, tinnitus, and a sensation of ear fullness. There may be progressive hearing loss and/or tinnitus between attacks. Patients may report sudden falls without loss of consciousness or vertigo, called **otolithic crises of Tumarkin**. The diagnosis is clinical, but audiometry may reveal fluctuations over time and/or progressive low-frequency hearing loss. Initial treatment includes low-salt diet and a diuretic. In refractory cases, labyrinthectomy or intratympanic gentamicin administration may be performed to ablate the inner ear.

Cogan's syndrome causes Ménière-like attacks and interstitial keratitis. The syndrome can be seen in association with systemic vasculitis, or may occur in isolation.

Vestibular migraine—Dizziness is common in migraine, but some patients have severe vertigo as the prominent feature of their migraines (**vestibular migraine**). Nystagmus of any type

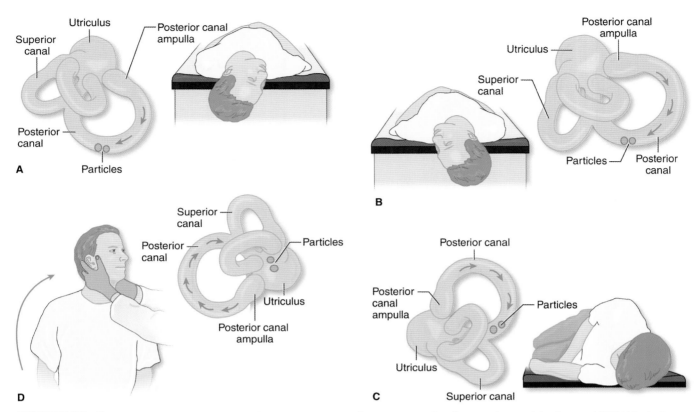

FIGURE 12–6 Epley maneuver. The stages of the Epley maneuver for a patient with right posterior semicircular canal BPPV (clockwise from A). See text for explanation. Reproduced with permission from Ropper A, Samuels M, Klein J: *Adams and Victor's Principles of Neurology*, 10th ed. New York, NY: McGraw Hill; 2014.

may be observed during or between episodes in patients with vestibular migraine. Some patients may have episodic vertigo without accompanying headache, in which case the diagnosis of vestibular migraine is one of exclusion when no alternative explanation can be found after appropriate evaluation. Acute and preventive treatment of vestibular migraine is the same as for migraine in general (see "Treatment of Migraine" in Ch. 26), although meclizine, an antiemetic, or a benzodiazepine may be added to the acute abortive regimen for treatment of vertigo during acute migraines.

Posterior circulation transient ischemic attack (TIA)— Posterior circulation TIA should be considered in patients with episodic vertigo with vascular risk factors or history concerning for vertebral artery dissection (e.g., recent trauma) (see "Transient Ischemic Attack" in Ch. 19). In patients with recurrent episodes of vertigo concerning for posterior circulation TIAs, vascular imaging of the head and neck should be obtained to evaluate the vertebrobasilar system.

An important and life-threatening non-neurologic etiology of unprovoked episodic dizziness to consider is cardiac arrhythmia.

REFERENCES

Drachman DA and Hart CW. An approach to the dizzy patient. *Neurol* 1972;22:323-334.

Kattah JC, Talkad AV, Wang DZ, Hsieh YH, Newman-Toker DE. HINTS to diagnose stroke in the acute vestibular syndrome: three-step bedside oculomotor examination more sensitive than early MRI diffusion-weighted imaging. *Stroke* 2009;40:3504-3510.

Newman-Toker DE. *Diagnosing dizziness in the emergency department: Why "What do you mean by 'dizzy'?" Should Not Be the First Question You Ask* [dissertation]. Baltimore, MD: The Johns Hopkins University, 2007.

Newman-Toker DE, Cannon LM, Stofferahn ME, Rothman RE, Hsieh YH, Zee DS. Imprecision in patient reports of dizziness symptom quality: a cross-sectional study conducted in an acute care setting. *Mayo Clin Proc* 2007;82:1329-1340.

Newman-Toker DE, Kerber KA, Hsieh YH, Pula JH, Omron R, Saber Tehrani AS, et al. HINTS outperforms ABCD2 to screen for stroke in acute continuous vertigo and dizziness. *Acad Emerg Med* 2013;20:986-996.

Facial Sensory and Motor Pathways & Approach to Facial Sensory and Motor Deficits

Cranial Nerves 5 & 7

CHAPTER

13

CHAPTER CONTENTS

TRIGEMINAL NERVE (CRANIAL NERVE 5)

Trigeminal Pathways

Disorders of the Trigeminal Nerve

FACIAL NERVE (CRANIAL NERVE 7)

Facial Nerve Pathways

Upper & Lower Motor Neuron Pattern Facial Weakness

TRIGEMINAL NERVE (CRANIAL NERVE 5)

The principal clinically relevant functions of the trigeminal nerve are facial somatic sensation and innervation of the muscles of mastication. The trigeminal nerve also innervates one palate muscle (tensor veli palitini) and one inner ear muscle (tensor tympani).

The trigeminal nerve supplies somatic sensation to the face, the inside of the mouth (although *not* taste), the sinuses, and most of the dura mater (including all supratentorial dura and the tentorium cerebelli; the rest of the posterior fossa dura mater is supplied by cranial nerve 10). The three divisions of the trigeminal nerve and the regions for which they supply sensation are:

1. Ophthalmic division (V_1): forehead, upper lid, upper half of cornea

2. Maxillary division (V_2): cheek, lower lid, lower half of cornea, roof of mouth, upper gums/teeth/lip

3. Mandibular division (V_3): lower gums/teeth/lip, lower jaw, anterior tongue

The muscles of mastication innervated by CN 5 are:

• Masseter
• Pterygoids
• Anterior belly of the digastric (the posterior belly of the digastric is innervated by 7)
• Mylohyoid (the stylohyoid is innervated by CN 7)

See Table 14–1 for a summary of the functions shared between CNs 5, 7, 9, and 10.

Trigeminal Pathways (Fig. 13–1)
Trigeminal Sensory Pathways

The facial sensory pathways of the trigeminal nerve are analogous to those for the body: All sensory information travels back to a ganglion, and pain and temperature sensation travel separately from other modalities. The sensory ganglion of CN 5 is called the **gasserian ganglion**, which resides in **Meckel's cave** (mnemonic: ganglion for cranial nerve **V** resides in Meckel's cave). The gasserian ganglion receives somatosensory input from the face and transmits that information to the brainstem at the level of the pons. Distal to the gasserian ganglion, the trigeminal nerve divides into three branches: ophthalmic (V_1), maxillary (V_2), and mandibular (V_3). V_1 and V_2 pass through the cavernous sinus, whereas V_3 does **not** pass though the cavernous sinus. V_1 exits the skull through the superior orbital fissure, V_2 through the foramen rotundum, and V_3 through the foramen ovale.

Proximal to the gasserian ganglion, the somatosensory information from CN 5 enters the brainstem at the level of the pons. Although the point of entry of CN 5 into the brainstem is at the level of the pons (as would be expected for the 5-6-7-8 schema described in Ch. 9), CN 5 has nuclei throughout the three levels of the brainstem. Light touch sensation from the face is transmitted primarily to the **main sensory nucleus of 5** (also called the **chief** or **principal sensory nucleus of 5**) at the level of entry in the pons, and the output from this nucleus crosses to join the medial lemniscus (carrying sensory information from the body), which ascends to the thalamus. Facial sensation information projects to the **ventral posterior medial (VPM) nucleus** of the

129

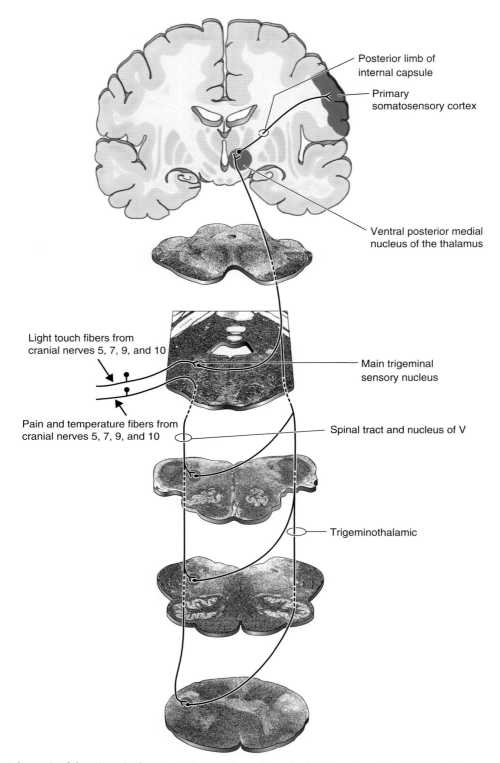

FIGURE 13–1 **Schematic of the trigeminal nerve pathways**. The pathway for facial proprioception including the mesencephalic nucleus of CN 5 is not shown here. Reproduced with permission from Martin J: *Neuroanatomy Text and Atlas*, 4th ed. New York, NY: McGraw Hill; 2012.

thalamus (recall sensation from the limbs and trunk travels to the ventral posterior lateral (VPL) nucleus of the thalamus; see Ch. 4). VPM projects to the somatosensory cortex in the postcentral gyrus.

Pain and temperature sensation from the face descend to the medulla in the **spinal tract of 5** (the facial analogue of the anterolateral tract) along with its associated **spinal nucleus of 5**. The spinal nucleus and tract of 5 extend as inferiorly as the upper cervical spine. The output of the spinal nucleus of 5 crosses to join the contralateral spinothalamic tract from the body and ascends to the ventral posterior medial (VPM) nucleus of the thalamus (pain and temperature sensation from the limbs and trunk travel to the VPL nucleus of the thalamus).

Jaw proprioception information is relayed to the **mesencephalic nucleus of 5** in the midbrain.

Trigeminal Motor Pathways

The **motor nucleus of 5** is medial to the main sensory nucleus of 5 in the dorsal pons. Unlike the common symptom of unilateral facial weakness in both central and peripheral nervous system diseases (see "Upper and Lower Motor Neuron Facial Weakness"), unilateral jaw weakness due to a focal lesion in the nervous system (e.g., a unilateral pontine lesion) is uncommon. This is in part due to the fact that the trigeminal motor nuclei receive bilateral cortical input, so unilateral hemispheric lesions such as strokes do not typically cause unilateral jaw weakness. However, bilateral jaw weakness may be seen in neuromuscular junction disorders (e.g., myasthenia gravis; see Ch. 29) and myopathies (see Ch. 30).

Brainstem Reflexes Involving the Trigeminal Nerve

The trigeminal nerve is involved in two brainstem reflexes, the corneal reflex and the jaw jerk reflex.

Corneal reflex—The corneal reflex is elicited by stimulating the cornea, which normally leads to reflex closure of the eyes. The trigeminal nerve is the afferent limb of the reflex (sensation from the cornea is carried by V_1), and the facial nerve (CN 7) is the efferent limb responsible for closure of the eye (by contraction of the orbicularis oculi muscle). The reflex is bilateral, so stimulating one cornea normally leads to bilateral closure of both eyes.

Jaw jerk reflex—The jaw jerk reflex is elicited by asking the patient to let the jaw hang slightly open, and then tapping on the upper chin gently with a reflex hammer. This reflex is mediated by the mesencephalic nucleus of 5 (afferent) and the motor nucleus of 5 (efferent). If the jaw jerk reflex is markedly brisk, this demonstrates upper motor neuron (central nervous system) pathology above the level of the spinal cord (i.e., in the brainstem or brain). The jaw jerk reflex is often tested in patients with upper motor neuron signs in the extremities to evaluate for signs of pathology superior to the spinal cord (i.e., to determine if the corticobulbar tracts are affected in addition to the corticospinal tracts).

Disorders of the Trigeminal Nerve

Facial Sensory Loss

Loss of facial sensation can occur due to a lesion in:

- The trigeminal nerve in the face, skull base, or cavernous sinus
- The trigeminal pathways in the dorsolateral brainstem (e.g., loss of pain and temperature sensation in the face is part

of lateral medullary syndrome along with contralateral loss of pain and temperature in the body, Horner's syndrome, ataxia, nausea, vomiting, vertigo, dysarthria, and dysphagia)
- VPM of the thalamus
- The subcortical white matter connecting VPM and somatosensory cortex
- The lateral postcentral gyrus (facial region of the somatosensory cortex)

Isolated facial sensory loss is most likely to be due to a lesion of the trigeminal nerve, the entry zone of the nerve in the pons, or a small cortical lesion because lesions at all other sites would likely cause other deficits due to involvement of adjacent structures:

- A brainstem lesion causing facial sensory loss will often also affect other cranial nerve nuclei.
- A cavernous sinus lesion causing facial sensory loss (which will only affect V_1 and V_2 divisions since V_3 does not pass through the cavernous sinus) will often also affect CNs 3, 4, and/or 6 (see Ch. 11).
- A thalamic lesion causing facial sensory loss will often also cause sensory loss beyond the face.
- A subcortical lesion causing facial sensory loss will often also affect additional adjacent sensory fibers representing other parts of the body.

Since the face and hand have the most cortical sensory representation, a common pattern of numbness for cortical, subcortical, and small thalamic lesions is contralateral face and hand numbness (**cheiro-oral** pattern).

Facial numbness due to an isolated trigeminal nerve lesion can be caused by:

- Malignancy: skull base tumor, cerebellopontine angle tumor, leptomeningeal metastasis
- Inflammatory disease: Sjögren's syndrome, sarcoidosis
- Spread of head and neck cancers along the trigeminal nerve (**perineural spread**), most commonly caused by squamous cell cancer of the skin on the face
- Dental pathology

Numb chin sign—Numbness of the chin (**numb chin sign**) should raise concern for metastatic malignancy affecting the mandibular (V_3) division of the trigeminal nerve in the skull base or the distal trigeminal branches in the mandible (usually the mental nerve, a branch of the inferior alveolar nerve, which is a branch of V_3). The numb chin sign may be the presenting feature of systemic malignancy or metastatic disease in a patient with known cancer. Breast cancer and lymphoma are among the most common malignancies causing the numb chin sign. When patients present with this symptom, history for other symptoms of malignancy should be elicited (e.g., weight loss, night sweats). The differential diagnosis includes dental etiologies and systemic causes of trigeminal neuropathy (e.g., Sjögren's syndrome, sarcoidosis). Evaluation should include panoramic dental x-ray, CT scan or bone scan of the jaw (to evaluate the mandible), CT scan of the head (to evaluate for a skull base lesion), and/or MRI of the brain with contrast (to evaluate the trigeminal nerve itself).

Trigeminal Neuralgia

In **trigeminal neuralgia**, brief lightening-like paroxysms of pain shoot through the face. These may be spontaneous or may be triggered by contacting the face (e.g., brushing the teeth). Trigeminal neuralgia is most commonly unilateral and most commonly affects the lower face (V_2 and/or V_3 regions). The condition may be idiopathic, or it can be caused by multiple sclerosis, a compressive vascular loop, any of the above-listed etiologies of trigeminal pathology, or it may begin after dental work (ostensibly due to irritation of the most distal branches of the trigeminal nerve).

If trigeminal neuralgia is present in a young woman and/or bilaterally, multiple sclerosis should be considered and MRI obtained. How can trigeminal neuralgia be caused by multiple sclerosis if multiple sclerosis is a central nervous system disease and the trigeminal nerves are peripheral nerves? When multiple sclerosis causes trigeminal neuralgia, the lesion is in the trigeminal entry zone in the pons, which is part of the central nervous system.

In idiopathic trigeminal neuralgia, facial sensation is generally normal. If facial sensation is diminished in a patient with trigeminal neuralgia, this is atypical and a structural lesion should be sought with neuroimaging.

Antiepileptics are used for pain control in trigeminal neuralgia, with the most supportive evidence being for carbamazepine. If neuroimaging reveals a vascular loop compressing the trigeminal nerve in a patient with trigeminal neuralgia, microvascular decompression can be considered if the patient does not respond to medications. In refractory cases of trigeminal neuralgia, surgical ablation of or radiotherapy to the gasserian ganglion may be considered.

FACIAL NERVE (CRANIAL NERVE 7)

The main clinically relevant function of the seventh cranial nerve is control of the facial musculature, although CN 7 has a number of additional functions:

- Parasympathetic:
  - Lacrimal and nasal glands
  - Submandibular and sublingual salivary glands (although the facial nerve passes through the parotid gland, it does not innervate it—CN 9 does)
  - Motor (beyond facial musculature): stapedius, posterior belly of the digastric (anterior belly of the digastric is innervated by CN 5)
  - Special sensory: taste to the anterior two thirds of the tongue (posterior one third is innervated by CN 9)
  - Sensory: somatic sensation for the external auditory meatus (shared with CNs 9 and 10)

See Table 14–1 for a summary of functions shared between CNs 5, 7, 9, and 10.

Facial Nerve Pathways

The seventh nerve nucleus is in the dorsal pons, and the nerve loops dorsally around the abducens (CN 6) nucleus before exiting anteriorly just lateral to the descending corticospinal tracts (see Fig. 9–1D). The "bump" on the dorsal pons where the seventh nerve loops around the CN 6 nucleus is called the **facial colliculus**. The nerve travels to and through the internal auditory canal with CN 8, then passes into the facial canal, finally emerging through the stylomastoid foramen to innervate the facial muscles after passing through the parotid. The nonmotor functions (sensory and visceral) are carried out by the **nervus intermedius**, which runs with the motor portion of the nerve but interacts with different brainstem nuclei related to sensory and visceral functions.

There are several important components of the facial nerve along its course in the skull before exiting the stylomastoid foramen to innervate the muscles of the face (Fig. 13–2). From proximal to distal:

- The **geniculate ganglion** is the main ganglion for all sensory and special sensory CN 7 functions (taste to anterior two thirds of the tongue, sensation around the ear).
- The **greater petrosal nerve** innervates the lacrimal and nasal glands (by way of the **sphenopalatine ganglion**, also known as the **pterygopalatine ganglion**).
- The **nerve to the stapedius** innervates the stapedius.
- The **chorda tympani** transmits taste from the anterior two thirds of the tongue and provides innervation to the salivary glands (submandibular and sublingual). Taste information travels to the **nucleus solitarius** in the medulla. (Mnemonic to recall that the nucleus solitarius is responsible for taste: nucleus soli**tastiest** [although note that taste is not the sole function of the nucleus solitarius, which also receives visceral afferent information; see Ch. 14]).

After exiting the stylomastoid foramen, subsequent branches of CN 7 are all motor: posterior auricular, digastric, stylohyoid, and the five branches to the facial muscles: temporal, zygomatic, buccal, mandibular, and cervical.

Upper & Lower Motor Neuron Pattern Facial Weakness (Figs. 13–3 & 13–4)

Just as the motor system for the extremities has upper motor neurons in the central nervous system and lower motor neurons in the peripheral nervous system, so too does the system for facial movements. Facial movements are mediated by the bilateral facial nerves (CN 7), which contain the lower motor neurons in this system. Just as for the body, each half of the face is controlled by the contralateral hemisphere: The left hemisphere face region of the motor cortex communicates with the right (contralateral)

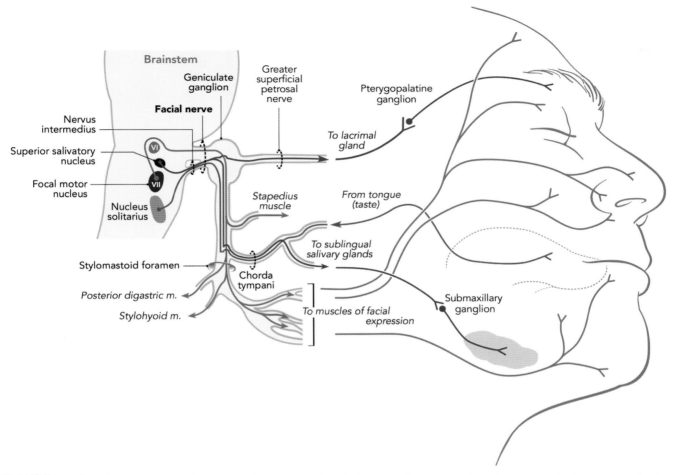

FIGURE 13–2 **Schematic of the facial nerve pathways**. Reproduced with permission from Martin T, Corbett J: *Practical Neuroophthalmology*. New York, NY: McGraw Hill; 2013.

CN 7 nucleus in the pons, which controls the muscles of the right side of the face; the right hemisphere face region of the motor cortex communicates with the left (contralateral) CN 7 nucleus in the pons, which controls the muscles of the left side of the face.

A lesion of the facial nerve will cause weakness of the whole face on that side: The patient will be unable to smile, puff the cheek, close the eye, raise the eyebrow, or wrinkle the forehead on the affected side (Fig. 13–5). Early on in a seventh nerve palsy, eye closure weakness may be subtle, and noted only if the patient fails to completely "bury" the eyelashes on attempted forceful eye closure. The nasolabial fold and forehead wrinkles may be diminished or absent on the affected side.

If facial weakness is due to an upper motor neuron lesion, only the lower face is affected: The patient is unable to smile on the affected side (contralateral to the brain lesion), but can still close the eye and raise the eyebrow. This is because the upper face is supplied not only by the contralateral hemisphere but also by the ipsilateral hemisphere. That is, each CN 7 contains the information from the contralateral motor cortex for the whole face and a "backup" for the upper face

from the ipsilateral hemisphere. So whereas a CN 7 lesion will prevent any input—ipsilateral or contralateral—from making it to the face, an upper motor neuron lesion will only remove its input to the contralateral facial nerve, but that facial nerve will still have its ipsilateral "backup" for the upper face. Why might there be a backup for the upper face? One possibility is that it is more important to protect the eye than to preserve the ability to smile—failure of eye closure can lead to corneal abrasion and ulceration.

Upper Motor Neuron Facial Weakness

Upper motor neuron facial weakness can be caused by a lesion in the motor cortex, subcortical white matter, or in the midbrain and upper pons before the upper motor neuron pathway has crossed to synapse with the contralateral CN 7 nucleus. Therefore, a lesion in the descending motor pathways (corticospinal tract and corticobulbar tract) anywhere superior to the midpons will cause contralateral weakness in both the face and the body. Once the lesion is in the CN 7 nucleus, CN 7 fascicle in the pons, or in the facial nerve itself, facial weakness will be in a lower motor neuron pattern (upper and lower facial weakness).

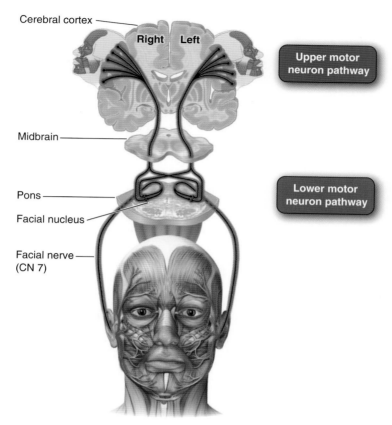

FIGURE 13-3 **Schematic of facial motor innervation.** See text for discussion.

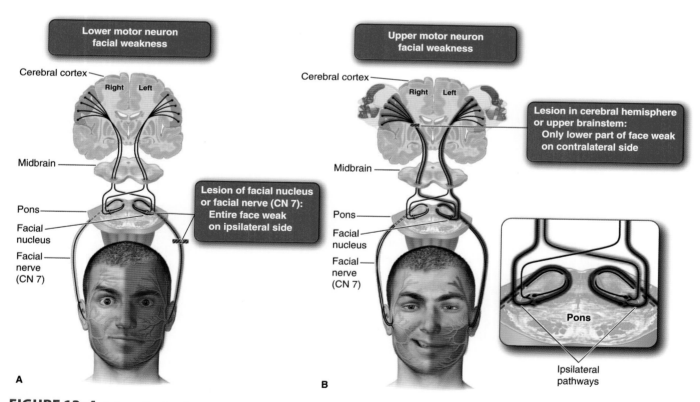

FIGURE 13-4 **Schematic showing upper and lower motor neuron pattern facial weakness. A:** A lesion of the facial nerve will cause weakness of both the upper face and lower face. **B:** A lesion of the motor cortex will cause contralateral lower facial weakness with preserved motor function of the upper face due to the ipsilateral "backup" to the upper face. (See text)

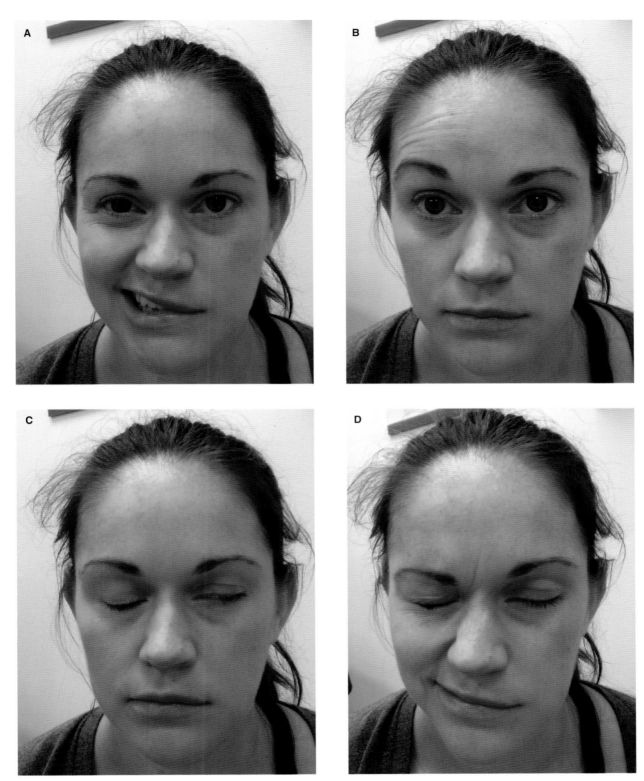

FIGURE 13–5 **Left-sided lower motor neuron pattern facial weakness (due to Bell's palsy). A:** When the patient attempts to smile, there is no movement of the left side of the face and the nasolabial fold is not visible on the left. The eye is slightly more open on the left. **B:** When the patient attempts to raise her forehead, the eyebrow elevates and the forehead wrinkles only on the right side. The flattening of the nasolabial fold on the left is again notable. **C:** On attempted gentle eye closure, the left eye does not close fully, and the sclera is seen as the eye elevates on attempted eye closure (Bell's phenomenon). **D:** When attempting to close the eyes more tightly, the eyelashes are "buried" on the right, but still fully visible on the left due to orbicularis oculi weakness.

Lower Motor Neuron Facial Weakness

Causes of lower motor neuron pattern facial weakness include:

- Bell's palsy, an idiopathic seventh nerve palsy (see "Bell's palsy").
- Infections: Lyme disease, HIV (especially at the time of seroconversion; see Ch. 20), Ramsay-Hunt syndrome.
- Inflammatory conditions: sarcoidosis, Guillain-Barré syndrome (facial weakness is common in Guillain-Barré syndrome, and is often bilateral; see Ch. 27).
- Tumor: At the cerebellopontine angle or in the internal auditory canal (e.g., vestibular schwannoma; see Ch. 24).
- Vascular: A stroke of the pons can affect the nucleus or fascicle of the seventh nerve causing a lower motor neuron pattern facial palsy in spite of the fact that the lesion is in the central nervous system (i.e., in the brainstem). When this occurs, there are often additional associated deficits, such as ipsilateral horizontal gaze palsy with dorsal lesions (due to the proximity of the CN 6 nucleus to the CN 7 nucleus) and/or contralateral weakness in the extremities with ventral lesions (if the not-yet-crossed descending corticospinal tract is affected—an example of the "crossed signs" of brainstem lesions; see Ch. 9).

All patients with facial nerve palsy should have an otoscopic examination to evaluate for vesicles in the ear that would suggest a diagnosis of **Ramsay-Hunt syndrome**, caused by varicella zoster virus (VZV) reactivation in the geniculate ganglion. Ramsay-Hunt syndrome is generally treated with steroids and antivirals.

Bell's palsy—Bell's palsy refers specifically to *idiopathic* facial nerve palsy (i.e., facial nerve palsy without an identifiable etiology). Bell's palsy is more common in patients with diabetes and during the third trimester of pregnancy. Facial weakness usually emerges over hours, and patients may report pain behind the ear, liquids dripping from one side of the mouth when drinking, and ocular irritation from inability to close the eye. Some patients report facial numbness as a way of describing the feeling of the face being weak, although true facial numbness due to trigeminal involvement is uncommon. If assessed, taste may be impaired on one half of the tongue on the side of the facial weakness (only if the nerve is affected proximal to the chorda tympani; this does not occur in all cases). Patients often report that sounds are louder on the affected side (**hyperacusis**) due to weakness of the stapedius muscle (which normally serves to dampen loud noises). Hyperacusis can be demonstrated by passing a vibrating tuning fork between the two ears, and noting if the patient finds it to be louder on the side of the facial weakness. Facial weakness in Bell's palsy may be incomplete at presentation, and if the lower face is predominantly affected, this can mimic an upper motor neuron pattern, leading to evaluation for stroke as the cause of facial weakness.

Most patients begin to recover from Bell's palsy by 1 month and recover completely over subsequent months. A short course of oral steroids can increase the degree and speed of recovery. Some practitioners treat Bell's palsy with antivirals (acyclovir) in addition to steroids based on the hypothesis that the condition may be caused by the herpes simplex virus (HSV), but the use of acyclovir is debated.

Neuroimaging is generally unnecessary in patients with Bell's palsy unless the patient does not improve or develops additional cranial nerve palsies. In patients with Bell's palsy who undergo neuroimaging, enhancement of the affected CN 7 may be observed.

Reduced blinking and impaired eye closure in Bell's palsy (as in any seventh nerve palsy) can cause corneal inflammation (exposure keratitis), which can lead to corneal ulceration. Therefore, an important supportive measure in patients with Bell's palsy is to protect the eye with artificial tears and patching.

As the facial nerve recovers, abnormal rewiring may lead to abnormal linking of facial movements, called **synkinesis**. Examples include linking of eye and mouth movements (squinting when smiling and vice versa) and linking of lacrimation and salivation (tearing while eating, a phenomenon called "crocodile tears").

Melkersson-Rosenthal syndrome—This is a rare syndrome characterized by recurrent seventh nerve palsy and facial/lip swelling, and patients have a fissured tongue. The disorder usually begins in childhood/adolescence, and the complete triad of symptoms may not be present in all cases.

Cranial Nerves 1, 9, 10, 11, & 12

CRANIAL NERVE 1 (OLFACTORY NERVE)

The olfactory nerves transmit smell information through the cribriform plate to the olfactory bulbs and tracts, which in turn transmit this information to the olfactory cortex in the medial temporal lobes. Smell information is the only sensory modality not transmitted to the thalamus prior to the cortex. In the case of smell, the information first arrives in the olfactory cortex, and is then transmitted to the medial dorsal nucleus of the thalamus.

Loss of smell is referred to as **anosmia**. Since the olfactory nerve fibers travel through the cribriform plate, and the olfactory tracts lie between the inferior surface of the frontal lobes and the skull base, these structures are susceptible to damage in head trauma and compression by skull base tumors (e.g., olfactory groove meningiomas). More common causes of impaired smell are sinus disease and upper respiratory infections, and rarer causes include **Kallman's syndrome** (anosmia and absence of gonadotropin-releasing hormone [GnRH] secreting neurons).

Anosmia may be part of the prodromal phase of neurodegenerative diseases (e.g., Parkinson's disease and other synucleinopathies; see Ch. 23). In this context, anosmia is noted more commonly in retrospect since it may be attributed to aging when initially present in isolation.

Another scenario in which smell plays a role in neurologic disease is in the olfactory auras associated with temporal lobe seizures: Patients may report a foul odor (e.g., "burning tires") that precedes temporal lobe seizure onset, presumably due to epileptic activity passing through medial temporal olfactory regions.

CRANIAL NERVE 9 (GLOSSOPHARYNGEAL) & CRANIAL NERVE 10 (VAGUS)

CNs 9 and 10 work together to supply the musculature of the pharynx (mostly supplied by CN 10) and transmit visceral afferent information from vascular baroreceptors, and each nerve also has additional individual functions listed below. CN 9 and CN 10 are discussed together since they are difficult to isolate clinically, and are commonly affected together since they both communicate with nuclei in the dorsolateral medulla, both pass through the jugular foramen, and they are adjacent throughout parts of the neck.

CN 9 supplies:

- One pharyngeal muscle: stylopharyngeus
- One gland: parotid
- One region of taste: posterior one third of the tongue
- One region of visceral sensation: carotid body
- Three small regions of somatic sensation: posterior one third of the tongue, pharynx (shared with CN 10), middle ear, and external auditory meatus (shared with CN 7 and CN 10)

The functions of CN 10 include:

- Motor supply to all muscles of the larynx and pharynx except tensor veli palitini (CN 5), mylohyoid (CN 5), stylohyoid (CN 7), stylopharyngeus (CN 9)
- Motor supply to one muscle of the tongue: palatoglossus (all others are innervated by CN 12)

- Somatic sensation from:
  - The dura mater of the posterior fossa aside from the tentorium (the sensory innervation to the rest of the dura including the tentorium is supplied by CN 5)
  - The pharynx (shared with CN 9)
  - The external auditory meatus (shared with CN 7 and CN 9)
- Visceral sensation from the aortic arch
- Visceral parasympathetic efferent supply to and afferent input from all of the viscera of the thorax and abdomen with the exception of the distal third of the GI tract and genitourinary organs (which receive their parasympathetic supply from sacral spinal cord levels S2–S4).
- Taste in the pharynx

There are several functions that are shared across cranial nerves CNs 5, 7, 9, and 10, which are summarized for comparison in Table 14–1. (Mnemonic for some of the miscellaneous muscles: the **t**rigeminal nerve innervates **t**ensor tympani and **t**ensor veli palitini; the **s**eventh nerve innervates **s**tylohoid and **s**tapedius.)

The laryngeal and pharyngeal motor input to CN 9 and CN 10 comes from the **nucleus ambiguus** in the dorsal medulla. Visceral motor supply that travels in CN 10 originates in the **dorsal motor nucleus of the vagus**. Afferent visceral information arrives with taste information to the **nucleus solitarius** (see Table 9–4).

Lesions of CN 10 can cause laryngeal and/or pharyngeal weakness. Laryngeal weakness can lead to softer voice (**hypophonia**), nasal voice, and guttural **dysarthria** (difficulty producing the consonants "G" and "K"). Pharyngeal weakness can cause difficulty swallowing (**dysphagia**).

On examination, CN 9 and CN 10 can be assessed by evaluating palate elevation and gag reflex. When there is unilateral palate weakness, the palate droops on the weak side and is pulled upward toward the stronger side. The gag reflex is mediated predominantly by CN 9 for the afferent limb (palate sensation) and predominantly CN 10 for the efferent limb (palate elevation).

Unilateral palate/larynx dysfunction can be caused by:

- **Brainstem pathology:** for example, posterior inferior cerebellar artery (PICA) stroke causing lateral medullary syndrome (causing unilateral palate/laryngeal dysfunction due to involvement of the nucleus ambiguus; other symptoms include vertigo, ataxia, Horner's syndrome, and/or crossed hemisensory loss [decreased pain/temperature sensation in the face ipsilateral to the lesion and body contralateral to the lesion])
- **Jugular foramen pathology:** for example, glomus jugulare tumor, which can affect CNs 9, 10, and 11
- **Local pathology in the neck:** for example, lymphadenopathy, carotid dissection
- **Complication of neck surgery:** for example, thyroid surgery or carotid endarterectomy

Isolated unilateral laryngeal dysfunction can also be caused by pathology in the upper thorax because the recurrent laryngeal nerve branch of the vagus nerve descends into the upper thorax before re-ascending to the larynx. Therefore, mediastinal, aortic, or apical lung pathology or cardiothoracic surgery can all cause recurrent laryngeal nerve dysfunction leading to hoarseness of the voice.

Bilateral laryngeal/pharyngeal dysfunction is commonly seen in motor neuron disease (e.g., amyotrophic lateral sclerosis [ALS]; see Ch. 28).

Glossopharyngeal Neuralgia

Glossopharyngeal neuralgia is the CN 9 analogue to trigeminal neuralgia (see Ch. 13). Lancinating neuralgic pain occurs in the throat and/or ear. Pain can be triggered by swallowing. Syncope occurs during attacks of glossophayngeal neuralgia in some cases due to altered visceral afferent transmission in CN 9. As in patients with trigeminal neuralgia, neuroimaging should be obtained to evaluate for the possibility of compression of CN 9 by a vascular loop (although most cases are idiopathic), and antiepileptics such as carbamazepine may be used for treatment.

CRANIAL NERVE 11 (SPINAL ACCESSORY)

CN 11 is a nerve derived from upper cervical roots that ascends to the foramen magnum and then leaves the skull through the jugular foramen with CN 9 and CN 10. CN 11 innervates two muscles: trapezius (which raises the shoulder) and sternocleidomastoid (which turns the head to the opposite side). CN 11 can be damaged unilaterally in the neck due to trauma or surgery or at the jugular foramen with CN 9 and CN 10 (e.g., by glomus jugulare tumor).

The upper motor neurons for control of the sternocleidomastoid are believed to be ipsilateral (rather than contralateral as for nearly all other muscles of the body), perhaps since the sternocleidomastoid turns the head to the contralateral side. Support for this idea comes from the observation that patients having seizures tend to turn the head away from the seizing hemisphere and toward the contralateral tonic–clonic motor activity (i.e., activation of the ipsilateral sternocleidomastoid causes the head to turn contralaterally).

CRANIAL NERVE 12 (HYPOGLOSSAL)

CN 12 (hypoglossal nerve) is a pure motor nerve innervating all muscles of the tongue except the palatoglossus (which is innervated by CN 10). The hypoglossal nuclei reside in the medulla, and as with other pure motor cranial nerves that innervate skeletal muscle, these nuclei are dorsal/posterior and midline (see Ch. 9). Just as with CN 7, each CN 12 nucleus receives input from the corticobulbar tracts originating in the

TABLE 14–1 Shared Functions Between Cranial Nerves 5, 7, 9, & 10.

Cranial Nerve	Glands of the Head and Neck	Taste	Baroreceptor Afferents	Muscles (not including the facial muscles innervated by CN 7)				Sensory to Dura Mater	Somatic Sensory to Tongue	Somatic Sensory to Ear
				Larynx	Mastication	Pharyngeal	Middle Ear			
CN 5					Temporalis Masseter Pteryogoids Anterior belly of digastric (All except posterior belly of digastric)	Tensor veli palitini Mylohyoid	Tensor tympani	Anterior and middle cranial fossa dura Tentorium	Anterior 2/3	
CN 7	Lacrimal Nasal Submandibular Sublingual (All except parotid)	Anterior 2/3 of tongue			Posterior belly of digastric	Stylohyoid	Stapedius			External ear
CN 9	Parotid	Posterior 1/3 of tongue	Carotid body/ sinus			Stylopharyngeus			Posterior 1/3	Middle ear
CN 10		Epiglottis/ pharynx	Aortic arch	All laryngeal muscles		All other pharyngeal muscles not innervated by CNs 5, 7, and 9		Posterior fossa dura aside from tentorium		External ear

contralateral motor cortex (these are the upper motor neurons in the system; the bilateral CN 12s contain the lower motor neurons). Unilateral tongue weakness causes the tongue to deviate to the weak side: when trying to protrude the tongue midline, the stronger side wins, pushing the tongue over to the weaker side. Weakness of the tongue can cause dysarthria, specifically for lingual sounds (e.g., difficulty producing the consonants "L," "D," and "T").

A unilateral hypoglossal nucleus, fascicle, or nerve lesion results in ipsilateral tongue weakness, causing deviation of the tongue toward the side of the lesion. Causes of CN 12 palsy include head and neck tumors, trauma, or surgery, as well as internal carotid artery dissection. In medial medullary syndrome (caused by infarct in the territory of the anterior spinal artery), the CN 12 fascicle (portion of the nerve still in the brainstem) and the descending (not-yet-crossed) corticospinal tract are affected, so there will be ipsilateral tongue weakness and contralateral body weakness. Bilateral tongue weakness with atrophy and fasciculations can be seen in motor neuron disease such as ALS (see Ch. 28).

A lesion of the corticobulbar tract (in the cortex, subcortical white matter, or brainstem superior to the hypoglossal nucleus in the medulla) results in contralateral tongue weakness, causing deviation of the tongue away from the side of the lesion. With a stroke affecting the motor cortex, for example, one will observe hemiparesis contralateral to the side of the hemispheric lesion, and the tongue will also be weak on the side of the hemiparesis. Therefore, the tongue will deviate toward the side of body weakness (which is away from the side of the hemispheric lesion). The reason for tongue deviation toward the weak side contralateral to a cortical lesion is not just simple crossed innervation: All tongue muscles are bilaterally innervated except genioglossus, the main tongue protruder, which is only innervated by the contralateral hemisphere. So the main muscle affected by a hemispheric lesion is the contralateral genioglossus, causing the tongue to protrude toward the weak side (overcome by the strong genioglossus on the normal side).

For summary tables of cranial nerve functions, cranial nerve nuclei functions, and cranial nerve-mediated reflexes, see Tables 9–2, 9–3, and 9–4.

The Peripheral Nervous System & Introduction to Electromyography/ Nerve Conduction Studies

INTRODUCTION TO ANATOMY & DISEASES OF THE PERIPHERAL NERVOUS SYSTEM

The peripheral nervous system includes the nerve roots, dorsal root ganglia, plexuses, and peripheral nerves. Nerve roots join to form plexuses (cervical plexus, brachial plexus, lumbosacral plexus), which give rise to peripheral nerves.

Individual peripheral nerves may be sensory, motor, autonomic, or mixed. Mixed nerves are two-way conduits: Efferent motor information travels from the spinal cord to the muscles and afferent sensory information travels in from the periphery to the spinal cord.

Efferent motor signals travel from the anterior horn cells (alpha motor neurons) into peripheral nerves by way of ventral roots. These are the lower motor neurons that are under the control of the corticospinal tracts (see Ch. 4).

Afferent sensory information travels from the peripheral nerves to dorsal root ganglia, and from dorsal root ganglia into the spinal cord by way of dorsal roots to enter the ascending sensory pathways (see Ch. 4).

Efferent peripheral nervous system sympathetic autonomic signals originate in the intermediolateral columns of the thoracic spinal cord, synapse in paraspinal ganglia, and then travel in postganglionic neurons to end organs.

The parasympathetic control of the organs of the thorax and most of the organs of the abdomen comes from the vagus nerve (cranial nerve 10), with the exception of the final third of the gastrointestinal tract, the bladder, and the reproductive organs, which receive parasympathetic input from nerves arising from nerve roots from sacral levels 2 through 4. The central control of the autonomic peripheral nervous system comes from hypothalamic-brainstem pathways.

Peripheral nervous system pathology can affect the roots (**radiculopathy**), dorsal root ganglia (**ganglionopathy**; also known as **sensory neuronopathy**), alpha motor neurons (**motor neuron disease**), brachial or lumbosacral plexus (**plexopathy**), or one or more peripheral nerves (**peripheral neuropathy**).

Localization of focal or multifocal peripheral nervous system findings requires determining whether a pattern of weakness, sensory disturbance, and/or reflex diminution/ absence can be explained by a problem with:

- A single nerve (**mononeuropathy**)
- A single root (**radiculopathy**)
- Multiple individual nerves (**mononeuropathy multiplex**)
- Multiple roots (**polyradiculopathy**)
- The brachial or lumbosacral plexus (**plexopathy**)

If a peripheral nervous system process is generalized rather than focal, clinical symptoms and signs can help to

TABLE 15-1 Clinical Features of Peripheral Nervous System Disorders.

	Key Clinical Feature	Focal versus Diffuse	Characteristics of Pain, if Present
Radiculopathy	Pain/sensory loss (dorsal root) Weakness (ventral root)	Focal symptoms limited to root distribution, often asymmetric	Radiating in root distribution
Ganglionopathy (Sensory neuronopathy)	Sensory ataxia	Diffuse, usually symmetric	If present, often burning in quality
Plexopathy	Weakness > sensory loss	Focal symptoms limited to involved limb	Depends on etiology
Mononeuropathy	Weakness and/or sensory loss	Focal symptoms limited to single nerve distribution	If present, in distribution of involved nerve
Mononeuropathy multiplex	Weakness and/or sensory loss	Multifocal, usually asymmetric	Present when vasculitis is etiology
Polyneuropathy	Weakness and/or sensory loss Paresthesias and/or pain	Diffuse, usually symmetric	If present, symmetric and usually begins distally

determine which level(s) of the peripheral nervous system is/are affected (i.e., polyneuropathy, polyradiculopathy, polyradiculoneuropathy, or ganglionopathy). The main symptoms of each category of peripheral nervous system disorder are listed in Table 15–1 and discussed in more detail in their respective sections in this chapter. Localization guides differential diagnosis since different types of pathologic processes can selectively affect different levels of the peripheral nervous system. Common causes of pathology at each level of the peripheral nervous system are listed in Table 15–2 and discussed in more detail below. Note that diabetes and HIV can cause a variety of different types of peripheral nervous system dysfunction.

ANATOMY & DISEASES OF NERVE ROOTS: RADICULOPATHY

Anatomy of Nerve Roots (Fig. 15–1)

In the cervical spine, each nerve root is numbered according to the cervical vertebra *above* which it exits: The C1 root exits above the C1 vertebra, the C2 root exits above the C2 vertebra (between C1 and C2), the C7 root exits above the C7 vertebra (between C6 and C7). The root exiting between C7 and T1 is labeled as the C8 root (although there is no C8 vertebra). This "resets" the numbering from T1 forward, so at the thoracic, lumbar, and sacral levels, roots are numbered by the level *below* which they exit: the T1 root exits below the T1 vertebra (between T1 and T2), the L1 root exits below the L1 vertebra (between L1 and L2), the S1 root exits below the S1 vertebra (between S1 and S2). The spinal cord ends at L1-L2, and the lumbar and sacral roots (the **cauda equina**) must descend inferiorly from the L1-L2 level to their corresponding neural foramina to exit. (See also Fig. 5-1.)

One of the most common causes of radiculopathy is intervertebral disc prolapse, which occurs most commonly at the cervical and lumbar levels where the spine is most mobile. At both cervical and lumbar levels, disc prolapse most commonly impinges on the nerve root whose number corresponds to the *inferior* vertebra of the pair of vertebrae surrounding the disc. For example, the disc between C5-C6 most commonly impinges on the C6 root, and the L4-L5 disc most commonly impinges on the L5 root. Note that because of the numbering scheme just described, this means that a herniated cervical disc compresses the root *at the level of exit*, whereas a herniated lumbar or sacral disc most commonly compresses the root that is going to exit *at the next level down*. For example, a herniated disc at C5-C6 typically compresses the C6 root, which exits between the C5 and C6 vertebral bodies. Most commonly, lumbar disc herniation impinges upon the root on the way down to the next level, called **posterolateral disc herniation**. Therefore, a herniated disc at L4-L5 most commonly compresses the L5 root, which is the root that is going to exit between the L5 and S1 vertebral bodies (the root that exits between L4 and L5 is the L4 root, which exits below its corresponding L4 vertebra). Less commonly, **far lateral disc herniation** can affect the root exiting at the level of the disc (e.g., L4-L5 disc affecting the L4 root) (see Fig. 17–3).

A few reference points are important in remembering which sensory dermatomes correspond to which nerve roots (Fig. 15–2):

- On the thorax and abdomen, the nipples are at the T4 level, the umbilicus at T10, and the waist line at L1.
- The upper extremity is supplied by C5-T2.
- The lower extremity is supplied by L1-S2.
- S3-S4-S5 supply the area around the anus, and S2-S3-S4 supply the genitalia.

The root supply of the upper and lower extremities is discussed in detail in Chapters 16 and 17.

TABLE 15–2 Etiologies of Peripheral Nervous System Disorders.

	Structural	Inflammatory	Infectious	Neoplastic	Toxic	Systemic Diseases	Hereditary
Radiculopathy	Disc disease Spondylosis Trauma	AIDP CIDP	Lyme disease CMV HSV2	Leptomeningeal Compressive		Ankylosing spondylitis Diabetic thoracic radiculopathy	
Ganglionopathy		Idiopathic inflammatory	HIV	Paraneoplastic	Vitamin B6 toxicity Platins	Sjögren's syndrome	
Plexopathy	Trauma Operative positioning	Parsonage-Turner Nondiabetic lumbo-sacral radiculopathy neuropathy		Infiltration Radiation-induced		Diabetic lumbosa-cral radiculoplexus neuropathy (Bruns-Garland syndrome)	Hereditary neuralgic amyotrophy
Mononeuropathy	Entrapment Trauma		Leprosy	Amyloidosis	Lead poisoning (radial nerve most common)	Diabetes Hypothyroidism	Hereditary neuropa-thy with liability to pressure palsies
Mononeuropathy multiplex		Primary nonsystemic vasculitic neuropathy Multifocal motor neuropathy	Leprosy HIV Hepatitis C	Neurolymphomatosis		Diabetes Systemic vasculitis Amyloidosis	Hereditary neuropa-thy with liability to pressure palsies
Generalized symmetric polyneuropathy		AIDP CIDP	HIV	Multiple myeloma Paraneoplastic	Chemotherapy Heavy metals Medications	Diabetes Vitamin B12 deficiency Uremia	Charcot-Marie-Tooth Hereditary sensory and autonomic neuropathy

Abbreviations: AIDP: acute inflammatory demyelinating polyradiculoneuropathy; CIDP: chronic inflammatory demyelinating polyradiculoneuropathy; CMV: cytomegalovirus; HIV: human immunodeficiency virus; HSV2: herpes simplex virus 2.

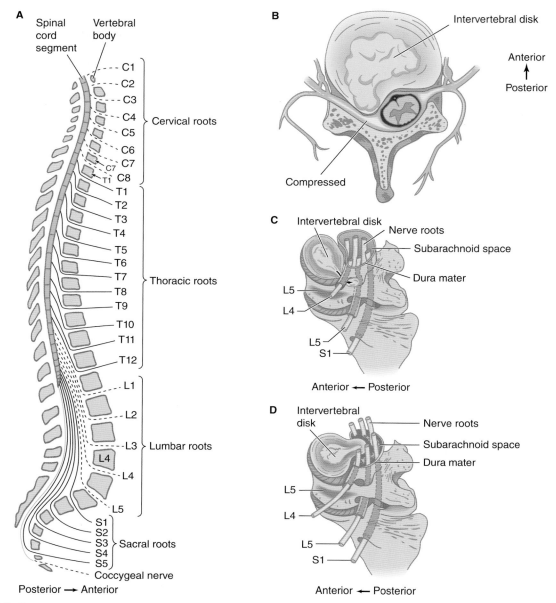

FIGURE 15–1 Schematic of the relationship of nerve roots to the spinal column. A: Sagittal view of the spine, showing cervical roots exiting above their corresponding vertebrae, whereas thoracic, lumbar, and sacral roots exit below their corresponding vertebrae. **B:** Axial view of disc herniation causing nerve root compression. **C:** Posterolateral lumbar disc herniation affecting the root exiting at the next level down (here, disc between L4 and L5 compresses L5 root). **D:** Central lumbar disc herniation affecting multiple roots of the cauda equina. Reproduced with permission from Aminoff M, Greenberg D, Simon R: *Clinical Neurology*, 9th ed. New York, NY: McGraw Hill; 2015.

Diseases of Nerve Roots (Radiculopathy)

Nerve roots can be affected by:

- Compression by local structures: disc, osteophyte
- Infection (radiculitis): Lyme disease, cytomegalovirus (CMV), herpes simplex virus 2 (HSV2), syphilis (along with the dorsal columns in tabes dorsalis)
- Inflammation: Guillain-Barré syndrome and chronic inflammatory demyelinating polyradiculoneuropathy (CIDP), both

of which are polyradiculoneuropathies (i.e., affect both roots and nerves)
- Malignancy: compression due to spine metastases or leptomeningeal metastases

Nerve roots may be affected in isolation or several roots may be involved simultaneously (**polyradiculopathy**). Nerve root irritation is generally painful, with pain radiating from the neck or back along the dermatome of the involved root. This may be accompanied by sensory loss in the same

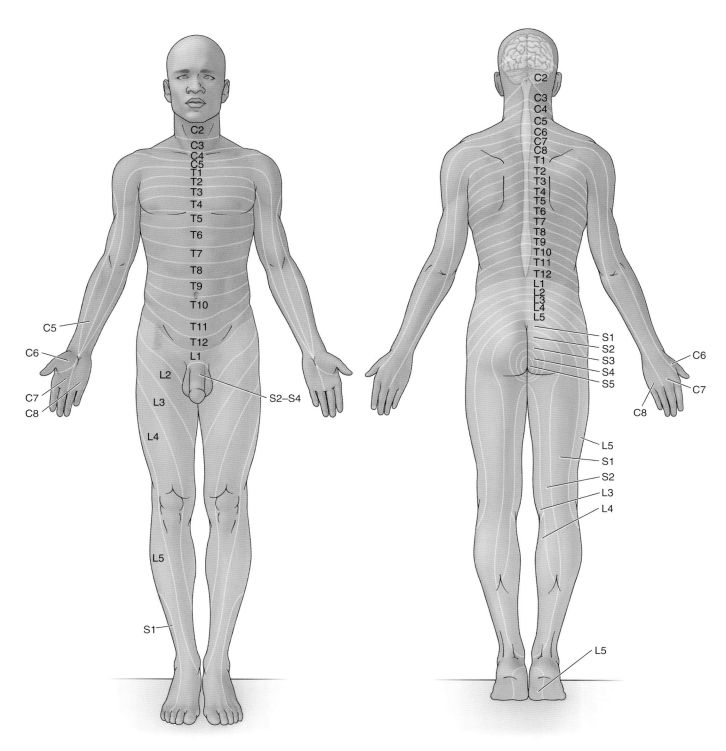

FIGURE 15–2 **Schematic of dermatomes.** Reproduced with permission from Martin J: *Neuroanatomy Text and Atlas*, 4th ed. New York, NY: McGraw Hill; 2012.

distribution. Depending on the root(s) involved, weakness and/or loss of reflexes may be observed. The specific distribution of these symptoms and signs is discussed for the upper and lower extremities in Chapters 16 and 17.

The most common cause of radiculopathy is compression due to degenerative disease of the spine leading to disc prolapse and osteophyte growth with spondylosis, which can cause **neural foraminal stenosis**, leading to compression of nerve roots. These changes can also lead to **central canal stenosis**, which can lead to spinal cord compression in the cervical spine (which can cause myelopathy; see Ch. 16), or compression of the roots of the cauda equina in the lumbar spine (which can cause neurogenic claudication; see Ch. 17). Other factors that may contribute to central canal stenosis are a congenitally small spinal canal and spondylolisthesis (displacement of one or more vertebral bodies in the antero-posterior plane, which can be caused by degenerative disease of the spinal column).

The cervical and lumbar regions of the spine are the most mobile, and so they are the most prone to wear and tear, which can lead to degenerative changes. The most common levels of radiculopathy due to degenerative changes are at the most mobile areas within these regions: C6-C7 (leading to C7 radiculopathy), C5-C6 (leading to C6 radiculopathy), L4-L5 (most commonly leading to L5 radiculopathy), and L5-S1 (most commonly leading to S1 radiculopathy).

Degenerative disease of the spine can also cause back or neck pain without causing radiculopathy or central canal stenosis. Neuroimaging for back or neck pain is generally only indicated in cases of intractable pain or progressive weakness for which surgery is under consideration, in patients with a history of or concern for malignancy (to evaluate for metastatic disease), or in patients with back/neck pain and fever (to evaluate for epidural abscess). In patients unable to undergo MRI, CT or CT myelography can be used. It should be noted that degenerative disc disease and spondylosis are often incidentally noted on MRI and may not be symptomatic, so clinical correlation between imaging, clinical history, and physical examination findings is essential.

Initial management of radiculopathy due to disc disease or spondylosis is nonsurgical unless there is a progressive motor deficit or intractable pain. When pain is the primary symptom, many patients will obtain relief with nonsteroidal anti-inflammatory drugs (NSAIDs) or acetaminophen (and/or a short course of oral steroids) and physical therapy. Patients who do not respond to these conservative measures within 1–2 months may be considered for epidural steroid injections. In patients with intractable pain in spite of 2–3 months of conservative measures or in patients with a progressive motor deficit, surgical intervention should be considered if there appears to be radiologic evidence of compressive radiculopathy that correlates with the patient's symptoms. Surgical intervention may lead to faster improvement than nonsurgical treatment in such cases, but many patients improve with conservative measures, and longer term outcomes may not differ significantly between patients who undergo surgery and those who do not. For patients with chronic back pain with minimal response to standard therapies, multidisciplinary pain management and complementary therapies such as yoga and acupuncture may be helpful.

Specific clinical features, diagnosis, and management of cervical and lumbar radiculopathy are discussed in Chapters 16 (upper extremity) and 17 (lower extremity).

DISEASES OF DORSAL ROOT GANGLIA: GANGLIONOPATHY (SENSORY NEURONOPATHY)

The dorsal root ganglia are the cell bodies of pseudounipolar neurons that transmit sensory information from the periphery to the spinal cord via the dorsal roots. The dorsal root ganglia can be affected in isolation causing the syndrome of **dorsal root ganglionopathy** (also known as **sensory neuronopathy**). Dorsal root ganglionopathy causes isolated sensory dysfunction (paresthesias, sensory loss, sensory ataxia, pain) with spared strength. However, gait and extremity movements may be severely impaired by sensory ataxia in spite of full force (see "Distinguishing cerebellar ataxia from sensory ataxia" in Ch. 8). Reflexes are usually absent. Burning pain and/or dysautonomia may be present in some cases.

The causes of dorsal root ganglionopathy include:

- Autoimmune disease: most commonly Sjögren's syndrome
- Paraneoplastic syndrome: most commonly due to anti-Hu antibodies (which are most commonly associated with small cell lung cancer)
- Medications: platinum-based chemotherapeutic drugs (platins), vitamin B6 toxicity
- Infection: most commonly HIV (though rare)
- Some cases are idiopathic

Immune-mediated causes are treated with immunomodulatory therapy.

DISEASES OF THE BRACHIAL OR LUMBOSACRAL PLEXUS: PLEXOPATHY

Pathology of the brachial plexus in the lower neck/axilla or lumbosacral plexus in the lower abdomen/pelvis leads to a pattern of weakness and/or sensory loss in an extremity that spans the distributions of multiple nerves and roots.

Causes of plexopathy include:

- Injury: traumatic injury, birth trauma (to the infant's brachial plexus or mother's lumbosacral plexus, or surgical injury)
- Malignant compression or infiltration
- Radiation therapy
- Inflammatory plexitis.

The most common causes of pathology of the brachial and lumbosacral plexuses are listed in Table 15–3 and discussed in detail for each extremity in Chapters 16 and 17.

DISEASES OF PERIPHERAL NERVES

The peripheral nerves can be affected individually (**mononeuropathy**), multiple individual nerves can be affected (**mononeuropathy multiplex**), or the peripheral nerves may be affected throughout the body (**polyneuropathy**).

TABLE 15–3 Etiologies of Brachial & Lumbosacral Plexopathies.

	Birth Trauma	Trauma	Surgery	Malignancy and Radiation Therapy	Inflammatory	Miscellaneous
Brachial Plexopathy	To infant	Shoulder injury Stinger (burner) syndrome	Sternotomy Axillary dissection Surgical positioning	Lung Breast Lymphoma	Parsonage-Turner syndrome	Rucksack paralysis
Lumbo-sacral Plexopathy	To mother	Pelvic injury	Pelvic surgery Hip surgery Lithotomy position	Colorectal Gynecologic Prostate Lymphoma Metastases	Diabetic lumbosacral radiculoplexus neuropathy (also known as diabetic amyotrophy, Bruns-Garland syndrome) Idiopathic lumbosacral radiculoplexus neuropathy	Retroperitoneal hematoma Psoas abscess

Mononeuropathy

Mononeuropathies most commonly occur due to compression/entrapment or trauma, but can rarely be caused by nerve infarct (vasculitic neuropathy; see "Vasculitic Neuropathy") or primary nerve tumor (e.g., schwannoma, neurofibroma; see "Tumors of the Peripheral Nervous System" in Ch. 24). The most common mononeuropathies are median neuropathy at the wrist (carpal tunnel syndrome), ulnar neuropathy at the elbow, and peroneal neuropathy at the fibular head/neck since these are the nerve segments most susceptible to external compression. The individual mononeuropathies of the upper and lower extremities are discussed in Chapters 16 and 17.

Mononeuropathy Multiplex

Mononeuropathy multiplex refers to the scenario in which multiple individual nerves are affected simultaneously or in sequence (e.g., a radial neuropathy followed by a peroneal neuropathy). Mononeuritis multiplex refers to the scenario in which mononeuropathy multiplex arises from an inflammatory etiology (e.g., vasculitic neuropathy).

The differential diagnosis for mononeuropathy multiplex includes:

- Vasculitic neuropathy (see below)
- Infections: leprosy, HIV, hepatitis C
- Malignancy: neurolymphomatosis or paraneoplastic neuropathy
- Multifocal motor neuropathy and multifocal acquired demyelinating sensory and motor neuropathy (MADSAM) (see Ch. 27)
- Hereditary neuropathy with liability to pressure palsies (HNPP) (see Ch. 27)
- Diabetes (although this more commonly causes a symmetric polyneuropathy)
- Amyloidosis (see Ch. 27)

All are discussed elsewhere except vasculitic neuropathy (see below).

Vasculitic Neuropathy

Vasculitis of the nerves causes nerve infarcts, resulting in painful, acute-onset mononeuropathies ("strokes" of the peripheral nerves). Vasculitic neuropathy commonly presents as classic mononeuropathy multiplex. However, if overlapping nerves are affected, vasculitic neuropathy may present as more confluent regions of sensorimotor deficits imitating polyneuropathy. Even in this more confluent presentation, vasculitic neuropathy more commonly presents asymmetrically, in contrast to polyneuropathy, which most commonly presents symmetrically.

Vasculitis affecting the peripheral nervous system is classified as either secondary to a systemic cause of vasculitis or as primary nonsystemic vasculitic neuropathy (i.e., vasculitis isolated to the peripheral nervous system). Systemic causes of vasculitis include:

- Primary systemic vasculitis: granulomatosis with polyangiitis (formerly called Wegener's granulomatosis) or eosinophilic granulomatosis with polyangiitis (formerly called Churg-Strauss syndrome)
- Systemic autoimmune disease: lupus, Sjögren's syndrome, rheumatoid arthritis, sarcoid
- Systemic infection: HIV, hepatitis B, hepatitis C (associated with cryoglobulinemia)

When vasculitic neuropathy is suspected, serologic studies should be sent to evaluate for systemic vasculitis (erythrocyte sedimentation rate [ESR], C-reactive protein [CRP], perinuclear antineutrophilic cytoplasmic antibody [p-ANCA], cytoplasmic antineutrophilic cytoplasmic antibody [c-ANCA]), systemic autoimmune diseases (antinuclear antibody [ANA], anti-Ro, anti-La), and viral infections (HIV, hepatitis B, hepatitis C, and cryoglobulins) that can cause vasculitis. Nerve conduction studies typically show signs of axonal loss (decreased amplitudes) since infarction leads to neuronal death leaving fewer axons to contribute to nerve conduction amplitude. Definitive diagnosis is made by nerve biopsy showing vasculitis. Treatment is with immunomodulatory therapy.

Polyneuropathy is discussed in Chapter 27. In contrast to mononeuropathies and mononeuropathy multiplex which tend to present asymmetrically, peripheral polyneuropathy most commonly presents symmetrically.

INTRODUCTION TO EMG & NERVE CONDUCTION STUDIES

Electromyography (EMG) and nerve conduction studies (NCS) serve several functions, including:

- Localization of symptoms and signs to particular roots and/or nerves and to particular sites along individual nerves (see Chs. 16 and 17)
- Distinction between axonal and demyelinating neuropathies (see Ch. 27)
- Distinction between diseases of nerve and diseases of muscle
- Diagnosis of diseases of the neuromuscular junction (see Ch. 29)

Nerve Conduction Studies (Fig. 15–3)

Compound Motor Action Potentials (CMAPs) & Sensory Nerve Action Potentials (SNAPs)

In nerve conduction studies, nerves are electrically stimulated through the skin, and the action potentials produced by this stimulus are recorded. If a motor nerve is stimulated, the response of the innervated muscle is observed, called the **compound muscle (or motor) action potential (CMAP)**. If a sensory nerve is stimulated, the response is recorded somewhere else along the nerve, called the **sensory nerve action potential (SNAP)**. For SNAPs, the nerve may be stimulated distally and recorded proximally (**orthodromic** stimulation; the same direction as normal sensory impulses travel), or the nerve may be stimulated proximally and recorded distally (**antidromic** stimulation; the opposite direction from the normal sensory transmission).

The three main features of CMAPs and SNAPs used in clinical diagnosis are **amplitude**, **distal latency**, and **conduction velocity**.[1] The amplitude predominantly reflects the integrity of axons in a nerve: the more axons, the higher the amplitude; the fewer axons the lower the amplitude. Therefore, *axonal* neuropathies will cause *decreased amplitudes* of CMAPs and/or SNAPs (mnemonic: **a**xonal neuropathies cause decreased **a**mplitudes). Note that since the CMAP is a measure of the muscle action potential, muscle diseases can also decrease CMAP amplitude.

Recall that myelin's function is to increase the speed of nerve transmission. Therefore, demyelination *decreases conduction velocity* and *prolongs distal latency* (i.e., conduction is

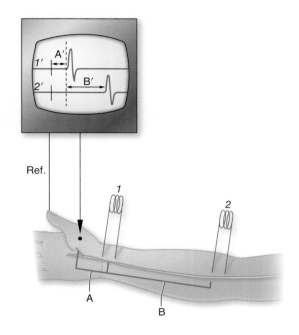

FIGURE 15–3 **Schematic of nerve conduction study.** Reproduced with permission from Ropper A, Samuels M, Klein J: *Adams and Victor's Principles of Neurology*, 10th ed. New York, NY: McGraw Hill; 2014.

slower, prolonging the time for nerve impulses to travel from proximal to distal).

Focal Slowing & Conduction Block

Demyelination can be focal, multifocal, or diffuse. In acquired etiologies of demyelination, the demyelination is generally focal or multifocal. For example, an acquired nerve injury (e.g., carpal tunnel syndrome at the wrist, ulnar neuropathy at the elbow) causes focal demyelination, and acquired immune-mediated demyelination (e.g., acquired immune demyelinating polyradiculoneuropathy [AIDP] or chronic inflammatory demyelinating polyradiculoneuropathy [CIDP]) causes multifocal demyelination. In most etiologies of inherited demyelination (e.g., Charcot-Marie-Tooth type 1), *all* myelin is abnormal, and so demyelination and resultant slowing of conduction velocity is *diffuse* (hereditary neuropathy with liability to pressure palsies is an exception; see Ch. 27). When demyelination is diffuse, conduction velocities are decreased *throughout* each individual affected nerve. If there is a focal region of a nerve that is demyelinated (e.g., the median nerve in the carpal

---

[1]The SNAP conduction velocity is determined by measuring the distance between the stimulating electrode and the recording site, and dividing this distance by the time it takes from stimulation to SNAP (**latency**). The CMAP requires transmission not only from the nerve to the muscle, but also across the neuromuscular junction, and this neuromuscular transmission also takes time. Therefore, in order to calculate the velocity with respect to transmission along only the motor nerve, the nerve is stimulated at two different locations, and the velocity is determined by the distance between these points divided by the difference between the time from the more proximal stimulation point to the CMAP and the more distal stimulation point to the CMAP (Fig. 15–3). This allows for analysis of transmission across the nerve, subtracting out the time related to transmission across the neuromuscular junction.

tunnel in carpal tunnel syndrome), there will be **focal slowing** across this region: when stimulating proximal to the lesion and recording distal to it, the focally demyelinated region will cause slowing of the nerve impulses. However, if both the stimulating and recording sites are distal to the abnormal region or both are proximal to it, conduction velocity should be normal. The finding of focal slowing allows for localization of a lesion along a particular nerve (e.g., the median nerve in the carpal tunnel; the ulnar nerve at the elbow).

Areas of focal or multifocal demyelination can also cause a phenomenon called **conduction block**. When conduction block is complete, stimulating a nerve proximal to a site of focal demyelination and recording distal to it will not result in any CMAP or SNAP. When conduction block is incomplete, the CMAP and/or SNAP *amplitude decreases* when compared to stimulating and recording distal or proximal to the demyelinated segment. Above, demyelinating neuropathies were described as causing a slowing of conduction velocity and axonal neuropathies as causing decreased amplitude, so why/how would a demyelinating process decrease the *amplitude* of CMAPs and/or SNAPs? In acquired demyelination, not all individual axons within a nerve are demyelinated. Therefore, when stimulating across a partially demyelinated region of a nerve, the normal axons conduct normally but the demyelinated axons do not. Since this results in fewer normally conducting axons, the amplitude decreases (there are other more complicated reasons for decreased amplitude in conduction block, which are beyond the scope here). Conduction block is more easily detected in motor nerves.

Again, note that *conduction block* and/or *focal slowing* suggest acquired demyelination (nerve injury or acquired demyelinating neuropathy; e.g., AIDP or CIDP), whereas *uniform* slowing throughout a given nerve suggests inherited demyelination (e.g., Charcot-Marie-Tooth disease).

Recall that sensory nerves travel to dorsal root ganglia, which give rise to the dorsal roots that enter the spinal cord. If the dorsal roots are affected in isolation (i.e., radiculopathy), SNAPs can be normal since the nerve itself may conduct normally even if its root is damaged. Motor neurons are continuous from the anterior horn of the spinal cord into the peripheral nerves in which they travel, so a problem anywhere along a motor nerve can lead to changes in CMAPs.

H Reflex

Although the dorsal root is not able to be tested directly with nerve conduction studies, it can be tested indirectly by way of the **H reflex**. The H reflex is an electrophysiologic test of the reflex arc, which is most commonly tested by examining the ankle reflex pathway: stimulating the tibial nerve (afferent sensory input to the reflex) and measuring the response in the soleus muscle. Since the impulse has to travel back through the nerve and dorsal root into the spinal cord, this allows for a measure of dorsal root function. If the tibial nerve has normal CMAP and SNAP amplitude and velocity

but the H reflex is absent (or has a prolonged latency), this suggests dysfunction of the S1 root or S1 level of the spinal cord. If there is a generalized peripheral neuropathy, this will affect afferent and efferent components of the H reflex, limiting interpretation.

F Wave

The proximal portion of motor neurons can be assessed by way of the **F wave**. If a supramaximal stimulus is given to a motor nerve, in addition to observing the CMAP, a subsequent wave called the F wave is observed. The F wave is the result of the stimulation also passing retrograde (antidromic) up the nerve (i.e., in the "wrong" direction), and stimulating the nerve to fire. Since this takes more time than the direct path down the nerve (i.e., orthodromic; in the "normal" direction), the F wave occurs after the CMAP. If the F wave is delayed (prolonged F wave latency) or absent in the setting of normal CMAPs, this signifies proximal motor nerve pathology or spinal cord pathology.

Abnormal F waves and H reflexes (prolonged latency or absence) are common early findings in Guillain-Barré syndrome (reflecting root involvement) (see Ch. 27).

In summary, using nerve conduction studies, individual nerves can be studied to determine the *site(s)* of nerve dysfunction (i.e., which nerve[s] and where along the nerve[s] if there is focal demyelination) and *type* of nerve dysfunction (i.e., axonal vs. demyelinating).

Electromyography (EMG) (Table 15–4)

EMG evaluates activity in individual muscles. EMG does not just detect primary muscle pathology, but can also detect changes in muscle caused by nerve disease (i.e., denervation and subsequent reinnervation). This latter function of EMG is important in localizing problems to a particular nerve or root: By examining which muscles show signs of denervation/reinnervation on EMG, it can be determined whether these muscles correspond to a particular nerve, root, or multiple nerves and/or roots.

The paraspinal muscles are the muscles innervated most proximally (closest to the spine). Therefore, EMG changes in these muscles suggest pathology at the root level.

EMG findings can be divided into those that occur with insertion of the EMG needle into the muscle (**insertional activity**), those that occur with the muscle at rest (**spontaneous activity**), and those that occur with patient activation of the muscle (**voluntary activity**). With voluntary activation, the **motor unit action potentials** (**MUAPs**) are analyzed for their amplitude, duration, whether their number of phases is increased (**polyphasia**), and the pattern in which they are recruited with increasing activation of the muscle by the patient (Table 15–4).

Insertional Activity

Some insertional activity is normal as the needle enters the muscle, but if this activity continues beyond the brief period of insertion, this is pathologic, although not specific: it can

TABLE 15–4 **EMG Findings in Muscle & Nerve Diseases.**

	Primary Muscle Disease	Primary Nerve Disease
Insertional activity	Increased (may be decreased with severe atrophy)	Increased (may be decreased with severe atrophy)
Spontaneous activity		
Fibrillation potentials	✓	✓
Positive sharp waves	✓	✓
Complex repetitive discharges	✓	✓
Fasciculation potentials		✓ (can also be a benign finding)
Myokymic discharges		✓
Myotonic discharges	✓	(rarely)
Voluntary activity: Motor unit action potentials		
Amplitude	Decreased	Increased
Duration	Decreased	Increased
Phases	Polyphasia	Polyphasia
Recruitment	Early	Reduced

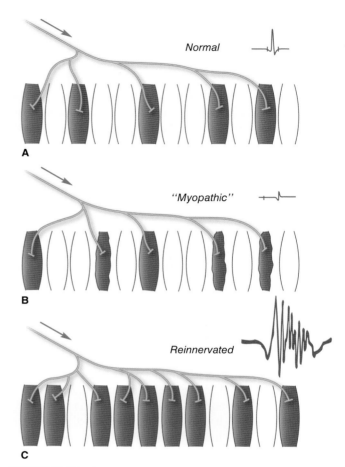

FIGURE 15–4 **Schematic of motor units in muscle and nerve disease.** See text for explanation. Reproduced with permission from Ropper A, Samuels M, Klein J: *Adams and Victor's Principles of Neurology*, 10th ed. New York, NY: McGraw Hill; 2014.

be seen in primary muscle pathology (e.g., myopathy) or in denervated muscle (i.e., neuropathy).

Spontaneous Activity

Muscle should normally be "silent" at rest, but pathology in either the muscles themselves or nerve pathology leading to denervation of muscles can lead to abnormal spontaneous activity detected on EMG. Types of spontaneous activity that may be observed include fasciculation potentials (which can also be a benign finding in normal muscle), fibrillation potentials, positive sharp waves, complex repetitive discharges, myokymic discharges, and myotonic discharges (Table 15–4). Of these, fasciculations and myokymic discharges are associated with *nerve* diseases, myotonic discharges are associated with *muscle* diseases, and fibrillation potentials, positive sharp waves, and complex repetitive discharges can occur with either muscle or nerve diseases. One instance in which myokymic discharges are particularly helpful is that they are present in radiation-induced plexopathy, distinguishing it from malignant infiltration of the plexus (which does not cause myokymic discharges; see Chs. 16 and 17).

Voluntary Activity

Motor unit action potential (MUAP) amplitude, duration, and phases (Fig. 15–4)—In primary muscle diseases, muscle

fibers are lost, and so corresponding MUAPs have *decreased amplitude and duration* (Fig. 15–4B).

In diseases affecting peripheral nerves, denervated muscle fibers are reinnervated by surviving axons after the acute period of denervation. Since surviving axons are taking over for axons lost to the disease process, these surviving axons must innervate a larger number of motor fibers than they did previously. Therefore, each nerve impulse leads to the simultaneous stimulation of more muscle fibers than before. This causes the resultant MUAPs to be larger (*increased amplitude*), longer (*increased duration*), and to have more complicated morphology with multiple phases (*polyphasia*) (Fig. 15–4C). Polyphasia can also be seen in muscle disease.

Motor unit action potential (MUAP) recruitment pattern (Fig. 15–5)—To increase muscular force, motor units can fire faster, or more motor units can be recruited (Fig. 15–5A). In diseases of motor nerves, there is loss of motor axons so there are fewer overall motor units to recruit (**reduced recruitment**). To generate adequate force, the existing units fire

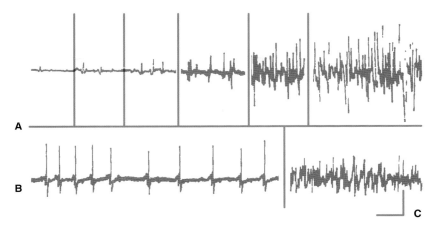

FIGURE 15–5 **Schematic of patterns of motor unit recruitment.** See text for explanation. Reproduced with permission from Ropper A, Samuels M, Klein J: *Adams and Victor's Principles of Neurology*, 10th ed. New York, NY: McGraw Hill; 2014.

more rapidly to compensate (Fig. 15–5B). In primary muscle diseases, the overall number of motor units is the same but there are fewer functioning muscle fibers in each motor unit. Therefore, to generate adequate force, more units are activated together early in muscle contraction, a pattern called **early recruitment** (Fig. 15–5C).

In patients with central nervous system causes of weakness (e.g., corticospinal tract lesion or poor effort), there are fewer motor units recruited, but they fire at a normal rate.

Repetitive stimulation to assess the neuromuscular junction is discussed with diseases of the neuromuscular junction in Chapter 29.

Radiculopathy, Plexopathy, & Mononeuropathies of the Upper Extremity

NEUROANATOMY OF THE UPPER EXTREMITY

The Nerve Root Supply of the Upper Extremity

In the cervical spine, nerve roots are numbered by the cervical level *above* which they exit: The C1 roots exit above the C1 vertebra, the C2 roots above the C2 vertebra (between C1 and C2), the C7 roots above the C7 vertebra (between C6 and C7). The roots exiting between C7 and T1 are the C8 roots (there is no C8 vertebra). This is different from the thoracic, lumbar, and sacral levels, where roots are numbered by the vertebral level *below* which they exit: The T1 roots exit below T1 (between T1 and T2), the L1 roots exit below L1 (between L1 and L2), the S1 roots exit below S1 (between S1 and S2) (see Fig. 15–1).

With respect to sensory dermatomes, the lateral upper arm is supplied by C5, the lateral forearm and lateral hand (including the thumb) is supplied by C6, the middle of the hand (including the middle finger) is supplied by C7, the medial hand (including the ring finger and the fifth finger) and medial forearm are supplied by C8, the medial upper arm is supplied by T1, and the axilla is supplied by T2; the index finger may be supplied by C6 or C7 (Fig. 16–1). On the dorsum of the arm/hand this same pattern is maintained. To remember this, trace around your own arm naming the dermatomes: On the arm with the palm facing upward, trace around the arm from lateral upper arm (C5) to lateral forearm (C6), around the hand from the thumb (C6) to the index and middle fingers (C7) to the ring and fifth fingers (C8), around to the medial forearm (C8) to the medial upper arm (T1) to the axilla (T2).

The Brachial Plexus

The nerve roots supplying the upper extremity (C5-T1) join to form the brachial plexus. The terminal branches of the brachial plexus are the nerves to the upper arm, forearm, and hand: the axillary, musculocutaneous, radial, ulnar, and median nerves. Nerves that arise from the plexus proximal to the terminal branches supply the shoulder muscles (long thoracic, suprascapular, subscapular nerves), pectoral muscles (medial and lateral pectoral nerves), and sensation to the medial upper arm and forearm (medial brachial cutaneous and medial antebrachial cutaneous nerves).

The best way to learn the brachial plexus is to draw it over and over again (Fig. 16–2). A mnemonic theme in drawing it is the theme of **threes**. Figure 16–2 is a schematic of the left brachial plexus, oriented with the left arm held out with the left hand on the right side of the page and the thumb up. In the arm, the radius/thumb side is considered lateral and the ulna/fifth finger side is considered medial.

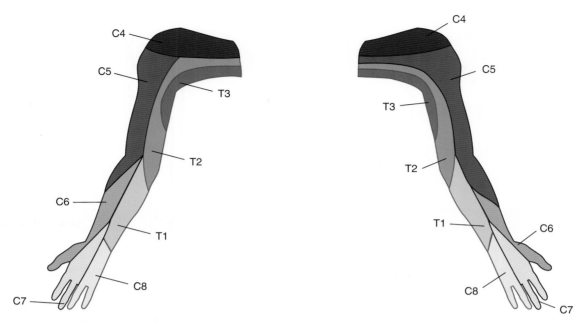

FIGURE 16–1 **Schematic showing dermatomes of the upper extremity.** The index finger may be supplied by C6 or C7; see also Fig. 15–2. Reproduced with permission from Waxman S: *Clinical Neuroanatomy*, 27th ed. New York, NY: McGraw Hill; 2013.

1. Draw **three** headless, armless, short-legged, long-bodied stick figures with the first and third having their small legs pointing to the left, and the middle one shorter and with the small legs pointing to the right (Fig. 16–2A).
2. Draw **three** lines in the shape of another headless, armless stick figure on its side with the legs connecting to the upper and lower lines and the "body" running parallel to those lines (Fig. 16–2B).
3. Draw **three** more lines: an X connecting the upper two horizontal lines, and a diagonal line connecting the bottom two (Fig. 16–2C).
4. Label the diagram from proximal (left of the diagram) to distal (right of the diagram): roots, trunks, divisions, cords, branches (nerves) (Fig. 16–2D):
   - The **roots** that make up the brachial plexus are C5, C6, C7, C8, and T1. These correspond to the five starting points on the left side of the diagram from top to bottom.
   - The segments before the X and diagonal line are the upper, middle, and lower **trunks**.
   - The X and the diagonal line are the anterior and posterior **divisions**, which join to form the three **cords**.
     - The three posterior divisions join to form the **posterior cord**.
     - The anterior divisions of the upper and middle trunks form the **lateral cord**.
     - The anterior division of the lower trunk forms the **medial cord**.
   (The posterior, medial, and lateral in the names of the cords are based on their anatomic relationship to the axillary artery.)

- The terminal **branches** are the five main nerves to the upper arm, forearm, and hand.
  - The terminal branches of the posterior cord are the **radial nerve** and the **axillary nerve**.
  - From top to bottom, the three terminal nerves originating from the sideways "M" shape are the **musculocutaneous nerve**, **median nerve**, and **ulnar nerve**.

Being able to reproduce this much from memory and knowing the muscles supplied by the terminal nerves will get you quite far in terms of localization to nerve(s), cord(s), trunk(s), and/or root(s). The next level of detail is the domain of neuromuscular experts.

Eleven additional nerves come off of the brachial plexus—nine of these can be remembered by several more rules of threes (Fig. 16–2E).

- **Three** nerves arise from roots:
  1. **Long thoracic** (C5-C7): innervates serratus anterior (weakness leads to scapular winging)
  2. **Nerve to the subclavius** (C5-C6): innervates subclavius (depresses the shoulder)
  3. **Dorsal scapular nerve** (C4-C5): innervates rhomboids (bring the scapula toward the back)
- **Three** nerves arise from the posterior cord:
  1. **Upper subscapular**: innervates subscapularis (internal rotation of the upper arm)
  2. **Lower subscapular**: innervates subscapularis and teres major (adducts and internally rotates the upper arm)
  3. **Thoracodorsal**: innervates latissimus dorsi (various movements of the shoulder)

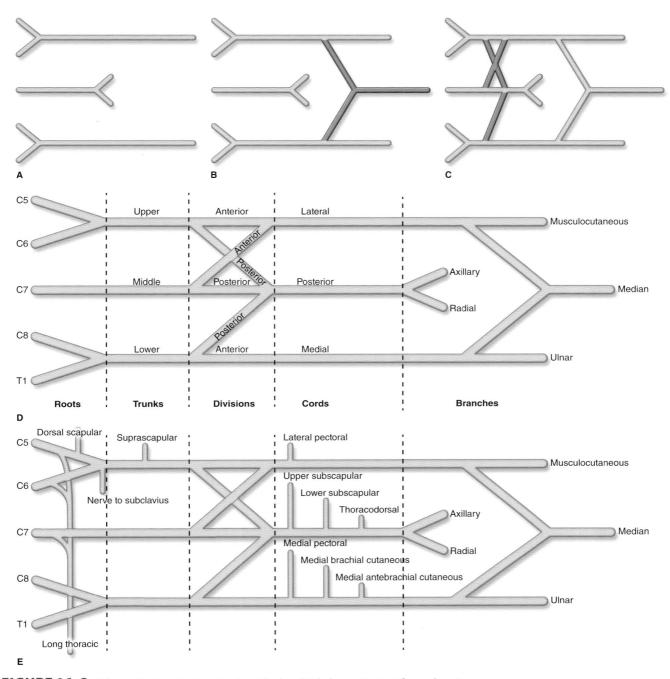

FIGURE 16–2 **Schematic showing how to draw the brachial plexus**. See text for explanation.

- **Three** nerves arise from the medial cord, all of which have *medial* in their names:
  1. **Medial pectoral**: innervates pectoralis major and minor (various movements of upper arm)
  2. **Medial brachial cutaneous**: sensation to medial upper arm
  3. **Medial antebrachial cutaneous**: sensation to medial forearm
- The last two nerves can be remembered by their relation to two other previously mentioned nerves:

1. There is a *medial* pectoral nerve from the medial cord, so there must be a **lateral pectoral nerve**, logically arising from the *lateral* cord (innervates pectoralis major).
2. There are *sub*scapular nerves, so there must be a **suprascapular nerve** (innervates supraspinatus and infraspinatus)—this nerve arises from the upper trunk, the only nerve to arise from a trunk. No nerves arise from divisions.

Drawings of the brachial plexus usually focus disproportionately on the complex web of trunks, divisions, and cords as is done here. This "web" is actually much shorter in length than the terminal nerves. The roots and trunks are located between the cervical spine and clavicle, the divisions are just posterior to the clavicle, the cords travel from just below the clavicle to the axilla, and the terminal nerves arise in the axilla. Therefore, pathology affecting the neck and upper chest can cause a plexopathy, whereas pathology in or distal to the axilla will usually affect one or more individual nerves.

The Anatomy of the Nerves of the Upper Extremity

The upper extremity can be divided into the upper arm, forearm, and hand. The thumb and fingers are moved by both intrinsic hand muscles and muscles in the forearm with tendon insertions in the fingers and thumb. To summarize the big picture (see Table 16–1 at the end of this chapter):

- The musculocutaneous nerve and axillary nerve *only* supply upper arm muscles (musculocutaneous: biceps, brachialis; axillary nerve: deltoid, teres minor).
- The radial nerve supplies muscles of the upper arm (triceps, brachioradialis) and forearm. Mnemonic: Radial nerve is the BEST: **b**rachioradialis, **e**xtensors, **s**upinator, and **t**riceps.
- All radial nerve–innervated *forearm* muscles control the wrist, fingers, and thumb except the supinator (which supinates the forearm). All radial nerve–innervated muscles *except* triceps, brachioradialis, and the long head of extensor carpi radialis are innervated by the **posterior interosseous nerve** branch of the radial nerve.
- All intrinsic hand muscles are innervated by the median and ulnar nerves. These two nerves also innervate forearm muscles, but do not innervate any upper arm muscles. All of the forearm muscles innervated by the median and ulnar nerves are involved in wrist, thumb, or finger movements *except* the median nerve–innervated pronator muscles (which pronate the forearm).

With respect to the wrist, fingers, and thumb, some important anatomic points are as follows (see Table 16–2 at the end of this chapter):

- All wrist, finger, and thumb extensors are radial nerve–innervated.
- All interossei are ulnar nerve–innervated.
- Where there is a division of labor between median and ulnar nerves, the median nerve innervates *lateral/radius/thumb–side* muscles and the ulnar nerve innervates *medial/ulna/fifth finger–side* muscles:
  - Flexor carpi radialis (median) vs flexor carpi ulnaris (ulnar)

- Flexor digitorum profundus 1 and 2 (median) vs flexor digitorum profundus 3 and 4 (ulnar)
- Lumbricals 1 and 2 (median) vs lumbricals 3 and 4 (ulnar)
- Flexor digitorum superficialis does not fit the above pattern: it is entirely innervated by the median nerve for all four digits.
- All nonextensor muscles of the fifth finger are ulnar nerve-innervated (abductor digiti minimi, opponens digiti minimi, flexor digiti minimi, flexor digitorum profundus, lumbrical 4) *except* the flexor digitorum superficialis (which is median nerve-innervated).

Each muscle of the upper extremity is innervated by a single nerve except the flexor pollicis brevis, which is innervated by both the median and ulnar nerves. However, each nerve is made up of multiple roots, most roots supply multiple nerves, and each muscle is generally supplied by more than one root. Table 16–3 (at the end of this chapter) shows the overlap of roots and nerves for the main clinically tested upper extremity muscles. This table can aid in differentiating between nerve and root lesions based on the pattern of weak muscles.

For example, axillary nerve pathology will cause weakened shoulder abduction (deltoid), but will spare shoulder external rotation (infraspinatus; suprascapular nerve) and internal rotation (subscapularis; subscapular nerve), whereas a C5 root lesion will weaken all of these actions (C5 input lost to axillary, suprascapular, and subscapular nerves). In a radial nerve palsy, the brachioradialis will be weak, but the biceps (musculocutaneous nerve) will remain strong, whereas a C6 root lesion will affect both the biceps and the brachioradialis (C6 input lost to musculocutaneous and radial nerves). A C7 root lesion would mimic a radial nerve lesion except that the brachioradialis (muscle and reflex) would be spared and shoulder adduction (latissimus dorsi) would be involved.

The muscles, nerves, and nerve roots associated with the commonly tested actions of the upper extremity are listed in Table 16–4 (categorized by action tested) and Table 16–5 (categorized by nerve tested) at the end of this chapter.

The movements of the thumb allow for three nerves to be tested: the median nerve for thumb abduction (abductor pollicis brevis; thumb out perpendicular to palm; Fig. 16–3A), the ulnar nerve for thumb adduction (adductor pollicis; thumb to palm; Fig. 16–3B), and the radial nerve for thumb extension (extensor pollicis longus and brevis; "thumbs up;" Fig. 16–3C). The opposition of the thumb and fifth finger is a median nerve–innervated action for the thumb (opponens pollicis) and an ulnar nerve–innervated action for the fifth finger (opponens digiti minimi).

Sensory Supply of the Hand (Fig. 16–4)

The region of sensation supplied by the median nerve includes the palmar surface of the thumb, index finger, middle finger,

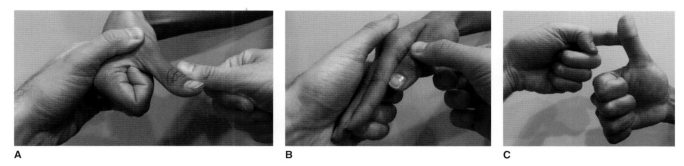

A   B   C

FIGURE 16–3 **Examination of three movements of the thumb to assess the three nerves innervating the hand. A: Assessment of abductor pollicis brevis (median nerve).** The patient is asked to rest the thumb on top of the closed fist and then to slide the thumb toward the midline "like a windshield wiper." Here, the left hand of the examiner prevents thumb extension while the right thumb of the examiner assesses the strength of thumb abduction. **B: Assessment of adductor pollicis (ulnar nerve).** The patient is asked to squeeze the thumb toward the palm and first finger "as if holding a dollar bill tightly between the thumb and hand," while the examiner tests the strength of adduction by trying to pull the thumb away from the hand. **C: Assessment of extensor pollicis longus and brevis (radial nerve).** The examiner asks the patient to give a "thumbs up" sign, and the examiner assesses the strength of thumb extension.

and lateral half (middle finger side) of the ring finger, and the palm proximal to the thumb and first two and a half fingers. The ulnar nerve supplies the rest of the palmar surface of the hand: the medial side (fifth finger side) of the ring finger, the fifth finger, and the palm immediately proximal to these. Although the ulnar nerve also supplies the dorsum of the hand corresponding to its palmar coverage (i.e., dorsal fifth finger and medial half of the ring finger), the median nerve's only sensory innervation on the dorsum of the hand is the dorsal finger tips and nail beds of the index, middle, and lateral half of the ring finger. The radial nerve (superficial sensory branch) covers the rest of the dorsum of the hand: the dorsal surface of the thumb, index finger, middle finger, lateral half of the ring finger up to the fingernails (which are supplied by the median nerve), and the dorsum of the hand proximal to these.

An important localization pearl is that the proximal thenar (thumb-side) palm, hypothenar (fifth-finger side) palm,

and dorsum of the hypothenar region are innervated by branches of the median and ulnar nerves that do not pass through the carpal tunnel (median nerve) or Guyon's canal (ulnar nerve) at the wrist. Therefore, in median and ulnar neuropathies at the wrist, these proximal regions of the hand will have intact sensation, whereas sensation will be impaired in lesions of the median or ulnar nerves proximal to the wrist (see "Median Neuropathy" and "Ulnar Neuropathy").

CERVICAL RADICULOPATHY & CERVICAL STENOSIS

Degenerative disease of the cervical spine can cause foraminal stenosis leading to radiculopathy and/or spinal canal stenosis leading to myelopathy (cervical stenosis).

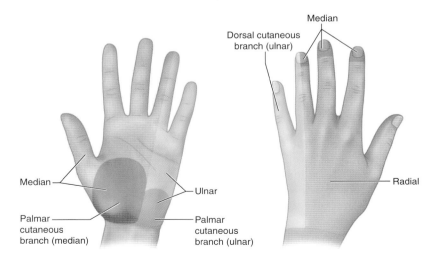

FIGURE 16–4 **Schematic showing sensory supply to the hand.**

Cervical Radiculopathy

The differential diagnosis for radiculopathy includes:

- Trauma: traumatic disc protrusion or root avulsion
- Degenerative disease of the spine: disc disease, spondylosis
- Neoplastic involvement of the roots: leptomeningeal metastases, neurolymphomatosis
- Infectious radiculitis: herpes simplex virus (HSV), cytomegalovirus (CMV), tabes dorsalis in syphilis, Lyme disease
- Inflammatory disease: acute and chronic inflammatory demyelinating polyradiculoneuropathy (AIDP and CIDP)

The most common cause of cervical radiculopathy is compression due to degenerative disc disease and/or spondylosis of the spine (**cervical spondylosis**). Disc material or osteophytes lead to neural foraminal stenosis, compressing nerve roots. The most common levels affected are C6-C7 (affecting the C7 root) and C5-C6 (affecting the C6 root), where the cervical spine is most mobile. The predominant symptom of cervical radiculopathy is neck pain that radiates in the distribution of the affected root(s) (see Fig. 16–1). In the affected dermatome(s), diminished sensation, diminished or absent reflexes (biceps and brachioradialis for C6, triceps for C7), and/or weakness (see Table 16–3) may be present depending on severity.

One examination maneuver to assess for radiculopathy as a cause of neck/upper extremity pain is **Spurling's maneuver**: The patient turns the head to the side of the pain and tilts the head back, and the examiner pushes down on top of the head. If radiating pain is reproduced by this maneuver, this is suggestive of cervical radiculopathy (if only local neck pain is reproduced, this is nonspecific).

If there is ambiguity between radiculopathy and neuropathy (e.g., C6 vs carpal tunnel syndrome or both, C8 vs ulnar neuropathy or both), EMG/nerve conduction studies can aid in localization. In pure radiculopathy (without concurrent neuropathy), sensory nerve action potentials (SNAPs) are *normal* because nerve conduction is measured distal to the dorsal root ganglion, and the dorsal root cannot be assessed by nerve conduction studies. EMG can be utilized to see if muscles with denervation changes are all referable to a single root as opposed to a nerve. Denervation changes in paraspinal muscles suggest radiculopathy because these muscles are innervated very proximally. (See Chapter 15 for discussion of EMG/nerve conduction studies.)

MRI can define the level(s) and degree of foraminal stenosis and can identify pathology other than disc disease/spondylosis (e.g., malignancy, inflammation; contrast should be administered if evaluating for these possibilities). MRI should be obtained in cases of intractable pain or progressive weakness for which surgery is under consideration, in patients with history of malignancy (to evaluate for metastatic disease), and in patients with back/neck pain accompanied by fever (to evaluate for epidural abscess). In patients

unable to undergo MRI, CT or CT myelography can be used. It should be noted that degenerative disc disease and spondylosis are often noted incidentally on MRI and may not be symptomatic, so clinical correlation between imaging and bedside findings is essential.

Initial management of cervical radiculopathy due to disc disease or spondylosis is nonsurgical unless there is intractable pain or a progressive motor deficit. When pain is the primary symptom, many patients will obtain relief with nonsteroidal anti-inflammatory drugs (NSAIDs) or acetaminophen (and/or a short oral steroid course) and physical therapy. Patients who do not respond to these conservative measures within 1–2 months can be considered for epidural steroid injection. In patients with intractable pain in spite of 2–3 months of conservative measures or in patients with progressive motor deficit, referral for surgical intervention may be considered.

Cervical Stenosis

Cervical spine disease can also cause myelopathy if the spinal cord is compressed (**central canal stenosis**). Patients present with gait disturbance, paresthesias, and/or weakness of the hands, and upper motor neuron signs in the upper and lower extremities (hyperreflexia, Babinski sign, Hoffmann sign, clonus, and/or spasticity). The patient may report electrical sensations shooting down the spine with forward flexion of the neck (**L'hermitte's sign**). Although L'hermitte's sign is classically associated with multiple sclerosis, it can be seen with cervical myelopathy due to any etiology. MRI reveals severe stenosis of the central canal and often demonstrates T2 hyperintensity in the spinal cord at the affected level(s) (Fig. 16–5). A characteristic "pancake-like" band of enhancement may be seen below the level of stenosis and may persist

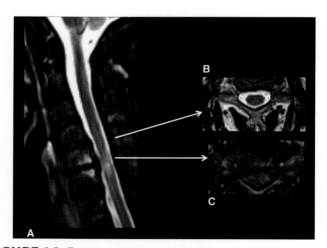

FIGURE 16–5 **MRI of the cervical spine in severe cervical stenosis (T2-weighted sequence). A:** Sagittal view of the cervical spine demonstrating severe stenosis at the C5-C6 level with T2 hyperintensity in the spinal cord at this level. An axial view at the C5-C6 level (**C**) shows complete loss of CSF signal surrounding the spinal cord as compared to the unaffected C4-C5 level (**B**).

after decompressive surgery (Flanagan et al., 2014). Cervical myelopathy due to degenerative spine disease is generally an indication for surgery.

BRACHIAL PLEXOPATHY

Pathology of individual plexus-derived nerves is discussed below. Brachial plexopathy is distinguished on examination by a combination of motor and/or sensory findings that cannot be attributed to specific individual nerves or roots, requiring localization to a cord, trunk, or multiple cords/trunks. Brachial plexopathy can be caused by pathology in the neck, upper chest, or axilla. Causes of brachial plexopathy include trauma (accidental injury, birth injury, surgical positioning), malignant compression/infiltration (most commonly breast or lung cancer), radiation therapy, and **Parsonage-Turner syndrome** (an inflammatory brachial plexitis also known as neuralgic amyotrophy; see "Parsonage-Turner Syndrome [Neuralgic Amyotrophy]").

Traumatic Brachial Plexopathy

Traumatic brachial plexopathy can occur due to:

- Injuries in which the shoulder is depressed, increasing traction on the upper brachial plexus between the neck and shoulder. Examples include motorcycle accidents in which the shoulder is the first point of contact with road, and birth canal trauma in which the infant's head is delivered before the shoulder and the infant's shoulder gets stuck (**shoulder dystocia**). With these types of injuries, the upper plexus (supplied by C5-C6) is affected leading to upper arm weakness with sparing of the hand (which is supplied largely by C8-T1), called **Erb-Duchenne palsy**.

- Injuries in which the axilla is stretched, causing traction on the lower brachial plexus. Examples include a patient's arm getting caught in a machine, a patient falling from a height and hanging on by the arm, or birth canal trauma in which there is traction on the arm of the infant. With these types of injuries, the lower plexus (supplied by C8-T1) is affected, leading to paralysis of the hand, but sparing of the upper arm (which is supplied largely by C5-C6), called **Klumpke palsy** (mnemonic: E and D are alphabetically before K, and Erb-Duchenne affects roots that are superior to Klumpke: C5-C6 for Erb-Duchenne palsy vs C8-T1 for Klumpke palsy).

- Penetrating injuries to the axilla.

- Surgical injury: axillary dissection, subclavian puncture, surgical positioning of arm, sternotomy causing compression of the brachial plexus.

- Compression: either sustained (e.g., backpack strap in **rucksack paralysis**) or forceful and transient (e.g., helmet of one football player impinges on the shoulder of another, called **stinger syndrome** or **burner syndrome**).

Neoplastic & Radiation-Induced Plexopathy

The brachial plexus is most susceptible to neoplastic compression near the lung apex (most commonly due to lung cancer [called a **Pancoast tumor** in this location]) and in the axilla (most commonly due to axillary lymph node disease due to breast cancer metastases or lymphoma). Compression or infiltration of the plexus is often painful and the lower plexus is more commonly affected, causing weakness predominantly in the hand. Since the sympathetic fibers to the face are supplied by C8-T1, malignant infiltration of the plexus may also cause Horner's syndrome (ptosis, miosis, and anhidrosis; see "Impaired Pupillary Dilation" in Ch. 10). Primary tumors of the plexus (e.g., neurofibroma or schwanomma) occur rarely (see Ch. 24). Contrast-enhanced MRI of the plexus can be used to look for evidence of tumor.

Radiation damage to the plexus can also cause a plexopathy, and the interval between radiation and development of symptoms can be as long as years in some cases, raising concern for tumor recurrence. Features more suggestive of radiation plexopathy are:

- Lack of pain (pain is a hallmark of neoplastic infiltration of the plexus)

- Upper plexus involvement (lower plexus involvement is more common in neoplastic infiltration of the brachial plexus)

- Myokymic discharges on EMG (not present in neoplastic infiltration of the brachial plexus)

Parsonage-Turner Syndrome (Neuralgic Amyotrophy)

Parsonage-Turner syndrome is an inflammatory brachial plexopathy that often occurs following a physiologic stress such as systemic infection, surgery, vigorous exercise, or childbirth. Severe axillary and/or shoulder pain is the initial symptom, and weakness in the arm subsequently emerges over hours to weeks. Weakness tends to involve upper plexus–innervated muscles (muscles of the shoulder and upper arm), although the lower plexus may be involved. Two nerves commonly affected in Parsonage-Turner syndrome are the long thoracic nerve (causing winging of the scapula) and the anterior interosseous nerve (causing weakness in flexion of the distal thumb, flexion of the distal index finger and middle finger, and forearm pronation). Sensory loss may be present, but weakness usually predominates. Rarely, bilateral findings can occur, usually asymmetrically. Most patients spontaneously recover completely over months to years. Analgesics and physical therapy are the key components of supportive management, and treatment with a short course of steroids may be considered. Recurrent attacks and family history suggest the rare inherited form of the condition (hereditary neuralgic amyotrophy, which is usually autosomal dominant due to mutation in *SEPT9* gene).

MONONEUROPATHIES OF THE UPPER EXTREMITY

Mononeuropathies of the upper extremities are most commonly caused by entrapment (due to pressure or overuse injury), surgical positioning, or upper extremity trauma. An acute-onset painful mononeuropathy without clear inciting factor should lead to consideration of nerve infarct as can be seen in vasculitic neuropathy (see Ch. 15).

Median Neuropathy

Carpal Tunnel Syndrome

The most common site of median nerve entrapment is in the carpal tunnel at the wrist (**carpal tunnel syndrome**) where the median nerve enters the hand along with the finger flexor tendons. Occupations and hobbies requiring repetitive wrist movements and/or sustained grip are common causes. Obesity, endocrinopathy (e.g., acromegaly, hypothyroidism), pregnancy, and arthritis are predisposing factors. Patients typically complain of pain and paresthesias in the hand, especially at night, and may report that shaking the hand relieves the symptoms. Although the median nerve sensory distribution only covers the palmar aspects of the thumb and first two and a half fingers (index, middle, and lateral half of ring finger) and the nail beds of these digits on the dorsum of the hand (see Fig. 16–4), it is not uncommon for patients to describe pain and/or paresthesias in the whole hand, and even ascending into the arm.

On examination, pinprick sensation may be diminished in the palmar aspect of the thumb, index finger, middle finger, and lateral half of the ring finger (i.e., middle finger side of the ring finger) compared to the palmar aspect of the fifth finger and medial half of the ring finger (i.e., fifth finger side of the ring finger). A very helpful localizing finding when present is diminished pinprick sensation that splits the ring finger: diminished on the middle finger side of the ring finger (median nerve supplied) compared to the fifth finger side (ulnar nerve supplied). Cervical radiculopathy (C6, C7, C8) can also cause sensory changes in the thumb and fingers, but will not cause the pattern of split sensory loss in the ring finger seen in median or ulnar neuropathy (see Figs. 16–1 and 16–4). Another helpful localizing sensory finding in median neuropathy at the wrist is the sparing of pinprick sensation over the proximal portion of the palm on the thumb side because this is innervated by the palmar cutaneous nerve, which is a median nerve branch that does not pass through the carpal tunnel.

When weakness is present in carpal tunnel syndrome, it is most commonly noted in the abductor pollicis brevis. This muscle can be isolated by asking the patient to slide the thumb toward the midline "like a windshield wiper" (abduction) against the examiner's thumb while the examiner isolates abduction by preventing thumb extension (see Fig. 16–3A). Weakness may be absent in mild cases of carpal tunnel syndrome. In advanced cases, atrophy of the thenar eminence may be present.

Tinel's sign can be elicited by tapping over the carpal tunnel and assessing for reproduction of the patient's symptoms. **Phalen's sign** can be elicited by having the patient flex the wrists and push the dorsal surfaces of the wrists together in a "reverse prayer" position for 30 seconds to see if symptoms are reproduced. These signs are not universally present in patients with carpal tunnel syndrome, and may be present in patients without the disorder, so they are both insensitive and nonspecific.

When patients present with pain and paresthesias in the hand and have sensory findings in the lateral hand and thumb, a distinction must be made between carpal tunnel syndrome and cervical radiculopathy. Radiculopathy typically causes neck pain and radiation of pain down the arm, although it may be hard to tease this apart from painful paresthesias in the hand extending up the arm that some patients describe in carpal tunnel syndrome. If abductor pollicis brevis weakness and sensory symptoms in the thumb are both present in isolation, this suggests carpal tunnel syndrome since the sensory supply of the thumb is C6, but the motor supply of abductor pollicis brevis is C8, and both C6 and C8 have more extensive sensory and motor distributions beyond the thumb.

EMG/nerve conduction studies can be used to confirm the diagnosis of carpal tunnel syndrome and assess the severity. The classic finding is slowing of median nerve conduction across the wrist. (Electro-diagnosis in carpal tunnel syndrome can be more challenging in patients with a **Martin-Gruber anastomosis**, a variant in which the median and ulnar nerves are connected.)

For mild cases of carpal tunnel syndrome, treatment is conservative, with rest from repetitive activities of the hand(s) and a wrist splint to avoid continued irritation of the median nerve. NSAIDs can be used for pain, with steroid injections sometimes used in severe cases. In moderate to severe cases, surgical release can lead to improvement. After surgery, pain may improve more rapidly than weakness or numbness, which may not improve completely depending on the duration and severity of symptoms at the time of surgery.

Median Neuropathy Proximal to the Carpal Tunnel

Referring to Table 16–1, note that all forearm muscles innervated by the median nerve are innervated *proximal* to the carpal tunnel. Therefore, weakness of flexion at the distal interphalangeal (DIP) joint (flexor digitorum profundus) of the index or middle finger or weakness of flexion at any of the proximal interphalangeal joints (flexor digitorum superficialis) suggests median nerve pathology proximal to the carpal tunnel. Referring to Figure 16–4, recall that the sensory supply of the thenar eminence is innervated by the palmar cutaneous branch of the median nerve, which does *not* pass through the carpal tunnel. Sensory loss on the thenar eminence is therefore another clue to a localization proximal to the carpal tunnel such as the proximal median nerve, brachial plexus, or C6 root.

Ligament of Struthers—This is a rare anatomic variant that can cause median nerve entrapment just above the elbow, leading to complete loss of median nerve function. The clinical findings are identical to median nerve pathology at its origin in the axilla (since the median nerve does not innervate any muscles proximal to the elbow), although pathology in the axilla often affects additional nerves of the brachial plexus.

Anterior Interosseous Nerve & Anterior Interosseous Neuropathy

The **anterior interosseous nerve** (**AIN**) is a pure motor branch of the median nerve that arises just distal to the elbow and innervates three muscles: pronator quadratus, flexor pollicis longus, and flexor digitorum profundus for the index and middle fingers. Since pronator teres (innervated by the median nerve, but not the AIN) also participates in pronation, the main findings in anterior interosseous neuropathy are loss of ability to flex the thumb and first two fingers at the DIP joint. This leads to inability to make the "OK sign" due to impaired flexion of the distal phalanges of the thumb and index finger. The AIN can be affected by trauma or surgical intervention in the proximal forearm (e.g., placement of a dialysis fistula) and is often one of the nerves affected in Parsonage-Turner syndrome.

Ulnar Neuropathy

The ulnar nerve can be palpated just superior to the medial epicondyle of the humerus: Plucking your ulnar nerve here will cause paresthesias in the medial hand, the basis of the "funny bone" phenomenon. The most common site of ulnar nerve entrapment is this location at the medial elbow, although compression can also occur at Guyon's canal at the wrist. Ulnar nerve entrapment at the elbow can occur due to direct compression (leaning on the elbow, sleeping on the elbow, coma), prolonged flexion (sleeping on the flexed elbow, practicing the violin), or years after elbow injury (**tardy ulnar palsy**). Entrapment at the wrist can be caused by prolonged pressure (e.g., after a long bicycle ride) or due to a ganglion cyst in Guyon's canal.

Patients with ulnar nerve entrapment at the elbow typically present with paresthesias in the palmar aspect of the fifth finger. Although the ulnar nerve travels through the arm and forearm, its sensory territory is *entirely distal to the wrist*. The sensory supply to the medial upper arm and forearm comes from the medial brachial cutaneous nerve and the medial antebrachial cutaneous nerves, which arise directly from the medial cord of the brachial plexus. Therefore, sensory deficits proximal to the wrist along the medial forearm suggest a lesion at the level of the medial cord, lower trunk, or C8 rather than ulnar neuropathy.

Sensory findings in ulnar neuropathy only occur distal to the wrist, involving the fifth finger, the medial half of the ring finger (the lateral half is median nerve-innervated), and the corresponding areas of the palm and dorsum of the hand. Notably, however, the region of the palm between the wrist and the ring finger and fifth finger, and the entire dorsal coverage of the fifth finger and medial portion of the ring finger are supplied by branches that do *not* pass through Guyon's canal (the palmar and dorsal cutaneous nerves; see Fig. 16–4). Therefore, sensation should be preserved in these regions in ulnar neuropathy at the wrist, but diminished in ulnar neuropathy at the elbow.

When ulnar neuropathy causes weakness, the following actions (muscles) are affected: finger abduction (dorsal interossei and abductor digiti minimi), finger adduction (palmar interossei), thumb adduction (adductor pollicis), and fifth finger opposition (opponens digiti minimi). A classic clinical sign demonstrating thumb adduction weakness is **Froment's sign**: A piece of paper is placed between the thumb and index finger, and the patient is asked to hold the paper while the examiner pulls. In ulnar neuropathy, the patient will flex the thumb and index finger (median nerve–innervated actions) into an "OK sign" to compensate for weak thumb adduction and index finger abduction (both ulnar nerve–innervated actions).

Flexor carpi ulnaris and flexor digitorum profundus for the ring finger and fifth finger are forearm muscles and so they are innervated proximal to the wrist. When weakness in these muscles is present due to ulnar neuropathy, this signifies ulnar neuropathy at the elbow rather than the wrist. Weakness in flexor digitorum profundus of the ring finger and fifth finger can be assessed by asking the patient to flex all four distal finger tips at the DIP joints against resistance. A difference in strength here as opposed to strength in flexor digitorum profundus of the index finger and middle finger allows for comparison of ulnar nerve–innervated muscles and median nerve–innervated muscles performing the same action. Patients with mild ulnar neuropathy may have no weakness if they present early in the course of the ulnar neuropathy, and may have sensory changes isolated to the fifth finger as the only symptom/sign.

Although a Tinel's sign at the elbow may be present in patients with ulnar nerve entrapment at the elbow, you will find that if you tap your own ulnar nerve hard enough at the medial epicondyle, a Tinel's sign may be produced, so this can be a nonspecific finding.

Nerve conduction studies are helpful in determining the site of ulnar nerve pathology if it is not clear clinically: slowing can be found either across the elbow or across the wrist. If the entrapment is located at the wrist, ultrasound or MRI should be performed to look for a ganglion cyst unless there is a clear history of occupational or hobby-related etiology of compression at the wrist.

With mild findings in ulnar neuropathy at the elbow, patients can be counseled not to lean on the elbow and not to sleep on the affected side, although the latter may be difficult given that it is generally not a conscious decision. A flexible elbow splint can prevent further irritation of the nerve by inhibiting elbow flexion, and wearing the splint at night can prevent involuntary flexion of the arm during sleep. The elbow can also simply be wrapped loosely in a towel at night to prevent flexion. Severe cases may require surgical release or ulnar nerve transposition surgery.

Radial Neuropathy

Mnemonic: the radial nerve is the "BEST": it innervates the **b**rachioradialis, **e**xtensors (all forearm, hand, and finger extensors), **s**upinator, and **t**riceps. The hallmark of a radial neuropathy is wrist drop due to weakness of wrist and finger extension. A key localizing feature is whether or not the triceps and its reflex are involved because the triceps is innervated proximal to the spiral groove of the humerus, and so it will only be involved in lesions proximal to this region (i.e., in the axilla). The radial nerve can be compressed in the axilla by the use of crutches (triceps will be affected since the nerve is affected proximal to the spiral groove), or in the upper arm by a humerus fracture or falling asleep with the arm in a position that compresses the radial nerve (e.g., draped over a chair; called "Saturday night palsy" since it can occur in the setting of alcohol intoxication).

The radial nerve does not innervate any intrinsic hand muscles—these are all innervated by the median and ulnar nerves. However, the examiner can be deceived into thinking that intrinsic hand muscles are involved in radial neuropathy if these muscles are not tested properly. Try it: Allow your wrist to flex limply forward and then try to abduct or flex your fingers. You will see that this is harder to do if the wrist is flexed compared to if the wrist is level, due to the tension in the fingers from the extensor tendons when the wrist is flexed. To test the intrinsic hand muscles in order to evaluate for additional weakness beyond radial nerve involvement in a patient with a wrist drop, the hand must be in a neutral position such as flat on a table.

Diagnosis of radial neuropathy is usually clinically evident based on the pattern of weakness, but EMG/nerve conduction studies can be performed if the site of compression is unclear, or for prognosis. Most compressive radial nerve palsies recover within weeks to months, and a wrist splint may be worn during the period of recovery to maximize function of the intrinsic muscles of the hand.

A small stroke in the hand area of the motor cortex (precentral gyrus) can imitate a radial nerve palsy (called pseudo-radial nerve palsy) since upper motor neuron pattern upper extremity weakness can disproportionately affect the extensors, triceps, and supinator, which are all radial nerve-innervated muscles. Additionally, acute-onset upper motor neuron lesions (e.g., stroke) generally cause hyporeflexia and flaccidity in the acute setting, similar to findings with a peripheral lesion. If a patient awakens with this pattern of arm weakness, the acuity of onset may be unclear. When uncertain, brain imaging should be obtained, especially in patients with vascular risk factors.

The radial nerve supplies sensation over the posterior and lower lateral upper arm and forearm (**posterior cutaneous nerve of arm**, **lower lateral cutaneous nerve of arm**), posterior forearm (**posterior cutaneous nerve of forearm**), and the dorsum of the index, middle, and lateral half of the ring finger up to the fingernail beds and dorsum of the hand from this region to the wrist (**superficial sensory branch**). On the dorsum of the hand, the superficial sensory branch of the radial nerve mirrors the median nerve's role on the front of the hand (except for the nail beds of the index finger, middle finger, and lateral half of the ring finger, which are the only median nerve–innervated sensory regions on the dorsum of the hand). The ulnar nerve provides sensation to both the palm and dorsum of the hand on the medial (ulnar) side, the fifth finger, and the medial half of the fourth finger.

Reviewing the sensory supply of the hand, the sensory supply to the palm is split between the median and ulnar nerves, and the dorsum of hand is split between radial and ulnar nerves except the fingernail beds of the index finger, middle finger, and lateral half of the ring finger, which are supplied by the median nerve (Fig. 16–4). Isolated involvement of the superficial sensory branch of the radial nerve (**Wartenberg's syndrome**) can therefore produce sensory symptoms over the dorsum of the hand including the thumb, index finger, middle finger, and lateral half of the ring finger, but will spare sensation in the nail beds of these fingers (median nerve-innervated) and in the dorsum of the fifth finger and the medial half of the ring finger (ulnar nerve-innervated). Isolated involvement of the superficial sensory branch of the radial nerve can be caused by compression of this nerve by handcuffs or an arm cast compressing the dorsal wrist.

Posterior Interosseous Nerve & Posterior Interosseous Neuropathy

The **posterior interosseous nerve** (**PIN**) is a pure motor branch of the radial nerve that supplies all radial nerve–innervated muscles except the triceps, brachioradialis, and extensor carpi radialis longus. The PIN can rarely be affected in isolation causing isolated weakness of finger and thumb extension and radial deviation of the wrist on wrist extension (due to weakness of extensor carpi ulnaris with preserved strength in extensor carpi radialis). Common causes of posterior interosseous neuropathy include trauma to the elbow and repetitive arm movements (occupational or hobby). A common site of entrapment is at the **arcade of Frohse**, a tendinous arch at the origin of the supinator muscle.

Axillary & Musculocutaneous Neuropathies

The axillary and musculocutaneous nerves have shorter courses than the other upper extremity nerves described thus far since they only innervate muscles in the upper arm. Although these nerves can rarely be involved in isolation (e.g., due to shoulder/upper arm trauma or surgical positioning), this is sufficiently uncommon that weakness in axillary nerve–innervated muscles (deltoid: shoulder abduction) or musculocutaneous nerve–innervated muscles (biceps: elbow flexion) requires a careful search for other involved muscle groups and consideration of a brachial plexopathy.

REFERENCE

Flanagan EP, Krecke KN, Marsh RW, Giannini C, Keegan BM, Weinshenker BG. Specific pattern of gadolinium enhancement in spondylotic myelopathy. *Ann Neurol* 2014;76:54-65.

TABLE 16–1 Innervation of the Upper Extremity.[a]

Nerve	Muscles			Sensory		
	Upper Arm	Forearm	Hand	Upper Arm	Forearm	Hand
Musculocutaneous nerve (C5-C6)	*Biceps* Brachialis				Lateral cutaneous nerve of forearm	
Axillary nerve (C5-C6)	Deltoid Teres minor			Upper lateral cutaneous nerve of arm		
Radial nerve (C5-T1)	*Triceps*	**S** *Brachioradialis* **P** Extensor carpi radialis longus **I** Extensor carpi radialis brevis **R** Extensor carpi ulnaris **A** Extensor digitorum communis **L** Extensor indicis proprius **G** Extensor digiti minimi **R** Extensor pollicis longus **O** Extensor pollicis brevis **O** Supinator **V** **E**	Posterior interosseous nerve	Posterior cutaneous nerve of arm Lower lateral cutaneous nerve of arm	Posterior cutaneous nerve of forearm	Superficial radial sensory nerve

Median nerve (C5-T1)

Pronator teres
Flexor carpi radialis
Flexor digitorum superficialis
Palmaris longus

Anterior interosseous nerve:
- Pronator quadratus
- Flexor pollicis longus
- Flexor digitorum profundus 1 and 2

CARPAL TUNNEL:
- Abductor pollicis brevis
- Flexor pollicis brevis[b]
- Opponens pollicis
- Lumbricals 1 and 2

Palmar cutaneous
Digital cutaneous

Ulnar nerve (C8-T1)

Flexor carpi ulnaris
Flexor digitorum profundus 3 and 4

GUYON'S CANAL:
- Adductor pollicis
- Flexor pollicis brevis[b]
- Opponens digiti minimi
- Flexor digiti minimi
- Abductor digiti minimi
- Palmar interossei
- Dorsal interossei
- Lumbricals 3 and 4

Palmar cutaneous
Dorsal cutaneous
Superficial terminal branch

[a]Muscles in **bold/italics** have associated reflexes (biceps, brachioradialis, and triceps).

[b]The flexor pollicis brevis muscle receives dual innervation from the median and ulnar nerves.

TABLE 16–2 Innervation of the Hand.

| | Wrist Flexors | | Forearm Finger Flexors | | Intrinsic Hand Muscles | | | |
					Thumb		Index, Middle, and Ring Fingers	Fifth Finger
Median nerve	Flexor carpi radialis	Palmaris longus	Flexor digitorum superficialis	Flexor digitorum profundus 1 and 2	Abductor pollicis brevis Opponens Pollicis	Flexor pollicis longus Flexor pollicis brevis[a]	Lumbricals 1 and 2	
Ulnar nerve	Flexor carpi ulnaris	Palmaris brevis		Flexor digitorum profundus 3 and 4	Adductor pollicis	Flexor pollicis brevis[a]	Lumbricals 3 and 4 Palmar and dorsal interossei	Abductor digiti minimi Opponens digiti minimi Flexor digiti minimi
	Wrist Extensors		**Forearm Finger Extensors**		**Extrinsic Muscles of the Thumb**			
Radial nerve	Extensor carpi radialis Extensor carpi ulnaris		Extensor digitorum communis Extensor indicis proprius Extensor digiti minimi		Abductor pollicis longus	Extensor pollicis longus Extensor pollicis brevis		

[a]The flexor pollicis brevis muscle receives dual innervation from the median and ulnar nerves.

TABLE 16–3 Root & Nerve Supply of the Muscles of the Upper Extremity.[a]

	C5	C6	C7	C8	T1
Axillary nerve	Deltoid	Teres minor			
Suprascapular nerve	Supraspinatus	Infraspinatus			
Long thoracic nerve		Serratus anterior			
Thoracodorsal nerve			Latissimus dorsi		
Musculocutaneous nerve	**Biceps**				
Radial nerve	**Brachioradialis**				
		Supinator			
		Extensor carpi radialis			
			Triceps		
			Extensor carpi ulnaris		
			Extensor pollicis		
			Extensor indicis proprius		
			Extensor digitorum communis		
Median nerve		Pronator teres			
		Flexor carpi radialis			
Ulnar nerve			Flexor digitorum superficialis		
				Pronator quadratus	
				Flexor digitorum profundus 1 and 2	
				Lumbricals 1 and 2	
				Abductor pollicis brevis	
				Flexor pollicis brevis	
				Flexor pollicis longus	
				Opponens pollicis	
				Flexor carpi ulnaris	
				Flexor digitorum profundus 3 and 4	
				Palmar and dorsal interossei	
				Lumbricals 3 and 4	
				Adductor pollicis	
				Opponens digiti minimi	
				Abductor digiti minimi	

[a]Muscles in bold have associated reflexes.

TABLE 16–4 Examination of the Upper Extremities by Action.

Action	Muscle	Nerve	Roots
Shoulder elevation	Trapezius	CN 11 (spinal accessory nerve)	
Abduction of upper arm (raising arm like a chicken wing)			
First 15–30 degrees	Supraspinatus	Suprascapular	C5-C6
Beyond 15–30 degrees	Deltoid	Axillary	C5-C6
Adduction of upper arm	Teres major	Lower subscapular	C5-C6
External rotation of upper arm	Infraspinatus	Suprascapular	C5-C6
	Teres minor	Axillary	C5-C6
Elbow flexion			
With forearm supinated	Biceps	Musculocutaneous	C5-C6
With forearm half-pronated (bottom of fist on table)	Brachioradialis	Radial	C5-C6
Elbow extension	Triceps	Radial	C7-C8
Wrist flexion	Flexor carpi radialis	Median	C6-C7
	Flexor carpi ulnaris	Ulnar	C8-T1
Wrist extension	Extensor carpi radialis	Radial	C6-C7
	Extensor carpi ulnaris	Radial	C7-C8
Four movements of the thumb			
Abduction (thumb out 90 degrees from palm/first finger)	Abductor pollicis brevis	Median	C8-T1
Opposition (thumb to fifth finger)	Opponens pollicis	Median	C8-T1
Adduction (thumb to side of index finger)	Adductor pollicis	Ulnar	C8-T1
Extension (thumbs up)	Extensor pollicis longus and brevis	Radial	C7-C8
Flexion of the fingers at the PIP joint	Flexor digitorum superficialis	Median	C7-C8-T1
Flexion of the fingers at the DIP joint			
Index and middle finger	Flexor digitorum profundus 1 and 2	Median	C8-T1
Ring and fifth finger	Flexor digitorum profundus 3 and 4	Ulnar	C8-T1
All extensors of fingers and thumb	Extensor digitorum communis	Radial	C7-C8
	Extensor indicis proprius		
	Extensor digiti minimi		
	Extensor pollicis longus		
	Extensor pollicis brevis		
Intrinsic non-thumb muscles of the hand (all ulnar except first and second lumbricals)			
Adduction of fingers	Palmar interossei	Ulnar	C8-T1
Abduction of fingers	Dorsal interossei	Ulnar	C8-T1
Flexion at the MCP joint while extending at PIP/DIP joints			
Index and middle finger	Lumbricals 1 and 2	Median	C8-T1
Ring and fifth finger	Lumbricals 3 and 4	Ulnar	C8-T1

Abbreviations: DIP: distal interphalangeal joint; MCP: metacarpal-phalangeal joint; PIP: proximal interphalangeal joint.

TABLE 16-5 Examination of the Upper Extremities by Nerve.

Nerve	Action	Muscle	Nerve Roots
Suprascapular nerve	Upper arm abduction first 15–30 degrees (raising arm like chicken wing)	Supraspinatus	C5-C6
	Upper arm adduction	Infraspinatus	C5-C6
Long thoracic nerve	Examine for scapular winging	Serratus anterior	C5-C6-C7
Axillary nerve	Abduction of upper arm (raising arm like a chicken wing)	Deltoid	C5-C6
Musculocutaneous nerve	Flexion at elbow of supinated forearm	Biceps	C5-C6
Radial nerve	Flexion at elbow of half-pronated forearm (fist on table)	Brachioradialis	C5-C6
	Extension of elbow	Triceps	C7-C8
	Extension of wrist in radial direction	Extensor carpi radialis	C6-C7
Posterior interosseous branch of radial nerve	Supination of forearm	Supinator	C6-C7
	Extension of wrist in ulnar direction	Extensor carpi ulnaris	C7-C8
	Extension of fingers	Extensor digitorum communis	C7-C8
		Extensor indicis proprius	C7-C8
		Extensor digiti minimi	C7-C8
		Extensor pollicis (longus and brevis)	C7-C8
Median nerve	Forearm pronation	Pronator teres	C6-C7
	Flexion of wrist in radial direction	Flexor carpi radialis	C6-C7
	Flexion of all fingers at PIP joint	Flexor digitorum superficialis	C8-T1
	Abduction of thumb (perpendicular to plane of palm)	Abductor pollicis brevis	C8-T1
	Thumb to fifth finger (thumb movement)	Opponens pollicis	C8-T1
	Flexion of index and middle fingers at MCP while extending at PIP/DIP joints	Lumbricals 1 and 2	C8-T1
Anterior interosseous branch of median nerve	OK sign	Flexor pollicis longus and flexor digitorum profundus 1	C8-T1
	Flexion of index and middle fingers at DIP joint	Flexor digitorum profundus 1 and 2	C8-T1
Ulnar nerve	Flexion of wrist in ulnar direction	Flexor carpi ulnaris	C8-T1
	Flexion of ring and fifth fingers at DIP joint	Flexor digitorum profundus 3 and 4	C8-T1
	Adduction of thumb to palm	Adductor pollicis	C8-T1
	Abduction of fingers (spreading fingers apart)	Dorsal interossei	C8-T1
	Adduction of fingers (holding fingers together)	Palmar interossei	C8-T1
	Fifth finger to thumb (fifth finger movement)	Opponens digiti minimi	C8-T1
	Flexion of fifth finger	Flexor digiti minimi	C8-T1
	Abduction of fifth finger	Abductor digiti minimi	C8-T1
	Flexion of ring and fifth fingers at MCP while extending at PIP/DIP joints	Lumbricals 3 and 4	C8-T1

Abbreviations: DIP: distal interphalangeal joint; MCP: metacarpal-phalangeal joint; PIP: proximal interphalangeal joint.

Radiculopathy, Plexopathy, & Mononeuropathies of the Lower Extremity

NEUROANATOMY OF THE LOWER EXTREMITY

Anatomy of the Nerve Roots of the Lower Extremity

At the thoracic, lumbar, and sacral levels, roots are numbered by the vertebral level *below* which they exit: The T1 roots exit below the T1 vertebra (between the T1 and T2 vertebrae), the L1 roots exit below the L1 vertebra (between the L1 and L2 vertebrae), and the S1 roots exit below the S1 vertebra (between the S1 and S2 vertebrae). The spinal cord ends at the L1-L2 vertebral level and the lumbar and sacral roots must therefore descend to reach the vertebral levels at which they exit. These descending roots are referred to as the **cauda equina** (see Fig. 15-1).

The sensory supply to the anterior thigh is covered by L1, L2, and L3 in three diagonal stripes running from proximal/lateral to distal/medial. L4, L5, and S1 cover the anterior shin in vertical stripes from medial to lateral: L4 covers the medial knee, medial shin, and instep; L5 covers the anterior and lateral shin and dorsum of the foot; and S1 the covers the distal lateral calf and lateral aspect and plantar surface of the foot (Fig. 17–1). A mnemonic way to remember the dermatomes of the lower extremity is to place your hands on your hips pointing inward/downward and then pat the thighs three times moving distally toward the knee (L1, L2, L3). From the

knee, point the hands directly downward toward the feet and pat the shins three times from medial to lateral (L4, L5, S1). This medial-to-lateral pattern continues on the foot with the medial foot (instep) supplied by L4, the lateral foot supplied by S1, and the majority of the dorsum of the foot supplied by L5 between the medial L4 and lateral S1 dermatomes.

The posterior middle thigh and calf are supplied by S1 (laterally) and S2 (medially), and the S1 and S2 dermatomes are bounded by L3-L4 medially and L5 laterally (see also Fig. 15-2).

To learn the motor actions controlled by each root, practice moving through the sequence of tested muscle groups from proximal to distal in front, then from proximal to distal in back, naming the roots as you move the associated muscles (Fig. 17–2): L2-L3 (hip flexion), L3-L4 (knee extension), L4-L5 (dorsiflexion of the foot), L5-S1 (hip extension), L5-S1 (knee flexion), S1-S2 (plantarflexion of the foot). All root pairs in the movement sequence are overlapping and in sequence, but note that L5-S1 is repeated for both hip extension and knee flexion. Hip adduction is supplied by L2-L4 and hip abduction predominantly by L5.

Anatomy of the Lumbosacral Plexus & the Nerves of the Lower Extremity

The lower extremity is supplied by nerve roots L1 through S3. These nerve roots converge to form the lumbosacral plexus,

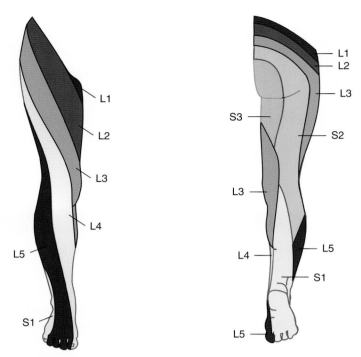

FIGURE 17–1 **Schematic showing dermatomes of the leg**. Reproduced with permission from Waxman *S: Clinical Neuroanatomy*, 27th ed. New York, NY: McGraw Hill; 2013.

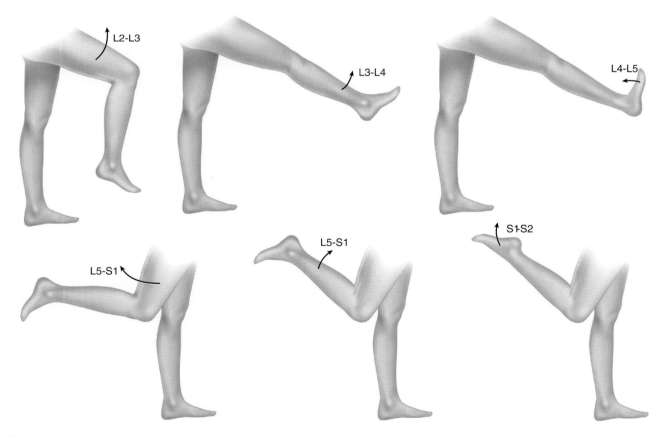

FIGURE 17–2 Schematic showing nerve roots supplying actions of the leg and foot.

which is divided into the lumbar plexus and the sacral plexus. Although diagrams of the lumbosacral plexus look equally as complex as those of the brachial plexus, localization is more straightforward since the foot is not as intricately controlled as the hand. Before going into the details, note that in general the lumbar plexus (L1-L4) only supplies muscles of the hip and thigh (though not all of them), and the sacral plexus (L4-S4) supplies all muscles distal to the knee (as well as muscles of the posterior and lateral hip and thigh that are not supplied by the lumbar plexus).

The L1-L4 roots supply the lumbar plexus, which innervates the muscles of the anterior and medial hip and thigh and provides sensory innervation to the anterior, medial, and lateral thigh, as well as the medial foot and shin. The sensory innervation of the medial foot and shin is supplied by the saphenous nerve, which is the only below-the-knee function of the lumbar plexus.

The functions of the lumbar plexus include (Table 17–1):

- Motor
  - **Femoral nerve**: iliopsoas (hip flexion) and quadriceps (knee extension and patellar reflex)
  - **Obturator nerve**: adductor muscles (hip/thigh adduction)
- Sensation
  - **Anterior thigh**: femoral nerve
  - **Medial thigh**: branches of the femoral and obturator nerves
  - **Lateral thigh**: lateral femoral cutaneous nerve
  - **Medial shin and foot**: saphenous nerve, a branch of the femoral nerve (Mnemonic to remember the origin of the saphenous nerve: sa**ph**enous nerve arises from **f**emoral nerve)

The lumbar plexus also supplies the ilioinguinal, iliohypogastric, and genitofemoral nerves, which supply the muscles of the lower abdominal wall and sensation in the inguinal region. These nerves are rarely affected clinically.

The L4-S4 roots supply the sacral plexus, which innervates all muscles below the knee as well as the muscles of the lateral and posterior thigh. The sensory supply of the sacral plexus covers the posterior thigh, and the shin, calf, and foot except for the medial shin/foot (supplied by the saphenous nerve from the lumbar plexus). The functions of the sacral plexus include (Table 17–1):

- Motor:
  - **Superior and inferior gluteal nerves**: gluteal muscles (superior gluteal nerve: gluteus medius and minimus (hip abduction); inferior gluteal nerve: gluteus maximus [hip extension])
  - **Sciatic nerve**: The sciatic nerve is composed of two component nerves that diverge at the level of the knee: the peroneal nerve and the tibial nerve. The sciatic nerve supplies the hamstring muscles, which are responsible for knee flexion (biceps femoris, semitendinosus, semimembranosus; all innervated by tibial division except the short head of the biceps femoris, discussed further below). The peroneal and tibial nerves supply all motor function below the knee, and all sensory function below the knee aside from the saphenous nerve territory (medial shin and foot).

  - **Peroneal nerve**: muscles of the lateral and anterior compartment of the shin/calf (tibialis anterior, peroneus longus, and brevis: ankle dorsiflexion and eversion; extensors of the toes)
  - **Tibial nerve**: muscles of the medial and posterior compartment of the shin/calf and intrinsic muscles of the foot (gastrocnemius, soleus, tibialis posterior: ankle plantar flexion and inversion; flexors of the toes)
- Sensation:
  - **Posterior thigh and calf**: posterior femoral cutaneous nerve
  - **Anterior and lateral shin and foot**: peroneal nerve
  - **Plantar surface of the foot**: tibial nerve branches

The overlap of roots and nerves for the main clinically tested lower extremity muscles is shown in Table 17–2. Muscle names in bold also have associated reflexes. The muscles are listed across from the nerve that supplies them and under the most prominent root supply (most muscles receive root supply from 1-3 adjacent nerve roots). This chart can aid in differentiating between nerve and root lesions based on the pattern of weak muscles.

The muscles, nerves, and nerve roots associated with the commonly tested actions of the lower extremity are listed in Table 17–3 (categorized by action tested) and Table 17–4 (categorized by nerve tested).

LUMBOSACRAL RADICULOPATHY & LUMBAR CANAL STENOSIS

Degenerative disease of the spine can lead to neural foraminal stenosis and central canal stenosis in the lumbar spine just as in the cervical spine. Just as in the cervical spine, foraminal stenosis can lead to radiculopathy. However, although central canal stenosis at the cervical and thoracic levels can lead to myelopathy, central canal stenosis in the lumbosacral region cannot cause myelopathy since the spinal cord ends at the beginning of the lumbar spine, with only the nerve roots of the cauda equina below the level of L2. Central canal stenosis in the lumbosacral region can therefore lead to compression of the nerve roots of the cauda equina (**lumbar stenosis**).

Lumbosacral Radiculopathy (Figs. 17–3 & 17–4)

L4-L5 and L5-S1 are the most commonly affected levels in lumbosacral radiculopathy. Due to the configuration of the descending roots of the cauda equina, the most common type of lumbosacral disc herniation (**posterolateral disc herniation**) affects the root whose number corresponds to the vertebral level below the herniated disc (e.g., L4-L5 disc affects

TABLE 17–1 Innervation of the Leg & Foot.

Nerve (Roots)	Muscles			Sensory		
	Thigh	Leg/Foot	Toes	Thigh	Calf/Shin	Foot
Femoral nerve (L2-L4)	Iliopsoas Quadriceps			Intermediate and medial cutaneous nerves of the thigh		Saphenous nerve (medial shin and foot)
Obturator nerve (L2-L4)	Adductors of thigh (longus, brevis, magnus, minimus)			Cutaneous branch (to medial thigh)		
Superior gluteal nerve (L4-S1)	Gluteus medius and minimus Tensor fasciae latae					
Inferior gluteal nerve (L5-S2)	Gluteus maximus					
Posterior femoral cutaneous nerve (S1-S3)				Posterior femoral cutaneous		
Lateral femoral cutaneous nerve (L2-L3)				Lateral femoral cutaneous		
Sciatic nerve (L5-S2)	Hamstrings:					
Peroneal nerve (L4-S1)	Short head of biceps femoris	Tibialis anterior Peroneus longus and brevis	Extensor hallucis longus and brevis Extensor digitorum longus and brevis		Lateral cutaneous nerve of calf	Sural nerve (lateral foot)
Tibial nerve (L5-S2)	Long head of biceps femoris Semimembranosus Semitendinosus	Gastrocnemius Soleus Tibialis posterior	Flexor digitorum longus and brevis Flexor hallucis longus and brevis			Medial and lateral plantar nerves Calcaneal nerve

TABLE 17–2 Root & Nerve Supply of Lower Extremity Muscles.[a]

	L2	L3	L4	L5	S1	S2
Femoral nerve	Iliopsoas					
			Quadriceps			
Obturator nerve	Hip/thigh adductors					
Superior gluteal nerve				Gluteus medius and minimus Tensor fasciae latae		
Inferior gluteal nerve				Gluteus maximus		
Sciatic nerve					Hamstrings	
Peroneal nerve			Tibialis anterior			
				Extensors of toes Peroneus longus/brevis		
Tibial nerve				Tibialis posterior		
					Gastrocnemius/Soleus Flexors of toes Intrinsic foot muscles	

[a]Muscles with associated reflexes are denoted in **bold**.

the L5 nerve root). This is "numerically" the same as in the cervical spine (disc herniation affects the root whose number corresponds to the more inferior vertebra of the pair of vertebrae surrounding the herniated disc), but the anatomic reason is different (see "Anatomy of nerve roots" in Ch. 15). In the less common **far lateral herniation**, compression of the root whose number corresponds to the superior of the two vertebrae may occur (i.e., L4-L5 disc affecting L4 nerve root) (Fig. 17–3).

The predominant symptom in lumbosacral radiculopathy is back pain radiating into the leg in the distribution of the affected root(s) (see Fig. 17–1). Diminished sensation in the affected dermatome(s), diminished or absent reflexes (e.g., ankle jerk for S1), and/or weakness may be present on examination depending on severity. The **straight leg raise test** is performed by lifting the patient's leg (flexing at the hip with the knee extended) with the patient in the supine position. This may reproduce the patient's symptoms of radiating pain in the leg being lifted or in the contralateral leg (**crossed straight leg raise test**) in patients with lumbar radiculopathy at L5 or S1 levels. The **reverse straight leg raise** test (extending the leg at the hip with the patient prone) may reproduce radiculopathy symptoms in patients with L3 or L4 radiculopathy. (Note that many patients report mild discomfort or "tightness" in the hamstring with these maneuvers, but a positive test requires reproduction of the radiating pain characteristic of radiculopathy.)

TABLE 17–3 Examination of the Lower Extremity by Actions.

Action	Muscle	Nerve	Roots
Hip flexion	Iliopsoas	Femoral	L2-L3
Hip extension	Gluteus maximus	Inferior gluteal	L5-S1
Hip abduction	Gluteus medius	Superior gluteal	L4-L5
Hip adduction	Adductors (longus, brevis, minimus, and magnus)	Obturator	L2-L3-L4
Knee extension	Quadriceps	Femoral	L3-L4
Knee flexion	Hamstrings	Sciatic	L5-S1
Dorsiflexion of foot	Tibialis anterior	Peroneal	L4-L5
Plantarflexion of foot	Gastrocnemius/soleus	Tibial	S1-S2
Inversion of foot	Tibialis posterior	Tibial	L5-S1
Eversion of foot	Peroneus longus and brevis	Peroneal	L5-S1
Extension of toes	Extensor hallucis longus	Peroneal	L5-S1
	Extensor digitorum longus and brevis	Peroneal	L5-S1
Flexion of toes	Flexor hallucis longus and brevis	Tibial	S1-S2
	Flexor digitorum longus and brevis	Tibial	S1-S2

TABLE 17–4 **Examination of the Lower Extremity by Nerve.**

Nerve	Action	Muscle	Nerve Roots
Femoral	Hip flexion	Iliopsoas	L2-L3
	Knee extension (including patellar reflex)	Quadriceps	L3-L4
Obturator	Thigh adduction	Adductors	L2-L3-L4
Superior gluteal	Abduction of thigh/hip	Gluteus medius	L4-L5
Inferior gluteal	Extension of thigh/hip	Gluteus maximus	L5-S1
Sciatic	Flexion of knee	Hamstrings	L5-S1
Peroneal (Mnemonic: Up and Out)	Dorsiflexion of foot	Tibialis anterior	L4-L5
	Eversion of foot	Peroneus longus and brevis	L5-S1
	Extension of toes	Extensor hallucis longus and brevis	L5-S1
		Extensor digitorum longus and brevis	L5-S1
Tibial (Mnemonic: Down and In)	Plantarflexion of foot (including ankle reflex)	Gastrocnemius/soleus	S1-S2
	Inversion of foot	Tibialis posterior	L5-S1
	Flexion of toes	Flexor digitorum longus and brevis	S1-S2
		Flexor hallucis longus and brevis	S1-S2

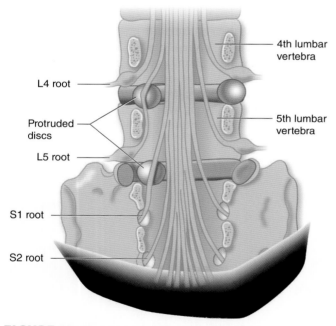

FIGURE 17–3 **Schematic of lumbosacral nerve root compression by disc prolapse.** The two disc bulges on the left of the image demonstrate how posterolateral disc protrusion compresses the root that will exit below the next vertebral body. Here, the L4-L5 disc compresses the L5 root and the L5-S1 disc compresses the S1 root. The disc bulge on the right side of the image shows how a far lateral disc herniation can affect the root exiting at the level of the disc. Here the L4-L5 disc compresses the L4 root. Far lateral lumbar disc herniation is much less common than posterolateral disc herniation. Reproduced with permission from Ropper A, Samuels M, Klein J: Adams and Victor's *Principles of Neurology*, 10th ed. New York, NY: McGraw Hill; 2014.

Similar to the case for cervical radiculopathy (see Ch. 16), neuroimaging of the lumbar spine is only indicated if there is intractable pain or progressive motor deficit, or if there is suspicion for malignancy or epidural abscess. Otherwise if there are no concerning features, a trial of conservative management (nonsteroidal anti-inflammatory drugs [NSAIDs] and/or acetaminophen and physical therapy) is indicated. Neuroimaging of the spine and referral for epidural steroid injection and/or surgical evaluation is considered only if symptoms worsen or are not responsive to conservative measures after several months. As with surgery for cervical radiculopathy, symptoms may improve more rapidly than with conservative management, but longer term outcomes may be similar.

Lumbar Canal Stenosis

In addition to foraminal stenosis, lumbar canal stenosis can occur due to degenerative disease of the lumbar spine (e.g., disc disease, spondylosis, and/or spondylolisthesis [anteroposterior displacement of one or more vertebrae]). Lumbar canal stenosis can result in compression of multiple lumbosacral roots, which can cause **neurogenic claudication**: pain, paresthesias, and/or weakness in the legs brought on by standing and walking that improves with rest. Vascular claudication can also lead to pain with exercise, but paresthesias or weakness would be atypical in vascular claudication. Symptoms of neurogenic claudication may be improved by leaning forward (e.g., resting on the shopping cart while walking) in addition to rest. Symptoms of neurogenic claudication may be better walking uphill as compared to downhill, because walking uphill requires leaning forward (relieving some pressure on the compressed roots) and walking downhill requires leaning backward (aggravating root compression). This is the opposite of what one would expect with vascular claudication (uphill requires more exertion, which would aggravate blood supply/demand mismatch, causing worsening symptoms in patients with vascular claudication).

In patients with neurogenic claudication, physical examination may be entirely normal unless the patient is asked to walk until symptoms emerge and then re-examined, at which point weakness may then be observed. MRI demonstrates stenosis of the lumbar canal due to disc disease, spondylosis, and/or spondylolisthesis with compression of nerve roots. With chronic stable mild symptoms, management is conservative, but with progressive or disabling symptoms, surgery should be considered.

Cauda Equina & Conus Medullaris Syndromes

When several roots of the cauda equina (lumbar and sacral nerve roots) are affected simultaneously, patients may develop sensory changes in the perineal region (saddle anesthesia), bowel and/or bladder dysfunction, radiating pain in the lower extremities, and/or lower extremity weakness. If the conus medullaris (distal portion of the spinal cord) is affected in isolation, bowel/bladder changes and non-radiating back pain may occur in the absence of lower extremity symptoms. Given the proximity of the conus medullaris to the roots of the cauda equina, both structures may be affected together. If there is concern for cauda equina or conus medullaris pathology, lumbosacral imaging is needed to determine the etiology. Potential pathology in this region includes compression by tumor or prolapsed disc, infection (e.g., epidural abscess, viral polyradiculitis, tuberculous arachnoiditis), neoplasm (e.g., leptomeningeal metastasis, neurolymphomatosis), and inflammatory diseases

(e.g., ankylosing spondylitis and sarcoidosis). Acute compressive cauda equina syndrome is a neurosurgical emergency. An uncommon tumor with a predilection for this region is **myxopapillary ependymoma** of the conus medullaris.

LUMBOSACRAL PLEXOPATHY

The lumbosacral plexus lies in the retroperitoneum and pelvis. Beyond being susceptible to the same categories of pathology as the brachial plexus (trauma, neoplastic compression/invasion, radiation injury, inflammatory conditions), the lumbosacral plexus can also be affected by infection (psoas abscess) and hematoma (retroperitoneal). The lumbosacral plexus is much less vulnerable to trauma than the brachial plexus, typically requiring major pelvic injury to be affected. Trauma during childbirth can affect the infant's brachial plexus as described in Chapter 16, but it is the mother's lumbosacral plexus that is subject to injury during labor. Gastrointestinal or genitourinary cancers and surgery or radiation for them can affect the lumbosacral plexus. As with brachial plexopathy, malignant infiltration tends to be painful whereas radiation therapy-induced lumbosacral plexopathy does not, and myokymic discharges on EMG are suggestive of radiation-induced plexopathy.

The lower-extremity inflammatory plexopathy analogue to Parsonage-Turner syndrome in the upper extremity (see "Parsonage-Turner Syndrome" in Ch. 16) is **lumbosacral radiculoplexus neuropathy**. This is most commonly seen in patients with diabetes (also called **diabetic amyotrophy** or **Bruns-Garland syndrome**), but can also be idiopathic. Lumbosacral radiculoplexus neuropathy begins with pain in the proximal lower extremity and then progresses to weakness of one or both lower extremities (when both lower extremities

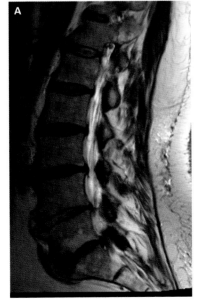
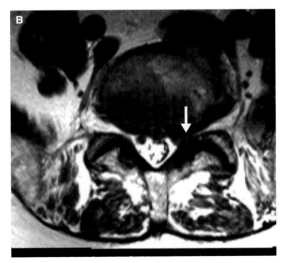

FIGURE 17–4 **MRI of lumbosacral disc herniation (T2-weighted). A:** Sagittal view demonstrating multilevel lumbar disc protrusions, most severe at L5-S1. **B:** Axial view demonstrating compression of the left S1 nerve root by the L5-S1 disc (**arrow**).

are involved, symptoms are typically asymmetric). When this occurs in diabetes, it often occurs at a time of good glycemic control and/or recent weight loss. Steroids and other immuno-modulatory therapy may be used for treatment of this condition. Recovery is often incomplete (unlike in Parsonage-Turner syndrome, which usually recovers completely over time).

Additional potential causes of lumbosacral plexopathy are hip surgery, psoas abscess, and retroperitoneal hematoma. A retroperitoneal hematoma can occur spontaneously in patients on anticoagulation, or due to complications of femoral artery catheterization or vascular surgery. A retroperitoneal hematoma may affect the femoral nerve in isolation (see "Femoral Neuropathy" below) or cause a plexopathy depending on its extent. Diagnosis is made by pelvic CT.

MONONEUROPATHIES OF THE LOWER EXTREMITY

The most common compressive neuropathies of the lower extremity are peroneal neuropathy (compression at the fibular head) and sciatic neuropathy (compression in the buttock). The nerves of the lumbar plexus (femoral, obturator, lateral femoral cutaneous) and the sciatic nerve can be injured by pelvic or hip trauma or surgery, or compressed by pelvic malignancy. The peroneal and tibial nerves can be injured due to knee trauma or surgery.

Femoral Neuropathy

The *femoral* nerve innervates two muscles associated with the *femur*: iliopsoas for hip flexion and quadriceps for knee extension (including the patellar reflex). The sensory coverage of the femoral nerve includes the anterior and medial thigh (intermediate and medial cutaneous branches) and the medial leg and foot by way of the saphenous nerve (Mnemonic: the sa**ph**enous nerve arises from the **f**emoral nerve). The femoral nerve passes through the iliopsoas and then beneath the inguinal ligament and can be injured at either site. Since the femoral nerve innervates the iliopsoas proximal to passing beneath the inguinal ligament, the presence of hip flexion weakness in addition to knee extension weakness and diminution/loss of the patellar reflex localizes a femoral neuropathy to the pelvis or retroperitoneum, whereas isolated knee extension weakness and loss of the patellar reflex with *spared* hip flexion strength suggests a more distal localization along the nerve.

An important aspect of the examination in patients with hip flexion and/or knee extension weakness is testing of hip adduction. The hip adductors are supplied by the obturator nerve, which is supplied by the L2 through L4 roots as is the femoral nerve. Therefore, hip flexion and/or knee extension weakness with *spared* hip adduction suggests femoral neuropathy (since the L2-L4 roots must be intact if obturator nerve function is intact), whereas hip flexion and/or knee extension weakness *and* hip adduction weakness suggest L2-L4 polyradiculopathy or lumbar plexopathy.

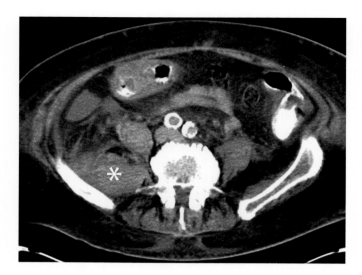

FIGURE 17–5   CT of the abdomen and pelvis demonstrating right psoas hematoma. This anticoagulated patient presented with back and hip pain and inability to walk, and was found to have an isolated femoral neuropathy on examination. The psoas hematoma is marked by an asterisk (*).

Causes of femoral neuropathy include pelvic or hip surgery or trauma, pelvic malignancy, and femoral catheterization procedures (which can injure the nerve in the inguinal region either directly or due to hematoma formation). In anticoagulated patients who develop back and leg pain and difficulty walking, signs of a femoral neuropathy should be sought on examination, which would suggest a psoas/retroperitoneal hematoma. The diagnosis of psoas/retroperitoneal hematoma can be made by CT of the pelvis (Fig. 17–5). Weakness and sensory changes beyond the femoral distribution in this context can occur with a more proximal retroperitoneal hematoma causing a lumbar plexopathy.

Obturator Neuropathy

Isolated obturator nerve injury is rare, but when it occurs, it causes weakness in hip adduction. Pelvic or hip trauma or surgery and childbirth are common etiologies. As described above, the obturator nerve shares root supply (L2-L4) with the femoral nerve, so weak hip adduction with sparing of hip flexion and knee extension suggests obturator neuropathy, whereas involvement of all of these actions (hip adduction, hip flexion, and knee extension) suggest L2-L4 polyradiculopathy or lumbar plexopathy.

Lateral Femoral Cutaneous Neuropathy (Meralgia Paresthetica)

The lateral femoral cutaneous nerve is a pure sensory nerve supplying the lateral thigh. Injury to the nerve causes numbness, paresthesias, and/or pain in this region, known as **meralgia paresthetica**. The nerve's position in the inguinal region adjacent to the anterior iliac spine makes it susceptible to injury from tight belts/pants especially in patients who are obese, rapidly gain weight (e.g., pregnancy), or rapidly lose weight.

Sciatic Neuropathy

The sciatic nerve is really the peroneal nerve and tibial nerve bundled together. It innervates the hamstring muscles (biceps femoris, semimembranosus, semitendonosus) that flex the knee, and then divides into the peroneal and tibial nerves in the popliteal fossa. The peroneal and tibial nerves control all movements of the foot and toes.

If there is a complete sciatic neuropathy, knee flexion and all movements of the foot will be weak. However, the sciatic nerve is often only partially affected, and in these patients, *the peroneal–innervated muscles are often affected in isolation* (or more affected than tibial nerve–innervated muscles). In such cases, sciatic neuropathy may be clinically indistinguishable from peroneal neuropathy. Peroneal neuropathy is most commonly due to compression at the fibular head (see "Peroneal Neuropathy" below). The short head of the biceps femoris is the only hamstring muscle innervated by the peroneal division of the sciatic nerve (the rest are innervated by the tibial portion), and so involvement of this muscle above the knee localizes the problem to the peroneal division of the sciatic nerve (as opposed to the most common site of compression of the peroneal nerve at the fibular head). However, the short head of the biceps femoris cannot be isolated clinically, so if a patient appears to have a peroneal neuropathy, the *short head of the biceps femoris* should be examined with electromyography (EMG) to look for denervation changes that would suggest localization to the peroneal division of the sciatic nerve proximal to the knee (see also "Approach to Foot Drop").

The sciatic nerve can be injured by pelvic or hip trauma or surgery, by an inappropriately placed gluteal injection, or by prolonged pressure on the buttock (e.g., supine due to intoxication or critical illness; pressure from sitting on the toilet seat or something in the back pants pocket). "Sciatica," referring to radiating pain down the back of the leg, is more commonly caused by radiculopathy affecting the S1 root rather than pathology of the sciatic nerve.

Peroneal Neuropathy

Peroneal neuropathy is the most common lower extremity mononeuropathy because the peroneal nerve is the lower extremity nerve most prone to compression. The most common site of compression is the head/neck of the fibula, where the nerve can be compressed due to frequent leg crossing (the leg on top is affected), prolonged bed-bound state, prolonged kneeling (usually occupational; e.g., flooring work), Baker's cyst, injury due to knee trauma or surgery, or rapid weight loss.

The peroneal nerve innervates the musculature of the anterior and lateral shin and foot: tibialis anterior (dorsiflexes the foot), peroneus longus and brevis (everts the foot), and the extensors of the toes. Mnemonic: The per**o**neal nerve brings the foot *up and out* (compared to the t**i**bial nerve, which brings the foot *down and in*). With respect to motor function of the foot, the peroneal nerve can be thought of as the lower extremity analogue of the radial nerve in the upper extremity in that it innervates all foot extensors. The peroneal nerve provides sensory supply to the lateral shin and dorsum of the foot.

The common peroneal nerve divides into the superficial and deep peroneal nerves that perform the individual components of the peroneal nerve functions listed above:

- The **superficial peroneal nerve** innervates the peroneus muscles (eversion) and provides sensation to the lateral calf and dorsum of the foot *except* the web space between the first two toes.
- The **deep peroneal nerve** supplies the tibialis anterior (dorsiflexion), the toe extensors, and sensation over the web space between the first two toes on the dorsum of the foot (mnemonic for the motor functions supplied by the deep peroneal nerve: *d*eep: *d*orsiflexion and *e*xtensors).

The superficial and deep peroneal nerves may be affected separately, impairing their individual functions, or together, impairing all peroneal nerve functions (common peroneal neuropathy). Common peroneal neuropathy leads to impaired dorsiflexion (foot drop) and foot eversion, but with spared plantarflexion and foot inversion (both tibial nerve functions). Numbness in common peroneal neuropathy may be present over the lateral calf and dorsum of the foot, although may be more limited in distribution over just the dorsum of the foot (since the sural nerve, which supplies the lateral calf, usually receives both peroneal and tibial input).

Tibial Neuropathy

The tibial nerve innervates the muscles of the posterior calf and plantar foot: gastrocnemius/soleus (plantarflexor), tibialis posterior (foot inversion), and all flexors of the toes. Mnemonic: The tibial nerve brings the foot down and in (compared to the peroneal nerve, which brings the foot up and out). The tibial nerve innervates the functions in the foot analogous to the combined functions of the median and ulnar nerves in the hand (flexors and intrinsic muscles of the hand/foot).

The tibial nerve is less commonly affected than the peroneal nerve since it is not as exposed as the peroneal nerve, but it can rarely be injured by knee trauma or a Baker's cyst in the popliteal fossa.

Tarsal Tunnel Syndrome

The most common site of tibial nerve compression (which is still rare) is at the tarsal tunnel, where the tibial nerve enters the foot with the flexor tendons of the toes under the medial malleolus (**tarsal tunnel syndrome**). Tarsal tunnel syndrome occurs most commonly in patients with prior ankle injury or arthritis of the ankle, but can rarely be caused by a ganglion cyst in the tarsal tunnel. The syndrome causes neuralgic pain

TABLE 17–5 Patterns of Weakness in Foot Drop Due to Lesions of the Peroneal Nerve, Sciatic Nerve, & L5 Root.

	Peroneal Nerve-Supplied Actions		Tibial Nerve-Supplied Actions	
	Dorsiflexion	**Eversion**	**Plantarflexion**	**Inversion**
Common peroneal neuropathy[a]	Weak	Weak	Spared	Spared
Sciatic neuropathy[b]	Weak	Weak	Weak	Weak
L5 radiculopathy	Weak	Weak	Spared	Weak

[a]Note that the divisions of the peroneal nerve may be affected in isolation: Isolated superficial peroneal neuropathy causes eversion weakness without dorsiflexion weakness; isolated deep peroneal neuropathy causes dorsiflexion weakness without eversion weakness. [b]Note that a sciatic neuropathy can preferentially affect the peroneal division, mimicking a common peroneal neuropathy (see text).

in the plantar foot, which may radiate proximally (just as patients with carpal tunnel syndrome sometimes report pain/paresthesias proximal to the site of entrapment). On examination, sensation may be decreased on the plantar surface of the foot and there may be a Tinel sign when tapping over the posterior medial malleolus (provocation of paresthesias over the plantar surface of the foot). There is usually no obvious weakness since the main toe flexors (whose tendons pass through the tarsal tunnel) are innervated proximal to the tarsal tunnel.

If a patient with tarsal tunnel syndrome does not respond to conservative treatment with NSAIDs, steroid injections can be considered. Surgery is reserved for intractable cases confirmed by EMG/nerve conduction studies demonstrating slowing across the tarsal tunnel and denervation of tibial nerve–innervated intrinsic foot muscles (e.g., adductors of toes).

APPROACH TO FOOT DROP

Foot drop refers to dorsiflexion weakness such that the foot "drops." This causes a steppage gait in which the patient lifts the foot very high off the ground to avoid tripping over the dropped foot and then slaps the foot down, since dorsiflexion cannot be used to soften the landing onto the heel as occurs in normal walking. Foot dorsiflexion (tibialis anterior) weakness can be caused by peroneal neuropathy, sciatic neuropathy, lumbosacral plexopathy, L5 radiculopathy, or a central lesion. Lumbosacral plexopathy will often cause more widespread lower extremity deficits, but foot drop may be the predominant manifestation of lesions at the other three peripheral localizations. Isolated common peroneal neuropathy causes foot drop and eversion weakness (loss of "up and out"), but does not affect plantarflexion or inversion (preserved "down and in") since these are tibial nerve–innervated functions. Inversion is a tibial nerve–innervated

function supplied by L5, but plantarflexion is a tibial nerve–innervated function supplied by S1-S2. Therefore, a foot drop with loss of both eversion and inversion but with spared plantar flexion suggests L5 radiculopathy (affecting both tibial nerve–innervated and peroneal nerve–innervated muscles). Loss of dorsiflexion, plantarflexion, inversion, and eversion suggests sciatic neuropathy (Table 17–5). In addition to weakness in various movements of the foot, L5 radiculopathy can also cause weakness of hip abduction.

As described above, sciatic neuropathy may be clinically indistinguishable from peroneal neuropathy, since the peroneal division of the sciatic nerve can be more susceptible to injury than the tibial division. In such cases, EMG can distinguish between sciatic and peroneal etiologies by looking for denervation of the *short head of the biceps femoris*, the only muscle innervated by the peroneal nerve above the fibular head (and the only hamstring muscle innervated by the peroneal division of the sciatic nerve). If there are denervation changes in the short head of the biceps femoris on EMG in a patient who appears to have a peroneal neuropathy, this localizes to the peroneal division of the sciatic nerve proximal to the fibular head (the fibular head is the more common site of peroneal nerve compression).

Foot drop can also be caused by a lesion affecting the foot area in the medial precentral gyrus (e.g., parasagittal meningioma). In such cases, there is often weakness beyond dorsiflexion in an upper motor neuron pattern (weak dorsiflexion, eversion, knee flexion, hip flexion; see Ch. 4) and upper motor neuron signs, but foot drop may be the predominant finding. Foot drop may also be a presenting feature of ALS, though physical examination and electrophysiologic findings generally extend beyond dorsiflexion weakness in this context (see Ch. 28).

During the period of recovery from foot drop (or for a foot drop not expected to recover), an ankle-foot orthosis can be used that maintains the foot in a more neutral position to restore the natural position of the foot during walking.

Seizures & Epilepsy

CHAPTER CONTENTS

DEFINITIONS & CAUSES OF SEIZURES & EPILEPSY

Seizures are caused by abnormal electrical discharges in the brain. Epilepsy is the condition of recurrent unprovoked seizures. The definition of "provoked" here is more precise than in common parlance and refers to *acute, reversible* provoking factors causing seizures. For example, acute hypoglycemia, alcohol withdrawal, high fever, and medication or drug toxicity are all acute reversible factors that can provoke seizures (Table 18–1). In these scenarios, the brain may be structurally normal, but exposure to the acute provoking factor leads

to seizures. When the cause is treated, the seizures typically improve and the patient is not necessarily at risk for future recurrent seizures.

Brain tumors, prior stroke, prior head trauma, prior CNS infection, and cortical malformations can all cause seizures, but these entities are neither acute nor reversible, and so recurrent seizures due to any of these causes are considered unprovoked. A patient with a brain tumor (or any of the prior CNS insults listed above) who has a first seizure has had the underlying potential seizure focus for some time. If no acute provoking factor is present (e.g., infection, metabolic derangement), one may ask why the patient seized on that particular day and not the day, week, or month before? Seizures in this context are considered to be *unprovoked* because they can occur at any time without any provoking factor, just like the unprovoked seizures of idiopathic genetic epilepsy syndromes. Therefore, patients with recurrent seizures due to brain tumors, prior trauma, prior stroke, prior neurosurgery, prior CNS infection, or any other irreversible underlying seizure focus (see Table 18–1) are considered to have epilepsy and should be treated as such.

Some causes of acute symptomatic (provoked) seizures such as acute stroke or hemorrhage, head trauma, or meningitis can increase the risk for development of epilepsy in the future since they can lead to irreversible brain damage, creating an epileptogenic focus.

EVALUATION OF PATIENTS WITH SEIZURES

A patient with seizure(s) will generally present for evaluation in one of three scenarios:

1. After a first seizure
2. With a history of seizures
3. Actively seizing

When a patient presents for evaluation after a seizure in any scenario, the goals of the clinical encounter are to determine the following:

- **Was the event truly a seizure?** The differential diagnosis for a transient alteration in neurologic function includes migraine, syncope, transient ischemic attack (TIA), cardiac arrhythmia, psychogenic nonepileptic seizure, and rare paroxysmal movement disorders (paroxysmal dyskinesias, episodic ataxias). A clear description of the event by witnesses should be obtained. The clinical features that can be used to aid in distinguishing between these are discussed below.
- **Were there any clear provoking factors?** A detailed medication and drug/alcohol history should be obtained, laboratory tests should evaluate for potential metabolic or infectious etiologies, and neuroimaging should be considered. If the patient has been on an antiseizure medication for prior seizures, it should be determined whether the patient is taking the medication(s) properly and consistently. Even patients with known epilepsy should be evaluated for potential provoking factors that may have caused them to have a seizure at that particular moment, such as an infection or a new medication that could lower the seizure threshold or alter the metabolism of their antiseizure medication(s).
- **Was this the first event or have there been others?** If there have been other prior events, was the patient ever evaluated for these? If so, was the patient ever on an antiseizure medication, and if so, did it help?
- **Are there any known risk factors for seizures?** These may include:
  - Prior stroke, head trauma, or CNS infection
  - Pediatric febrile seizures
  - Other first-degree relative(s) with seizures
  - Abnormal gestation, birth, or cognitive development
- **Has there been emergence of any neurologic deficit prior to or since the onset of seizure(s) to suggest a focal lesion (e.g., progressive weakness, numbness, visual changes, personality/cognitive changes)?**

TABLE 18–1 Causes of Provoked Seizures & Epilepsy.

Causes of Acute Provoked Seizures	Causes of Epilepsy
Acute brain pathology:	**Structural brain lesions:**
• Acute stroke or intracranial hemorrhage	• Intracranial tumor
• Acute head trauma	• Cortical malformation
• Acute infectious meningitis/encephalitis	• Vascular malformation
• Autoimmune encephalitis	• Prior stroke or intracranial hemorrhage
• Posterior reversible encephalopathy syndrome (PRES) (see Ch. 19)	• Prior head trauma
• Cerebral venous sinus thrombosis/cortical vein thrombosis (see Ch. 19)	• Prior infection (meningitis/encephalitis) or chronic infection (neurocysticercosis)
Metabolic derangements, including:	• Neurodegenerative disease
• Hypo- or hyperglycemia	**Genetic epilepsy syndromes** (see Table 18–3)
• Hyponatremia	
• Hypocalcemia	
• Hypomagnesemia	
Medications, including:	
• Bupropion	
• Tramadol	
• Fluoroquinolones	
• Cephalosporins	
• Carbapenems	
• Isoniazid	
Drugs/drug withdrawal	
• Alcohol	
• Cocaine	
Systemic illness	
• Systemic infection with fever	
• Renal failure	

CLINICAL FEATURES OF SEIZURES

The clinical manifestations (or **semiology**) of seizures depend on the area(s) of the brain from which seizure activity arises and/or to which this activity spreads. Seizures are classified as having **focal** onset, **generalized** onset, or unknown onset.

Focal (Partial) Seizures

Focal seizures are classified by whether there is preserved awareness (formerly called simple partial seizures) or impaired awareness (formerly called complex partial seizures), and whether the first manifestation is a motor feature or not. The clinical manifestations depend on the origin of seizure activity within the brain and can include focal motor symptoms (tonic-clonic movements, automatisms, posturing, head and/or eye deviation); focal sensory symptoms (paresthesias that tend to spread over seconds); visual, auditory, or olfactory hallucinations; autonomic symptoms; cognitive/behavioral changes; and/or psychic phenomena such as déjà vu (a sense of already having experienced a new place or event), jamais vu (a sense of never having been in a familiar place or situation), or a sense of fear. The aura that may precede a seizure arises from a focal origin of seizure activity before it spreads to involve other regions of the brain. A seizure may begin focally and evolve to a bilateral tonic-clonic seizure (called focal to bilateral tonic-clonic; formerly called secondarily generalized).

Postictal weakness (**Todd's paralysis**) may occur in the limb(s) affected by seizure activity. If a seizure is unwitnessed and a patient is found with focal postictal weakness, the patient may be initially thought to have had a stroke. Therefore, seizure with subsequent postictal paralysis should be considered in the differential diagnosis of acute stroke and TIA and vice versa.

Generalized Seizures

Generalized seizures are characterized by impaired consciousness and bilateral motor manifestations if motor manifestations are present. Motor manifestations can be **tonic** (stiffening of involved body parts), **clonic** (rhythmic movements), **tonic-clonic** (mix of tonic and clonic), **myoclonic** (brief jerks), or **atonic** (loss of postural tone causing drop attacks). Rarely, seizures of frontal origin can produce more complex motor manifestations (e.g., bicycling, pelvic thrusting). Self-injury (e.g., tongue bite, shoulder dislocation), bladder/bowel incontinence, and altered level of consciousness commonly occur with generalized tonic-clonic seizures.

A **postictal state** is common after a generalized seizure, and is characterized by altered consciousness, which can range from confusion to coma depending on the severity and length of preceding seizure activity. In a patient with altered level of consciousness following seizure(s), continued nonconvulsive seizures may be occurring and must be distinguished from a postictal state. Subtle signs such as twitching of the eyes or eyelids, gaze deviation, or twitching of the extremities can be clues to nonconvulsive seizures, but overt clinical manifestations may be absent, and only electroencephalography (EEG) can definitively distinguish between ongoing electrographic seizure activity and a postictal state. Therefore, it is prudent to consider EEG monitoring after prolonged seizures with continued altered state of consciousness.

If a patient is found comatose or confused without clear cause and recovers without specific intervention, unwitnessed seizure with a subsequent postictal state should be considered in the differential diagnosis.

Absence seizures are generalized seizures characterized by brief periods of altered awareness in which patients are unable to communicate or engage with the environment. They may be accompanied by automatisms. Absence seizures occur primarily in the context of childhood-onset epilepsy syndromes.

Distinguishing Seizures From Other Transient Neurologic Events

When available, eyewitness accounts of what happened during a possible seizure can be helpful in distinguishing seizures from other transient neurologic events. However, in many instances, the distinction remains challenging based on historical clues alone.

Distinguishing Seizure From Syncope

In a patient who presents after an unexplained loss of consciousness, some features of the clinical history may be more suggestive of seizure as opposed to syncope. Although a few tonic-clonic jerks or brief posturing may be seen in syncope, sustained tonic-clonic activity is suggestive of seizure. However, if a patient has syncope in a chair or other position in which they cannot become immediately supine, more sustained motor activity may be observed. Tongue biting (particularly on the lateral tongue) is more common in seizure, but can be caused by syncope if the patient hits the chin/jaw when falling. Urinary and/or fecal incontinence is more commonly seen with seizures than with syncope, although in a patient who becomes orthostatic en route to the bathroom to urinate, the full bladder may empty during syncope. After syncope, patients generally return rapidly to consciousness (unless syncope leads to head trauma causing more sustained loss of consciousness), whereas a more prolonged state of confusion or altered consciousness is more characteristic of seizure with a postictal state. Patients who have had a syncopal episode may recall the feelings of presyncope preceding the event (e.g., feeling of "blacking out," "becoming warm all over"), whereas patients with seizures may recall a preceding aura (e.g., foul odor, sense of déjà vu) or have no recollection of the event whatsoever. Although some practitioners obtain a serum prolactin level as part of the diagnostic workup to distinguish seizure from syncope, this test is neither sensitive nor specific—it can be normal after seizure and it can be elevated after syncope, so it does not reliably distinguish seizure from syncope.

Distinguishing Seizure From Transient Ischemic Attack

Seizures generally cause "positive" symptoms (i.e., abnormal movements, paresthesias, visual phenomena), whereas transient ischemic attacks (TIAs) generally cause "negative" symptoms (i.e., weakness, loss of sensation, visual field deficits). The symptoms of both seizures and TIAs may arise suddenly and improve gradually over minutes to hours. With recurrent events, seizures are more likely to be stereotyped, whereas TIAs are more likely to be varied (unless the TIAs are all due to a particular stenotic vessel, in which case TIAs may also be stereotyped). If a patient has vascular risk factors, this may lead one to err on the side of evaluating for causes of TIA (see "Transient Ischemic Attack" in Ch. 19) when the clinical history is ambiguous, but prior stroke can also be a risk factor for seizure. Therefore, when in doubt, it is prudent to consider evaluating for causes of TIA and causes of seizure in parallel.

Distinguishing Seizure From Migraine With Aura

Both migraine and seizure can produce "positive" focal symptoms (e.g., paresthesias, visual auras), although those of migraine tend to evolve/spread over minutes, whereas those of seizures generally evolve/spread over seconds. Migraine does not lead to alterations in level of consciousness, although it can cause mild confusion in some patients. A headache is a common (but not universal) accompaniment to migraine with aura, but a headache can also be a component of a seizure aura or postictal state.

Distinguishing Seizures From Psychogenic Nonepileptic Seizures

Psychogenic nonepileptic seizures (PNES; formerly called pseudo-seizures) may be a manifestation of a functional neurologic disorder (previously referred to as conversion disorder). Clinical features suggestive of PNES rather than epileptic seizures include prolonged bilateral movements that are asynchronous and/or flailing (as opposed to rhythmic tonic-clonic movements in seizures, though note that frontal lobe seizures can cause atypical movements such as pelvic thrusting), preservation of consciousness (e.g., preserved ability to communicate or respond to external stimuli despite bilateral motor activity, or recall of event after it is over; generalized bilateral tonic-clonic seizure activity will be accompanied by altered state of consciousness with no recall of event), forced eye closure during episodes (eyes are generally open during epileptic seizures), episodes occurring exclusively during periods of wakefulness and/or with others present (while epileptic seizures can occur during wakefulness, onset during sleep is common), episodes provoked by stress or other emotional circumstances, and continued events in spite of multiple antiseizure medications (though this can also occur in refractory epilepsy). However, patients with epilepsy can have both seizures and PNES, and patients with underlying psychiatric conditions can have seizures. The only definitive way to diagnose events as being nonepileptic is to obtain prolonged video

EEG monitoring that captures events and their electrographic correlates to determine if the EEG demonstrates seizures or remains normal. PNES is treated with cognitive-behavioral therapy.

As should be clear from the above discussion, it can be very challenging to distinguish between seizures and other types of paroxsymal spells based on history alone. The diagnosis of seizures is sometimes even difficult when the clinician is observing an event or abnormal movements in a patient in coma. The gold standard is continuous EEG to capture an event or during an ongoing or fluctuating state of altered consciousness to see if there is associated electrographic evidence of seizure activity. However, some deep foci of seizure activity may not be apparent on surface EEG, so even this is not perfectly sensitive to determine whether an event is epileptic or not.

ELECTROENCEPHALOGRAPHY (EEG) IN THE EVALUATION OF SEIZURES

There is a growing encyclopedia of EEG findings and associated acronyms, which can broadly be divided into five categories:

1. Normal variants not associated with epilepsy but of unclear significance (e.g., small sharp spikes, wicket spikes)
2. Findings associated with focal or global cerebral pathology but not necessarily with epilepsy (e.g., focal or generalized slowing, triphasic waves, frontal intermittent rhythmic delta activity [FIRDA])
3. Interictal epileptiform discharges indicating cortical irritability and risk of seizures (e.g., spikes, sharp waves, spike-and-slow-wave discharges, periodic lateralized discharges [PLDs, formerly called PLEDs], generalized periodic discharges [GPDs, formerly called GPEDs], lateralized rhythmic delta activity [LRDA])
4. Seizures
5. Artifact, which can be due to:
   - Patient factors (e.g., blinking, movements)
   - Technical factors (e.g., electrocardiographic [ECG] artifact, interference from electrical hospital equipment, issues with EEG leads)

EEG is most useful in the following scenarios:

- Determining if a particular type of event is a seizure (e.g., versus PNES) by capturing EEG data during a typical event (usually requires continuous EEG monitoring)
- Determining if a patient with an altered level of consciousness is having nonconvulsive seizures contributing to the altered state of consciousness (also usually requires continuous EEG monitoring to capture intermittent seizure activity) (see "Nonconvulsive Status Epilepticus")
- Determining whether a patient with seizures has a particular electrographic signature of a certain epilepsy syndrome so as to guide prognosis and management

- Determining the risk of future seizures in patients after first seizure (see "Evaluation and Management of Patients After a First Seizure")
- Precise localization of a seizure focus if patients are being considered for epilepsy surgery (see "Refractory [Drug-Resistant] Epilepsy")

EEG may be obtained as a routine EEG (generally 20 minutes of recording) or as continuous EEG (hours to days of monitoring). The routine EEG is often obtained to assess for interictal epileptiform discharges (see point 3 on the previous page) in patients who have had one or more episodes concerning for seizure. The sensitivity of a single 20-minute routine EEG recording to detect interictal epileptiform discharges is only around 50%, although sensitivity can be increased by performing the EEG in the sleep-deprived state, performing EEG within 24 hours of a seizure event, or repeating EEG on multiple occasions. Notably, a small proportion of the population may have epileptiform discharges of no clinical significance, and a number of medications can also cause EEG abnormalities. Therefore, the absence of epileptiform discharges does not "exclude" epilepsy and their presence does not "confirm" epilepsy. Seizures and epilepsy are clinical diagnoses and EEG findings must be interpreted in light of the clinical history. If a patient has had paroxysmal events and there is a strong clinical suspicion that the patient has had seizures, a normal EEG should not necessarily dissuade the clinician from treating these as seizures. Similarly, if the clinician has a strong suspicion that the events are not seizures (e.g., syncope, migraine), an epileptiform finding on routine EEG should not necessarily dissuade the clinician from that impression.

What remains uncertain is how much the clinician should weight the routine EEG in a patient for whom the history of the events is difficult to interpret/classify. For example, if an otherwise healthy patient presents with recurrent, discrete, clinically ambiguous episodes (e.g., "feeling foggy" for a few minutes every few months), a normal EEG does not exclude the possibility that these are seizures, and an abnormal interictal EEG does not confirm that they are seizures. If the events are frequent enough, the gold standard is to capture events during inpatient video EEG monitoring. An intermediate step is at-home ambulatory EEG for 24–48 hours. However, even when extended EEG monitoring captures a spell, deep seizure foci can be missed with surface recordings. If the events are rare, a few days of inpatient monitoring may be hard to justify since the likelihood of capturing an event may be low. Ultimately, in patients whose events are difficult to classify, infrequent, and in whom the EEG is normal (or ambiguous), a decision must be made in collaboration with the patient as to whether to attempt treatment with an antiseizure medication as a potential diagnostic and therapeutic maneuver.

EVALUATION & MANAGEMENT OF PATIENTS AFTER A FIRST SEIZURE

In a patient who presents after a first seizure, an effort should be made to determine whether the seizure was provoked. This requires a careful medication and drug history, laboratory evaluation (including electrolytes and toxicology screen), and neuroimaging (MRI with contrast preferred; arterial and/or venous imaging may be considered depending on clinical context). Lumbar puncture should be considered if there is concern for CNS infection or inflammatory disease (e.g., autoimmune encephalitis). Epilepsy-protocol MRI generally includes coronal views of the hippocampi to look for asymmetries in size or signal characteristics on T2/FLAIR (fluid-attenuated inversion recovery) sequences that may suggest an underlying focus for temporal lobe epilepsy (**mesial temporal sclerosis**) (Fig. 18–1).

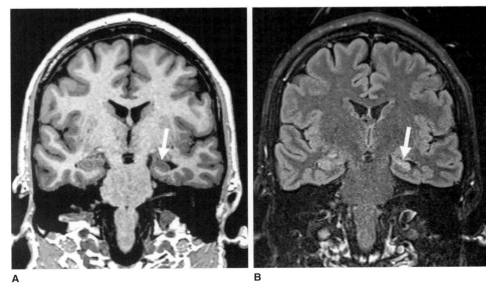

FIGURE 18–1 **Mesial temporal sclerosis demonstrated on MRI. A:** Coronal T1-weighted image showing asymmetric hippocampi (smaller left hippocampus). **B:** Coronal FLAIR image showing increased signal in the left hippocampus. Reproduced with permission from Ropper A, Samuels M, Klein J: Adams and Victor's *Principles of Neurology*, 10th ed. New York, NY: McGraw Hill; 2014.

It should be noted that seizures can produce transient MRI abnormalities, most commonly diffusion restriction (on DWI/ADC sequences) and/or T2/FLAIR hyperintensity in the cortex, splenium, and/or thalamus (Fig. 18–2). Diffusion restriction on MRI can also be caused by acute stroke (see "Diffusion-Weighted Imaging and Apparent Diffusion Coefficient MRI Sequences" in Ch. 2). The pattern of diffusion restriction due to seizure can be distinguished from stroke in that seizure-related diffusion restriction is often limited to the cortex, can span multiple vascular territories, and the ipsilateral thalamus may also be involved in the absence of signal change in the white matter between the thalamus and involved cortex.

If a clear acute, reversible etiology of a patient's seizure is identified (e.g., hypoglycemia, meningitis, drug intoxication or withdrawal, posterior reversible encephalopathy syndrome) and the patient has returned to normal with treatment of this underlying provoking condition, antiseizure medication (ASM) treatment is not necessarily indicated. EEG is not particularly helpful in this scenario since patients are generally not treated with ASMs for acute provoked seizures whether the EEG is abnormal (which it may be immediately after a seizure) or not. If there were multiple and/or difficult-to-control seizures due to an underlying acute reversible provoking factor, a short course of ASMs may be maintained and later tapered. Some clinicians perform an EEG before deciding to taper an ASM in this setting, and so prefer to have a baseline EEG to which to compare it.

If there is a structural lesion identified in a patient with a first seizure (e.g., tumor, vascular malformation, cortical malformation), long-term ASM treatment is generally indicated. In such patients, an acute factor that provoked the seizure at that particular time should be sought (e.g., infection, electrolyte abnormality), but may be absent. Even if a patient with a structural lesion is found to have a reversible provoking factor (e.g., infection) that may have triggered the first seizure, the structural lesion creates high risk for future recurrence of seizures, warranting ASM therapy.

If no acute provoking factor of a first seizure is evident, neuroimaging reveals no structural etiology, and there is no prior history of risk factors for seizure (e.g., prior stroke), an EEG should be obtained to evaluate for electrographic abnormalities that may suggest a seizure focus.

Should a patient with an acute unprovoked seizure with no structural cause be treated with an ASM? The Multicentre Trial for Early Epilepsy and Single Seizures (MESS) addressed this question (Marson et al., 2005). In this study, about 1400 patients who had an unprovoked seizure were randomized to immediate ASM therapy or deferred ASM therapy (deferred until deemed appropriate by the treating physician). Although immediate therapy increased the length of time to subsequent seizures and decreased the length of time to achieving a 2-year period of remission compared to deferred treatment, there were no differences in seizure freedom at 5 years, quality of life, or severe adverse events between the groups. There were slightly more minor adverse drug events in the immediate initiation group.

A follow-up study using the MESS data determined that the patients at lowest risk for recurrent seizure are those patients who have had only a single seizure, have a normal neurologic examination and no history of developmental delay or learning disability, and have a normal EEG (Kim et al., 2006). The 5-year seizure risk in these low-risk patients in this study was

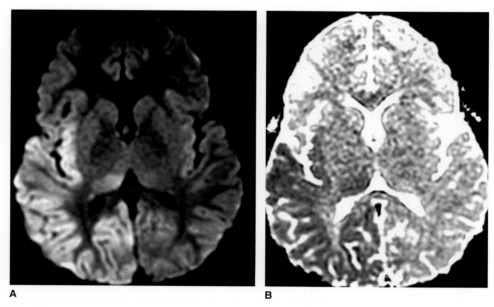

A   **B**

FIGURE 18-2 Diffusion restriction due to status epilepticus. Diffusion-weighted imaging (DWI) (**A**) and apparent diffusion coefficient (ADC). (**B**) MRI sequences demonstrating cortical diffusion restriction in the right occipital and temporal lobes as well as in the right thalamus. The pattern of diffusion restriction is not confined to a single vascular territory (spans middle cerebral artery [MCA] and posterior cerebral artery [PCA] territories) and involves only the cortex and thalamus.

about 30%, and did not differ significantly between immediate and deferred treatment strategies. However, if any of these factors was present (i.e., there had been more than one seizure prior to presentation, the neurologic examination was abnormal or there was developmental delay or learning disability, or the EEG was abnormal), the risk of delaying ASM treatment (on seizure recurrence and time to remission) was significant.

Medium-risk patients were defined as those having only one of these factors (i.e., two to three seizures *or* an abnormal neurologic examination or history of developmental delay or learning disability *or* an abnormal EEG). Medium-risk patients had a 35% 1-year risk of seizure recurrence (and a 56% risk of seizure recurrence by 5 years) with deferred treatment compared to a 24% risk at 1 year (and 39% risk at 5 years) with immediate treatment. High-risk patients were defined as having more than one of the factors listed above or four or more prior seizures; they had a 59% seizure recurrence risk at 1 year (and 73% at 5 years) with deferred treatment compared to a 36% seizure recurrence risk at 1 year (and 50% at 5 years) with immediate treatment (Kim et al., 2006).

Therefore, according to these data, after an unprovoked seizure with no structural etiology, medium-risk or high-risk patients should be treated immediately with long-term ASM therapy. A similar conclusion was drawn in the International League Against Epilepsy (ILAE) 2014 definition of epilepsy: A patient may be defined as having epilepsy after a single unprovoked seizure if their risk of a second seizure was at least 60% (Fisher et al., 2014). Guidelines from the AAN and AES also cite a first unprovoked nocturnal seizure as being high risk for subsequent seizures (Krumholz et al., 2015). So after a first unprovoked seizure, the following patients should be considered at high risk of subsequent seizures and likely warrant ASM therapy:

- Structural lesion (brain tumor, prior stroke, prior trauma)
- Abnormal EEG (including but not limited to evidence of an epilepsy syndrome)
- Nocturnal seizure

The only patient group with a first unprovoked seizure for whom the "to treat immediately or not to treat immediately" dilemma arises is low-risk patients (defined as patients with a single unprovoked seizure, a normal examination and no prior history of developmental delay or learning disability, and a normal EEG) with no structural etiology on neuroimaging. Treatment decisions in such cases must be individualized in collaboration with the patient, presenting the risk of future events and the risks and benefits of treatment. Some low-risk patients will prefer to initiate a medication immediately due to fear of the consequences of a second seizure (risk of injuries, risk of further prolonging the period during which the patient cannot drive). Some low-risk patients will prefer to defer medication initiation since even if the patient has a second unprovoked seizure in the future after which medication initiation would then be recommended, the patient will have gained the maximum medication-free period in this scenario.

Counseling After a First Seizure

After a first unprovoked seizure, whether being treated or not, patients should be counseled on safety. Patients with active epilepsy or who have just had a first seizure should be counseled not to drive, operate heavy machinery, work at heights or near fire, bathe/swim alone, or participate in any other activity during which a seizure could lead to significant injury or death. Laws vary from state to state with respect to the seizure-free period necessary before driving, so local regulations should be consulted. The recommended seizure-free period for driving (6–12 months in most U.S. states) can be used as a rough guide for avoidance of other potentially risky activities.

OUTPATIENT MANAGEMENT OF EPILEPSY

Determining an Antiseizure Medication Regimen for a Patient With Epilepsy

Some epilepsy syndromes may respond to (or may be worsened by) particular antiseizure medications (ASMs). For example, valproate is first-line therapy for many idiopathic genetic generalized epilepsy syndromes, with the exception of childhood absence epilepsy for which ethosuximide is first-line therapy. Carbamazepine is particularly effective for partial (focal) seizures, but may worsen idiopathic genetic generalized epilepsy syndromes such as childhood absence epilepsy. Some ASMs may be contraindicated in particular patient populations. For example, valproate should be avoided in women of child-bearing age due to teratogenicity. Valproate should also be avoided in patients with mitochondrial disease and children under 2 years old due to increased risk of hepatotoxicity.

Beyond these scenarios, the treatment of epilepsy is largely empiric: The clinician seeks the ideal ASM or combination of ASMs that controls the patient's seizures with no (or minimal) side effects. An initial ASM choice for an adult with epilepsy is often chosen based on potential drug interactions, side effect profile, and whether or not there is a need for rapid titration and/or IV administration (Table 18–2).

Antiseizure Medications & Drug–Drug Interactions

The older ASMs phenobarbital, phenytoin, carbamazepine, and valproate have the most drug–drug interactions. Phenobarbital, phenytoin, and carbamazepine are enzyme inducers, lowering the levels of other medications. Valproate is an enzyme-inhibitor, increasing the levels of other medications. Therefore, these drugs would be suboptimal for patients on multiple medications, especially if a patient is being treated with warfarin or chemotherapy. The inducers phenobarbital, phenytoin, and carbamazepine can also decrease the effectiveness of oral contraceptives. Oral contraceptives can decrease lamotrigine levels.

TABLE 18-2 Characteristics of Commonly Used Antiseizure Medications (ASMs).

	Channel of Action	Most Common Indication, If Specific (Otherwise Broad Spectrum)	Unique Adverse Effects[a]	Significant Drug–Drug Interactions	IV Formulation Available	Other
Brivaracetam	SV2A	Focal seizures			Yes	
Cannabidiol	Multiple	Lennox-Gastaut Dravet Tuberous sclerosis				
Carbamazepine (CBZ)	Na$^+$	Focal seizures	Hyponatremia	Inducer (decreases levels of other medications)		• Also used for trigeminal neuralgia, mania • Auto-induction: leads to falling levels after several weeks • Risk of Stevens-Johnson higher with HLA-B1502 (more common in Asian patients)
Cenobamate	Na$^+$	Focal seizures	• DRESS • QT Shortening	Inducer (decreases levels of other medications)		
Clobazam	GABA	Focal seizures				
Clonazepam	GABA					
Eslicarbazepine	Na$^+$	Focal seizures	Hyponatremia			
Ethosuximide (ESX)	Ca^{++}	Absence seizures				
Felbamate	Multiple		• GI symptoms • Aplastic anemia			
Gabapentin (GBP)	Ca^{++}	Focal seizures	• Peripheral edema			Used for neuropathic pain
Lacosamide (LCM)	Na$^+$		Cardiac (PR prolongation)		Yes	
Lamotrigine (LTG)	Na$^+$		Avoid in patients with cardiac disease	LTG levels decreased by oral contraceptives		• Used as mood stabilizer • Safest in pregnancy
Levetiracetam (LEV)	SV2A		Psychiatric		Yes	
Oxcarbazepine (OXC)	Na$^+$	Focal seizures	Hyponatremia	Inducer		
Perampanel	AMPA		Psychiatric			
Phenobarbital (PB)	GABA			Inducer (decreases levels of other medications)	Yes	

Drug	Mechanism	Clinical use	Adverse effects	Enzyme effect	Level monitoring	Notes
Phenytoin (PHT)	Na$^+$		Purple glove syndrome with IV	Inducer (decreases levels of other medications)	Yes	When assessing levels, use corrected if low albumin
Pregabalin	Ca^{++}	Focal seizures				Also used for neuropathic pain
Primidone	GABA			Inducer (decreases levels of other medications)		
Rufinamide	Na$^+$	Lennox-Gastaut	QT shortening			
Topiramate (TPM)	Multiple		• Nephrolithiasis • Weight loss • Word finding difficulty • Paresthesias in distal extremities			Used for migraine
Valproate (VPA)	Multiple	Broad spectrum including Idiopathic genetic epilepsy syndromes	• Weight gain • Tremor • Parkinsonism • Hyperammonemia • *Most teratogenic	Inhibitor (increases levels of other medications)	Yes	Also used for migraine and mood stabilization
Vigabatrin	GABA	• Focal seizures • Infantile spasms in Tuberous sclerosis	• Visual field defects			
Zonisamide (ZNS)	Multiple		Nephrolithiasis			

[a]Life-threatening adverse affects such as hepatotoxicity, bone marrow toxicity, teratogenicity, and Stevens-Johnson syndrome can occur with nearly all ASMs, as can neurologic adverse affects such as dizziness, nystagmus, mental cloudiness. Osteoporosis also occurs with many ASMs.

Side Effects & Toxicities of Antiseizure Medications

Nearly all ASMs can cause dizziness, double vision, sedation, and/or behavioral changes, although these symptoms are generally more pronounced with the older agents (phenobarbital, phenytoin, carbamazepine, and valproate) and are less common with newer agents. These side effects may be dose limiting but are generally not dangerous to the patient.

Life-threatening toxicities that can occur with many of the ASMs include hepatic toxicity, hematologic abnormalities (agranulocytosis, aplastic anemia), and Stevens-Johnson syndrome (a severe drug-induced cutaneous and mucosal reaction that can be fatal). Several ASMs can also increase risk for osteoporosis. Due to all of these potential toxicities, initiation of most ASMs requires evaluation with baseline complete blood count (CBC), hepatic and renal function tests, and calcium and vitamin D levels. For most ASMs, these laboratory tests are generally followed serially after initiation to evaluate for any signs of toxicity or changes in hepatic or renal function that could require a change in dosage.

The highest risks of Stevens-Johnson syndrome are with phenytoin, phenobarbital, carbamazepine, and lamotrigine. The risk of Stephens-Johnson syndrome with carbamazepine is higher in Asian patients with a particular HLA type (HLA-B*1502), so this should be screened for before starting carbamazepine in Asian patients. Although the risk of Stevens-Johnson syndrome is commonly believed to be highest with lamotrigine, the current practice of initiating the medication with a slow uptitration has decreased this risk, and the risk is in fact present with all ASMs. Any patient started on an ASM should be instructed to stop the medication immediately and seek medical evaluation should a rash develop. Explaining to parents of children initiating an ASM to report the development of any rash is particularly important since children frequently develop rashes of various sorts. The rash of Stevens-Johnson can begin quite innocuously and might not raise concern unless parents are instructed to watch for it.

Carbamazepine, oxcarbazepine, and eslicarbazepine can cause hyponatremia, so serum sodium should be followed in patients on these ASMs. Lacosamide can cause PR interval prolongation, and cenobamate and rufinamide can cause QT interval shortening, so a baseline ECG should be obtained before initiating the medication and another ECG should be obtained in follow up to evaluate for any ECG changes. Lamotrigine may also cause arrythmias in patients with underlying heart disease according to in vitro data. Topiramate and zonisamide can increase the risk of nephrolithiasis. Levetiracetam and perampanel can have psychiatric adverse effects, so should be used in caution in patients with psychiatric conditions; psychiatric changes (depression, irritability, aggressiveness) should be screened for in patients taking these medications. Valproate has the highest associated risk of fetal malformations when taken by pregnant women, and topiramate and phenobarbital also carry high risks of teratogenicity, so these three ASMs should be avoided in women of child-bearing age. Lamotrigine and levetiracetam appear to have the lowest risk of fetal malformations when used in pregnant women (see "Epilepsy & Pregnancy"). Many ASMs require dose modification for patients during pregnancy and the postpartum period, as well as in patients with renal and/or hepatic dysfunction.

In addition to potential toxicities, some ASMs have additional properties that may influence their use. Valproate and topiramate are effective for migraine prophylaxis, and could be considered in patients with both migraine and epilepsy. Valproate can cause weight gain and topiramate can cause weight loss, so the latter might be preferred if a patient seeks to lose weight. Valproate has the highest rate of fetal malformations and should be avoided in women of child-bearing age. Valproate and lamotrigine both have mood-stabilizing properties, whereas levetiracetam, brivaracetam, and perampanel can cause irritability and depression, so the former two may be preferred in patients with psychiatric comorbidities while the latter three should generally be avoided. Lacosamide may be suboptimal in patients with cardiac conduction system disease due to the risk of PR interval prolongation.

Phenobarbital, phenytoin, valproate, lacosamide, and levetiracetam can all be administered intravenously if a patient cannot take oral medications.

Whichever medication is chosen, it should generally be initiated at the lowest dose and slowly uptitrated with the goal of seizure control and tolerability.

Drug levels are most commonly followed for phenytoin and valproate, although they may be used for other medications to assess for adherence or to establish a baseline level to follow during pregnancy or when another medication will be initiated that may interact with the original medication. Phenytoin levels need to be corrected for low albumin levels.

Antiseizure Medication Titration & Combination

At each follow-up visit, a patient on ASMs should be assessed for whether seizure frequency has improved and whether there are side effects of the ASM(s). If there is neither improvement nor side effects, one should also determine if the patient is taking the medication properly. If there is uncertainty about this, drug levels can be obtained. After initiation of ASM therapy, one of four scenarios generally occurs:

1. At a certain dose of an ASM, seizures are well controlled without significant side effects: The patient's epilepsy is successfully controlled.

2. The maximal dose of an ASM is reached, but seizure frequency is unchanged or not sufficiently diminished, or side effects are intolerable. A different ASM should be initiated and uptitrated. The first ASM should be off-titrated if it was ineffective or not tolerated, and this should be done gradually to avoid rebound/withdrawal seizures.

3. The maximal dose of an ASM is reached with partial but incomplete control of seizures. A second medication should be initiated and uptitrated. If the combination of medications is highly effective, it may be unclear whether

the advantage was achieved by the new ASM or the combination of ASMs. If seizures are well controlled, slow down-titration or off-titration of the original medication can be considered under close observation since monotherapy is ideal when possible.

4. A submaximal dose of an ASM leads to improved but incomplete seizure control but with intolerable side effects. Dose reduction to the previously tolerated dose is necessary with addition of a second ASM and uptitration of this second agent. Depending on the success of introduction of the second ASM, the first may be slowly off-titrated, as in the prior two scenarios.

One particular situation of which to be aware in ASM titration is that of carbamazepine autoinduction: carbamazepine induces its own metabolism, and so as a result, the initial effectiveness may decrease around 6 weeks to 2 months after initiating the medication, requiring a dose increase.

Refractory (Drug-Resistant) Epilepsy

In one study, about half of patients with epilepsy became seizure free for 1 year with the first attempted ASM, but of those who did not, only about a quarter responded to the second attempted ASM regimen, and returns only diminished further when attempting treatment with a third regimen (Kwan and Brodie, 2000; Chen et al., 2018). While some patients' seizures may be controlled with complex regimens of more than two ASMs, if seizures are not controlled after adequate trials of two well-tolerated ASMs (individually or together), the patient is considered to have refractory (drug-resistant) epilepsy. Such patients should be considered for epilepsy surgery, thermal ablation, neuromodulation (vagus nerve stimulation, responsive neurostimulation, deep brain stimulation), and/or the ketogenic diet.

If surgical resection of the epileptic focus is under consideration, precise localization of the seizure focus is undertaken with MRI or nuclear medicine study (ictal single photon emission computed tomography [SPECT] or interictal positron emission tomography [PET]) and intracranial EEG (also called electrocorticography) using subdural grids and strips or more minimally invasive implantation of stereo-EEG electrodes. Intracranial EEG is used both to map epileptic foci and to delineate functional regions of normal cortex (e.g., language, motor function) to assist in surgical planning. An additional test that may be performed is the Wada test, which uses sodium amytal or sodium amobarbital injected into each carotid sequentially to selectively temporarily "silence" one hemisphere at a time so as to test cognitive function attributable to that hemisphere in order to predict potential postsurgical deficits.

Tapering Off Antiseizure Medications in Seizure-Free Patients

In patients who have been seizure free for 2 years, the question often emerges as to whether ASMs can be titrated off. A gradual taper can be attempted, explaining to the patient that there is about a 40% risk of seizure recurrence, and that the risk is greatest during the period of off-titration. Therefore, during this period, the patient should not drive, should not swim or bathe unaccompanied, and should not work at heights. If a patient has a seizure during the taper, lifelong ASM therapy is generally warranted. Some practitioners perform an EEG before considering tapering off ASMs to compare to prior EEGs in order to guide this decision. Epilepsy can be considered resolved in patients with childhood epilepsy syndromes (see Table 18–3) that are self-limited to a particular age range and in patients who have not had a seizure in 10 years including 5 years with no ASM treatment (Fisher et al., 2014).

SPECIAL SCENARIOS IN THE MANAGEMENT OF SEIZURES & EPILEPSY

Childhood-Onset Seizures

A number of epilepsy syndromes arise in infancy or childhood that have particular clinical and electrographic features, some of which respond to specific treatments (Table 18–3). Other causes of seizures in infants include:

- In utero or peripartum stroke, hemorrhage, or infection
- Inborn errors of metabolism
- Brain malformations

Pediatric Febrile Seizures

If a child presents with seizures and fever, this should lead to consideration of meningitis, encephalitis, or cerebral malaria (in endemic regions). However, in children up to about 5 years of age, seizures may occur in the setting of fever without CNS infection. Pediatric febrile seizures in this context are referred to as simple or complex. A pediatric febrile seizure is classified as a **simple febrile seizure** if it is generalized, lasts less than 15 minutes, and occurs less than once in 24 hours. With simple febrile seizures, the risk of future development of epilepsy is not felt to be significantly elevated and so such patients generally do not require further evaluation with respect to the seizures (i.e., EEG is generally not necessary), and ASM treatment is not generally indicated.

However, if any of the above criteria for simple febrile seizure are not met (i.e., pediatric febrile seizures that are focal, last more than 15 minutes, and/or occur more than once in 24 hours), these are considered to be **complex febrile seizures**. Complex febrile seizures are associated with an increased risk of future febrile seizures and development of epilepsy. EEG may be considered in cases of complex febrile seizures to evaluate for an underlying epileptic focus or a signature of an underlying epilepsy syndrome. Prophylactic ASM treatment may be considered in some patients with complex febrile seizures if EEG is suggestive of an underlying epilepsy syndrome.

For children with either simple or complex febrile seizures, parents should be provided with rectal diazepam to be

TABLE 18–3 Pediatric Epilepsy Syndromes.

	Age of Onset	Seizure Type	Other Clinical Features	EEG Features	Treatment
Ohtahara syndrome	0–3 months	• Tonic • Spasms • Other	Often fatal before age 1	Burst suppression	Often refractory to ASMs
Dravet syndrome (Severe myoclonic epilepsy of infancy)	0–1 year	Various, often prolonged	• Developmental regression • SCN1A mutation (sodium channel)	May be normal initially, later slowing & epileptiform discharges	• VPA • Clobazam • Cannabidiol • Stiripentol • Fenfluramine
West syndrome	0–1 year	Infantile spasms	Developmental delay/intellectual disability; often secondary to underlying cause	Hypsarrhythmia	• ACTH • Vigabatrin
Doose syndrome (Myoclonic astatic epilepsy)	1–5 year	• Myoclonic-astatic (drop attacks) • Various	Intellectual development may be normal or impaired	May be normal initially; later spike/wave & slowing	• ASMs • Ketogenic diet
Lennox-Gastaut Syndrome	3–10 years (Peaks 3–5 years)	• GTC • Atonic (drop attacks) • Atypical absence	Intellectual disability	Slow spike/wave (2–2.5 Hz)	VPA, cannabidiol
Landau-Kleffner Syndrome	2–10 years (Peaks 5–7 years)	• Any type (some patients do not have seizures)	Pure word deafness with preserved hearing; other progressive language deficits	• Temporal/temporoparietal spikes • Spike/wave during sleep	• ASMs • Steroids • Surgery
Rasmussen encephalitis	1–15 years	• Focal motor/epilepsia partialis continua	Progressive unilateral hemisphere atrophy with contralateral hemiparesis; associated with antibody to GluR3 (glutamate receptor)	Focal epileptiform discharges	• Immunomodulatory therapy • Hemispherectomy
Panayiotopoulos syndrome	1–15 years	Eye deviation, vomiting, autonomic features (sweating, pallor, salivation)	Normal development; usually remits	Occipital spikes	• ASMs • Usually remits after teenage years
Childhood epilepsy with centrotemporal spikes (aka Benign Rolandic epilepsy, BECTS)	2–13 years	Nocturnal focal motor seizures of mouth with drooling, aphasia	Usually spontaneously remits	Centrotemporal spikes	Spontaneously remits (though can be treated until then)
Childhood absence epilepsy	3–10 years	Brief absence seizures		3-Hz spike/wave during seizures	• Ethosuximide • VPA • (Note: CBZ may worsen absence epilepsy)
Juvenile myoclonic epilepsy (JME)	12–18 years	• GTC • Absence • Myoclonic	Myoclonic jerks in AM	4–6 Hz spike/wave	VPA

Abbreviations: ACTH: adrenocorticotropic hormone; ASMs: antiseizure medications; EEG: electroencephalography; GTC: generalized tonic-clonic seizure; VPA: valproic acid.

administered if a subsequent febrile seizure occurs and lasts longer than 5 minutes.

Seizures in Patients With HIV

When seizures occur in an HIV-positive patient, CNS opportunistic infection should be considered (see "Opportunistic Infections of the Nervous System in HIV/AIDS" in Ch. 20). Limited data on interactions between ASMs and antiretrovirals are summarized in a 2012 American Academy of Neurology guideline statement (Birbeck et al., 2012). In general, this guideline recommends that enzyme-inducing ASMs be avoided in patients on antiretrovirals when possible. Particular interactions highlighted in the guideline include the following:

- Phenytoin appears to decrease lopinavir and ritonavir levels and may require dose augmentation of these antiretrovirals.
- Valproate may increase zidovudine levels and may require a dose reduction of zidovudine.
- Atazanavir/ritonavir appears to decrease lamotrigine levels and may require a dose increase of lamotrigine.

Epilepsy & Pregnancy

One of the most feared adverse effects of ASMs is teratogenicity. The background risk of major congenital malformations in the general population is about 1%–3%. The ASM that augments this risk the most is valproate, with a rate of major congenital malformations of 10%–20%. Topiramate and phenobarbital also carry relatively high risks of teratogenicity compared to other ASMs. Lamotrigine and levetiracetam appear to be the safest ASMs in pregnancy, and the risks associated with other ASMs fall in between. ASMs also increase the risk of neurodevelopmental disorders, with the highest risk again coming from valproate. Higher ASM doses and ASM polytherapy increase the risk of both congenital malformations and neurodevelopmental disorders.

If a woman with epilepsy plans to become pregnant, the ideal scenario would be if her ASM(s) could be tapered off. If the patient has been seizure free for 2 years or more, tapering off of ASMs can be considered to see if she can tolerate being off ASMs for several months before conception. However, this is rarely feasible in practice, and the majority of patients will require ASM therapy through pregnancy. Every effort should be made to limit the number of ASMs and the dosage of ASMs in pregnant women, trying to find the minimal effective regimen before conception. If a patient's seizures have been controlled on a highly teratogenic ASM (valproate, topiramate, or phenobarbital), a cross-titration to a lower risk ASM should be considered before conception.

If a patient becomes pregnant while already on ASMs (including valproate or topiramate), titration to a different medication regimen should *not* be attempted for several reasons: seizures during this period could be harmful to the fetus (as well as the mother), the period of neurulation during which teratogenic risk may be highest has often already passed by the time the pregnancy is apparent, and cross-titration of ASMs will lead to greater exposure to multiple ASMs during the period of cross-titration.

All women of child-bearing age on ASMs should be given folic acid to lower the risk of teratogenicity (especially neural tube defects) should they become pregnant. If a woman on ASMs becomes pregnant and was not on folic acid, this should be initiated immediately, since folic acid reduces the risk of neurodevelopmental disorders and major congenital malformations.

ASM levels should be obtained before pregnancy and followed closely since changes in metabolism and volume of distribution may require dose readjustment to maintain the desired therapeutic ASM levels during pregnancy. After delivery, dose adjustment of ASMs is often necessary again since metabolism and volume of distribution return to pre-pregnancy states.

Some practitioners advocate for the use of daily vitamin K beginning 1 month before delivery in pregnant women on ASMs to prevent hemorrhagic disease of the newborn since vitamin K levels in the fetus may be reduced by enzyme-inducing ASMs, although this practice is debated.

Breastfeeding while on ASMs is not felt to be harmful to the newborn and should be encouraged, though infants should be monitored for sedation if the mother is taking phenobarbital, primidone, or benzodiazepines.

Antiseizure Medication Prophylaxis for At-Risk Patients Who Have Not Had Seizures

There are only a few scenarios in which a brief course of prophylactic ASM therapy is utilized in a patient who has not yet had a seizure:

- For 7 days after severe head trauma to reduce the risk of early seizures (although this has no effect on whether the patient will develop epilepsy later)
- For 7 days after a craniotomy (although this practice is debated)
- After aneurysmal subarachnoid hemorrhage until the aneurysm is secured, since the patient is at risk for seizures and seizures could increase the risk of rebleeding (although this practice is debated)

For most other scenarios in which one might consider seizure "prophylaxis," there are no data to support the practice. ASMs are generally *not* given to patients with a brain tumor, stroke, hemorrhage, or meningitis unless they have a seizure, since the risks of ASM toxicities and interactions with other medications may outweigh the benefits.

STATUS EPILEPTICUS

Status epilepticus is defined as 5 or more minutes of continuous seizures, or repeated seizures without return to consciousness between them.

Three aspects of management for status epilepticus must be pursued in parallel: management of the "ABCs" (i.e., medical stabilization of the patient), treatment of seizures, and search for an underlying cause.

1. **Management of the "ABCs" (airway, breathing, circulation).** Ongoing seizures are a medical emergency in addition to a neurologic emergency. Both seizures and sedative medications used to treat them can lead to respiratory compromise and cardiovascular instability. Continuous oxygen saturation monitoring and cardiovascular monitoring are essential and intubation/mechanical ventilation may be necessary.

2. **Treatment of seizures in status epilepticus.** The usual algorithm for the treatment of status epilepticus is as follows:

   - Serial doses of benzodiazepines (IV lorazepam, IV diazepam, or IM midazolam) are administered (glucose and thiamine are generally given as well at this stage; see below).

   - If seizures continue after adequate benzodiazepine dosing, a second-line agent is initiated, most commonly (fos)phenytoin, leviteracetam, valproate, or phenobarbital. A recent trial found no difference in outcome between fosphenytoin, levetiracetam, and valproate, with seizure cessation in about 50% of patients with any of these medications (Kapur et al., 2019 and Chamberlain et al., 2020 [ESETT trial]).

   - If seizures continue, the patient is considered to be in *refractory status epilepticus*, and should be intubated and coma should be induced with pentobarbital, midazolam, propofol, or thiopental. Note that this step is generally only taken for generalized convulsive seizures but not for focal motor status epilepticus; use of these measures in nonconvulsive status epilepticus is debated (see "Nonconvulsive Status Epilepticus"). Continuous EEG monitoring is initiated at this point to guide degree of sedation (either seizure suppression or burst suppression) and success of therapy. A daily maintenance ASM is also initiated, usually the same ASM that was used in the prior step.

   - Induced coma is generally maintained for approximately 24 hours. Sedatives are then slowly weaned under continuous EEG monitoring to determine whether seizures have resolved or whether further therapy is necessary. If seizures persist after this 24 hour period of anesthesia, this is referred to as *super-refractory status epilepticus*. Treatment involves additional ASMs and/or sedative agents, ketamine, hypothermia, ketogenic diet, immunotherapy (if there is concern for an autoimmune etiology), electroconvulsive therapy, transcranial magnetic stimulation, and/or surgical intervention (if a seizure focus can be identified).

3. **Search for an underlying cause.** Evaluation for hypoglycemia, electrolyte abnormalities, drug intoxication or withdrawal, structural lesion, or an infectious or inflammatory etiology of status epilepticus should proceed in parallel with treatment of status epilepticus. In patients with a history of epilepsy, status epilepticus may be provoked by an acute systemic insult or low ASM levels. Glucose and thiamine are generally given immediately to patients in status epilepticus: If hypoglycemia is present, it must be reversed rapidly; if there is no hypoglycemia, there is little harm in empirically treating for this possibility. Thiamine is given with glucose so as to prevent development of Wernicke's encephalopathy in potentially at-risk patients (see "Wernicke's Encephalopathy" in Ch. 22).

Patients with no clear cause of refractory status epilepticus (i.e., no history of epilepsy, acute provoking factor, or structural lesion) are classified as having NORSE (new-onset refractory status epilepticus); if this syndrome is preceded by fever, it is called FIRES (febrile infection-related epilepsy syndrome). New-onset super refractory status epilepticus is referred to as NOSRSE. Although no etiology is found in many cases, patients should be evaluated for autoimmune antibody-mediated syndromes (e.g., anti-NMDA receptor encephalitis) and CNS infection (Matthews et al., 2020).

Nonconvulsive Status Epilepticus

Nonconvulsive status epilepticus (NCSE) refers to seizure activity without frank convulsions. Subtle motor signs (e.g., eye deviation or nystagmus, eyelid or facial twitching, extremity twitching) may be present, but some patients may only have alterations in level of consciousness ranging from confusion to coma. The diagnosis is made definitively by noting electrographic seizure activity on EEG. Continuous EEG for at least 24 hours is generally required to evaluate for NCSE, since seizures may be intermittent. If the EEG is ambiguous (i.e., epileptiform discharges but without clear evidence of seizure), a benzodiazepine trial can be undertaken to see if there is both electrographic and clinical improvement in response to benzodiazepine administration.

NCSE should be considered in patients who fail to recover consciousness after one or more seizures. NCSE should also be considered in the differential diagnosis of altered mental status and coma since up to 20% of comatose patients in intensive care units may have evidence of NCSE when monitored with continuous EEG. It remains unclear whether poor outcomes in critically ill patients with NCSE are significantly ameliorated by treating NCSE aggressively, since poor outcomes may be more a reflection of the underlying cause of NCSE rather than NCSE itself. Therefore, although attempts should be made to control NCSE with ASMs while treating the underlying cause, anesthetic agents are less commonly used for NCSE as compared to their regular use for convulsive status epilepticus.

REFERENCES

Birbeck GL, French JA, Perucca E, Simpson DM, Fraimow H, George JM, et al. Evidence-based guideline: antiepileptic drug selection for people with HIV/AIDS. *Neurol* 2012;78:139-145.

Chamberlain JM, Kapur J, Shinnar S, Elm J, Holsti M, Babcock L, et al. Efficacy of levetiracetam, fosphenytoin, and valproate for established status epilepticus by age group (ESETT): a double-blind, responsive-adaptive, randomised controlled trial. *Lancet* 2020;395:1217-1224.

Chen Z, Brodie MJ, Liew D, Kwan P. Treatment outcomes in patients with newly diagnosed epilepsy treated with established and new antiepileptic drugs: a 30-year longitudinal cohort study. *JAMA Neurol* 2018;75(3):279-286.

Fisher RS, Acevedo C, Arzimanoglou A, Bogacz A, Cross JH, Elger CE, et al. ILAE official report: a practical clinical definition of epilepsy *Epilepsia* 2014;55(4):475-482.

Kapur J, Elm J, Chamberlain JM, Barsan W, Cloyd J, Lowenstein D, et al. Randomized trial of three anticonvulsant medications for status epilepticus. *N Engl J Med* 2019;381(22):2103-2113.

Kim LG, Johnson TL, Marson AG, Chadwick DW, MRC MESS study group. Prediction of risk of seizure recurrence after a single seizure and early epilepsy: further results from the MESS trial. *Lancet Neurol* 2006;5:317-322.

Krumholz A, Wiebe S, Gronseth GS, Gloss DS, Sanchez AM, Kabir AA, et al. Evidence-based guideline: management of an unprovoked first seizure in adults: Report of the Guideline Development Subcommittee of the American Academy of Neurology and the American Epilepsy Society. *Neurol* 2015;84(16):1705-1713.

Kwan P, Brodie MJ. Early identification of refractory epilepsy. *NEJM* 200;342:314-319.

Marson A, Jacoby A, Johnson A, Kim L, Gamble C, Chadwick D, et al. Immediate versus deferred antiepileptic drug treatment for early epilepsy and single seizures: a randomised controlled trial. *Lancet* 2005;365:2007-2013.

Matthews E, Alkhachroum A, Massad N, Letchinger R, Doyle K, Claassen J, et al. New-onset super-refractory status epilepticus: a case series of 26 patients. *Neurol* 2020;95(16):e2280-e2285.

Vascular Diseases of the Brain & Spinal Cord

CHAPTER

19

The brain and spinal cord can be affected by a variety of conditions related to the vascular system:

- Ischemic stroke: lack of blood flow to a portion of the brain (or more rarely the spinal cord)
- Intracranial or spinal hemorrhage at five possible sites:
  - Epidural hematoma: between the skull or spine and dura
  - Subdural hematoma: between the dura and arachnoid
  - Subarachnoid hemorrhage: between the arachnoid and brain or spinal cord
  - Intraparenchymal (intracerebral) hemorrhage: in the brain itself (or less commonly hemorrhage into the spinal cord [hematomyelia])
  - Intraventricular hemorrhage (within the ventricular system of the brain)
- Cerebral venous sinus thrombosis

- Vascular malformations
- Vasculopathies, including vasculitis and reversible cerebral vasoconstriction syndrome (RCVS)

OVERVIEW OF ISCHEMIC STROKE & INTRACEREBRAL HEMORRHAGE

The term **stroke** refers to the clinical scenario in which a patient is "struck" by a sudden-onset neurologic deficit localizable to the brain (or more rarely the spinal cord; see "Vascular Disease of the Spinal Cord"). The vascular conditions that are collectively referred to as stroke (or cerebrovascular accident) include ischemic stroke and intracerebral hemorrhage (ICH). ICH is sometimes referred to as "hemorrhagic stroke." Although subarachnoid hemorrhage is sometimes included as a cause of stroke, its clinical presentation and management are distinct from ischemic stroke and ICH. Although both ischemic stroke and ICH can present similarly, their management differs. Although the potential etiologies of ischemic stroke and ICH overlap, there are unique causes of each that must be considered.

Ischemic stroke and ICH both present with sudden-onset focal neurologic deficits, but ICH is more commonly accompanied by headache, nausea/vomiting, and depressed level of consciousness at onset due to increased intracranial pressure and brain displacement from mass effect of the hematoma. However, ischemic stroke may also present with headache, nausea/vomiting, and/or depressed level of consciousness depending on the size and location of the area of ischemia, so distinction between ischemic stroke and ICH often cannot be made on clinical grounds alone. Therefore, a CT scan is necessary for diagnosis as soon as stroke is suspected.

Acute management of ischemic stroke and acute management of ICH share many aspects of supportive care but differ with respect to two parameters: coagulation and blood pressure (Table 19–1). In acute ischemic stroke, the goals are to decrease thrombosis (thrombolysis, antiplatelet agents, or in some instances anticoagulation) and allow autoregulation of blood pressure (to restore/maintain tissue perfusion). In acute ICH, the goals are to stop bleeding (reversal of anticoagulation, administration of clotting factors) and reduce blood pressure (to decrease the likelihood of hematoma expansion).

Aside from these two parameters, the majority of acute supportive management and subsequent supportive care is shared between ischemic stroke and ICH:

- Electrocardiogram (ECG) and cardiac monitoring (to evaluate for myocardial infarction or arrhythmia, which can cause or be caused by stroke).
- Evaluation of swallowing and prevention of aspiration.
- Control of blood glucose to avoid hypoglycemia or hyperglycemia.
- Maintenance of euthermia (by treating fever and underlying infection if it occurs).
- Treatment of seizures if they occur (more common with ICH as compared to ischemic stroke).
- Evaluation for and management of elevated intracranial pressure.
- Early mobilization.
- Deep venous thrombosis (DVT) prophylaxis. Pharmacologic DVT prophylaxis can be started immediately after

ischemic stroke unless tissue plasminogen activator (tPA) is administered (in which case it is delayed 24 hours). However, pharmacologic DVT prophylaxis is generally not started until 24–48 hours after ICH. Mechanical prophylaxis can begin immediately after either type of stroke.

- Physical therapy, speech therapy, and/or occupational therapy.

ISCHEMIC STROKE

The types of neurologic deficits seen with ischemic stroke depend on the size and location of the infarct. A small infarct may cause symptoms so mild that the patient does not present for medical attention. This is borne out by the frequency with which evidence of a prior infarct is noted on a CT scan performed for other reasons in a patient with no known prior clinical history of stroke. However, a small infarct in the internal capsule or anterior pons could lead to contralateral hemiplegia. The stroke syndromes caused by infarction in the various vascular territories are discussed in Chapter 7 (see "Clinical Syndromes Associated with Cerebral Vascular Territories" in Ch. 7).

Transient Ischemic Attack

A transient ischemic attack (TIA) was initially defined as stroke symptoms that last for less than 24 hours. However, the increased sensitivity of MRI with diffusion-weighted imaging (DWI) has demonstrated that many patients with transient stroke symptoms have actually had small strokes. Therefore, TIA is now defined as transient stroke symptoms that resolve completely without evidence of infarction on MRI. Most TIAs last for minutes to about an hour, and those that last longer often have evidence of infarction on DWI even if symptoms resolve completely. The risk of subsequent stroke after TIA can be estimated by the ABCD2 score (Johnston et al., 2007):

- **A**ge: 1 point if ≥60
- **B**lood pressure: 1 point if ≥140/90 mm Hg at time of presentation
- **C**linical symptoms of TIA
  - 2 points for unilateral weakness or
  - 1 point for speech disturbance without weakness or
  - 0 points for any other symptoms without weakness or speech disturbance
- **D**iabetes: 1 point if present
- **D**uration of TIA: 2 points for ≥60 minutes, 1 point for 10–59 minutes. 0 points if <10 minutes

A score of 1–3 yields a 2-day and 7-day stroke risk of approximately 1%, a score of 4–5 yields a 2-day stroke risk of approximately 4% and a 7-day stroke risk of approximately 6%, and a score of 6–7 yields a 2-day stroke risk of approximately 8% and a 7-day stroke risk of approximately 11% (Johnston et al., 2007). Some practitioners use this score to determine whether evaluation for etiology of TIA should

TABLE 19–1 Comparison of Acute Management of Ischemic Stroke Versus Intracerebral Hemorrhage.

	Coagulation	Blood Pressure
Ischemic stroke	**Reduce** (thrombolysis, antiplatelets)	**Permissive hypertension** (autoregulation)
Intracerebral hemorrhage	**Increase** (reversal of coagulopathy, administration of clotting factors)	**Decrease**

proceed as an inpatient or can be performed in rapid outpatient follow up. Evaluation for etiology and stroke prevention after TIA are discussed with secondary prevention of stroke below.

Etiology of Ischemic Stroke

Understanding the potential etiologies of ischemic stroke allows for an understanding of the acute management, evaluation for etiology, and secondary prevention of ischemic stroke (Table 19–2). Any pathophysiologic process that disrupts blood supply to one or more regions of the brain can cause ischemic stroke. Anatomically, the blood supply to the brain begins in the left ventricle of the heart, travels through the aorta to the cervical vessels (carotid arteries and vertebral arteries), and ultimately passes through the cerebral arterial system. Pathology at any of these levels can lead to ischemic stroke, as can diseases of the blood itself. Therefore, the initial evaluation for stroke etiology (discussed in more detail below) must evaluate:

- The arteries:
  - Ultrasound, CT angiogram (CTA), MR angiogram (MRA), or digital subtraction angiography
  - Evaluation for risk factors for arterial disease: blood pressure, blood glucose, lipids, smoking status
- The heart: cardiac monitoring and echocardiogram
- If clinically indicated, the blood; for example, for hypercoagulability or sickle cell disease

TABLE 19–2 Etiologies of Ischemic Stroke.

Vascular Causes of Stroke	Cardiac Causes of Stroke	Hematologic Causes of Stroke
Arterial disease	**Cardiac sources of embolism**	• Hypercoagulable state
• Atherosclerosis	• Atrial fibrillation	• Sickle cell anemia
• Cervical artery dissection	• Left ventricular failure	• Hyperviscosity
• Vasculopathy	• Myocardial infarction	• Intravascular lymphoma
• Radiation-induced	• Endocarditis	
• Inherited (e.g., CADASIL)	• Infectious	
• Vasculitis	• Inflammatory	
• Primary CNS vasculitis	• Thrombotic (e.g., due to malignancy)	
• Secondary CNS vasculitis (e.g., infectious)	• Cardiac tumor	
• Vasospasm		
Venous disease	**Other cardiac causes of stroke**	
• Venous sinus thrombosis	• Cardiac arrest	
• Cortical vein thrombosis	• Patent foramen ovale (due to paradoxical embolism)	

Arterial Disease as a Cause of Ischemic Stroke

Diseases of the cerebral vasculature that can lead to ischemic stroke include:

- Atherosclerosis and thromboembolic disease of the arteries
- Lipohyalinosis of small penetrating arteries (small vessel disease)
- Carotid or vertebral artery dissection
- Cerebral vasospasm (e.g., reversible cerebral vasoconstriction syndrome [RCVS] or secondary to subarachnoid hemorrhage)
- Vascular compression by an external mass (e.g., a neck tumor compressing one of the carotids)
- Vasculopathy, including vasculitis, radiation-induced vasculopathy, moyamoya

Atherosclerosis and thromboembolic disease as a cause of ischemic stroke—**Thrombosis** refers to local formation of a clot in the lumen of a blood vessel. **Embolism** refers to passage of material from a more proximal source to a more distal location. In the case of the cerebral arteries, embolism may arise from the heart, the aortic arch, the cervical vessels (the carotid arteries or vertebral arteries), or from the venous circulation if there is a patent foramen ovale (see "Secondary Stroke Prevention in Patients With Patent Foramen Ovale"). Atherosclerosis is the main cause of thrombotic disease of the cervical and cerebral blood vessels. Risk factors for atherosclerosis include hypertension, diabetes, hyperlipidemia, and smoking. Embolism from the carotid arteries or vertebral arteries to a more distal cerebral vessel is referred to as **artery-to-artery embolism** (e.g., from the internal carotid artery to the middle cerebral artery). Stroke can also be caused by embolism of thrombotic material from the heart to the cerebral blood vessels (see "Cardiac Causes of Ischemic Stroke"). If a patient has a patent foramen ovale, embolism from the venous circulation can cause stroke (**paradoxical embolism**). Rare causes of cerebral embolism not due to thromboembolism include air embolism, fat embolism, and amniotic fluid embolism.

Lipohyalinosis of small penetrating arteries as a cause of ischemic stroke—Chronic hypertension can lead to thickening of the walls of the small penetrating arteries (small vessel disease), which can predispose to lacunar infarcts in the deep subcortical regions (internal capsule or thalamus) or the anterior pons (see "Lacunar Strokes" in Ch. 7).

Cervical artery dissection as a cause of ischemic stroke—Cervical artery dissection is a tear between the layers of the wall of the cervical vessels (i.e., carotids or vertebral arteries). It is a common cause of stroke in the young and can be caused by head or neck trauma (which may be major or so minor that it cannot be recalled), chiropractic manipulation, and collagen disorders (e.g., Ehlers-Danlos, fibromuscular dysplasia).

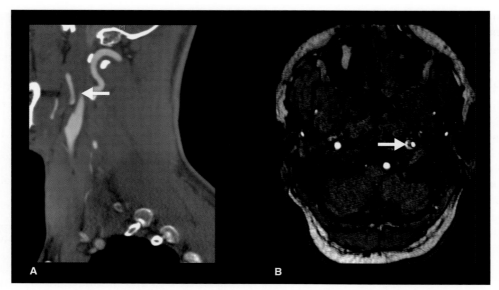

FIGURE 19–1 **Internal carotid artery dissection. A:** CT angiogram of the neck in sagittal view demonstrating "flame-shaped" appearance of internal carotid artery dissection (**arrow**). **B:** T1-weighted axial MRI with fat saturation demonstrating "crescent" appearance of intramural hematoma in left internal carotid artery dissection (**arrow**).

Cervical artery dissection can present as TIA or stroke, or may present with local symptoms such as neck pain, headache, and in the case of carotid artery dissection, lower cranial nerve palsies (cranial nerves 9–12) and/or Horner's syndrome (in the case of internal carotid dissection only ptosis and miosis will be seen, but no anhidrosis because sweating fibers travel with the external carotid; see "Impaired Pupillary Dilatation" in Ch. 10). The risk of stroke is highest in the first week after dissection, and some patients may have multiple TIAs or strokes during this period. A dissected vessel has a flame-shaped appearance on CTA (Fig. 19–1A), and a crescentic intramural hematoma can be visualized on T1-weighted fat saturation MRI (Fig. 19–1B). Secondary stroke prevention in patients with TIA or stroke due to cervical artery dissection is discussed below (see "Secondary Stroke Prevention in Patients With Cervical Artery Dissection").

Vasospasm as a cause of ischemic stroke—Vasospasm can be caused by:

- Local irritation of the blood vessels by subarachnoid hemorrhage or meningitis
- Failure of cerebral autoregulation, which can be seen in posterior reversible encephalopathy syndrome (PRES; see "Posterior Reversible Encephalopathy Syndrome") and eclampsia/postpartum angiopathy
- Drugs such as cocaine and marijuana, and medications such as selective serotonin reuptake inhibitors (SSRIs) and sympathomimetic-containing cold medications can cause reversible cerebral vasoconstriction syndrome (RCVS; see "Reversible Cerebral Vasoconstriction Syndrome")

Vasculopathy and vasculitis as a cause of ischemic stroke—Beyond atherosclerosis, there are a number of other causes of vasculopathy that can cause ischemic stroke, including:

- Radiation-induced vasculopathy (see "Neurotoxicity of Radiation Therapy" in Ch. 24)
- Reversible cerebral vasoconstriction syndrome (RCVS), which can cause stroke or hemorrhage (most commonly subarachnoid hemorrhage when hemorrhage occurs)
- Moyamoya (which can be primary or secondary)
- Cerebral autosomal dominant arteriopathy with subcortical infarcts and leukoencephalopathy (CADASIL) and cerebral autosomal recessive arteriopathy with subcortical infarcts and leukoencephalopathy (CARASIL)
- Vasculitis: blood vessel inflammation that may be primary or secondary (e.g., secondary to infection or to a systemic vasculitic syndrome)

These and other vasculopathies are discussed below (see "Rarer Causes of Ischemic Stroke: Vasculopathies, Vasculitis, and Genetic Disorders")

Cardiac Causes of Ischemic Stroke

Cardiac causes of stroke include:

- Atrial fibrillation: clot formation due to stasis in the left atrium (especially the left atrial appendage) leads to cerebral embolism
- Cardiac valvular disease (and mechanical cardiac valves)
- Left ventricular failure with dilated left ventricle: clot formation due to stasis in the left ventricle leads to cerebral embolism

- Myocardial infarction: due to development of left ventricular thrombus (mural thrombus)
- Infective endocarditis with septic embolization
- Nonbacterial thrombotic endocarditis (marantic endocarditis) with embolization, which can be caused by:
  - Inflammatory endocarditis in rheumatologic disease (e.g., Libman-Sacks endocarditis in lupus)
  - Malignancy causing thombus formation on cardiac valves (most common with mucin-secreting adenocarcinomas)
- Cardiac tumors on which thrombus may form (e.g., fibroelastoma, atrial myxoma, metastasis)
- Patent foramen ovale, which can serve as a conduit for thrombus formed in the venous circulation to find its way to the arterial system and cause stroke.
- Cardiac arrest with hypoxic-ischemic injury. The gray matter is most sensitive to hypoxia, so hypoxic-ischemic injury can cause diffuse infarction of the cortex and/or basal ganglia (Fig. 19–2).

Hematologic Causes of Acute Ischemic Stroke

Problems with the blood itself can also lead to stroke:

- Hypercoagulable states, which may be inherited (e.g., factor V Leiden mutation, prothrombin gene mutation, protein C deficiency, protein S deficiency, antithrombin III deficiency) or acquired (e.g., antiphospholipid antibodies, hypercoagulability of malignancy, disseminated intravascular coagulation)
- Sickle cell anemia
- Hyperviscosity, which can be caused by polycythemia vera and Waldenström's macroglobulinemia
- Intravascular lymphoma

Initial Evaluation of a Patient With Acute Ischemic Stroke

The goal of the initial evaluation of a patient with a sudden-onset neurologic deficit is to establish whether the diagnosis is stroke and exclude potential "mimics" such as seizure/postictal state, migraine, unwitnessed head trauma, hypoglycemia or other acute metabolic abnormality, or intoxication. If a seizure is unwitnessed, the postictal confusion and/or Todd's paralysis can mimic stroke. A migraine aura occurring for the first time may mimic stroke, especially before the classic headache emerges. Although acute metabolic derangements often present with global neurologic deficits rather than focal ones, focal findings can occur in the setting of hyperglycemia. Trauma and intoxications are generally apparent from the history and examination, but may require collateral information and toxicology screening (especially if a patient is simply "found down"). If a patient presents with acute left arm and face tingling, evaluation for myocardial infarction should be undertaken, since chest pain may not be a prominent feature of cardiac ischemia in older patients or patients with impaired pain perception due to diabetic neuropathy.

For any acute-onset neurologic deficit, monitoring of all vital signs is essential, and ECG, blood sugar, basic chemistries, complete blood count, and coagulation profile should be obtained while clinical evaluation is undertaken.

In practice, when acute stroke is suspected, history and examination are often performed en route to a CT scan since the use of thrombolytic treatment (IV tPA) or catheter-based mechanical thrombectomy for acute ischemic stroke requires rapid exclusion of alternative diagnoses (most importantly intracerebral hemorrhage) within a narrow time window from symptom onset. If CT reveals an alternative diagnosis

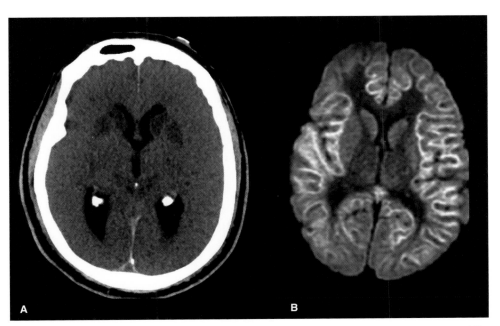

FIGURE 19–2 **Neuroimaging in hypoxic-ischemic injury caused by cardiac arrest. A:** Axial CT demonstrating diffuse sulcal effacement and symmetric hypodensity of the basal ganglia. **B:** Axial DWI MRI demonstrating diffuse cortical and bilateral basal ganglia diffusion restriction.

such as intracranial hemorrhage, the diagnostic and treatment approach shift accordingly.

Other important tests to obtain in addition to CT when considering thrombolytic therapy are serum platelets, plasma thromboplastin (PT), and partial thromboplastin time (PTT) to evaluate for a coagulopathy that would be a contraindication to such treatment. CTA is used to assess for large vessel occlusion potentially amenable to mechanical thrombectomy. CT perfusion (CTP) is used to evaluate for tissue that is ischemic but not yet infarcted (**ischemic penumbra**), which is potentially salvageable with early reperfusion if mechanical thrombectomy is performed (see "Mechanical Thrombectomy"). Serum creatinine should be measured to assess the safety of IV contrast needed for CTA/CTP, but in patients with no history of renal disease, guidelines recommend that contrast studies need not be delayed while awaiting serum creatinine.

Neuroimaging Findings in Acute Ischemic Stroke

The CT scan may show no abnormalities in the acute setting of acute ischemic stroke since the CT hypodensity caused by ischemic stroke can take up to 12 hours to emerge. In some cases, however, subtle findings related to vessel occlusion or early ischemia may be seen on noncontrast CT in the acute setting: a hyperdense vessel (a sign of clot and/or slow flow in the vessel) (Fig. 19–3), blurring of the gray–white junction/sulcal effacement (Fig. 19–3), and, in middle cerebral artey (MCA) stroke, hypodensity of the insular ribbon (Fig. 19–4A). Early parenchymal hypodensity may be more easily visible when changing the window setting to 30-30 (Fig. 19–4B). If the clinical impression is that the patient is having an ischemic stroke, the CT scan does not reveal an alternative explanation for the patient's symptoms, and

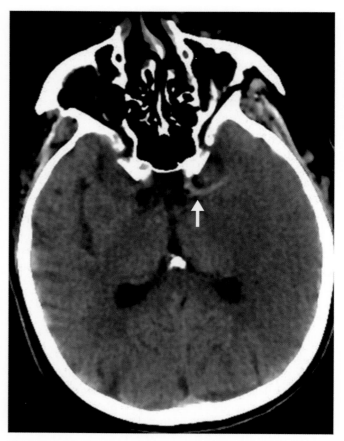

FIGURE 19–3 Early signs of ischemia on noncontrast CT imaging I: hyperdense vessel and sulcal effacement. Axial noncontrast CT demonstrating hyperdense left MCA (**arrow**) and diffuse sulcal effacement with loss of gray–white differentiation in the left MCA territory.

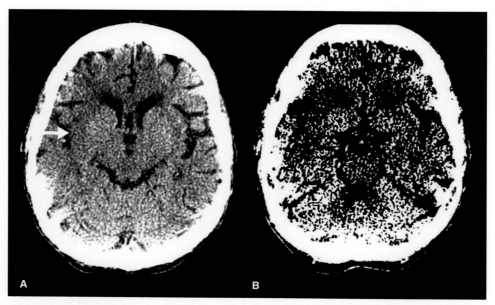

FIGURE 19–4 Early signs of ischemia on noncontrast CT imaging II: loss of the insular ribbon. A: Axial noncontrast CT demonstrating hypodensity of the right insular cortex (**arrow**; compare to the left insular cortex). **B:** The same slice as in (**A**), windowed to 30-30, more clearly demonstrating hypodensity in the region of the right insula.

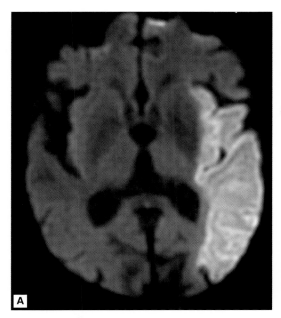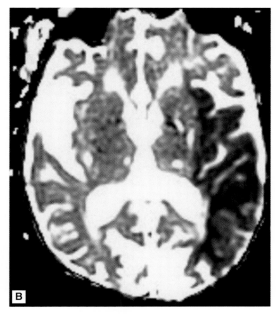

FIGURE 19–5 **Diffusion-weighted imaging (DWI) and apparent diffusion coefficient (ADC) MRI in acute ischemic stroke.** Axial DWI (**A**) and ADC (**B**) demonstrate diffusion restriction in the territory of the left MCA.

the time of onset of symptoms is well established with the patient having presented within the 3-hour (or in some cases 4.5-hour) window, the patient can be considered for thrombolytic therapy if there are not contraindications (see "Thrombolysis" below).

MRI with diffusion weighted imaging (DWI) and apparent diffusion coefficient (ADC) sequences can demonstrate ischemic stroke within less than an hour after onset, and so MRI is much more sensitive than CT in the acute setting. Acute ischemic strokes appear bright on DWI and dark on ADC (Fig. 19–5). CTA can be performed to look for arterial occlusion that may be apparent before signs of tissue ischemia are visible on CT (Fig. 19–6). CT perfusion can demonstrate the **ischemic penumbra** (tissue that is ischemic but not yet infarcted). However, these studies take longer and may not be accessible acutely, and neither is required for the administration of IV tPA in the appropriate clinical setting. CTA and MRI may be performed acutely to determine whether a patient is a candidate for catheter-based intervention (see "Mechanical Thrombectomy" below).

Ischemic strokes do not become visible on fluid-attenuated inversion recovery (FLAIR) imaging until about 6 hours from onset, so a stroke visible on diffusion sequences that is not yet visible on FLAIR is generally less than 6 hours from onset. ADC darkness is generally present for several days before normalizing, although DWI brightness may persist for approximately 7–10 days.

Although DWI/ADC sequences are believed to be the gold standard in stroke diagnosis, it should be noted that false negatives do occur (6.8% false negative rate per Edlow et al., 2017), especially with posterior fossa strokes, small strokes, and/or if the MRI is obtained very early after symptom onset.

Subacute strokes (about 1 week to 1 month old) can demonstrate enhancement on postcontrast CT or MRI (Fig. 19–7). This radiographic appearance may be mistaken for tumor if there is no clear clinical history of stroke, but subacute stroke can be radiologically distinguished from tumor in several ways:

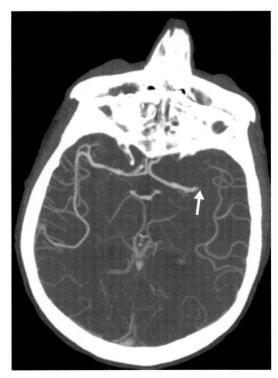

FIGURE 19–6 **CT angiography (CTA) in acute ischemic stroke.** Axial CTA demonstrating cut-off of the left MCA with distal reconstitution.

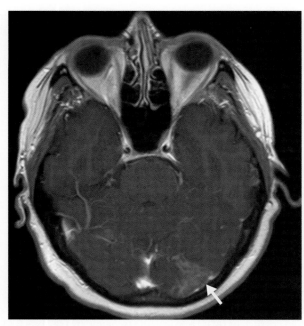

FIGURE 19–7 Contrast enhancement in subacute stroke.
Axial postcontrast T1-weighted MRI demonstrating wedge-shaped enhancement in the left MCA-PCA borderzone, consistent with subacute ischemic stroke.

subacute strokes typically conform to a vascular territory, and usually demonstrate no or minimal surrounding edema or mass effect on surrounding structures as would be seen with tumors. In ambiguous cases, serial imaging should be performed to see if the lesion expands as would be expected with tumor, or develops volume loss (encephalomalacia) as would be expected with infarction.

Initial Treatment of Acute Ischemic Stroke

Since ischemic stroke is due to decreased blood supply to a region of the brain, the goal of treatment is restoration of brain perfusion. The two ways in which this is achieved are thrombolysis and mechanical thrombectomy. If the patient does not meet criteria for these interventions, permissive hypertension (also called blood pressure autoregulation) can maintain brain perfusion, and in select cases, induced hypertension may be considered (see "Permissive Hypertension [Blood Pressure Autoregulation] & Induced Hypertension in the Treatment of Acute Ischemic Stroke").

Thrombolysis

Time window—Thrombolysis restores perfusion by aiding in the dissolution of occlusive thrombus. IV tissue plasminogen activator (IV tPA, also known as alteplase) is currently used, though there is increasing evidence that tenecteplase may be equally effective. The time window for IV tPA is up to 4.5 hours since the patient's last known well time, meaning the last time the patient was observed normal before the onset of stroke symptoms. The time window was previously only extended from 3 to 4.5 hours from last known well time for patients younger than 80 years, without combined history of stroke and diabetes, who are not on an anticoagulant (even if INR [international normalized ratio] is subtherapeutic), and who do not have a very large stroke (defined as National Institutes of Health [NIH] stroke scale score > 25 or > 1/3 MCA territory) (based on ECASS III). However, recent guidelines recommend administration of IV tPA up to 4.5 hours after onset of ischemic stroke symptoms for most patients, noting uncertainty of benefit in patients with NIHSS greater than 25 (AHA/ASA guidelines, 2019).

Some patients present with an unknown last seen well time (e.g., awakening with stroke deficits, called "wake up strokes"). In such patients, an estimation of time of onset can be made with MRI: since ischemic stroke does not cause FLAIR changes until about 6 hours, if there is DWI evidence of stroke but no FLAIR evidence of stroke, the stroke has occurred within the past 6 hours. Patients with wake-up stroke, unknown last seen well time, and DWI positive/FLAIR negative strokes on MRI appear to benefit from tPA (WAKE-UP trial, 2018).

Contraindications—The main risk of thrombolysis is symptomatic intracranial hemorrhage, which occurs in up to 6% of ischemic stroke patients treated within the standard time window. The risk of hemorrhage is much lower in patients treated with tPA who are ultimately not found to have had an ischemic stroke (e.g., when migraine mimics stroke). Beyond presenting outside the time window, the main contraindications to IV tPA administration for ischemic stroke are those that would increase the risk of bleeding:

- Blood pressure greater than 185/110 mm Hg, although tPA can be administered if blood pressure can be brought to and sustained below this level with antihypertensive treatment
- Coagulopathy: intrinsic or due to therapeutic anticoagulation; tPA contraindicated if INR greater than 1.7, PT greater than 15 seconds, platelets less than 100,000/mm^3, use of novel oral anticoagulant (apixaban, dabigatran, edoxaban, rivaroxaban) within the prior 48 hours
- Intracranial vascular malformation or aneurysm
- Prior intracerebral hemorrhage
- Recent major surgery or trauma (within 14 days)
- Recent systemic (e.g., gastrointestinal) hemorrhage (within 21 days)
- Recent stroke or head trauma (within 3 months)
- Aortic dissection
- Endocarditis

Many of these contraindications were established based on exclusion criteria for clinical trials, and risk/benefit must be determined for each individual patient depending on the precise nature of the contraindication and the severity of the potential deficits from an untreated stroke.

Complications—After undergoing thrombolysis, patients must be monitored closely for 24 hours for symptoms/signs of intracerebral hemorrhage. Blood pressure is maintained below 180/105 to reduce the risk of hemorrhagic complications. In patients with no clinical evidence of hemorrhage during this period, a CT scan is generally obtained 24 hours after IV tPA administration to evaluate for any asymptomatic hemorrhage. No antiplatelet agents or anticoagulants are administered during the 24-hour period after tPA administration, but may be administered after 24 hours if there is no clinical or radiologic evidence of intracranial hemorrhage. If symptomatic intracerebral hemorrhage occurs, IV tPA should be stopped (if infusion is incomplete), systolic blood pressure should be reduced below 180 mm Hg (see "Permissive Hypertension [Blood Pressure Autoregulation] & Induced Hypertension in the Treatment of Acute Ischemic Stroke"), and coagulopathy should be addressed with cryoprecipitate or antifibrinolytic agents (aminocaproic acid or tranexamic acid).

Another post-tPA complication to be aware of is orolingual angioedema. This is typically unilateral (on the side of the deficits; contralateral to the infarcted region), and patients on ACE inhibitors are at higher risk. If severe, intubation may be necessary, and treatment includes steroids, diphenhydramine, and ranitidine or famotidine.

Mechanical Thrombectomy

Mechanical thrombectomy is a catheter-based procedure through which clot can be extracted using either a stent retriever or aspiration device. If a patient has evidence of a catheter-accessible large vessel occlusion seen on CTA (e.g., distal internal carotid or proximal MCA), mechanical thrombectomy should be considered, and can be performed even if IV tPA has already been given. The standard time window for mechanical thrombectomy is up to 6 hours since last seen well time (Goyal et al., 2016), but intervention can be considered in an expanded time window up to 24 hours since last seen well time in select patients who have demonstrable salvageable tissue at risk (ischemic but not yet infarcted, i.e., penumbra) (DEFUSE 3 [2018] and DAWN [2018] trials). The DEFUSE 3 trial demonstrated benefit of mechanical thrombectomy over medical therapy between 6 to 16 hours in patients with NIHSS greater than 6 and mismatch between ischemic core and penumbra based on automated image analysis (on CT perfusion or DWI MRI). The DAWN trial demonstrated benefit between 6 to 24 hours in patients with NIHSS greater than 10 and mismatch between clinical severity and infarct volume on neuroimaging.

The time window for mechanical thrombectomy in the posterior circulation is less well established; catheter-based therapies may be considered up to 12–24 hours after onset of stroke in the posterior circulation.

Complications of mechanical thrombectomy include groin hematoma at the catheter insertion site and arterial dissection, but the risk of intracerebral hemorrhage is lower than with tPA alone, so the majority of tPA contraindications do not apply.

Given the longer time window and fewer contraindications to mechanical thrombectomy compared to IV tPA, mechanical thrombectomy could in principle be available to a greater number of stroke patients than tPA, but can only be performed by specialized providers/centers requiring appropriate mechanisms of triage to such centers, for example, through telestroke programs.

Permissive Hypertension (Blood Pressure Autoregulation) & Induced Hypertension in the Treatment of Acute Ischemic Stroke

Patients with acute ischemic stroke are often hypertensive at presentation, which may be a physiologic response to attempt to restore/maintain perfusion of ischemic brain tissue through collaterals. For the first 24 hours after ischemic stroke, it is recommended that the blood pressure be allowed to autoregulate for this reason (permissive hypertension). Guidelines suggest allowing autoregulation up to 220/120 mm Hg if thrombolytic therapy is not given, or up to 180/105 mm Hg if thrombolysis is given, if systemically tolerated. Therefore, if a patient is taking oral antihypertensive agents at the time of acute ischemic stroke, these are generally withheld for the first 24 hours after stroke. After 24 hours, blood pressure is generally gradually lowered unless there is evidence of clinical worsening.

In some cases of large vessel occlusion (e.g., internal carotid or proximal MCA), patients may be noted to have worsening of their neurologic deficits at lower blood pressures, and improvement at higher blood pressures. This may occur with spontaneous fluctuation of blood pressure or with a trial of raising the blood pressure with a bolus of IV fluids when the blood pressure is lower than on initial presentation. In such blood pressure-dependent patients, maintaining the patient's blood pressure above the threshold at which symptoms improve (e.g., with phenylephrine) may be beneficial (Rordorf et al., 2001; Hillis et al., 2003).

Antiplatelets & Anticoagulants in the Treatment of Acute Ischemic Stroke

All patients with acute ischemic stroke who do not receive tPA should receive aspirin within 48 hours. In patients who receive tPA, aspirin is generally initiated 24 hours after this if there has been no tPA-related hemorrhage. The IST and CAST trials demonstrated that aspirin administration within the first 48 hours after acute ischemic stroke reduced the risk of a second in-hospital stroke and increased survival to hospital discharge in spite of a small increased risk of ICH (IST trial, 1997; CAST trial, 1997; Chen et al., 2000). Aspirin is also an effective long-term secondary prevention medication (see "Antiplatelet Agents for Secondary Stroke Prevention"). In patients with minor stroke (who do not require anticoagulation for atrial fibrillation), a short course (21 days) of dual antiplatelet therapy (clopidogrel plus aspirin) is more effective than a single agent alone in preventing early recurrent ischemic stroke in the first 90 days (CHANCE trial, 2013; POINT trial, 2018; combined analysis Pan et al., 2019;

for further discussion see "Antiplatelet Agents for Secondary Stroke Prevention").

Although it was previously common practice to treat acute ischemic stroke patients with intravenous heparin, the IST trial suggested that risks of this treatment outweigh the benefits. The only situation in which acute anticoagulation is supported by data and guidelines at time of stroke is when stroke is due to venous sinus thrombosis (see "Cerebral Venous Sinus Thrombosis & Cortical Vein Thrombosis"). Other scenarios in which practitioners may treat acute ischemic stroke with anticoagulation are listed below, but it should be noted that many of these uses of anticoagulation for acute stroke are debated by practitioners and in the literature:

- Acute basilar artery thrombosis
- Artery-to-artery embolism from carotid stenosis while awaiting carotid endarterectomy (there are some data to support this from a subgroup analysis from the TOAST trial [Adams et al., 1999]).
- Acute cervical artery dissection (carotid or vertebral); however, a large meta-analysis (Kennedy et al., 2012) and a single small randomized controlled trial (CADISS trial, 2015) suggest that there is no difference in outcome between patients treated with antiplatelets vs anticoagulation (see "Secondary Stroke Prevention in Patients With Cervical Artery Dissection").
- Cardioembolism from atrial fibrillation, especially if the stroke occurs in a patient with known atrial fibrillation who has been off anticoagulation (e.g., for a minor surgical procedure) or is subtherapeutically anticoagulated. However, the risks and benefits of anticoagulation in the acute setting remain unclear. A delay in initiating (or resuming) anticoagulation is often considered if the stroke is moderate in size or larger, given that the daily risk of ischemic stroke from atrial fibrillation is felt to be less than the daily risk of hemorrhagic conversion of the stroke (The daily stroke risk in a patient with atrial fibrillation is roughly equivalent to the yearly stroke risk associated with the patient's CHADS2 score divided by 365, though may be higher in the immediate post-stroke period). Note that anticoagulation is recommended for *long-term* secondary stroke prevention in patients with stroke caused by atrial fibrillation (see "Anticoagulation for Secondary Stroke Prevention").

Surgical Interventions in the Treatment of Acute Ischemic Stroke

In patients with large strokes of the cerebellum or large MCA strokes, stroke-related cerebral edema can raise intracranial pressure, which puts the patient at risk for herniation. In addition to hyperosmolar therapy (see "Hyperosmolar Therapy in the Treatment of Acutely Elevated Intracranial Pressure" in Ch. 25), surgery to decompress the edematous brain may be considered. For patients with large cerebellar strokes, suboccipital craniectomy is often performed and can

lead to dramatic improvement. For patients with large MCA strokes, decompressive hemicraniectomy (removal of a skull flap on the side of the stroke to accommodate the swollen hemisphere) within 48 hours after stroke onset can be lifesaving and may improve outcomes (DECIMAL trial, 2007; DESTINY trial 2007; HAMLET trial, 2009; DESTINY II, 2014). However, many patients will have their lives saved only to survive with significant disability (see Ropper, 2014 for a cleverly titled editorial on the subject, "Hemicraniectomy: To Halve or Halve Not"). Therefore, decisions about whether to pursue this measure in patients with large MCA strokes must be individualized.

Supportive management measures for patients with ischemic stroke are discussed at the beginning of the chapter (see "Overview of Ischemic Stroke & Intracerebral Hemorrhage").

Readers are encouraged to consult the latest AHA/ASA Guidelines for the Early Management of Patients With Acute Ischemic Stroke for up-to-date recommendations (and note the very helpful supplemental tables that provide concise summaries of trials cited in the guidelines).

Evaluation for Etiology of Ischemic Stroke

Since the etiology of stroke most commonly involves either the intracranial vasculature, cervical vasculature, heart, and/or the effects of common atherosclerotic risk factors on these structures, the initial evaluation for stroke etiology assesses each of these:

- The patient should be screened for modifiable risk factors: hypertension, diabetes (by serum glucose or hemoglobin A1c), hyperlipidemia (by serum lipids), smoking, and/or excessive alcohol use.
- The intracranial and cervical vasculature can be assessed by MRA, CTA, or digital subtraction angiography; the carotid arteries can also be evaluated with Doppler ultrasound. Time of flight MRA (which uses a measure of blood flow rather than contrast) may exaggerate the degree of stenosis compared to CTA or carotid ultrasound (since decreased flow may give the impression of decreased lumen caliber).
- The heart should be evaluated by transthoracic echocardiogram to evaluate for thrombus, left atrial dilatation (which may be associated with atrial fibrillation), and valvular vegetation (although transesophageal echocardiogram is more sensitive to assess for vegetation). Cardiac monitoring should also be performed to look for atrial fibrillation. If atrial fibrillation is not observed with in-hospital monitoring and there is not another clear etiology of stroke, prolonged cardiac monitoring (e.g., 14–30 days) should be performed.

If the etiology of the stroke remains unclear after the above evaluation (**cryptogenic stroke**) or stroke occurs in a young patient, an expanded stroke evaluation is often undertaken. This may include:

- Prolonged cardiac monitoring with an implantable cardiac monitor should be strongly considered for embolic-appearing strokes of unclear etiology (CRYSTAL AF, 2014).
- Agitated saline (bubble) study during the echocardiogram to look for patent foramen ovale (PFO). If a PFO is found, a search for DVT is undertaken with Doppler ultrasound of the lower extremities and MR venography (MRV) of the pelvis to evaluate for thrombosis of the pelvic veins (which may be caused by **May-Thurner syndrome**: iliac vein thrombosis due to compression of the left common iliac vein by the right common iliac artery).
- Evaluation for a hypercoagulable state: antiphospholipid antibodies (anti–cardiolipin antibodies, lupus anticoagulant, beta-2 glycoprotein antibody) and genetic mutations (protein C or S deficiency, antithrombin III deficiency, factor V Leiden, prothrombin gene mutation). Of these, only the antiphospholipid antibodies are associated with both arterial and venous thromboembolism. The others are primarily associated with venous thromboembolism, and so could only potentially cause a stroke if a PFO or other shunt between the venous and arterial circulations is present.
- Screen for malignancy by positron emission tomography (PET) scan or CT chest/abdomen/pelvis since malignancy can lead to a hypercoagulable state.
- Lumbar puncture to look for signs of an inflammatory or infectious etiology if vasculopathy is suggested on vascular imaging (e.g., primary central nervous system [CNS] vasculitis, secondary vasculitis due to infection such as varicella zoster virus).
- Transesophageal echocardiogram to look for infectious, inflammatory, or neoplastic valvular lesions, atrial clot, or aortic atherosclerosis.
- Blood cultures if there is concern for infectious endocarditis.

In spite of the many potentially exotic causes of stroke in the young, the most common causes remain the mundane ones: vascular risk factors, arrhythmia, and cervical artery dissection.

Secondary Prevention of Ischemic Stroke

Primary stroke prevention refers to modification of risk factors to prevent a first stroke. *Secondary* stroke prevention refers to modifying risk factors after stroke or TIA to reduce the risk of a subsequent stroke. Stroke secondary prevention measures include the following:

- Hypertension should be controlled by diet, exercise, and if necessary, antihypertensive medications. Antihypertensive medications are generally initiated if BP is more than or equal to 140/90, though a target of less than 130 may be considered in patients with lacunar stroke (SPS3 [2013] showed a nonsignificant decrease in recurrent ischemic stroke and significant decrease in intracerebral hemorrhage with this lower BP target compared to SBP < 140).
- Hyperlipidemia should be controlled by diet, exercise, and statin therapy (if LDL ≥ 100 mg/dL).

- Blood sugar in patients with diabetes should be controlled by diet, exercise and if necessary, medications.
- Patients should be aided in quitting smoking and reducing excessive alcohol intake.
- Patients should be on an antiplatelet agent (unless they require anticoagulation; see "Antiplatelet Agents for Secondary Stroke Prevention" and "Anticoagulation for Secondary Stroke Prevention").
- Patients with atrial fibrillation should be anticoagulated with warfarin or a novel oral anticoagulant (apixaban, rivaroxaban, dabigatran, edoxaban) unless there is a contraindication to anticoagulation, in which case an antiplatelet agent may be used.
- Patients with symptomatic moderate or severe carotid stenosis should be considered for intervention with carotid endarterectomy or carotid artery stenting (see "Secondary Stroke Prevention in Patients With Carotid Artery Stenosis").
- Patients with hypercoagulable states may require anticoagulation.

Antiplatelet Agents for Secondary Stroke Prevention

An antiplatelet agent is indicated for secondary ischemic stroke prevention in all patients who have had a TIA or ischemic stroke unless they are already receiving antithrombotic therapy with anticoagulation. The choices are aspirin, clopidogrel, dipyridamole, and ticagrelor, alone or in combination. Whether or not the dose of aspirin matters is debated; some practitioners believe that some patients may require higher doses of aspirin than other patients for adequate platelet inhibition. A number of studies have compared antiplatelet agents alone and in combination. The combination of dipyridamole and aspirin may be more effective for secondary stroke prevention than aspirin alone (EPSP2 trial, 1996; ESPRIT trial, 2006), but the side effect of headache, expense compared to aspirin, and twice daily dosing have led to dipyridamole/aspirin being less commonly used than aspirin alone.

Combined treatment with aspirin and clopidogrel is not more effective than either alone in *long-term* secondary stroke prevention, and bleeding risk is increased compared to either alone (MATCH trial, 2004; CHARISMA trial, 2006; SPS3 trial, 2012). However, use of aspirin and clopidogrel together is beneficial compared to aspirin alone when used for the first 21 days following TIA or small ischemic stroke in preventing recurrent stroke in the *short-term* (outcomes measured at 90 days) (CHANCE trial, 2013; POINT trial, 2018). CHANCE and POINT differed in several ways. CHANCE used a loading dose of 300 mg of clopidogrel and maintained clopidogrel as monotherapy after the first 21 days of dual antiplatelet therapy, while POINT used a loading dose of 600 mg of clopidogrel and maintained dual antiplatelet therapy for 90 days. Although both trials showed reduction in recurrent ischemic stroke within 90 days with dual antiplatelet therapy compared to monotherapy, CHANCE showed no increase in hemorrhage risk with dual antiplatelet therapy vs. aspirin alone, whereas POINT showed an increased risk of hemorrhage. The combined results demonstrate a benefit of 21 days of dual antiplatelet therapy after TIA or small ischemic stroke (pooled analysis of CHANCE and POINT: Pan et al., 2019). The combination of ticagrelor and aspirin for 30 days after mild/moderate stroke (NIHSS5) or TIA also improves short-term outcomes (at 30 days) compared to aspirin alone, though higher rates of severe bleeding occur with ticagrelor and aspirin compared to aspirin alone (THALES trial, 2020).

The other scenario in which dual antiplatelet therapy for secondary stroke prevention is considered is in patients with stroke due to symptomatic intracranial stenosis (i.e., stroke in the territory of a stenotic intracranial vessel), based on results from the medical management group in the SAMMPRIS trial (2014) (see "Secondary Stroke Prevention in Patients With Intracranial Arterial Stenosis"). In SAMMPRIS, maximal medical therapy (which included 90 days of aspirin and clopidogrel) was superior to stenting, but there was no comparison of dual antiplatelet therapy to antiplatelet monotherapy.

In patients who have a TIA or stroke while already on an antiplatelet agent, some practitioners change from one antiplatelet to another or change the antiplatelet dose, although there are no data to guide such decisions.

One review of the complex array of data on antiplatelet agents for secondary stroke prevention sums up the topic with a tongue-in-cheek haiku expressing that being on *an* antiplatelet agent is most important, but that it may matter less which one(s): "For stroke prevention, / use an antiplatelet drug. / Treat hypertension" (Kent and Thaler, 2008).

Anticoagulation for Secondary Stroke Prevention

If atrial fibrillation is diagnosed, anticoagulation with warfarin or a novel oral anticoagulant (apixaban, rivaroxaban, dabigatran, edoxaban) is indicated for secondary stroke prevention unless there is a strong contraindication; in such patients an antiplatelet agent is used. Although anticoagulation for long-term secondary prevention has been studied in a variety of other scenarios such as noncardioembolic stroke (WARSS trial, 2001) and intracranial arterial stenosis (WASID trial, 2005), no benefit has been seen and increased risk of hemorrhage has been observed. However, these trials utilized warfarin; novel oral anticoagulants (which have a lower risk of intracranial hemorrhage) have not been studied in these specific contexts. Use of novel oral anticoagulants for secondary prevention after embolic stroke of undetermined source (ESUS) has shown no benefit beyond aspirin and increased bleeding risk compared to aspirin (NAVIGATE ESUS, 2018 [rivaroxaban vs aspirin]; RESPECT ESUS, 2019 [dabigatran vs aspirin]).

Scenarios aside from atrial fibrillation in which anticoagulation for secondary ischemic stroke prevention is often utilized include:

- Hypercoagulable states, whether genetic (e.g., protein C or S deficiency, antithrombin III deficiency, factor V Leiden, prothrombin gene mutation) or acquired (e.g., antiphospholipid antibodies, hypercoagulability of malignancy).
- Low cardiac ejection fraction due to cardiomyopathy. The WARCEF trial of warfarin versus aspirin in patients with low ejection fraction found that the benefit of anticoagulation for *primary* stroke prevention was outweighed by the risk of major hemorrhage (driven primarily by GI hemorrhage with no difference in intracranial hemorrhage; WARCEF trial, 2012). However, anticoagulation may be considered for *secondary* stroke prevention after a stroke occurs in a patient with a low ejection fraction.
- Left ventricular thrombus
- Stroke due to venous sinus thrombosis (see "Cerebral Venous Sinus Thrombosis & Cortical Vein Thrombosis").

Many practitioners advocate waiting 2–4 weeks from the time of an ischemic stroke before initiating anticoagulation if the size of the stroke is moderate or large to decrease the risk of hemorrhagic conversion of the ischemic stroke.

Secondary Stroke Prevention in Patients With Carotid Artery Stenosis

Carotid stenosis may be treated by carotid endarterectomy or carotid artery stenting to prevent further stroke in certain circumstances. Carotid stenosis is considered to be *symptomatic* if the stenosis is found ipsilateral to a stroke or a TIA in the anterior cerebral artery (ACA) territory or middle cerebral artery (MCA) territory (or posterior cerebral artery [PCA] territory if there is a fetal PCA; see "Arterial Supply of the Cerebral Hemispheres" in Ch. 7). If carotid stenosis is severe (70%–99%) and symptomatic, carotid intervention reduces the risk of subsequent stroke sufficiently to warrant the risks of intervention. With moderate (50%–69%) symptomatic stenosis, the initial trials showed a benefit of carotid intervention in men but not women, although the benefit was less than for severe stenosis. However, given advances in risk factor modification since these trials were performed, management of symptomatic moderate carotid stenosis is now debated. Mild symptomatic stenosis (<50%) and carotid occlusion are not considered indications for intervention (NASCET trial, 1991; VACS trial, 1991; ECST trial, 1998; Rothwell et al., 2003).

If carotid stenosis is discovered incidentally with no prior stroke or TIA referable to that carotid, it is considered to be *asymptomatic*. Intervention is not recommended for mild or moderate asymptomatic stenosis. Although there may be benefit to intervening in asymptomatic severe stenosis for primary stroke prevention, clinical trials addressing this (VACS trial, 1993; ACAS trial 1995; ACST trial, 2004) were performed before the advent of modern medical management (including statins), so the benefit of intervention in this scenario is now debated. Some practitioners recommend intervention for asymptomatic carotid stenosis greater than 80%, but evaluate patients with asymptomatic stenosis less than 80% with serial ultrasounds (and/or evaluation for embolic signals with transcranial Doppler ultrasound [TCD] per ACES trial, 2010) and recommend intervention only if there is progression of stenosis or the patient has a stroke or TIA (making the carotid symptomatic). Another scenario in which asymptomatic severe carotid stenosis may be intervened upon is in a patient undergoing cardiac surgery to reduce the risk of perioperative stroke, although this is also debated.

The choice between carotid endarterectomy and stenting depends on patient-specific characteristics: endarterectomy may be preferred for older patients, and stenting for younger patients (CREST trial, 2010), due to higher periprocedural stroke rates with stenting requiring living longer to achieve the long-term benefit of intervention. In patients in whom surgical risk is high (e.g., severe cardiac disease), stenting is often preferred.

Secondary Stroke Prevention in Patients With Symptomatic Intracranial Arterial Stenosis

Although procedural intervention can be effective in patients with symptomatic extracranial arterial disease, severe symptomatic intracranial arterial stenosis does not appear to improve with procedural intervention. The SAMMPRIS trial demonstrated that aggressive medical management (including statins and 90 days of dual antiplatelet therapy with aspirin and clopidogrel) was superior to MCA stenting for secondary stroke prevention in patients with symptomatic MCA stenosis (SAMMPRIS trial, 2014). Therefore, some practitioners utilize dual antiplatelet therapy in patients with stroke or TIA due to intracranial arterial stenosis based on the results in the medical management group in this study.

The WASID trial demonstrated that there was no benefit—and increased risk—of anticoagulation with warfarin for intracranial stenosis as compared to antiplatelet therapy (WASID trial, 2005).

Secondary Stroke Prevention in Patients With Patent Foramen Ovale

In about 25% of the population, the foramen ovale that connects the right and left atria in the fetal circulation fails to close after birth, leaving a **patent foramen ovale** (**PFO**). Through this conduit from the venous circulation to the arterial circulation, a venous clot can pass to the left heart and cause cerebral embolism (**paradoxical embolus**). A classic clinical history for paradoxical embolism is a stroke that occurs after the Valsalva maneuver (e.g., straining during a bowel movement), since the Valsalva maneuver increases right to left cardiac flow if a PFO is present.

In patients with stroke of unknown etiology (**cryptogenic stroke**), there is a higher prevalence of PFO. Therefore, in patients with cryptogenic stroke, evaluation for a PFO with agitated saline (bubble) study during the echocardiogram should be considered. If a PFO is found, the patient should be evaluated for a source of paradoxical embolism. The main sites to evaluate for DVT are the legs (with Doppler ultrasound) and the pelvis (with MRV). If a venous clot is discovered, anticoagulation is utilized and a search for a cause of hypercoagulability is pursued. If no venous clot is discovered in a patient with PFO and stroke, an antiplatelet agent is generally used for secondary stroke prevention, and percutaneous PFO closure may be considered if: no

alternative stroke mechanism can be identified, the patient is under 60 years (though PFO closure may be considered in patients older than 60 with no identified risk factors for stroke), and there is a large shunt through the PFO and/or associated atrial septal aneurysm (RESPECT, 2017; CLOSE, 2017; REDUCE, 2017; DEFENSE-PFO, 2018; AAN practice advisory: Messé et al., 2020). Percutaneous PFO closure carries a risk of atrial fibrillation, though this complication is usually transient. The RoPE score can be used to help predict whether a PFO is more likely to be causative or incidental, using parameters of stroke risk factors (hypertension, diabetes, prior stroke/TIA, smoking), stroke location (cortical), and age; PFO is more likely to be causative in younger patients with fewer risk factors and cortical location of stroke (Kent et al., 2013).

Secondary Stroke Prevention in Patients With Cervical Artery Dissection

For secondary stroke prevention in patients with stroke or TIA due to cervical artery dissection, antiplatelet agents and anticoagulation appear to be equivalent in large meta-analyses (Kennedy et al., 2012) and one small clinical trial (CADISS trial, 2015; 1-year follow up CADISS trial, 2019), although appropriate therapy has been debated. Stroke recurrence risk after dissection-related stroke is low (2% at 3 months; 2.5% at 1 year), making it challenging to perform an adequately powered trial. Most retrospective data are for carotid dissection with very limited data for vertebral artery dissection, though CADISS included patients with vertebral dissection in addition to those with carotid artery dissection. Some practitioners avoid anticoagulation if a dissection extends intracranially due to risk of subarachnoid hemorrhage if an intracranial dissection were to rupture. Others argue that if there is no subarachnoid hemorrhage at the time of diagnosis of dissection, it is unlikely to occur and so anticoagulation may be safe (Metso et al., 2007). Treatment is generally maintained for 3–6 months with follow-up imaging to assess for recanalization or persistent occlusion of the vessel. Patients who are anticoagulated are generally switched to an antiplatelet agent after an initial period of anticoagulation.

There are no data to guide appropriate *primary* preventive management of patients who develop cervical artery dissection and present with local symptoms (e.g., neck pain, Horner's syndrome, cranial nerve 9–12 palsies), but have not yet had a stroke or TIA. Some studies suggest that the risk of stroke in these patients in the acute setting is quite high (Biousse et al., 1995), leading some practitioners to use anticoagulation as primary prevention in the acute period if a cervical artery dissection is diagnosed in a patient with local symptoms only (i.e., no stroke or TIA), although others utilize antiplatelet agents.

A dissecting aneurysm (**pseudoaneurysm**) may develop in a dissected vessel over time, but this finding generally does not have any clinical significance with respect to outcome.

Rarer Causes of Ischemic Stroke: Vasculopathies, Vasculitis, & Genetic Disorders

Moyamoya

Moyamoya is the Japanese term for "puff of smoke," which refers to the angiographic appearance of a "cloud" of collateral vessels that develop in response to stenosis of the distal internal carotid artery, proximal MCA, and/or proximal ACA unilaterally or bilaterally. Moyamoya *disease* refers to an idiopathic (presumed genetic) etiology that usually presents in childhood, whereas moyamoya *syndrome* denotes that moyamoya physiology has developed in response to another cause of vessel occlusion (e.g., prior radiation treatment, infectious or inflammatory vasculitis, sickle cell disease, atherosclerosis) or an associated underlying condition (e.g., Down's syndrome or a neurocutaneous syndrome such as neurofibromatosis). Patients can present with TIA, ischemic stroke, or hemorrhage. TIA may be provoked by exertion or hyperventilation, possibly due to a "steal" phenomenon from the stenosed vessel and its collateral network. Diagnosis is made by angiography (CTA, MRA, or digital subtraction angiography), which demonstrates characteristic vessel occlusion and the "puff of smoke" of the collateral network.

Treatment of moyamoya can include surgical procedures that directly or indirectly link the extracranial and intracranial circulations to bypass the stenotic vessel in order to increase blood flow to the affected hemisphere(s). Direct linkage of the extracranial and intracranial circulations can be achieved through extracranial-intracranial (EC-IC) bypass: the superficial temporal artery (a branch of the external carotid artery) is connected to the MCA. Indirect linkage of the extracranial and intracranial circulations can be achieved by placing the superficial temporal artery in contact with the dura mater to promote neovascularization (**synangiosis**).

Cerebral Vasculitis

CNS vasculitis can be primary (primary vasculitis/angiitis of the central nervous system) or secondary. Secondary CNS vasculitis can be due to infection (e.g., varicella zoster virus, *Aspergillus*, meningovascular syphilis, bacterial meningitis) or due to systemic vasculitis (e.g., granulomatosis with polyangiitis [formerly called Wegener's granulomatosis], eosinophilic granulomatosis with polyangiitis [also known as Churg-Strauss syndrome]). Giant cell arteritis (also known as temporal arteritis), which classically presents with headache, visual loss, scalp pain, and jaw claudication, can rarely present with vasculitis of the vertebral arteries leading to posterior circulation strokes.

Primary CNS vasculitis can only be diagnosed definitively by brain biopsy. The symptoms and laboratory features of primary CNS vasculitis are all nonspecific: headache, subacute cognitive decline, strokes, inflammatory cerebrospinal fluid (CSF), and/or any of a number of diverse (and also nonspecific) MRI findings (strokes, mass lesions, white matter hyperintensities, vessel irregularities, and/or contrast enhancing lesion[s]). Headache and inflammatory CSF are so common in the disorder that the diagnosis is unlikely if they are not present, but both findings of course have broad differential diagnoses.

Clinicians may latch onto a diagnosis of CNS vasculitis when vascular irregularities are observed on MRA, CTA, or conventional angiogram, but these radiologic abnormalities only indicate the presence of a vascul*opathy*, which has a differential diagnosis far broader than vasculitis (e.g., atherosclerosis, reversible cerebral vasoconstriction syndrome [RCVS]). Since treatment of primary CNS vasculitis requires cyclophosphamide, if this diagnosis is being considered, biopsy confirmation is essential to avoid unnecessary risks of this medication without a definitive diagnosis.

Susac Syndrome

Susac syndrome is an autoimmune vasculopathy characterized by the triad of encephalopathy, branch retinal artery occlusion, and sensorineural hearing loss. Lesions in the central corpus callosum are characteristic (Fig. 19–8), but additional nonspecific white matter lesions are also common and may lead to misdiagnosis as multiple sclerosis. CSF is typically inflammatory. Patients may not present with all three elements of the triad, but will most often develop them within months of onset. In patients in whom the diagnosis is suspected but not all aspects of the triad are clinically present, laboratory testing (i.e., MRI, fluorescein angiogram, audiometry) may reveal subclinical evidence of other elements of the triad.

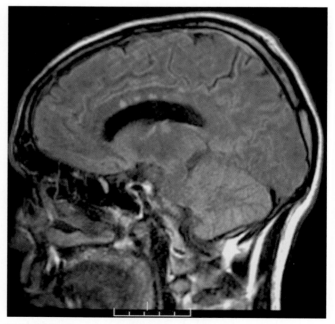

FIGURE 19–8 Susac syndrome. Sagittal FLAIR MRI demonstrating lesions in the mid-portion of the corpus callosum. (Reproduced with permission from Ropper AH, Samuels MA, Klein JP, et al: *Adams and Victor's Principles of Neurology*, 11th ed. New York, NY: McGraw Hill; 2019.)

Anti-endothelial cell antibodies have been described in association with the disorder. Treatment is with immunomodulatory therapy. The disease may be monophasic or relapsing.

Intravascular Lymphoma

Intravascular large B-cell lymphoma is a rare lymphoma that develops within the lumens of small and medium blood vessels. It is a multisystem disorder, but the presenting features may be neurologic due to strokes caused by lymphomatous occlusion of cerebral blood vessels. These are most commonly small vessel subcortical strokes. Strokes may be clinically apparent as acute-onset deficits, or the accumulation of small subclinical subcortical strokes may lead to a presentation with subacute cognitive decline. Any level of the nervous system may be involved, including myelopathy and neuropathy concurrent with or independent of brain involvement. Diagnosis often requires biopsy of affected nervous system tissue, although biopsy of skin lesions (if there is skin involvement) or random skin biopsy may be diagnostic in some cases. Treatment is with combination chemotherapy including anti–B-cell therapy with rituximab.

Cerebral Autosomal Dominant Arteriopathy with Subcortical Infarcts and Leukoencephalopathy (CADASIL) & Cerebral Autosomal Recessive Arteriopathy with Subcortical Infarcts and Leukoencephalopathy (CARASIL)

Cerebral autosomal dominant arteriopathy with subcortical infarcts and leukoencephalopathy (CADASIL) is an inherited CNS vasculopathy that causes migraines, strokes, and progressive neuropsychiatric dysfunction leading to dementia. MRI in CADASIL demonstrates a subcortical leukoencephalopathy (confluent T2/FLAIR hyperintensity in the white matter) with characteristic extension into the white matter of the anterior temporal lobes (Fig. 19–9) (this region can also be similarly affected in myotonic dystrophy; see "Myotonic Dystrophy" in Ch. 30). Diagnosis of CADASIL is made by genetic testing (mutation of the *NOTCH3* gene on chromosome 19) or skin biopsy to evaluate blood vessels in the skin. There is no definitively proven stroke-prevention strategy, although any coexisting vascular risk factors for stroke should be well controlled, and many patients are given aspirin.

A recessive and much less common form of the disorder (CARASIL) is caused by mutation in the *HTRA1* gene on chromosome 10. It is similar in clinical and radiologic presentation to CADASIL, but affected patients additionally have premature alopecia and lumbar spondylosis.

Mitochondrial Encephalopathy With Lactic Acidosis & Stroke-like Episodes (MELAS)

Patients with mitochondrial encephalopathy with lactic acidosis and stroke-like episodes (MELAS) may present with transient neurologic stroke-like episodes, generally before age 40. On neuroimaging, the stroke-like episodes in MELAS cause signal changes that are typically isolated to the cortex and do not conform to individual vascular territories. Accumulation of cerebral damage due to stroke-like episodes leads to encephalopathy. Migraines and seizures are common. Patients typically have other features of mitochondrial disease including short stature, deafness, myopathy, and lactic acidosis. MELAS is associated with mitochondrial mutation *A3243G*. Acute stroke-like episodes may resolve with administration of L-arginine, and prophylactic administration may reduce the frequency of stroke-like episodes (Koga et al., 2005).

Fabry Disease

Fabry disease is an X-linked lysosomal storage disease due to a mutation in the *GLA* gene (which leads to deficiency of

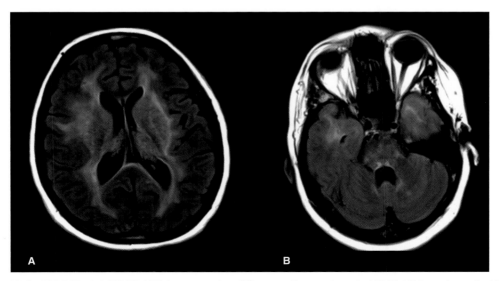

FIGURE 19–9 **MRI in CADASIL.** Axial FLAIR MRI demonstrating diffuse, confluent subcortical T2/FLAIR hyperintensity (**A**) extending into the anterior temporal lobes (**B**).

the lysosomal enzyme alphagalactosidase). It causes painful limb paresthesias (due to small fiber neuropathy and often exacerbated by high or low temperatures), angiokeratomas of the skin (most commonly in the lower abdomen and groin), corneal opacities, renal disease, cardiac disease, and strokes. Treatment involves enzyme replacement (alphagalactosidase) and addressing systemic manifestations.

Long-term Sequelae of Ischemic Stroke: Recrudescence, Seizures, & Cognitive Impairment

Recrudescence

Patients who have had a prior stroke may present with reemergence of resolved deficits or worsening of baseline deficits in the setting of infection or other systemic illness, a phenomenon known as **recrudescence.** Any patient with a prior stroke is at risk for another, and so recurrent stroke is the primary differential diagnosis in this setting. However, it would be somewhat unlikely to have a stroke in the exact same territory with the exact same deficits as a prior stroke, so when patients present with worsening of prior deficits, they should be evaluated for an infection or metabolic abnormality that could be a cause of recrudescence.

Post-stroke Seizures

Prior stroke is a common cause of epilepsy in older adults. Seizures generally emerge about 6 months to 1 year after infarct and require treatment with antiepileptic medications to prevent recurrence. An acute precipitant of seizures should be sought (e.g., infection, electrolyte abnormality, new medication; see Table 18–1), though may not be present. Seizures at the time of presentation of an acute ischemic stroke are uncommon (though more common if the stroke is due to

venous sinus thrombosis or cortical vein thrombosis), but are more common in the setting of acute ICH.

Post-stroke Cognitive Impairment

Cerebrovascular disease can affect cognition due to stroke(s) in regions such as the hippocampus, thalamus, or frontal lobe(s), and/or can cause progressive cognitive impairment due to accumulation of chronic subcortical ischemic disease (see "Vascular Dementia" in Ch. 23).

INTRACEREBRAL HEMORRHAGE

Intracerebral hemorrhage (ICH) presents with sudden-onset focal neurologic deficits, as does acute ischemic stroke. Compared to ischemic stroke, however ICH is more often accompanied by one or more of the following clinical features (Runchey and McGee, 2010):

- Headache
- Nausea/vomiting
- Depressed level of consciousness at onset (due to displacement of brain tissue by the hematoma and/or intraventricular extension of hemorrhage)
- Extreme hypertension (diastolic pressure > 110 mm Hg)
- Seizures at presentation

Any of these findings can also occur in the setting of ischemic stroke, and so definitive diagnosis requires CT. On CT, acute blood is hyperdense and visible at presentation (Fig. 19–10); this is in contrast to acute ischemic stroke, in which CT scan may be normal at presentation (see "Neuroimaging Findings in Acute Ischemic Stroke"). Vascular imaging (e.g., CTA or MRA) should be performed to assess for a vascular malformation that may require surgical intervention.

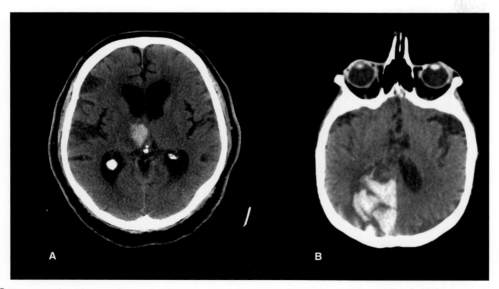

FIGURE 19–10   Intracerebral hemorrhage. Axial noncontrast CT images demonstrating thalamic hemorrhage consistent with hypertensive hemorrhage (**A**), and occipital lobar hemorrhage consistent with cerebral amyloid angiopathy-related hemorrhage (**B**).

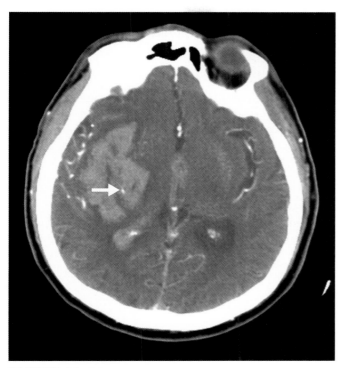

FIGURE 19-11 **Spot sign in intracerebral hemorrhage.** Axial postcontrast CT demonstrating punctate focus of enhancement within an intraparenchymal hemorrhage.

If one or more spots of contrast is seen in the hematoma (**spot sign**), this is associated with a higher risk of hematoma expansion (Goldstein et al., 2007) (Fig. 19–11).

Acute Management of Intracerebral Hemorrhage

ICH expansion occurs most commonly in the first 24 hours, and within that period, most commonly within the first 6 hours. Acute management of ICH is geared toward prevention of hematoma expansion by lowering the blood pressure and reversing any coagulopathy if present. Intravenous antihypertensive infusion (typically with nicardipine) guided by intra-arterial blood pressure monitoring is often necessary. Warfarin should be reversed with vitamin K, administration of fresh frozen plasma, and/or prothrombin complex concentrate; heparin should be reversed with protamine; dabigatran should be reversed with idarucizumab; rivoraxaban and apixaban should be reversed with andexanet alfa; IV tPA should be reversed with cryoprecipitate or antifibrinolytic agents (aminocaproic acid or tranexamic acid).

The degree to which blood pressure should be lowered remains unclear: It appears to be safe to lower systolic blood pressure as low as 140 mm Hg, but it remains uncertain whether lowering blood pressure that much improves outcomes as opposed to only lowering systolic blood pressure to less than 180 mm Hg (INTERACT2 trial, 2013; ATACH-2 Trial, 2016). Note that ATACH-2 achieved lower blood pressures in the first few hours of treatment and had a higher

rate of renal adverse events in the first 7 days in the less than 140 mm Hg group. Furthermore, patients in ATACH-2 who presented with systolic blood pressure greater than 220 mm Hg had greater risk of neurologic deterioration with intensive blood pressure control (goal < 140 mm Hg) than with standard blood pressure control (goal < 180) (Qureshi et al., 2020). Current guidelines recommend reduction of systolic blood pressure to 140 mm Hg if presenting systolic blood pressure is 150–220 mm Hg (Hemphill et al., 2015), but guidance is less precise on blood pressure target if presenting systolic blood pressure is greater than 220 mm Hg. Less aggressive targets (e.g., <180 mm Hg) may be considered in this latter scenario.

Patients with acute ICH must be monitored closely in an intensive care unit setting with CT scan repeated for any change in neurologic examination. CT scans are typically repeated 6 hours after the initial scan and then at 24 hours to look for any evolution in the ICH. Electroencephalography (EEG) should be considered to evaluate for nonconvulsive seizures in patients whose examination appears to be worse than would be expected for the location and/or extent of hemorrhage, although thalamic and intraventricular hemorrhages can lead to fluctuations in level of consciousness without causing seizures.

In patients with large cerebellar ICH (>3 cm), surgical evacuation of the hematoma can be lifesaving. Although supratentorial hematoma evacuation does not appear to improve overall outcomes, it may be considered in patients with ICH close to the cortical surface (STICH trial, 2005; STICH 2 trial, 2013) or ICH that expands with rapid clinical deterioration in patients with a reasonable chance of recovery. Although an initial study of minimally invasive surgery to evacuate ICH did not show significant benefit in outcome over standard medical care (MISTIE III trial, 2019), there was a suggestion that greater volume of reduction of ICH was more likely to lead to benefit, and further trials are ongoing.

General supportive measures for ICH are discussed in the beginning of the chapter (see "Overview of Ischemic Stroke & Intracerebral Hemorrhage"), and are similar to those for ischemic stroke, except that pharmacologic DVT prophylaxis is generally not initiated until 24–48 hours after ICH (pneumatic compression stockings should be used throughout hospitalization).

Etiologies of Intracerebral Hemorrhage

The causes of ICH include:

- Chronic hypertension. Hypertensive hemorrhage has a predilection for the deep brain structures (basal ganglia, thalamus, and deep subcortical white matter), the anterior pons, and the cerebellum. These are sites of perforating vessels that appear particularly susceptible to damage due to chronic hypertension. Lobar hemorrhage may also be caused by hypertension.

- Cerebral amyloid angiopathy (CAA): CAA-related hemorrhages are most commonly lobar (see "Cerebral Amyloid Angiopathy").

- Head trauma.
- Coagulopathy (inherited, acquired, or due to anticoagulant use) or thrombocytopenia (e.g., disseminated intravascular coagulation [DIC], thrombotic thrombocytopenia purpura [TTP], acute leukemia).
- Rupture of a vascular malformation (e.g., aneurysm, arteriovenous malformation, cavernous malformation).
- Hemorrhage into an ischemic stroke (**hemorrhagic conversion**), which is more common with embolic strokes, septic emboli in endocarditis, and strokes in the PCA territory.
- Cerebral venous sinus thrombosis (see "Cerebral Venous Sinus Thrombosis & Cortical Vein Thrombosis").
- Cocaine (due to acute hypertension).
- Hemorrhagic cerebral metastases. The metastatic tumors reported to be most susceptible to hemorrhage are melanoma, renal cell carcinoma, thyroid cancer, and choriocarcinoma. However, since lung metastases are far more common than any of these, the most common hemorrhagic brain metastases are due to lung cancer. Since acute blood may make the radiologic detection of an underlying mass difficult, contrast-enhanced CT or MRI may be repeated several months after ICH if there is suspicion for an underlying mass.

Cerebral Amyloid Angiopathy

The same amyloid protein that accumulates in the brain in Alzheimer's disease can accumulate in cerebral blood vessels, a condition known as **cerebral amyloid angiopathy (CAA)**. CAA may coexist with Alzheimer's disease, but the two can occur independently. Like Alzheimer's, CAA is predominantly a disease of older individuals. Amyloid deposition in blood vessels leads to increased risk of ICH. CAA-related ICH is most commonly lobar hemorrhage (as compared to the deep hemorrhages that occur with hypertension). In CAA-related ICH, additional asymptomatic lobar microhemorrhages are often noted on gradient echo (GRE) and susceptibility-weighted (SWI) MRI sequences with a predilection for the gray–white junction of the occipital lobes (Fig. 19–12). Convexal subarachnoid hemorrhage (i.e., in the sulci) can also occur, leading to superficial siderosis. Risk of CAA-related hemorrhage is increased in patients with the ε4 and ε2 alleles of the *APOE* gene.

CAA most commonly presents as lobar ICH, though some patients may present with **amyloid spells** (also called CAA-related transient focal neurologic episodes; for discussion see Smith et al., 2021). These spells are brief, transient episodes of focal sensory or motor deficits that spread from one region of the body to another (along adjacent regions of the motor/sensory homunculus, e.g., from face to arm). Rarely, transient visual or language deficits may occur. Amyloid spells are believed to be related to convexal subarachnoid hemorrhage that may induce cortical spreading depression. Amyloid spells should be considered in the differential diagnosis for TIA and seizure in older patients, especially if the MRI demonstrates microhemorrhages and/or cortical superficial siderosis suggestive of CAA.

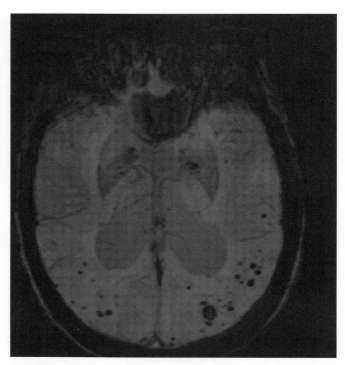

FIGURE 19–12 **MRI in cerebral amyloid angiopathy.** Axial GRE MRI demonstrating multiple microhemorrhages at the gray–white junction, predominantly in the occipital lobes.

The diagnosis of CAA should be considered in patients over age 55 with lobar ICH without another clear cause of ICH (considered "possible CAA"), and is especially likely in that setting if there is superficial siderosis and/or additional lobar microhemorrhages limited to the cortex/juxtacortical regions on GRE/SWI sequences (considered "probable CAA"; definite diagnosis requires histologic diagnosis) (Modified Boston Criteria: Linn et al., 2010). Patients with ICH due to CAA are at high risk for recurrent ICH. Some practitioners recommend avoidance of anticoagulation in such patients (though a patient with CAA-related ICH and a mechanical valve may be an exception to this recommendation), and recommend using antiplatelets only if there is a strong indication (Eckman et al., 2003).

A rare variant of CAA is **CAA-related inflammation**. In this condition, patients present with subacute cognitive decline and/or seizure, and imaging reveals asymmetric inflammatory lesions (T2/FLAIR hyperintensities) and multiple microhemorrhages (Fig. 19–13). Cerebrospinal fluid may be inflammatory and marked clinical improvement with steroids may be observed. The clinical course may be monophasic, relapsing, or progressive.

Resuming Anticoagulation After Anticoagulation-Associated Intracerebral Hemorrhage

In patients with anticoagulant-associated hemorrhage, the question often arises as to if and when to reinitiate

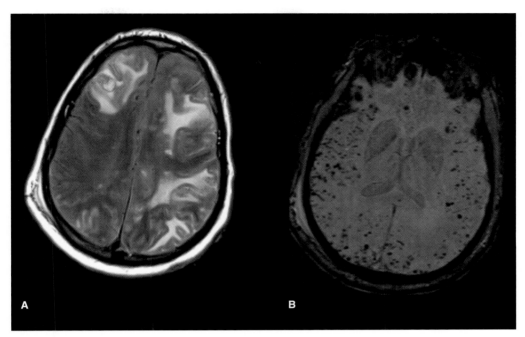

FIGURE 19–13 **MRI in cerebral amyloid angiopathy-related inflammation. A:** FLAIR MRI demonstrating asymmetric subcortical T2/FLAIR hyperintensity. **B:** GRE MRI demonstrating diffuse lobar microhemorrhages.

anticoagulation. This is a scenario for which there are no randomized controlled trial data, requiring a careful balance of the perceived benefit of anticoagulation weighed against the perceived risk of anticoagulation. The highest risk scenario for being off of anticoagulation is in patients with a mechanical prosthetic cardiac valve in the mitral position, and so anticoagulation is often reinitiated within days after ICH in patients with mechanical valves.

Management of pulmonary embolism and other systemic thrombosis (e.g., DVT, limb ischemia) in patients with recent ICH depends on how long it has been since the ICH, the risk to the other organs of not anticoagulating (e.g., has pulmonary embolism led to right heart strain?), and whether other potential interventions for thrombosis aside from systemic anticoagulation could be performed (e.g., can inferior vena cava filter be placed in the case of DVT? Can a local procedure such as thrombectomy or local anticoagulant infusion be performed for limb ischemia? Should left atrial appendage closure be considered for a patient with atrial fibrillation?)

All such decisions must take each individual patient's clinical scenario into account from both the ICH perspective (i.e., lobar vs deep, time since ICH) and the thrombosis perspective (i.e., differing risks of *not* anticoagulating in the setting of mechanical valve, DVT, pulmonary embolism, atrial fibrillation).

Although atrial fibrillation substantially elevates the risk for ischemic stroke, it has a relatively low daily risk of ischemic stroke (the percentage stroke risk per year associated with the patient's CHADS2 score divided by 365). Therefore, after an ICH in a patient with atrial fibrillation, anticoagulation is often held for several weeks. With respect to the risks

of anticoagulation from the ICH perspective, one decision analysis suggests that the risk of ICH recurrence after lobar CAA-related hemorrhage with anticoagulation outweighs the benefits of stroke prevention in the setting of atrial fibrillation, whereas the risk of ICH recurrence after deep/hypertensive hemorrhage may be outweighed by the benefit of anticoagulation in patients with a high risk of recurrent ischemic stroke (i.e., high CHADS2 score) (Eckman et al., 2003). Two recent meta-analyses suggest that resumption of anticoagulation after ICH in patients with atrial fibrillation may be safer than it is generally considered, but these studies may be confounded by selection bias (Biffi et al., 2017; Korompoki et al., 2017). Note that both of these studies and the decision analysis mentioned above only evaluated warfarin. In patients who have suffered warfarin-associated ICH and are considered at high risk for thromboembolic events from atrial fibrillation so as to warrant resumption of anticoagulation, one approach is to use a novel oral anticoagulant since risk of ICH is significantly lower with these agents compared to warfarin.

CENTRAL NERVOUS SYSTEM VASCULAR MALFORMATIONS

CNS vascular malformations are abnormal collections of blood vessels that can present with hemorrhage, seizure, and/or focal deficits, or may be discovered incidentally if neuroimaging is obtained for another indication. Diagnosis of the type of vascular malformation can often be made by radiologic characteristics (Table 19–3, Figs. 19–14, 19–15, 19–16, 19–17). In patients with ICH without a clear etiology (i.e., not clearly

TABLE 19–3 Features of Central Nervous System Vascular Malformations.

	Capillary Telangiectasia	Developmental Venous Anomaly (DVA)	Cavernous Malformation	Arteriovenous Malformation (AVM)
Vascular structures	Capillaries	Veins	Capillaries	Arteriovenous (no capillaries)
Intervening brain tissue	Yes, normal	Yes, normal	No	Yes, abnormal
Hemorrhage risk	Rare	<1%/year	1%–3%/year	About 3%/year, but depends on various factors (see text)
Clinical	Usually benign incidental finding	Usually benign incidental finding	Can be incidental but may cause hemorrhage, seizure, focal deficits	Risk of hemorrhage, seizure, focal deficits
Imaging	Hypointense on GRE/SWI, enhancement on postcontrast Most common location is pons	Identified on postcontrast images or in venous phase of angiography	"Popcorn" appearance on T2 MRI Usually not visualized on angiography	"Tangle" of vessels on angiography

Abbreviation: MRI: Magnetic resonance imaging.

due to hypertension, anticoagulant use, probable CAA) and no clear vascular lesion on CTA or MRA, digital subtraction angiography should be performed to evaluate for a vascular malformation.

Arteriovenous malformations (AVMs) are the vascular malformations most likely to cause ICH and are the best studied with respect to the risk of ICH. Risk factors for hemorrhage due to an AVM include prior ICH, deep location, deep venous drainage, and older age. Treatment can include surgical excision, catheter-based endovascular embolization, or radiation therapy. Intervention is generally pursued if an AVM ruptures causing ICH, but management for unruptured AVMs is less straightforward. The ARUBA trial (2014; long-term follow up reported in 2020) found no benefit of procedural intervention and medical management (e.g., treatment of seizures) versus medical management alone for unruptured AVMs, but intervention may be considered if hemorrhage risk is high and surgical risk is acceptable.

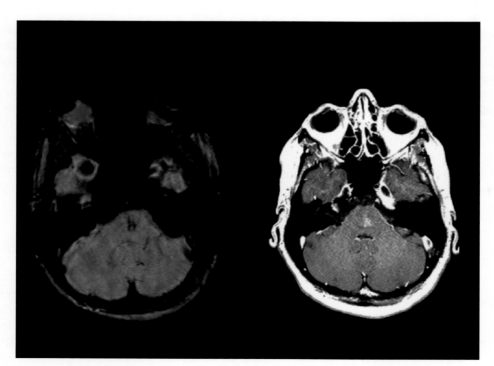

FIGURE 19–14 **Capillary telangiectasia.** GRE sequence showing hypointensity in pons (A) with corresponding contrast enhancement on T1 postcontrast sequence (B).

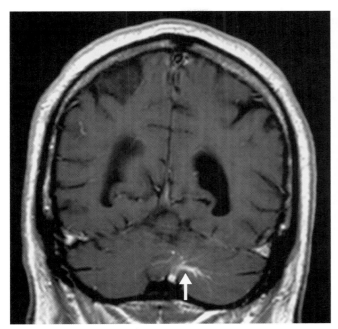

FIGURE 19–15 Developmental venous anomaly. Coronal postcontrast MRI demonstrating developmental venous anomaly of the inferior medial left cerebellum (arrow). (Reproduced with permission from Ropper A, Samuels M, Klein J: *Adams and Victor's Principles of Neurology*, 10th ed. New York, NY: McGraw Hill; 2014.)

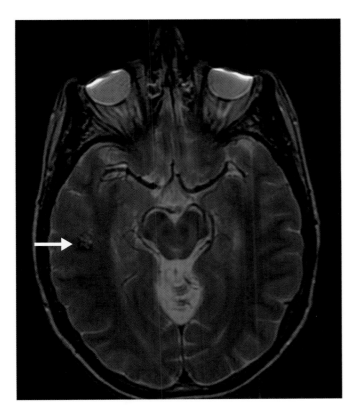

FIGURE 19–16 Cavernous malformation. Axial T2-weighted MRI demonstrating "popcorn" appearance of a right temporal cavernous malformation.

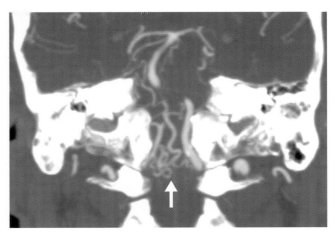

FIGURE 19–17 Arteriovenous malformation. Coronal CT angiogram demonstrating arteriovenous malformation arising from the vertebrobasilar system.

Surgical risk is measured by the Spetzler-Martin scale, which predicts higher risk of postoperative neurologic deficits or death if an AVM is larger, in eloquent cortex, and/or deep (Spetzler and Martin, 1986).

SUBARACHNOID HEMORRHAGE

Subarachnoid hemorrhage (SAH) can be caused by:

- Aneurysm rupture or bleeding from other types of vascular malformations
- Head trauma
- Venous sinus thrombosis or cortical vein thrombosis
- Reversible cerebral vasoconstriction syndrome (RCVS)
- Cerebral amyloid angiopathy (CAA)

SAH in one or a few adjacent sulci (**convexal SAH**) is suggestive of trauma, cortical vein thrombosis, reversible cerebral vasoconstriction syndrome (RCVS), or CAA as an etiology (Fig. 19–18A).

SAH in the basal cisterns and/or more widely distributed is concerning for aneurysm rupture unless there is a clear history of trauma (Fig. 19–18B).

Aneurysmal Subarachnoid Hemorrhage

SAH due to rupture of an intracranial aneurysm leads to death in about half of patients, with a significant percentage dying before they reach the emergency room. Patients present with an acute-onset headache that is maximal at onset (thunderclap headache), classically the "worst of their life." Headache can be isolated or may be accompanied by meningismus, nausea/vomiting, cranial nerve palsies, altered consciousness (from confusion to coma), and/or seizures. Some patients report a prior severe "sentinel headache" in the preceding weeks.

Diagnosis is generally made by noncontrast CT scan, which is extremely sensitive within the first day after symptom onset, but sensitivity decreases with time from the initial

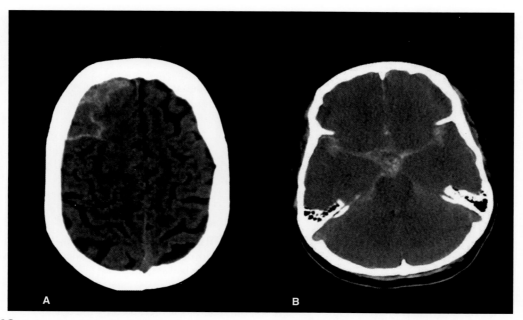

FIGURE 19–18 Subarachnoid hemorrhage. Axial noncontrast CT images demonstrating: **A:** Convexal (sulcal) subarachnoid hemorrhage in the right frontal lobe in a patient with reversible cerebral vasoconstriction syndrome. **B:** Diffuse cisternal subarachnoid hemorrhage in a patient with a ruptured intracranial aneurysm.

hemorrhage and with smaller hemorrhage volumes. If CT is negative and suspicion is high, lumbar puncture should be performed to evaluate for blood products. SAH must be differentiated from blood in the CSF due to traumatic lumbar puncture. CSF findings suggestive of SAH are the persistence of a similar quantity of red blood cells over several tubes and **xanthochromia**. Xanthochromia refers to a change in CSF color (most sensitively detected by spectrophotometry) signifying blood breakdown in the CSF, demonstrating that blood has been in the CSF for longer than the time of lumbar puncture. If suspicion for SAH remains high despite normal CT and normal or equivocal lumbar puncture results, angiography should be performed. If there is CT or lumbar puncture evidence of SAH but angiography is unrevealing, angiography is generally repeated after 1–2 weeks. Although the sensitivity of CTA continues to improve, digital subtraction angiography remains the gold standard for diagnosis of intracranial aneurysms.

Prevention & Management of Neurologic Complications of Subarachnoid Hemorrhage (Table 19–4)

Patients with aneurysmal SAH should be monitored in an ICU setting for complications of SAH due to ruptured aneurysm. Neurologic complications include rebleeding, seizures, hydrocephalus (due to blockage of CSF flow by subarachnoid blood), vasospasm (due to irritation of the blood vessels by subarachnoid blood), and delayed cerebral ischemia.

Definitive treatment of a bleeding aneurysm to prevent rebleeding is with surgical clipping or endovascular therapy. If surgical intervention must be delayed for more than 2–3 days, aminocaproic acid may be administered in

this period to reduce the risk of rebleeding. If the patient is on an antiplatelet or anticoagulant, this should be held and anticoagulants should be reversed as in patients with ICH. Until the aneurysm is secured, blood pressure should be controlled to reduce rebleeding risk, but the precise blood pressure goal has not been clearly established. After an aneurysm is secured, blood pressure is generally allowed to autoregulate to prevent hypoperfusion and/or vasospasm.

TABLE 19–4 Prevention & Management of Neurologic Complications of Subarachnoid Hemorrhage.

Complication	Prevention	Treatment
Rebleeding	Surgical/endovascular intervention Aminocaproic acid if aneurysm cannot be secured immediately Blood pressure control	
Hydrocephalus		Extraventricular drain
Vasospasm/ Delayed cerebral ischemia	Nimodipine Maintenance of euvolemia	IV vasopressors, inotropes Intra-arterial intervention (vasodilators, balloon angioplasty)
Seizures	Antiepileptic drug prophylaxis can be considered (debated)	Antiepileptic drug if seizures occur

If seizures occur in the setting of SAH, they should of course be treated. Some practitioners administer prophylactic antiepileptics to prevent seizures, although this practice is debated in patients who have not had seizures.

If hydrocephalus is present, an external ventricular drain (EVD) is usually placed.

Delayed cerebral ischemia due to cerebral arterial vasospasm can occur between 3 days and 3 weeks after SAH. This may manifest as new focal deficits or change in level of consciousness. Vasospasm can be screened for by transcranial Doppler ultrasound (TCD), which may reveal increased flow velocity (due to arterial narrowing) before clinical signs of ischemia appear. Nimodipine (a calcium channel blocker) improves outcomes, though the mechanism does not appear to be decrease in vasospasm. If delayed cerebral ischemia occurs, treatment options include intravenous vasopressors/inotropes and intra-arterial therapies (vasodilators or balloon angioplasty).

Non-neurologic complications of SAH include hyponatremia (due to syndrome of inappropriate secretion of antidiuretic hormone [SIADH] and/or cerebral salt wasting), cardiac arrhythmias, heart failure, and neurogenic pulmonary edema. Cardiopulmonary complications of SAH are likely due to the sympathetic surge induced by cerebral injury. Supportive measures include maintenance of euglycemia, euthermia, and euvolemia, as well as prevention of DVT. For DVT prophlyaxis, mechanical prophylaxis is generally utilized until 24 hours after securing of the aneurysm, after which prophylactic anticoagulation may be used.

Perimesencephalic Subarachnoid Hemorrhage (Fig. 19–19)

SAH restricted to the cisterns immediately surrounding the brainstem (predominantly the interpeduncular and prepontine cisterns) is only rarely associated with aneurysm (<10% of cases) and has a far more benign prognosis compared to aneurysmal SAH. If this pattern of SAH is found, patients generally still undergo angiography to look for aneurysm.

Unruptured Intracranial Aneurysms

Screening for intracranial aneurysms in asymptomatic patients is generally only undertaken in patients with two or more first-degree relatives with aneurysms, but is sometimes also considered in patients with a genetic predisposition to aneurysms (e.g., polycystic kidney disease, Ehlers-Danlos syndrome). Such patients are generally screened every 5 years with MRA or CTA.

With increasing use of MRA and CTA, incidental aneurysms are identified with increasing frequency. Risk of rupture is correlated with increasing aneurysm size (lower risk with aneurysms <7 mm), site (lower risk with anterior circulation (lowest in cavernous carotid); highest risk with posterior circulation), growth on subsequent imaging, and prior history of aneurysm rupture (i.e., from another aneurysm). These factors along with patient factors (e.g., age, comorbidities) are considered in determining the risk/benefit of intervention (with surgical clipping or endovascular coiling) versus observation with serial imaging. Smoking, hypertension, and use of cocaine can all increase risk of rupture, so these modifiable risk factors must be addressed if present.

In patients with unruptured aneurysms, the question often arises as to whether antiplatelets and anticoagulants are safe. Although these medications are unlikely to increase the risk of rupture, if rupture were to occur, resulting SAH could be worsened. In general, aspirin is considered safe, but anticoagulation requires a careful assessment of the risks and benefits of use in each individual patient. For example, accepting the risk of the use of anticoagulants may be unavoidable with a mechanical heart valve or large pulmonary embolism, but risk stratification by CHADS2 score in patients with atrial fibrillation may lead to a more complex

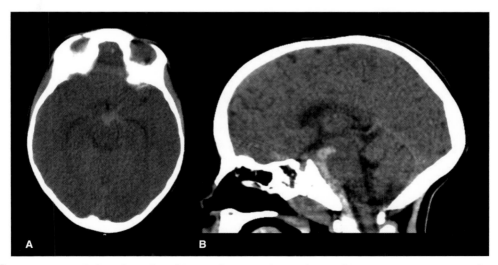

FIGURE 19–19 **Perimesencephalic subarachnoid hemorrhage.** Axial (**A**) and sagittal (**B**) noncontrast CT images demonstrating subarachnoid hemorrhage isolated to the region anterior to the brainstem.

analysis of risk and benefit depending on the size and location of the aneurysm.

INTRAVENTRICULAR HEMORRHAGE

Intraventricular hemorrhage (IVH) can occur as a complication of ICH or SAH, or it can occur in isolation (Fig. 19–20). The differential diagnosis for the etiology of IVH is similar to ICH and SAH: coagulopathy, trauma, bleeding from a vascular malformation or aneurysm, and extension from ICH. Due to blockage of CSF flow, IVH typically presents with symptoms of elevated intracranial pressure: headache, nausea/vomiting, and altered level of consciousness. Blood pressure should be controlled and coagulopathy reversed if present, just as in ICH. Placement of an extraventricular drain (EVD) is often necessary due to development of hydrocephalus. Some patients may ultimately need ventriculoperitoneal shunting for persistent impaired CSF resorption due to blood in the ventricular system. The use of intraventricular administration of tPA to lyse intraventricular clot was studied in CLEAR III (2017) and did not demonstrate improved clinical outcomes, although there was a suggestion of benefit in patients whose intraventricular clot burdens were reduced more than 80%.

SUBDURAL HEMATOMA

Subdural hematoma (SDH) occurs due to tearing of bridging veins that run between the brain and the dura. Head trauma is the most common cause of acute SDH. In older adults with brain atrophy (leading to greater tension on the bridging veins) or in patients on anticoagulation, the trauma necessary to cause SDH may be so minor that it cannot be recalled by the patient.

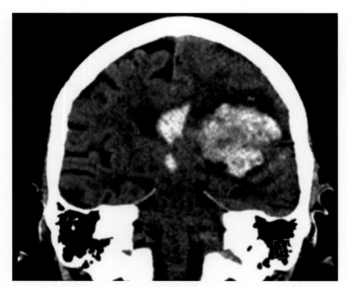

FIGURE 19–20 Intraventricular hemorrhage. Coronal non-contrast CT image of a left hemispheric intraparenchymal hemorrhage with extension into the left lateral ventricle and third ventricle.

Unlike most cerebrovascular conditions that develop suddenly, SDH may also develop more insidiously (**chronic SDH**) after minor trauma (e.g., in patients who are elderly and/or on anticoagulation) or in the setting of intracranial hypotension (see "Decreased Intracranial Pressure [Intracranial Hypotension]" in Ch. 25). Chronic SDH can present with subacute headache, alterations in consciousness, focal deficits, and/or seizures. Some patients have fluctuating symptoms found ultimately to be due to seizures by EEG monitoring, but in some patients, these fluctuations have no electrographic correlate and may be due to transient ischemia or cortical spreading depression induced by the SDH (for review and discussion, see Levesque et al., 2020).

Acute SDH appears as a crescent-shaped hyperdensity on CT (blood filling the space between the dura and the brain) (Fig. 19–21A). With chronic SDH, there may be different radiographic densities in the subdural space due to blood products of varying ages. Chronic SDH can develop into a **hygroma**, a fluid collection without obvious blood products in the subdural space.

The decision of whether to surgically drain an acute traumatic SDH depends on the size of the SDH and the degree of resultant midline shift, as well as the clinical state of the patient (Glasgow Coma Scale [GCS] and pupil symmetry). Pupillary asymmetry or a decline in GCS by 2 or more points from the time of trauma to the time of evaluation in a patient with SDH are generally indications for surgery no matter what the size of the SDH. An acute SDH of 10 mm or more or with 5 mm or more of SDH-induced midline shift is generally considered an indication for surgical drainage irrespective of neurologic examination findings. Size of SDH and clinical state are also used to determine candidates for surgical drainage in patients with chronic SDH.

EPIDURAL HEMATOMA

Epidural hematoma (EDH) is almost always caused by head trauma. Normally, the dura is fixed to the skull with no true epidural "space." This is in contrast to the subdural space, which is a true space between the brain and the dura. Head trauma leading to damage to the middle meningeal artery is the most common etiology of EDH. As arterial blood accumulates, it "dissects" the dura away from the skull, leading to a lens-shaped collection of blood on neuroimaging (Fig. 19–21B). It may be this pathophysiology that accounts for the "lucid interval" between head trauma and decline in consciousness that occurs in some patients with EDH: The arterial blood must reach a certain volume/pressure to overcome the adherence of the dura to the skull, and when it does, the hematoma rapidly expands, raising intracranial pressure. However, this lucid interval is not always present in patients with EDH.

Similar to SDH, size of the EDH and clinical state determine which patients require urgent operative drainage. Surgical evacuation is generally necessary for EDH greater than 30 mL regardless of clinical state, or EDH with coma (GCS < 9) or pupil asymmetry.

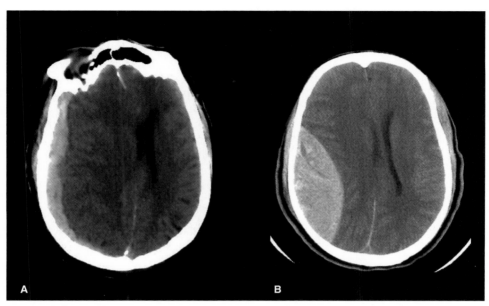

FIGURE 19–21 **Subdural and epidural hematoma.** Axial noncontrast CT images demonstrating: **A:** Right-sided subdural hematoma ("crescent" shaped). **B:** Right-sided epidural hematoma ("lens" shaped).

CEREBRAL VENOUS SINUS THROMBOSIS & CORTICAL VEIN THROMBOSIS

Venous sinus thrombosis (VST) should be considered in patients with unexplained progressive headache, especially if symptoms or signs of elevated intracranial pressure are present (e.g., nausea, vomiting, headache worse when supine, papilledema, sixth nerve palsy/palsies [see "Symptoms and Signs of Increased Intracranial Pressure" in Ch. 25]), although patients may present with isolated headache. Patients may also present with seizures, ischemic stroke, ICH, or SAH.

Diagnosis of VST is made definitively by demonstrating venous occlusion on dedicated venous imaging (MRV or CTV; Fig. 19–22), but should be suspected on nonvascular noncontrast CT or MRI in the following scenarios:

- Diffuse cerebral edema without trauma
- ICH that is parasagittal (caused by thrombosis of the superior sagittal sinus), bithalamic (caused by thrombosis of the internal cerebral veins), temporo-occipital (caused by transverse sinus thrombosis), or juxtacortical (caused by cortical vein thrombosis)
- ICH with edema out of proportion to the size of the hemorrhage
- Convexal SAH (i.e., in the cerebral convexities; also called sulcal SAH)
- Thrombosed cortical vein (hyperdensity on CT or clot seen on GRE/SWI MRI sequences)
- Hyperdensity over one of the sinuses on noncontrast CT (**cord sign**)
- Lack of flow in the posterior superior sagittal sinus on contrast-enhanced CT (**empty delta sign**)

MRV and CTV can reveal thrombosed venous sinuses, but irregularity of the sinuses due to normal structures can be misleading (e.g., arachnoid granulations, asymmetries due to unilateral transverse sinus hypoplasia). When in doubt, contrast-enhanced MRI can be used to look for filling defects in the venous sinuses. Diffuse pachymeningeal enhancement may also sometimes be seen in VST due to engorged dural veins (though other causes of diffuse pachymeningeal enhancement should also be considered such as inflammatory/infectious meningitis or intracranial hypotension). Cortical vein thrombosis can be notoriously difficult to diagnose with MRV and CTV given the small caliber of cortical veins; radiological clues listed above should raise suspicion for this diagnosis, and digital subtraction angiography may be considered.

VST can be caused by CNS or sinus infection, or any etiology of a hypercoagulable state including:

- Oral contraceptive use
- Pregnancy/peripartum period
- Systemic malignancy
- Systemic inflammatory disease (e.g., inflammatory bowel disease, lupus)
- Genetic hypercoagulable state (factor V Leiden, prothrombin gene mutation, protein C deficiency, protein S deficiency, antithrombin III deficiency)
- Antiphospholipid antibody syndrome
- Nephrotic syndrome
- Dehydration

Treatment is with anticoagulation. Anticoagulation is thought to be safe and effective even if there is ICH secondary to VST (Einhaupl et al., 1991; de Brujin and Stam, 1999; meta-analysis: Stam et al., 2002). If patients worsen in spite of anticoagulation, endovascular interventions can be considered,

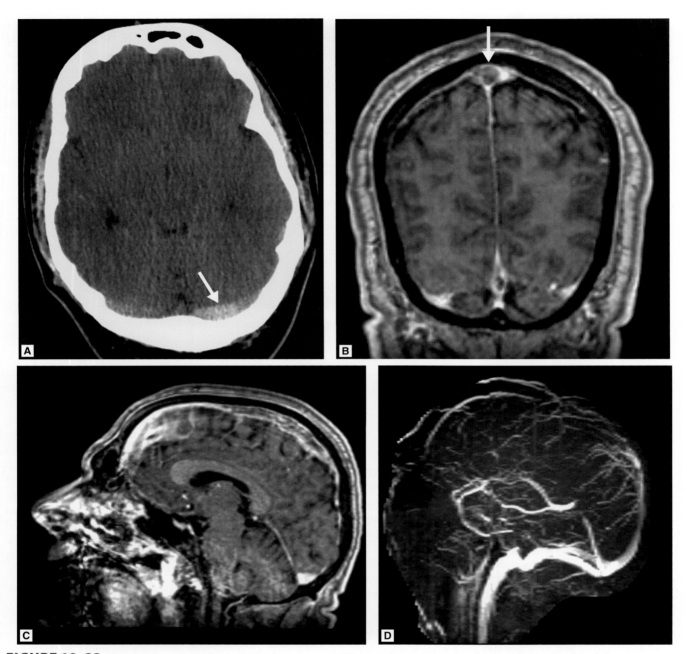

FIGURE 19–22 **Venous sinus thrombosis. A:** Axial noncontrast CT image demonstrating cord sign in the region of the left transverse sinus (**arrow**). **B**: Coronal T1-weighted postcontrast MRI demonstrating lack of filling of the superior sagittal sinus (**arrow**). **C:** Sagittal T1-weighted postcontrast MRI demonstrating lack of filling of the superior sagittal sinus. **D:** Sagittal MRV, demonstrating lack of filling of the superior sagittal sinus.

although data are limited. In cases of extensive thrombosis with elevated intracranial pressure, management of intracranial pressure is required (see "Treatment of Acutely Elevated Intracranial Pressure" in Ch. 25).

An evaluation for a hypercoagulable state should be undertaken in all patients with VST unless there is another clear ongoing underlying trigger (e.g., malignancy) that would warrant life-long anticoagulation whether a specific hypercoagulable abnormality is found or not. It should be

noted that some of the components of the hypercoagulable evaluation can be abnormal in the setting of anticoagulation and/or thrombosis, confounding interpretation when evaluated in the acute setting. For example, protein C and protein S are lowered by warfarin; antithrombin III is lowered by heparin.

If an ongoing irreversible hypercoagulable state is discovered during evaluation, life-long anticoagulation may be necessary (e.g., active malignancy, clotting disorder).

This is generally not necessary for provoked VST (e.g., peripartum, dehydration, trauma, CNS/sinus infection), for which anticoagulation is usually maintained for 3–6 months.

OTHER CEREBROVASCULAR DISORDERS

Posterior Reversible Encephalopathy Syndrome

Posterior reversible encephalopathy syndrome (PRES) is a condition named for the most common and most prominent location of radiographic changes (posterior), usual clinical course (reversible), and one of the component clinical features (encephalopathy). However, the radiographic changes may extend beyond the posterior of the brain; the syndrome can include seizures, headache, and/or visual changes with or independent of encephalopathy; and in rare cases the disorder can result in ischemia or hemorrhage resulting in irreversible disability. The classic syndrome is one in which a patient develops headache, seizure, visual changes, and/or altered mental status with characteristic neuroimaging changes consisting of subcortical T2/FLAIR white matter hyperintensities in the occipital lobes in the MCA-PCA borderzone territories (see "Watershed [Borderzone] Territories" in Ch. 7) that resolve when the underlying cause is treated (Fig. 19–23). Etiologies of PRES include:

- Hypertensive emergency
- Eclampsia
- Immunosuppressive agents (e.g., tacrolimus, cyclosporine)
- Chemotherapeutic agents (e.g., bortezomib)

There is a broad spectrum of neuroimaging changes in this condition beyond the classic appearance described above, including contrast enhancement, vascular narrowing on MRA or CTA, cerebral ischemia/hemorrhage, and/or signal changes in the anterior circulation (a common pattern is in the MCA-ACA watershed/borderzone territories; see "Watershed [Borderzone] Territories" in Ch. 7), brainstem, cerebellum, and/or gray matter (cortex and/or deep gray).

Treatment is of the underlying cause: lowering blood pressure in hypertensive emergency; magnesium, lowering blood pressure, and delivery of the baby in eclampsia; and removal of the offending agent in medication-induced PRES. If seizures occur, these should be treated with antiseizure medications, but if the underlying cause is identified and treated, prolonged treatment with antiseizure medications is generally not necessary beyond a short course while the underlying cause is treated.

Reversible Cerebral Vasoconstriction Syndrome (RCVS)

Reversible cerebral vasoconstriction syndrome (RCVS) (also called Call-Fleming syndrome) is a condition of reversible vasospasm of the intracranial arteries, as the name suggests. Patients most commonly present with isolated thunderclap headache (sudden-onset, maximal-at-onset), although focal features and/or seizures may be seen if the condition causes ischemic stroke or hemorrhage. When intracranial hemorrhage occurs, it is most commonly convexal SAH (see Fig. 19–18A). Vasospasm is apparent on vascular imaging, which has the appearance of alternating constriction and dilation of vessels in a "sausage-link"–like (or "beaded") appearance (Fig. 19–24). The most common causes of RCVS include:

- Drugs: marijuana, cocaine, amphetamines
- Medications: selective serotonin reuptake inhibitors (SSRIs) and over-the-counter cold medicines with sympathomimetics (e.g., pseudoephedrine)
- Postpartum period (postpartum angiopathy), which can occur with or without preeclampsia/eclampsia
- PRES: the two conditions may co-occur

Treatment involves discontinuation of the underlying drug or medication trigger if one is identified. Some practitioners treat RCVS with nimodipine, verapamil, and/or magnesium. Most patients recover completely both clinically and radiologically within days to weeks after symptom onset.

Superficial Siderosis

Superficial siderosis refers to chronic subarachnoid bleeding leading to deposition of blood products around the brainstem, cranial nerves, and cerebellum. The classic symptoms are insidious development of hearing loss (due to involvement of cranial nerve 8), ataxia (due to cerebellar involvement), and motor dysfunction with upper motor neuron signs (due to involvement of the descending corticospinal tracts). MRI reveals low T2 signal surrounding the circumference of the brainstem and cerebellum with evidence of blood surrounding these structures on SWI/GRE sequences. Causes include prior head or spine trauma, arteriovenous malformation, and CNS tumors, although, in many cases, no clear cause is determined. Some practitioners consider treatment of superficial siderosis with iron chelators, though this is often ineffective. Although CAA can cause siderosis, it is typically limited to the cortical sulci rather than affecting the brainstem/cerebellum and therefore does not typically cause the classic clinical features of superficial siderosis described here.

VASCULAR DISEASE OF THE SPINAL CORD

Many of the same types of vascular pathology that occur in the brain can also occur in the spinal cord, although much less commonly. This includes ischemic stroke, epidural hematoma, spinal cord hemorrhage, and vascular malformations.

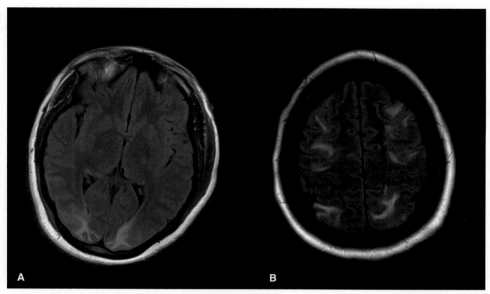

FIGURE 19–23 **Posterior reversible encephalopathy syndrome (PRES).** Axial FLAIR MRI demonstrating subcortical T2/FLAIR hyperintensity in the white matter of the MCA-PCA boderzones (**A**) and the MCA-ACA borderzones (**B**).

Ischemic Stroke of the Spinal Cord

Ischemic stroke of the spinal cord presents with sudden-onset myelopathy. The main differential diagnosis is acute spinal cord compression, and urgent imaging is needed to evaluate for the latter since surgical intervention is often necessary in acute cord compression. Spinal cord infarction most commonly occurs in the setting of aortic disease (rupture of aortic aneurysm or complication of surgical repair of aortic aneurysm). A rarer etiology of spinal cord infarction is **fibrocartilaginous embolism**, in which disc fragments are thought to embolize to the spinal vasculature after trauma or exertion. Fibrocartilaginous embolism typically presents with acute back pain in addition to myelopathy.

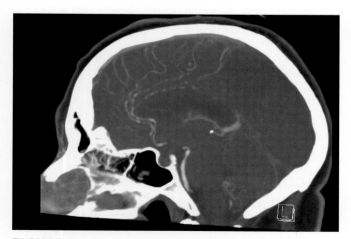

FIGURE 19–24 **Reversible cerebral vasoconstriction syndrome (RCVS).** Sagittal CT angiogram, demonstrating diffuse irregularity ("beading") of the anterior cerebral arteries.

The spinal cord is supplied by the anterior spinal artery and paired posterior spinal arteries (all of which originate from the vertebral arteries). The anterior spinal artery is fed by radicular arteries that branch from the aorta along the length of the spinal cord. The largest radicular branch and one of the most vulnerable to damage in abdominal aortic surgery is the **artery of Adamkiewicz**, normally found at the level of the lower thoracic spine (at about T10). The anterior spinal circulation is vulnerable to disruption, which most commonly occurs due to aortic pathology or aortic surgery. Anterior spinal artery territory infarction typically presents as bilateral lower extremity weakness and loss of pain and temperature sensation with preserved proprioception and vibration sense (see "Anterior Cord Syndrome" in Ch. 5). There is also a watershed territory between the anterior and posterior circulations in the central cord, and central cord infarction can occur with global hypoperfusion.

MRI with diffusion-weighted imaging (DWI) sequences may demonstrate spinal cord infarction, but DWI is not as sensitive in the spinal cord as it is for cerebral infarction. Given the rarity of spinal cord infarction, appropriate treatment is not well established. Based on the pathophysiology, perfusion should be maintained by avoiding hypotension, and some practitioners utilize lumbar CSF drainage to enhance spinal cord perfusion.

Spinal Hemorrhage

Hemorrhage into the spinal cord (**hematomyelia**) or its surroundings (epidural, subdural, subarachnoid) can be caused by spinal trauma, anticoagulation, or bleeding from a spinal vascular malformation. The most common compartment for spinal hemorrhage is the epidural space. A spinal epidural hematoma can result from trauma or as a complication of spinal surgery or epidural administration of anesthesia. Epidural hematoma is generally easily identified on CT as a hyperdensity in the spinal canal. Treatment is surgical evacuation.

Spinal Dural Arteriovenous Fistula

The most common arteriovenous (AV) malformation of the spine is the spinal dural AV fistula (AVF), which typically presents with a progressive myelopathy that may fluctuate over time spontaneously and/or with exertion. Spinal dural AVF most commonly occurs in older men. MRI typically reveals diffuse spinal cord edema and prominent posterior flow voids (Fig. 19–25). Longitudinal contrast enhancement of the spinal cord may be seen, and may be discontinuous with an intervening nonenhancing segment of the cord (**missing piece sign;** Zalewski et al., 2018). The malformation itself may sometimes be visualized with MRA. The myelopathy may worsen if steroids are administered, which may occur if the initial clinical impression is that cord edema seen on MRI represents transverse myelitis rather than venous congestion

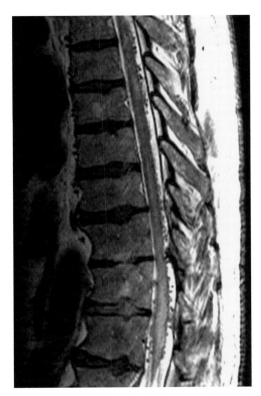

FIGURE 19–25 **Spinal dural arterio-venous fistula.** Sagittal T2-weighted MRI of the spine demonstrating cord edema (T2 hyperintensity) and multiple flow voids (hypointense "spots") in the CSF space posterior to the spinal cord. (Reproduced with permission from Ropper A, Samuels M, Klein J: *Adams and Victor's Principles of Neurology*, 10th ed. New York, NY: McGraw Hill; 2014.)

from an AVF. Definitive diagnosis requires spinal angiogram, and treatment may be surgical or catheter-based. Spinal dural AVF is an important underrecognized and treatable cause of progressive myelopathy.

REFERENCES

ACAS trial Executive Committee for the Asymptomatic Carotid Atherosclerosis Study. Endarterectomy for asymptomatic carotid artery stenosis. *JAMA* 1995;273:1421–1428.

ACST trial Halliday A, Mansfield A, Marro J, Peto C, Potter J, Thomas DJ, et al. MRC Asymptomatic Carotid Surgery Trial (ACST) Collaborative Group. Prevention of disabling and fatal strokes by successful carotid endarterectomy in patients without recent neurological symptoms: randomised controlled trial. *Lancet* 2004;363:1491–1502.

ACES trial Markus HS, King A, Shipley M, Topakian R, Cullinane M, Reihill S, et al. Asymptomatic embolisation for prediction of stroke in the Asymptomatic Carotid Emboli Study (ACES): a prospective observational study. *Lancet Neurol* 2010;9(7):663–671.

Adams HP, Bendixen BH, Leira E, Chang KC, Davis PH, Woolson RF, et al. Antithrombotic treatment of ischemic stroke among patients with occlusion or severe stenosis of the internal carotid artery: A report of the trial of Org 10172 in acute stroke treatment (TOAST). *Neurol* 1999;53:122–125.

AHA/ASA Acute Ischemic Stroke Guidelines Powers WJ. Guidelines for the Early Management of Patients With Acute Ischemic Stroke: 2019 Update to the 2018 Guidelines for the Early Management of Acute Ischemic Stroke: A Guideline for Healthcare Professionals From the American Heart Association/American Stroke Association. *Stroke* 2019;50(12):e344–e418.

ARUBA trial 2014 Mohr JP, Parides MK, Stapf C, Moquete E, Moy CS, Overbey JR, et al. Medical management with or without interventional therapy for unruptured brain arteriovenous malformations (ARUBA): a multicentre, non-blinded, randomised trial. *Lancet* 2014;383(9917):614–621.

ARUBA trial 2020 Mohr JP, Overbey JR, Hartmann A, von Kummer R, Salman RA, Kim H, et al. Medical management with interventional therapy versus medical management alone for unruptured brain arteriovenous malformations (ARUBA): final follow-up of a multicentre, non-blinded, randomised controlled trial. *Lancet Neurol* 2020;19(7):573–581.

ATACH 2 trial Qureshi AI, Palesch YY, Barsan WG, Hanley DF, Hsu CY, Martin RL, et al. Intensive blood-pressure lowering in patients with acute cerebral hemorrhage. *N Engl J Med* 2016;375(11):1033–1043.

Biffi A, Kuramatsu JB, Leasure A, Kamel H, Kourkoulis C, Schwab K, et al. Oral anticoagulation and functional outcome after intracerebral hemorrhage. *Ann Neurol* 2017;82(5):755–765.

Biousse V, D'Anglejan-Chaillon J, Toboul PJ, Amarenco P, Bousser MG. Time course of symptoms in extracranial carotid artery dissections: a series of 80 patients. *Stroke* 1995;26:235–239.

CADISS trial CADISS trial investigators. Antiplatelet treatment compared with anticoagulation treatment for cervical artery dissection (CADISS): a randomised trial. *Lancet Neurol* 2015;14:361–367.

CADISS trial 2019 Markus HS, Levi C, King A, Madigan J, Norris J. Antiplatelet therapy vs anticoagulation therapy in cervical artery dissection: The Cervical Artery Dissection in Stroke Study (CADISS) Randomized Clinical Trial Final Results. *JAMA Neurol* 2019;76(6):657–664.

CAST trial CAST (Chinese Acute Stroke Trial) Collaborative Group. CAST: randomized placebo-controlled trial of early aspirin use in 20,000 patients with acute ischemic stroke. *Lancet* 1997;349:1641–1649.

CHANCE trial Wang Y, Wang Y, Zhao X, Liu L, Wang D, Wang C, et al. Clopidogrel with aspirin in acute minor stroke or transient ischemic attack. *N Engl J Med* 2013;369:11–19.

CHARISMA trial Bhatt DL, Fox KA, Hacke W, Berger PB, Black HR, Boden WE, et al. Clopidogrel and aspirin versus aspirin alone for the prevention of atherothrombotic events. *N Engl J Med* 2006;354:1706–1717.

Chen ZM, Sandercock P, Pan HC, Counsell C, Collins R, Liu LS, et al. Indications for early aspirin use in acute ischemic stroke: a combined analysis of 40,000 randomized patients from the Chinese Acute Stroke Trial and the International Stroke Trial. *Stroke* 2000;31:1240–1249.

CLEAR III trial Hanley DF, Lane K, McBee N, Ziai W, Tuhrim S, Lees KR, et al. Thrombolytic removal of intraventricular haemorrhage in treatment of severe stroke: results of the randomised, multicentre, multiregion, placebo-controlled CLEAR III trial *Lancet* 2017;389(10069):603–611.

CLOSE trial Mas JL, Derumeaux G, Guillon B, Massardier E, Hosseini H, Mechtouff L, et al. Patent foramen ovale closure or anticoagulation vs. antiplatelets after stroke. *N Engl J Med* 2017;377:1011–1021.

CLOSURE I trial Furlan AJ, Reisman M, Massaro J, Mari L, Adams H, Albers G, et al. Closure or medical therapy for cryptogenic stroke with patent foramen ovale. *N Engl J Med* 2012;366:991–999.

CREST trial Brott TG, Hobson RW, Howard G, Roubin GS, Cark WM, Brooks W, et al. Stenting versus endarterectomy for treatment of carotid-artery stenosis. *N Engl J Med* 2010;363:11–23.

CRYSTAL AF trial Sanna T, Diener HS, Passman RS, Lazzaro VD, Bernstein RA, et al. Cryptogenic stroke and underlying atrial fibrillation. *N Engl J Med* 2014;370:2478–2486.

DAWN trial Nogueira RG, Jadhav AP, Haussen DC, Bonafe A, Budzik RF, Bhuva P, et al. Thrombectomy 6 to 24 hours after stroke with a mismatch between deficit and infarct. *N Engl J Med* 2018;378:11–21.

de Brujin SF, Stam J. Randomized, placebo-controlled trial of anticoagulant treatment with low-molecular-weight heparin for cerebral sinus thrombosis. *Stroke* 1999;30(3):484–488.

DECIMAL trial Vahedi K, Vicaut E, Mateo J, Kurtz A, Orabi M, Guichard J, et al. Sequential-design, multicenter, randomized, controlled trial of early decompressive craniectomy in malignant middle cerebral artery infarction (DECIMAL Trial). *Stroke* 2007;38(9):2506–2517.

DEFENSE-PFO Lee PH, Song JK, Kim JS, Heo R, Lee S, Kim DH, et al. Cryptogenic stroke and high-risk patent foramen ovale: the DEFENSE-PFO trial. *J Am Coll Cardiology* 2018;71:2335–2342.

DEFUSE trial Albers GW, Marks MP, Kemp S, Christensen S, Tsai JP, Gutierrez SO, et al. Thrombectomy for stroke at 6 to 16 hours with selection by perfusion imaging. *N Engl J Med* 2018;378:708–718.

DESTINY trial Jüttler E, Schwab S, Schmiedek P, Unterberg A, Hennerici M, Witzik J, et al. Decompressive Surgery for the Treatment of Malignant Infarction of the Middle Cerebral Artery (DESTINY): a randomized, controlled trial *Stroke* 2007;38:2518–2525.

DESTINY II trial Jüttler E, Unterberg A, Woitzik J, Bosel J, Amiri H, Sakowitz OW, et al. Hemicraniectomy in older patients with extensive middle-cerebral-artery stroke. *N Engl J Med* 2014;370:1091–1100.

ECASS III trial Hacke W, Kaste M, Bluhmki E, Brozman M, Davalos A, Guidetti D, et al. Thrombolysis with alteplase 3 to 4.5 hours after acute ischemic stroke. *N Engl J Med* 2008;359:1317–1329.

Eckman MH, Rosand J, Knudsen KA, Singer DE, Greenberg SM. Can patients be anticoagulated after intra-cerebral hemorrhage? A decision analysis. *Stroke* 2003;34:1710–1716.

ECST trial European Carotid Surgery Trialists' Collaborative Group. Randomised trial of endarterectomy for recently symptomatic carotid stenosis: final results of the MRC European Carotid Surgery Trial (ECST) *Lancet* 1998;35:1379–1387.

Edlow BL. Diagnosis of DWI-negative acute ischemic stroke: a meta-analysis. *Neurol* 2017;89(3):256–262.

Einhäupl KM, Villringer A, Meister W, Mehraein S, Garner C, Pellkofer M, et al Heparin treatment in sinus venous thrombosis. *Lancet* 1991 Sep 7;338(8767):597–600.

ESPRIT trial ESPRIT Study Group. Aspirin plus dipyridamole versus aspirin alone after cerebral ischaemia of arterial origin (ESPRIT): randomised controlled trial. *Lancet* 2006;367:1665–1673.

ESPS2 trial Diener HC, Cunha L, Forbes C, Silvenius JS, Mets P, Lowenthal A. European Stroke Prevention Study 2. Dipyridamole and acetylsalicylic acid in the secondary prevention of stroke. *J Neurol Sci.* 1996;143:1–13.

Goldstein JN, Fazen LE, Snider R, Schwab K, Greenberg SM, Smith EE, et al. Contrast extravasation on CT angiography predicts hematoma expansion in intracerebral hemorrhage. *Neurology* 2007;68:889–894.

Goyal M, Menon BK, van Zwam WH, Dipple, DWJ, Mitchell PJ, Demchuk AM, et al. Endovascular thrombectomy after large-vessel ischaemic stroke: a meta-analysis of individual patient data from five randomised trials. *Lancet* 2016;387(10029):1723–1731.

HAMLET trial Hofmeijer J, Kappelle LJ, Algra A, Amelink GJ, van Gijn J, van der Worp HB, et al. Surgical decompression for space-occupying cerebral infarction (The Hemicraniectomy After Middle Cerebral Artery Infarction with Life-Threatening Edema Trial [HAMLET]): a multicentre, open, randomised trial. *Lancet Neurol.* 2009;8:326–333.

Hillis AE, Ulatowski JA, Barker PB, Torbey M, Ziai W, Beauchamp NJ, et al. A pilot randomized trial of induced blood pressure elevation: effects on function and focal perfusion in acute and subacute stroke. *Cerebrovasc Dis* 2003;16:236–246.

INTERACT 2 trial Anderson CS, Heeley E, Huang Y, Wang J, Stapf C, Delcourt C, et al. Rapid blood-pressure lowering in patients with acute intracerebral hemorrhage. *N Engl J Med* 2013;368:2355–2365.

IST trial International Stroke Trial Collaborative Group. The International Stroke Trial (IST): a randomised trial of aspirin, subcutaneous heparin, both, or neither among 19,435 patients with acute ischemic stroke. *Lancet* 1997;349:1569–1581.

Johnston SC, Rothwell PM, Nguyen-Huynh MN, Giles MF, Elkins JS, Bernstein AL, et al. Validation and refinement of scores to predict very early stroke risk after transient ischaemic attack. *Lancet* 2007;369:283–292.

Kennedy F, Lanfranconi S, Hicks C, Reid J, Gompertz P, Price C, et al. Antiplatelets vs anticoagulation for dissection CADISS nonrandomized arm and meta-analysis *Neurol* 2012;79:686–689.

Kent DM, Thaler DE. Stroke prevention—insights from incoherence *N Engl J Med* 2008;359:1287–1289.

Kitsios GD, Thaler DE, Kent DM. Potentially large yet uncertain benefits: a meta-analysis of PFO closure trials. *Stroke* 2013;44:2640–2643.

Knudsen KA, Rosand J, Karluk K, Greenberg SM. Clinical diagnosis of cerebral amyloid angiopathy: validation of the Boston criteria. *Neurol* 2001;56:537–539.

Koga Y, Akita Y, Nishioka J, Yatsuga S, Povalko N, Tanabe Y, et al. L-arginine improves the symptoms of strokelike episodes in MELAS. *Neurol* 2005;64:710–712.

Korompoki E, Filippidis FT, Nielsen PB, Giudice AD, Lip GYH, Kuramatsu JB, et al. Long-term antithrombotic treatment in intracranial hemorrhage survivors with atrial fibrillation. *Neurol* 2017;89(7): 687–696.

Levesque M et al., Nonepileptic, Stereotypical, and Intermittent Symptoms (NESIS) in Patients With Subdural Hematoma: Proposal for a New Clinical Entity With Therapeutic and Prognostic Implications. *Neurosurgery* 87:96–103, 2020.

Linn J, Halpin A, Demaerel P, Ruhland J, Giese AD, Dichgans M, et al. Prevalence of superficial siderosis in patients with cerebral amyloid angiopathy. *Neurol* 2010;74(17):1346–1350.

MATCH trial Diener HC, Bogousslavsky, Brass LM, Cimminiello C, Csiba L, Kaste M, et al. Aspirin and clopidogrel compared with clopidogrel alone after recent ischaemic stroke or transient ischaemic attack in high-risk patients (MATCH): randomised, double-blind, placebo-controlled trial. *Lancet* 2004;364:331–337.

Messé SR, Gronseth GS, Kent DM, Kizer JR, Homma S, Rosterman L, et al. Practice advisory update summary: Patent foramen ovale and secondary stroke prevention. *Neurol* 2020;94:876–885.

Metso TM, Metso AJ, Helenius J, Haapaniemi E, Salonen O, Porras M, et al. Prognosis and safety of anticoagulation in intracranial artery dissections in adults. *Stroke* 2007;38:1837–1842.

MISTIE III trial Hanley DF, Thompson RE, Rosenblum M, Yenokyan G, Lane K, McBee N, et al. Efficacy and safety of minimally invasive surgery with thrombolysis in intracerebral haemorrhage evacuation (MISTIE III): a randomised, controlled, open-label, blinded endpoint phase 3 trial. *Lancet* 2019;393(10175):1021–1032.

NASCET trial North American Symptomatic Carotid Endarterectomy Trial Collaborators. Beneficial effect of carotid endarterectomy in symptomatic patients with high-grade carotid stenosis. *N Engl J Med* 1991;325:445–453.

NAVIGATE ESUS trial Hart RG, Sharma M, Mundl H, Kasner SE, Bangdiwala SI, Berkowitz SD, et al. Rivaroxaban for stroke prevention after embolic stroke of undetermined source. *N Engl J Med* 2018;378:2191–2201.

PC trial Meier B, Kalesan B, Mattle HP, Khattab AA, Hildick-Smith D, Dudek D, et al. Percutaneous closure of patent foramen ovale in cryptogenic embolism. *N Engl J Med* 2013;368:1083–1091.

POINT trial Johnston SC, Easton JD, Farrant M, Barsan W, Conwit RA, Elm JJ, Clopidogrel and aspirin in acute ischemic stroke and high-risk TIA. *N Engl J Med* 2018;379:215–225.

REDUCE trial Sondergaard L, Kasner SE, Rhodes JF, Andersen G, Iversen HK, Nielsen-Kudsk JE, et al. Patent foramen ovale closure or antiplatelet therapy for cryptogenic stroke. *N Engl J Med* 2017;377:1033–1042.

RESPECT ESUS trial Diener HC, Sacco RL, Easton JD, Granger CB, Bernstein RA, Uchiyama S, et al. Dabigatran for prevention of stroke after embolic stroke of undetermined source. *N Engl J Med* 2019; 380:1906–1917.

RESPECT trial Carroll JD, Saver JL, Thaler DE, Smalling RW, Berry S, MacDonald LA, et al. Closure of patent foramen ovale versus medical therapy after cryptogenic stroke. *N Engl J Med* 2013;368:1092–1100.

RESPECT trial Saver JL, Carroll JD, Thaler DE, Smalling RW, McDonald LA, Marks DS, et al. Long-term outcomes of patent foramen ovale closure or medical therapy after stroke. *N Engl J Med* 2017;377(11):1022–1032.

Ropper AH. Hemicraniectomy—to halve or halve not. *N Engl J Med* 2014;370:1159–1160.

Rothwell PM, Eliasziw M, Gutnikov SA, Fox AJ, Taylor DW, Mayberg MR, et al. Analysis of pooled data from the randomized controlled trials of endarterectomy for symptomatic carotid stenosis. *Lancet* 2003;361:107–116.

Rordorf G, Koroshetz WJ, Ezzeddine MA, Segal AZ, Buonanno FS. A pilot study of drug-induced hypertension for treatment of acute stroke. *Neurol* 2001;56:1210–1213.

Runchey S, McGee S. Does this patient have a hemorrhagic stroke? Clinical findings distinguishing hemorrhagic stroke from ischemic stroke. *JAMA* 2010;303:2280–2286.

SAMMPRIS trial Derdeyn CP, Chimowitz MI, Lynn MJ, Fiorella D, Turan TN, Janis LS, et al. Aggressive medical treatment with or without stenting in high-risk patients with intracranial artery stenosis (SAMMPRIS): the final results of a randomised trial. *Lancet* 2014;383:333–341.

Smith EE, Charidimou A, Ayata C, Werring DJ, Greenberg SM, et al. Cerebral amyloid angiopathy-related transient neurologic episodes. *Neurol* 2021;97:231–238.

Spetzler RF, Martin NA. A proposed grading system for arteriovenous malformations. *J Neurosurg* 1986 Oct;65(4):476–483.

SPS3 trial SPS3 investigators. Effects of clopidogrel added to aspirin in patients with recent lacunar stroke *N Engl J Med* 2012;367:817–825.

Stam J, De Bruijn SF, DeVeber G. Anticoagulation for cerebral sinus thrombosis. *Cochrane Database Syst Rev* 2002;(4):CD002005.

STICH trial Mendelow AD, Gregson BA, Fernandes HM, Murray GD, Teasdale GM, Hope DT, et al. Early surgery versus initial conservative treatment in patients with spontaneous supratentorial intracerebral haematomas in the International Surgical Trial in Intracerebral Haemorrhage (STICH): a randomised trial. *Lancet* 2005:365:387–397.

STICH II trial Mendelow AD, Gregson BA, Rowan EN, Murray GD, Gholkar A, Mitchell PM, et al. Early surgery versus initial conservative treatment in patients with spontaneous supratentorial lobar intracerebral haematomas (STICH II): a randomised trial. *Lancet* 2013:382:397–408.

THALES trial Johnston SC et al. Ticagrelor and Aspirin or Aspirin Alone in Acute Ischemic Stroke or TIA. *N Engl J Med* 2020;383:207–217.

TOAST trial TOAST Investigators. Low molecular weight heparinoid, ORG 10172 (danaparoid), and outcome after acute ischemic stroke: a randomized controlled trial. The Publications Committee for the Trial of ORG 10172 in Acute Stroke Treatment (TOAST) Investigators. *JAMA* 1998;279:1265–1272.

VACS trial (asymptomatic carotid stenosis) Hobson RW, Weiss DG, Fields WS, Goldstone J, Moore WS, Towne JB, et al.

Efficacy of carotid endarterectomy for asymptomatic carotid stenosis. The Veterans Affairs Cooperative Study Group. *N Engl J Med* 1993;328:221–227.

VACS trial (symptomatic carotid stenosis) Mayberg MR, Wilson SE, Yatsu F, Weiss DG, Messina L, Hershey LA, et al. Carotid endarterectomy and prevention of cerebral ischemia in symptomatic carotid stenosis. Veterans Affairs Cooperative Studies Program 309 Trialist Group. *JAMA* 1991;266:3289–3294.

WARCEF trial Homma S, Thompson JL, Pullicino PM, Levin B, Freudenberger RS, Teerlink JR, et al. Warfarin and aspirin in patients with heart failure and sinus rhythm. *N Engl J Med* 2012;366:1859–1869.

WARSS trial Mohr JP, Thompson JL, Lazar RM, Levin B, Sacco RL, Furie KL, et al. A comparison of warfarin and aspirin for the prevention of recurrent ischemic stroke. *N Engl J Med* 2001;345:1444–1451.

WASID trial Chimowitz MI, Lynn MH, Howlett-Smith H, Stern BJ, Hertzberg VS, Frankel MR, et al. Comparison of warfarin and aspirin for symptomatic intracranial arterial stenosis. *N Engl J Med* 2005;352:1305–1316.

Zalewski N, Rabinstein AA, Brinjikji W, Kaufmann TJ, Nasr D, Ruff MW, et al. Unique gadolinium enhancement pattern in spinal dural arteriovenous fistulas. *JAMA Neurol* 2018;75(12):1542–1545.

Infectious Diseases of the Nervous System

CHAPTER CONTENTS

Neurologic infections can be classified by clinical syndrome/ localization (e.g., meningitis vs encephalitis vs myelitis vs radiculitis) and by the type of infection (e.g., viral, bacterial, tuberculous, fungal, parasitic). This chapter is organized by clinical syndrome, with each section organized into subsections by the type of infection. At the end of the chapter, the neurologic manifestations of HIV/AIDS are discussed. Table 20–1 provides a summary of the most common types of clinical syndromes caused by each pathogen or group of pathogens.

MENINGITIS

Meningitis (inflammation of the meninges) can be caused by:

- Infection: most commonly bacterial, viral, fungal, or tuberculous; rarely parasitic
- Immune-mediated: for example, sarcoidosis, rheumatoid arthritis, granulomatosis with polyangiitis (formerly called Wegener's granulomatosis), IgG4-related disease, anti-GFAP astrocytopathy (meningoencephalitis

TABLE 20–1 Neurologic Syndromes Caused by Infections.

	Acute Meningitis	Subacute/ Chronic Meningitis	Acute Encephalitis	Vasculitis	Dementia	Focal Brain Lesion(s)	Cranial Nerve Palsies	Spinal Disease	Radiculitis	Neuropathy	Myositis
Bacteria	✓			✓ (with meningitis)		✓ (abscess)	✓ (in Listeria rhombencephalitis)	✓ (epidural abscess)			✓
Viruses	✓		✓	VZV HIV	HIV	PML	HIV VZV (Ramsay-Hunt)	✓ (myelitis)	CMV HSV-2	HIV	✓
Fungi		✓		Aspergillus; others in setting of meningitis		✓	✓ (with meningitis)				
Tuberculosis		✓		✓ (with meningitis)		Tuberculoma	✓ (with meningitis)	✓ (Pott's disease, spinal meningitis)	✓ (Arachnoiditis)		
Syphilis		✓		✓	✓		✓ (with meningitis)	✓ (Tabes dorsalis)			
Lyme disease			Very rarely				Most commonly CN 7	Very rarely	✓	✓	
Parasites	✓	✓		✓		✓		✓			✓

Abbreviations: CN: cranial nerve; HSV: herpes simplex virus; PML: progressive multifocal leukoencephalopathy; VZV: varicella zoster virus.

or meningoencephalomyelitis; 25% have underlying neoplasm, most commonly ovarian teratoma), Vogt-Koyanagi-Harada (uveitis, vitiligo, alopecia, hearing loss)

- Medications (chemical meningitis): nonsteroidal anti-inflammatory drugs (NSAIDs), intravenous immunoglobulin (IVIg), trimethoprim-sulfamethoxazole
- Neoplasm: leptomeningeal metastases (also called carcinomatous meningitis), rupture of dermoid or epidermoid cyst, paraneoplastic (anti-GFAP, see above)

Most infectious meningeal processes predominantly affect the leptomeninges (arachnoid and pia), whereas most inflammatory processes predominantly affect the pachymeninges (dura mater), although there can be simultaneous involvement of both the pachymeninges and leptomeninges in both types of processes (see Fig. 2–10 and accompanying discussion "Contrast-enhanced Neuroimaging" in Ch. 2). Carcinomatous meningitis typically refers to leptomeningeal metastases (see "Leptomeningeal Metastases" in Ch. 24). Dural metastases also occur (most commonly with prostate and breast cancer).

Bacterial meningitis and viral meningitis tend to be acute in onset and evolution, whereas fungal meningitis, tuberculous meningitis, inflammatory meningitis, and carcinomatous meningitis are more commonly subacute or chronic in onset and evolution.

Viral meningitis and chemical meningitis are sometimes referred to as **aseptic meningitis**.

Bacterial Meningitis

Bacteria can infect the meninges by spreading from sinus infections or inner ear infections, spreading hematogenously from remote sites of infection, or infecting the meninges directly in the setting of open head trauma or neurosurgery.

The most common causes of bacterial meningitis vary with age and immunocompetence. In infants less than 1 month of age, *Listeria*, *Escherichia coli*, and *Streptococcus agalactiae* (group B) are most common (mnemonic: **less** than 1 month of age: *Listeria*, *E. coli*, *Strep. agalactiae*). In children and adults, *Streptococcus pneumoniae* and *Neisseria meningitidis* are most common. *Listeria* should be considered in patients who are older than age 50 or immunocompromised (e.g., HIV, immunosuppressive therapy). In addition to meningitis, *Listeria* may cause involvement of the brainstem (**rhombencephalitis**), producing cranial nerve and cerebellar deficits. *Haemophilus influenzae* should be considered in children, although this is now rare due to widespread vaccination in childhood. In the setting of open head trauma or neurosurgery, *Staphylococcus aureus* and gram-negative bacteria should be considered.

Head trauma does not need to be open to create a passage for entry of bacteria from outside: Basilar skull fracture can create a communication between the meninges and the outside world. A skull defect should be considered as a cause of bacterial meningitis if a patient with prior neurosurgery or head trauma presents with cerebrospinal fluid (CSF) leak (clear fluid from the nose or ears) and/or recurrent meningitis. CSF can be distinguished from nasal secretions by testing fluid for beta-2-transferrin (present in CSF but not mucus) or for glucose (present in CSF but not mucus, although CSF glucose may be extremely low in bacterial meningitis, limiting utility of this test).

Clinical Features of Bacterial Meningitis

Bacterial meningitis can be rapidly fatal, so prompt diagnosis and treatment are crucial. The classic features are fever, neck stiffness, headache, and altered mental status, although a systematic review found that fewer than half of patients have all of these symptoms at presentation (Attia et al., 1999). Additional symptoms can include photophobia and nausea/vomiting. Purpuric rash may be seen with *Neisseria* meningitis.

Meningitis should be considered as a possibility in any patient with fever and headache, although many systemic illnesses that cause fever may also cause some degree of headache. A particularly high index of suspicion for meningitis must be maintained in the elderly, who may have minimal or no fever, and whose neck stiffness may be attributed to osteoarthritis (erroneously or appropriately, but misleadingly in either case if the patient has meningitis). Additionally, careful consideration of meningitis is important in febrile infants, in whom mental status may be difficult to assess.

The classic signs of Kernig and Brudzinski are highly specific when present, but unfortunately quite insensitive (Attia et al., 1999). Both signs demonstrate meningismus by causing traction on the inflamed meninges. The Kernig sign is performed by flexing the hip and then extending the knee with the patient in the supine position. If pain prohibits extension of the knee, this is a positive sign (mnemonic: to look for **K**ernig's sign: extend the **k**nee). The Brudzinski sign is performed by flexing the patient's head: If the patient flexes at the hips and knees, this is a positive sign.

Treatment of Bacterial Meningitis

In most medical texts (including this one), diagnosis of a disease is generally discussed before treatment. In contrast, when discussing bacterial meningitis, *treatment* is discussed first because if bacterial meningitis is being considered, treatment should be rapidly initiated before/while pursuing diagnostic evaluation since delayed initiation of antibiotic treatment—even by hours—leads to poorer outcomes. Therefore, antibiotics should *not* be delayed while awaiting lumbar puncture. CSF cultures remain positive up to hours after initiation of antibiotics, and protein, glucose, and cell count abnormalities persist up to several days following initiation of antibiotics. The theoretical concern that antibiotics should be delayed so as not to alter the CSF results is unfounded, and so antibiotic treatment should be given as soon as possible if bacterial meningitis is in the differential diagnosis. Blood cultures are positive in a large proportion of patients with acute bacterial meningitis and can be drawn at the time of antibiotic administration.

In adults with presumed community-acquired bacterial meningitis, recommended empiric treatment is with a third-generation cephalosporin (ceftriaxone or cefotaxime) to cover *N. meningitidis* and *S. pneumoniae* and vancomycin to cover potentially resistant strains of *S. pneumoniae*. Ampicillin should be added to cover for *Listeria* if the patient is younger than 1 month, older than 50 years, or immuncompromised. Some practitioners recommend initiating ampicillin in all patients since a patient's immune status may not be known at the time of presentation. If there has been prior neurosurgery or penetrating trauma, empiric treatment is with vancomycin and cefepime, ceftazidime, or meropenem (in place of ceftriaxone or cefotaxime) to expand gram-negative coverage to include *Pseudomonas*. In patients with penicillin/beta-lactam allergy, regimens may include fluoroquinolones, chloramphenicol, and/or trimethoprim-sulfamethoxazole. Antibiotic treatment can be narrowed once the culture and sensitivity data from the CSF become available. If there is concern for encephalitis in addition to meningitis based on the clinical picture, acyclovir should be added empirically to treat possible herpes simplex virus (HSV) encephalitis (see "Herpes Simplex Virus Encephalitis") while awaiting CSF results and neuroimaging.

Steroids (dexamethasone) are generally also administered in parallel with antibiotics for bacterial meningitis, beginning before or with the first dose of antibiotics (Brouwer et al., 2015). Dexamethasone has a mortality benefit in adult patients with *S. pneumoniae* meningitis and children with *H. influenzae* meningitis, and some practitioners discontinue steroids if CSF cultures reveal an alternative pathogen. However, a mortality benefit for dexamethasone in the treatment of acute meningitis was not found in low-income countries, a finding attributed to higher prevalence of HIV and malnutrition, late presentation (due to limited access to health care), not all patients in the studies ultimately having bacterial

meningitis (limited diagnostics), and inadequate resources for supportive care of critical illness (Brouwer et al., 2015).

Lumbar Puncture in Bacterial Meningitis

As discussed above, antibiotics should be administered immediately if there is concern for bacterial meningitis, and lumbar puncture (LP) should not delay initiation of empiric therapy.

Head CT should be considered before LP if the diagnosis of meningitis/encephalitis itself is in question or if the patient is felt clinically to be at risk for a mass lesion (abscess) or diffuse cerebral edema that could raise the risk of herniation with LP. CT should be considered before LP in patients with focal deficit, seizure, papilledema, depressed mental status, immunocompromise, intracranial mass lesion, or age greater than 60 (Hasbun et al., 2001).

The classic CSF findings in bacterial meningitis are elevated opening pressure, extremely elevated protein (generally >100 mg/dL), extremely elevated white blood cell (WBC) count (>100 cells/mm^3, but often in the 1000s) with neutrophil predominance, and decreased glucose (<40% of serum glucose, but often much lower) (Table 20–2). CSF culture is used to diagnose the particular bacterial organism and determine antibiotic sensitivity.

The multiplex PCR BioFire FilmArray Meningitis/Encephalitis panel assesses for several bacterial (*S. pneumoniae*, *S. agalactiae*, *N. meningitidis*, *L. monocytogenes*, *H. influenzae*, *E. coli*), viral (HSV-1, HSV-2, HHV-6, VZV, CMV, enterovirus, human parechovirus), and fungal (*Cryptococcus neoformans* and *Cryptococcus gattii*) causes of meningitis/encephalitis simultaneously. It is considered highly sensitive and specific for bacteria and viruses tested (though false positives and false negatives do occur), but less sensitive for *Cryptococcus* for which cryptococcal antigen is more sensitive

TABLE 20–2   Cerebrospinal Fluid Findings in Central Nervous System Infections.

	Protein (mg/dL)	Glucose (mg/dL)	WBCs (cells/µL)	Other
Bacterial	100s–1000s	<40% serum glucose (often much lower)	100s–10,000s (Neutrophilic predominance early, lymphocytic later)	Gram stain and culture
Viral	50–100s	Usually normal, though can be decreased in mumps, CMV, HSV2, LCMV, arboviruses	100s–1000 (Typically lymphocytic predominance)	Viral PCRs (except for VZV for which IgG is more sensitive, and arboviruses for which IgM is more sensitive) RBCs may be present in HSV
Fungal	100–500	Low	100s–1000 (Typically lymphocytic predominance, though eosinophils may be seen)	Cryptococcal antigen most sensitive for cryptococcus Antigen and antibody tests used for endemic mycoses Culture + (1,3)-β-D-glucan used for *Candida*
Tuberculosis	100–1000	Low	100s–500 (Typically lymphocytic predominance)	PCR (Xpert), culture

Abbreviations: HSV: herpes simplex virus; PCRs: polymerase chain reactions; RBCs: red blood cells; VZV: varicella zoster virus; WBCs: white blood cells.

than PCR. Therefore, if there is high suspicion for a particular infection and multiplex PCR is negative, individual testing for the pathogen in question should be pursued. Additionally, multiplex PCR does not provide antibiotic sensitivity data.

Complications of Bacterial Meningitis

The differential diagnosis for an acute neurologic change in a patient with bacterial meningitis includes:

- Seizures, including nonconvulsive seizures, for which continuous EEG may be necessary to make a diagnosis (see "Nonconvulsive status epilepticus" Ch. 18)
- Acute ischemic stroke due to infectious vasculitis (see "Infectious CNS Vasculitis")
- Venous sinus thrombosis (see "Cerebral Venous Sinus Thrombosis and Cortical Vein Thrombosis" in Ch. 19)
- Cerebral edema (management of elevated intracranial pressure is discussed in Ch. 25)
- Abscess formation (intracerebral or subdural empyema), which may require surgical drainage (see "Bacterial Focal Brain Lesions")

Chronic complications in patients with bacterial meningitis can include:

- Hearing loss
- Epilepsy
- Cognitive impairment
- Hydrocephalus

Isolation of Patients With Bacterial Meningitis & Prophylaxis of Contacts

While awaiting microbiologic diagnosis, patients should be placed on droplet precautions (mask and face protection for providers), but only patients with *N. meningitidis* meningitis require isolation and droplet precautions and prophylaxis of close contacts. If *N. meningitidis* is found to be the etiology, close contacts should receive a single dose of intramuscular ceftriaxone or 2 days of rifampin.

Viral Meningitis

A large number of viruses can cause viral meningitis including herpes simplex viruses (HSV) 1 and 2, enteroviruses, arboviruses, HIV, varicella zoster virus (VZV), and lymphocytic choriomeningitis virus (LCMV). Viral meningitis presents similarly to bacterial meningitis with headache, fever, neck stiffness, and photophobia, but is typically less severe than bacterial meningitis and does not usually cause alterations in consciousness (unless there is an associated encephalitis). Viral meningitis is one type of aseptic meningitis, a term used to describe meningitis with no growth on CSF bacterial culture.

Aseptic meningitis may occur at the time of HIV seroconversion, so patients with viral meningitis should be screened for HIV risk factors (see "HIV Seroconversion Syndromes Involving the Nervous System").

Mollaret's meningitis refers to recurrent viral meningitis, most commonly caused by HSV-2 (the HSV strain that causes genital herpes).

In viral meningitis, CSF protein and WBC count are generally elevated (but not to the degree seen in bacterial meningitis), and glucose is usually normal, though low glucose may be seen in meningitis caused by mumps, HSV2, LCMV, arboviruses (see Table 20–2). The CSF WBCs are classically predominantly lymphocytes, although neutrophils may be present early in viral meningitis. Precise diagnosis of the viral pathogen is made by CSF polymerase chain reaction (PCR). The multiplex PCR BioFire assay assesses for seven viruses (see above), but note that false negatives for HSV and enterovirus have been reported with this assay. Care is supportive with the exception of HSV and VZV meningitis, which are treated with IV acyclovir.

Fungal Meningitis

Fungal meningitis most commonly affects patients who are immunocompromised (e.g., due to HIV infection or immunosuppressive medications), although immunocompetent patients can be affected. The presentation is typically more subacute than with viral or bacterial meningitis, emerging over days to weeks. Headache is almost always present, but the inflammatory aspects of meningitis such as fever and neck stiffness may be minimal or even absent if the patient develops fungal meningitis in the setting of immunocompromise. Therefore, a high index of suspicion for potential fungal meningitis must be maintained in patients who develop headaches while on chronic immunosuppressive therapy or in the setting of diseases causing immunocompromise (e.g., HIV). Cranial nerve palsies and seizures may also be seen, especially in advanced cryptococcal meningitis. Strokes in the basal ganglia may occur due to infectious involvement of penetrating lenticulostriate arteries at the base of the brain.

Cryptococcal Meningitis

Cryptococcus neoformans is the most common cause of fungal meningitis in patients who are immunocompromised. *Cryptococcus gattii* can affect immunocompetent patients and is endemic in the Pacific Northwest. Due to meningeal inflammation caused by cryptococcal meningitis, cranial nerve palsies, deep infarcts (due to involvement of penetrating vessels), and communicating hydrocephalus can develop. Hydrocephalus can lead to rapid changes in mental status that often improve with large-volume LP to relieve intracranial pressure. In severe cases, LP may be required daily, and patients may ultimately require ventriculoperitoneal shunting.

CSF in fungal meningitis demonstrates increased protein and WBC count with decreased glucose, but not typically to the extreme values seen in bacterial meningitis (Table 20–2). The most sensitive diagnostic tests for *Cryptococcus* are CSF cryptococcal antigen and CSF cryptococcal culture. Cryptococcal antigen is sensitive and rapid, but not available in many areas of the world most affected by AIDS and accompanying central nervous system (CNS) opportunistic infections. Cryptococcal culture is sensitive and more widely available, but results return much less rapidly. India ink stain is not as sensitive as either test. Although *C. neoformans* and *C. gattii* PCR are included in the BioFire assay, note that PCR is less sensitive than cryptococcal antigen, and so false negatives may be seen.

MRI may show hydrocephalus, meningeal enhancement, mass lesions (cryptococcomas), and/or dilated perivascular spaces with a soap bubble appearance that represent gelatinous pseudocysts.

Treatment of cryptococcal meningitis begins with amphotericin and flucytosine induction therapy, followed by fluconazole until the CD4 count is greater than 200 cells/mm^3 for 6 months.

Other Fungal Causes of Meningitis

Other fungi that can cause meningitis include the endemic mycoses and *Candida*. Although *Aspergillus* can rarely cause meningitis, it more commonly causes infarction or mass lesions (see "Fungal Focal Brain Lesions").

The endemic mycoses are dimorphic fungi including *Coccidioides* (Southwest United States, Central and South America), *Histoplasma* (Mississippi and Ohio River regions, Central and South America, Southern Africa, Southeast Asia), and *Blastomyces* (Mississippi and Ohio River regions, Great Lakes region). These organisms can affect immunocompetent individuals, causing meningitis that may be preceded by or concurrent with pulmonary involvement, though isolated neurologic involvement can occur without systemic disease. Abscess may complicate meningitis. Diagnosis is made by CSF antigen and antibody testing. Treatment is with amphotericin and azoles for *Histoplasma* and *Blastomyces* meningitis, but azole therapy alone is used for *Coccidioides* meningitis.

Candida meningitis can occur in patients who are immunocompromised, post-neurosurgery, or in patients with VP shunts. Diagnosis is by CSF culture; (1,3)-D-glucan may be positive but is not specific to *Candida*. Treatment is with amphotericin and flucytosine, and infected VP shunts should be removed.

Tuberculous Meningitis

Like fungal meningitis, tuberculous meningitis presents more insidiously than viral and bacterial meningitis, typically over weeks. The clinical presentation can include any of the classic features of meningitis (headache, fever, meningeal signs, altered mental status), and may also include cranial nerve palsies. As in cryptococcal meningitis, hydrocephalus and subcortical infarcts in the basal ganglia may develop. Although evidence of concurrent or prior pulmonary tuberculosis may be seen on chest x-ray, many patients develop tuberculosis meningitis without systemic involvement.

Neuroimaging may demonstrate hydrocephalus, basal ganglia infarcts, and/or meningeal enhancement. CSF profile is similar to that in fungal meningitis with moderate elevations in WBC count (lymphocytic predominance) and protein, and diminished glucose with values less extreme than in bacterial meningitis (Table 20–2). Unfortunately, CSF culture is insensitive, and molecular testing (Xpert MTB/RIF) is often not widely available in areas of highest incidence. Therefore, in areas of high incidence and limited diagnostic resources, empiric treatment is often initiated in the following scenarios: patients who present with meningitis and a CSF pattern inconsistent with bacterial meningitis, patients who fail to improve with treatment of bacterial meningitis, or in HIV-infected patients who have a CD4 count greater than 200 cells/mm^3 (making *Cryptococcus* unlikely) or who do not respond to treatment for cryptococcal meningitis.

Treatment generally consists of 2 months of a four-drug regimen (isoniazid, rifampin, pyrazinamide, and ethambutol) followed by an additional prolonged course of isoniazid and rifampin. Corticosteroids are often added during the initial 2 months. In patients with coexisting HIV infection who are not already on antiretroviral therapy, it may be necessary to defer initiation of antiretrovirals until after an initial period of treatment of tuberculous meningitis due to the risk of **immune reconstitution inflammatory syndrome** (IRIS) (see "Immune Reconstitution Inflammatory Syndrome").

Tuberculosis can also cause focal brain lesions (**tuberculoma**) and disease of the spine (**Pott's disease**), which are discussed below (see "Tuberculous Focal Brain Lesions" and "Tuberculosis of the Spine").

Lyme Meningitis & Other Manifestations of Neuroborreliosis

Lyme disease is caused by the spirochete *Borrelia* (*B. burgdorferi* is the most common species in the United States) transmitted by the *Ixodes* tick. Neurologic manifestations of Lyme are referred to as neuroborreliosis. Lyme meningitis may be preceded by the target rash typical of the disease or other types of rash, although not all patients develop a rash, or may not have noticed it (e.g., if on the back).

Other neurologic manifestations of Lyme disease that can occur early in the illness include seventh nerve palsy (or less commonly other cranial nerve palsies) and radiculoneuritis (which can mimic Guillain-Barré syndrome clinically, but with a lymphocytic pleocytosis in the CSF). Meningitis, cranial nerve palsy, and radiculoneuritis can occur individually or together, and may occur in the same time period as systemic features of Lyme disease such as arthritis and carditis. The combination of meningitis and radiculitis—meningoradiculitis—is referred to as Bannwarth's syndrome, and is more common in Europe. Rarer neurologic manifestations of Lyme include mononeuritis multiplex, encephalitis, and myelitis.

Diagnosis of Lyme is made by serum antibodies: positive ELISA and positive Western blot for both IgM (2 or more out of 3 bands) and IgG (5 or more out of 10 bands), though serology may be negative in early infection. Since the antibodies may pass from the serum to CSF, CSF:serum antibody index is used to evaluate for intrathecal Lyme antibody production rather than relying merely on the presence of CSF antibodies to diagnose neuroborreliosis. CSF antibodies (and elevated CSF:serum antibody index) can persist in treated patients, but patients with active CNS Lyme will have pleocytosis and elevated protein on CSF analysis. Neurologic involvement by Lyme is generally treated with oral doxycycline or IV ceftriaxone, with IV therapy reserved for severely affected patients (e.g., severe meningitis or rare instances of encephalitis or myelitis) (Lantos et al., 2020).

Syphilitic Meningitis & Other Manifestations of Neurosyphilis

Syphilis can affect the nervous system in the first years of the disease (early neurosyphilis) or many years after initial infection (late neurosyphilis). Early neurosyphilis affects the meninges, causing syphilitic meningitis; this may be complicated by stroke (meningovascular syphilis). Late neurosyphilis can present with tabes dorsalis (see "Other Infectious Conditions of the Spine") and dementia (called general paresis).

Diagnosis of syphilis relies on two types of tests: nontreponemal tests (RPR and VDRL) and treponemal tests (FTA-ABS, TPPA, and immunoassay-based tests). In patients with early neurosyphilis (meningitis/meningovascular syphilis), serum nontreponemal and treponemal tests are nearly always positive, and CSF VDRL is highly specific though relatively insensitive (reported sensitivities range from approximately 30%–70%). In patients with meningitis and/or stroke who have positive serum testing for syphilis, lymphocytic pleocytosis and elevated protein are highly suggestive of neurosyphilis even in the setting of negative CSF VDRL (given that it is not adequately sensitive). In such patients, CSF treponemal testing can be performed (FTA-ABS), though its interpretation is challenging: It can be positive simply due to transfer from blood due to CSF (especially if LP is bloody) and remains positive even in treated patients. However, if both CSF VDRL and CSF treponemal tests are negative, neurosyphilis is extremely unlikely to be the diagnosis.

In late neurosyphilis (tabes dorsalis and general paresis), serum RPR and VDRL may be negative but serum treponemal tests are nearly always positive. The approach to CSF analysis is the same as above: CSF VDRL is diagnostic but insensitive; CSF treponemal tests can be considered in patients in whom CSF VDRL is negative, but positivity does not necessarily reflect neurosyphilis due to passive blood-to-CSF transfer; negative CSF VDRL and negative CSF treponemal tests essentially rule out neurosyphilis.

Treatment of neurosyphilis is with high-dose IV penicillin G. Response to treatment is generally followed with lumbar puncture at 6 month intervals until the CSF parameters and VDRL normalize.

Parasitic Meningitis

Eosinophilic meningitis should raise suspicion for a parasitic infection, but CSF eosinophilia can also be seen in some fungal infections (e.g., coccidioidomycosis) and when hematologic malignancy involves the CNS.

Naegleria fowleri causes an acute, fulminant, often fatal meningoencephalitis called primary amebic meningoencephalitis. *Naegleria fowleri* is acquired through exposure to infested fresh water by swimming, water sports, or rarely nasal irrigation with contaminated tap water. Diagnosis is made by CSF wet mount or PCR. The optimal treatment regimen is uncertain due to the rarity of the condition, but often involves combinations of antiparasitic, antifungal, and antibacterial agents.

Angiostrongylus cantonensis is acquired by eating infected seafood or contaminated sea plants. It is endemic in Southeast Asia, Pacific Islands, and Caribbean. It generally causes a relatively mild meningitis. Diagnosis is by CSF PCR, and treatment is with steroids and supportive care.

VIRAL ENCEPHALITIS

Encephalitis (inflammation of the brain) can be caused by:

- Infection: most commonly viral
- Inflammation:

  - Postinfectious: for example, acute disseminated encephalomyelitis (ADEM; see "Acute Disseminated Encephalomyelitis" in Ch. 21)
  - Antibody-mediated: for example, anti-NMDA (*N*-methyl-D-aspartate) receptor encephalitis (see "Paraneoplastic Syndromes of the Nervous System" in Ch. 24)

Due to direct brain involvement in encephalitis, altered mental status and seizures may be present early in the course of the illness in addition to headache and fever, while meningeal signs are generally absent (unless there is a combined meningoencephalitis).

A large number of viruses can cause encephalitis including herpes simplex virus (HSV), varicella zoster virus (VZV), enteroviruses, and arboviruses (e.g., mosquito-borne: West Nile virus, Eastern equine encephalitis virus, St. Louis encephalitis virus, dengue virus; tick-borne: Powassan), cytomegalovirus (CMV), Epstein-Barr virus (EBV), and human herpes virus-6 (HHV-6). CMV, EBV, and HHV-6 encephalitis typically occur only in patients who are immunocompromised, with HHV-6 occurring almost exclusively in patients who have undergone bone marrow transplant.

MRI changes suggestive of particular viral encephalitides are discussed below. HSV, VZV, CMV, HHV-6, and enteroviruses are diagnosed by CSF PCR, and the arboviruses are most sensitively diagnosed by CSF IgM.

HSV, VZV, CMV, and HHV-6 have specific treatment (IV acyclovir for HSV and VZV; ganciclovir and foscarnet for

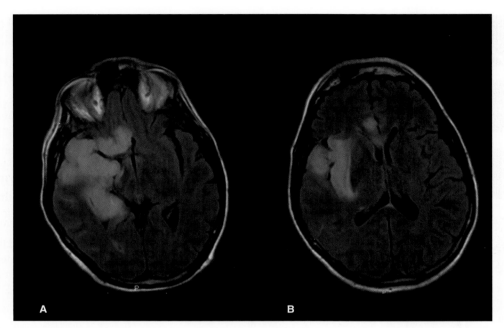

FIGURE 20–1 **HSV encephalitis.** Axial FLAIR MRI demonstrating T2/FLAIR hyperintensity in the right medial and anterior temporal lobe (**A**), inferior frontal lobe (**A**), and insula (**B**).

CMV and HHV-6), whereas care is supportive for other viral encephalitides.

Herpes Simplex Virus (HSV) Encephalitis

HSV encephalitis is the most common viral encephalitis and can be rapidly fatal. Therefore, there must be a low threshold for empiric treatment with IV acyclovir in any patient presenting with a potential infectious encephalitis. HSV encephalitis is most commonly caused by HSV-1 in adults and HSV-2 in infants, though both adults and infants can develop encephalitis from either HSV-1 or HSV-2. HSV encephalitis presents similarly to other viral encephalitides with headache, altered mental status, and/or seizures. MRI demonstrates unilateral or bilateral T2/FLAIR hyperintensities limited to limbic regions (medial temporal lobe, insula, inferior frontal lobes) (Fig. 20–1). Hemorrhagic foci, diffusion restriction, and contrast enhancement may be seen. CSF shows a viral pattern (Table 20–2), and CSF red blood cell (RBC) count may be increased due to the hemorrhagic nature of the infection. Temporal lobe lateralized periodic discharges (LPDs) may be present on EEG. Definitive diagnosis is made by CSF HSV PCR. CSF HSV PCR may be negative early in the course of the illness, so a negative test does not exclude the diagnosis, and the test should be repeated if clinical suspicion is high. Treatment is with IV acyclovir.

Rarely, HSV encephalitis can relapse. Another course of acyclovir should be administered and the patient should be evaluated for anti-NMDA receptor antibodies, since there is emerging evidence that relapse may be immune-mediated by the mechanism of anti-NMDA receptor antibodies (Armangue et al., 2014) (see "Autoimmune Limbic Encephalitis" in Ch. 24).

Varicella Zoster Virus (VZV) Encephalitis

VZV can cause encephalitis in individuals who are immunocompetent or immunocompromised, and may be more severe in patients who are immunocompromised. VZV can cause CNS vasculitis in addition to encephalitis, leading to infarction with focal deficits. Although VZV meningitis and encephalitis may be diagnosed by CSF VZV PCR, VZV vasculitis and myelitis are diagnosed more sensitively by CSF IgG than by CSF PCR. VZV encephalitis is treated with IV acyclovir, and if there is an associated vasculitis, addition of steroids may be considered (see "Infectious CNS Vasculitis").

Arboviral Encephalitis

Many of the arboviral encephalitides have specific geographic distributions (e.g., Eastern equine encephalitis: east coast of United States; Japanese encephalitis in East/South Asia; dengue in Central/South America, Africa, Asia; Powassan in Northeast US, Great Lakes region, Canada), although some are now present globally (e.g., West Nile virus). In addition to headache, fever, altered mental status, and seizures, arboviral encephalitides are often accompanied by movement disorders such as tremor and/or parkinsonism. West Nile virus can also cause an acute flaccid paralysis due to involvement of the spinal cord gray matter. MRI of the brain in arboviral encephalitides can reveal symmetric T2/FLAIR hyperintensities in the deep gray matter (basal ganglia and thalamus) (Fig. 20–2). Unlike most other viral CNS infections for which CSF PCR is used for diagnosis, the arboviral encephalitides are diagnosed by CSF IgM, and some patients will have a neutrophilic

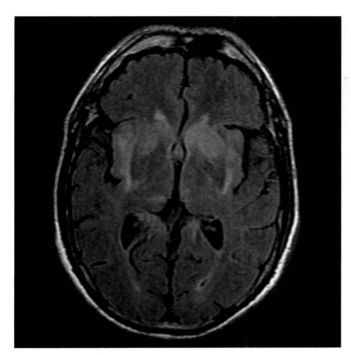

FIGURE 20–2 **Eastern equine encephalitis.** Axial FLAIR MRI demonstrating T2/FLAIR hyperintensity in the basal ganglia bilaterally.

pleocytosis rather than a lymphocytic pleocytosis in the CSF. Treatment is supportive.

Rabies

Rabies is acquired from contact with an infected animal (dog and bat bites are most common). Encephalitic and paralytic forms (flaccid paralysis) can be seen. Fear of water (hydrophobia) may be seen with the encephalitic form. Once the disease has affected the nervous system, it is fatal, so post-exposure prophylaxis is essential in potentially exposed patients, and pre-exposure vaccine should be offered to at-risk individuals.

Cytomegalovirus (CMV) & Human Herpes Virus-6 (HHV-6) Encephalitis

CMV and HHV-6 encephalitis typically occur only in patients who are immunocompromised. CMV encephalitis can occur in patients with CD4 less than 50, and patients often also have other concurrent complications of CMV infection (e.g., retinitis, colitis, radiculitis). On neuroimaging, CMV typically causes periventricular white matter changes and ependymal enhancement.

HHV-6 encephalitis occurs almost exclusively in patients who have undergone bone marrow transplant patients. MRI demonstrates T2 hyperintensities in the medial temporal lobes.

CMV and HHV-6 are diagnosed by CSF PCR and treated with ganciclovir and/or foscarnet.

FOCAL INFECTIOUS BRAIN LESIONS

Focal infectious brain lesions should be considered in the differential diagnosis for any patient with acute to subacute onset of focal neurologic symptoms/signs, especially if accompanied by fever or occurring in immunocompromised patients. Headache and seizures are common accompanying features.

Bacterial Focal Brain Lesions
Cerebral Abscess

Bacterial brain abscesses can arise due to direct spread of bacteria from adjacent compartments (e.g., sinusitis), open skull trauma, neurosurgery, or hematogenous spread from another site of infection (e.g., endocarditis). Neuroimaging reveals a ring-enhancing lesion with surrounding edema, and the center of the abscess often demonstrates diffusion restriction (Fig. 20–3). If abscess is suspected, blood cultures should be

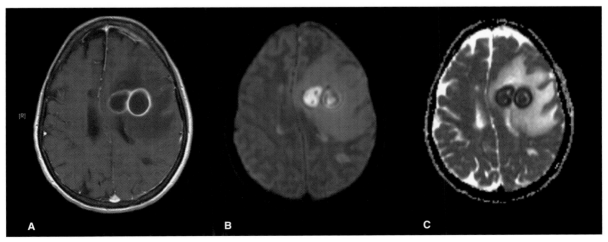

FIGURE 20–3 **Cerebral abscess.** Axial MRI demonstrating ring-enhancing lesions on T1-weighted postcontrast sequence (**A**), and DWI hyperintensity (**B**) with ADC hypointensity (**C**) consistent with diffusion restriction.

drawn and empiric antibiotics that include anaerobic coverage should be initiated immediately. Surgical aspiration or evacuation is usually necessary. If a clear source of infection is not evident from the patient's history, the patient should be evaluated for endocarditis, cranial infections (e.g., sinus, mastoid), and other potential systemic sources of infection.

Epidural Abscess & Subdural Empyema

Like cerebral abscesses, bacterial infection of the epidural space (**epidural abscess**) or subdural space (**subdural empyema**) can also arise due to trauma, neurosurgery, or local spread of infection from other cranial compartments. Treatment is with antibiotics (including anaerobic coverage as with brain abscess) and surgical drainage.

Viral Focal Brain Lesions

Progressive multifocal leukoencephalopathy (**PML**) caused by JC virus infection can be seen in HIV-infected patients (with CD4 <200 cells/mm^3), patients immunosuppressed after organ transplantation, and patients receiving immunomodulatory therapies such as natalizumab (see "Long-term Treatment of Relapsing-Remitting Multiple Sclerosis" in Ch. 21). Focal or multifocal neurologic deficits emerge subacutely, with symptoms/signs depending on the site(s) of lesions.

Neuroimaging in PML reveals juxtacortical T2/FLAIR hyperintensity respecting the boundary between gray and white matter (Fig. 20–4A). The middle cerebellar peduncle is another common site of involvement, leading to presentation with ipsilateral ataxia (Fig. 20–4B). Lesions typically do not cause any mass effect or contrast enhancement, except in the setting of immune reconstitution inflammatory syndrome

(IRIS) in which contrast enhancement may be seen (see "Immune Reconstitution Inflammatory Syndrome"). Diagnosis is made based on clinical features and context, radiologic findings, and PCR confirmation of JC virus infection in the CSF.

Treatment for PML is an area of active investigation, with recent small studies demonstrating possible benefit with the immune checkpoint inhibitor pembrolizumab (Cortese et al., 2019) and donor-derived BK-virus specific T cells (Muftuoglu et al., 2018). Some practitioners treat patients with mirtazapine based on case reports suggesting possible clinical benefit (mirtazapine blocks 5-HT2A receptors, which are thought to be the means of JC virus entry into glial cells). In patients who develop PML due to natalizumab therapy, the drug is removed with plasmapheresis, although this raises the risk of development of IRIS (see "Long-term Treatment of Relapsing-Remitting Multiple Sclerosis" in Ch. 21).

Fungal Focal Brain Lesions

Mucormycosis affects patients who are immunocompromised, diabetic, have elevated serum iron (e.g., hemochromatosis, deferoxamine therapy), or who use IV drugs. **Rhinocerebral mucormycosis** is the term given to extension of infection from the sinuses into the orbit and cavernous sinuses causing ocular motor palsies and other cranial neuropathies. Mucormycosis can also rarely cause a focal brain abscess (most commonly in the basal ganglia). Angioinvasion can cause stroke or hemorrhage. Treatment is with amphotericin and surgical debridement of sinus involvement when present, but prognosis is often poor when there is brain involvement.

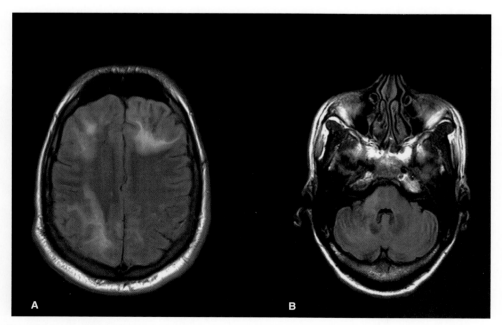

FIGURE 20–4 **Progressive multifocal leukoencephalopathy.** Axial FLAIR MRI demonstrating multifocal juxtacortical T2/FLAIR hyperintensities without mass effect (**A**) and T2/FLAIR hyperinensity in the right middle cerebellar peduncle (**B**).

Aspergillus can also cause fungal brain abscess in immunocompromised patients, and like mucormycosis, can also lead to angioinvasion causing stroke or hemorrhage. Treatment is with voriconazole.

As described above, cryptococcal lesions known as **cryptococcomas** can occur. These are most common in the setting of cryptococcal meningitis and occur most commonly in the basal ganglia (see "Cryptococcal Meningitis").

Tuberculous Focal Brain Lesions

Tuberculomas are focal tuberculous granulomas which may evolve into tubercular abscesses. They appear as ring-enhancing lesions on contrast-enhanced neuroimaging. Treatment is generally with antituberculosis therapy and steroids, with surgery only being necessary in cases with significant mass effect or those complicated by hydrocephalus that does not respond (or does not respond adequately) to antituberculosis treatment.

Parasitic Focal Brain Lesions

Toxoplasmosis

Toxoplasmosis can occur in immunosuppressed patients with CD4 less than 100 cells/mm^3. It causes one or more focal brain lesions with predilection for the basal ganglia and/or deep white matter, leading to subacute development of contralateral hemiparesis, contralateral movement disorder, and/or confusion. Brain imaging reveals one or more ring-enhancing lesions with surrounding edema (Fig. 20–5).

In immunocompromised patients, the main differential diagnosis for subcortical ring-enhancing lesions is toxoplasmosis versus primary CNS lymphoma, which can resemble each other clinically (subacute focal/multifocal deficits) and radiologically (subcortical ring-enhancing lesion[s]). If a patient does not have a positive serum toxoplasmosis IgG, this makes the possibility of toxoplasmosis unlikely. However, since the antibody is positive in a significant proportion of the population, IgG positivity does not confirm a diagnosis of CNS toxoplasmosis. Definitive distinction between toxoplasmosis and primary CNS lymphoma can only be made by biopsy, so the usual approach is to treat for toxoplasmosis (sulfadiazine [or clindamycin if sulfa allergy] and pyrimethamine) and follow the patient clinically and radiologically. Steroids should be avoided during this phase if possible, since this can lead to clinical/radiologic improvement of lymphoma as well, obscuring the diagnosis. If there is clinical and radiographic improvement after several weeks of empiric toxoplasmosis therapy, the diagnosis of toxoplasmosis is presumed. If there is no improvement, biopsy should be considered to make a definitive diagnosis.

Neurocysticercosis

Neurocysticercosis (NCC) is one of the most common causes of acquired epilepsy in the world. NCC is endemic in Central/South America, Asia, and Africa, but seen worldwide due to migration from endemic areas. The *Taenia solium* tapeworm can be acquired from eating undercooked pork. The eggs of the parasite are shed in the stool, and it is the eggs that find their way to the brain to cause NCC. The eggs are transmitted by the fecal–oral route by autoinoculation or from one individual to another. This means that a patient does not have to eat pork to acquire NCC, a patient only has to shake hands with someone who has the tapeworm and is shedding eggs. The eggs most commonly go to the brain, ventricular system, or subarachnoid space (called **racemose cysts** when in the subarachnoid space), but can also go to the spine or eyes.

The most common presentation of NCC is seizures, although intraventricular or infratentorial subarachnoid cysts can also cause hydrocephalus. Patients may present many

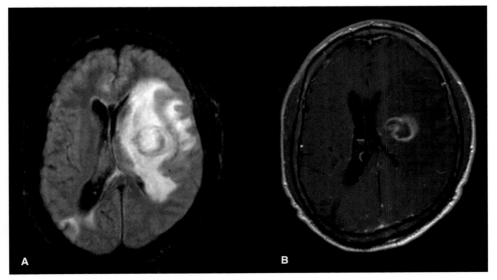

FIGURE 20–5 **Toxoplasmosis. A:** Axial FLAIR MRI demonstrating left frontal lesion surrounded by extensive edema causing mass effect on the left lateral ventricle. **B:** Axial T1-weighted postcontrast MRI demonstrating that the lesion in **A** is ring enhancing.

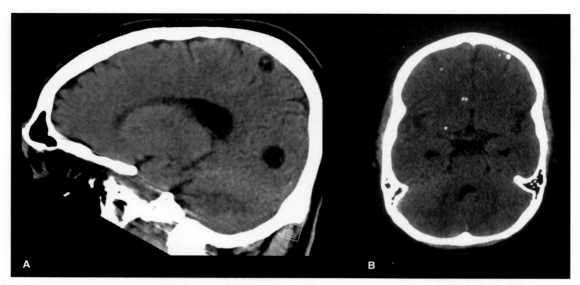

FIGURE 20–6 **Neurocysticercosis. A:** Vesicular neurocysticercosis. Sagittal noncontrast CT demonstrating cystic hypodensities in the superior parietal lobe and occipital lobe with a central hyperdensity (scolex) in the parietal lesion. **B:** Calcified neurocysticercosis. Axial noncontrast CT demonstrating multiple punctate hyperdensities in the bilateral frontal lobes consistent with calcified neurocysticercosis.

years after infection, so NCC should be a consideration in patients from endemic areas, even if they have lived outside of an endemic area for a prolonged period.

In the brain parenchyma, NCC passes through several stages with different radiologic manifestations: a vesicular stage (cyst with central hyperdensity, called a **scolex**), colloidal and granular stages (cyst with surrounding enhancement and edema), and finally a calcified stage (Fig. 20–6).

Treatment depends on the stage, location, and number of cysts. At any stage of NCC, if seizures are present, they should be treated with antiseizure medications. Antiparasitic treatment (albendazole and/or praziquantel) is used for the stages during which the parasites are active (vesicular, colloidal, and granular, but *not* the calcified stage), and steroids are administered in parallel with antiparasitic treatment to reduce the inflammatory response to cysts dying as a result of antiparasitic treatment. Albendazole is used alone (with steroids) if there are two or fewer viable cysts, and albendazole is combined with praziquantel (and steroids) if there are more than two viable cysts. A longer course of antiparasitic treatment may be necessary for racemose cysts, which can be harder to eliminate. For intraventricular or subarachnoid cysts, surgical removal and/or shunting may be necessary in some cases to treat hydrocephalus. Patients should be screened for ocular NCC with fundoscopy prior to treatment; although rare, this condition can worsen with antiparasitic therapy and requires surgical removal prior to initiation of antiparasitics. Given that patients from endemic regions could also have latent tuberculosis or strongyloides that could worsen with steroids, patients should be screened for tuberculosis (chest x-ray, purified protein derivative [PPD] test) and given empiric strongyloides treatment (ivermectin) prior to initiating steroids.

Rarely, innumerable cysts can be seen, a scenario referred to as **neurocysticercotic encephalitis** (Fig. 20–7). This form

of NCC is more common in young women. The burden of cysts in neurocysticercotic encephalitis is so high that antiparasitic treatment can provoke a massive inflammatory response leading to cerebral edema. Therefore, antiparasitic treatment

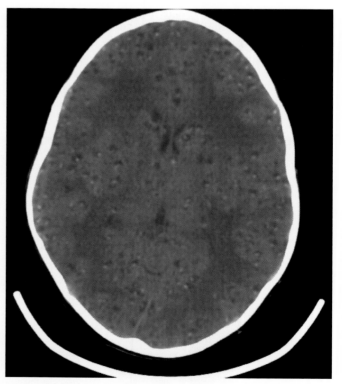

FIGURE 20–7 **Cysticercotic encephalitis.** Axial noncontrast CT demonstrating innumerable cystic hypodensities with central hyperdensities, consistent with vesicular neurocysticercosis. The extensive burden of lesions represents cysticercotic encephalitis.

should *not* be used for this form of the infection, only steroids (and antiseizure medications if seizures occur).

Granulomatous Amebic Encephalitis

Granulomatous amebic encephalitis can be caused by *Acanthamoeba* species or *Balamuthia mandrillaris*. Although referred to as "encephalitis," the condition is caused by multifocal CNS lesions, leading to subacute onset of focal or multifocal deficits. *Acanthamoeba* predominantly affects patients who are immunocompromised, whereas *Balamuthia* can affect immunocompetent individuals. Both organisms can cause preceding or concurrent skin findings; in *Balamuthia* infection, the skin lesion is most commonly on the nose. Neuroimaging demonstrates one or more ring-enhancing lesion(s). Diagnosis is often made by biopsy demonstrating organisms. Data on treatment are limited, and combinations of antiparasitic, antifungal, and antibacterial agents are often used.

Other Parasitic Focal Brain Lesions

A number of other parasitic diseases in endemic areas can cause focal brain lesions including schistosomiasis, echinococcosis, paragonimiasis, and Chagas disease. Schistosomiasis of the brain often demonstrates a unique "arborized" pattern of enhancement (i.e., both nodular and linear enhancement) on MRI (Fig. 20–8).

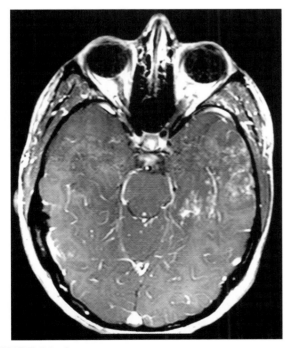

FIGURE 20–8 Schistosomiasis. Axial T1 post-contrast MRI demonstrating 'arborized' pattern of enhancement in the left temporal lobe. (Reproduced with permission from Ropper AH, Samuels MA, Klein JP, et al: *Adams and Victor's Principles of Neurology*, 11th ed. New York, NY: McGraw Hill; 2019.)

Infectious CNS Vasculitis

Infectious vasculitis leading to stroke can be caused by HIV, VZV, meningovascular syphilis (months to years after initial infection), mucormycosis, *Aspergillus*, and bacterial, tubercular, or fungal meningitis. VZV, *Mucor*, and *Aspergillus* infectious vasculitis occur almost exclusively in immunocompromised patients. Treatment is of the underlying infection. Some practitioners add steroids in patients with VZV vasculitis.

Infectious Cranial Neuropathies

Seventh nerve palsy may be a presenting feature of Lyme disease or HIV seroconversion (see "HIV Seroconversion Syndromes Involving the Nervous System"), and may occur in isolation or in combination with involvement of cranial nerve 8 in **Ramsay-Hunt syndrome** (VZV reactivation in the geniculate ganglion causing accompanying vesicular rash in the ear and/or on the palate).

The lower cranial nerves are commonly affected in diphtheric neuropathy (see "Diphtheric Neuropathy").

Tuberculous meningitis and cryptococcal meningitis can also cause accompanying cranial nerve palsies, as can leprosy (see "Leprosy").

Botulism causes multiple cranial neuropathies (see "Infection at the Neuromuscular Junction: Botulism").

Infectious optic neuropathies can be caused by *Bartonella* (cat scratch disease; associated with neuroretinitis and a macular star on fundoscopy), syphilis, and rarely by Lyme disease.

INFECTIONS OF THE SPINE

Infections of the spine can occur in various anatomical locations:

- Epidural space (spinal epidural abscess)
- Spinal meninges (spinal meningitis)
- Spinal cord itself (infectious myelitis, spinal cord abscess)
- Spinal interneurons (tetanus)
- Anterior horns of the spinal cord (poliomyelitis)
- Vertebrae (Pott's disease in tuberculosis, osteomyelitis)

Spinal Epidural Abscess

Spinal epidural abscess can occur due to hematogenous spread from a systemic source of infection, IV drug use, local spread from spinal osteomyelitis, exposure of the epidural space due to spinal surgery or trauma, or spontaneously in patients with diabetes, alcohol use disorder, and/or immunocompromise. Symptoms include fever, back pain, and rapidly progressive myelopathy. Diagnosis is made by MRI and treatment includes urgent surgical intervention and broad-spectrum antibiotics.

Spinal Meningitis

Spinal meningitis refers to inflammation of the spinal meninges and can occur concurrently with or independent of cerebral meningitis. Two common causes of spinal meningitis are tuberculosis and syphilis.

Infectious Myelitis

Acute Viral Myelitis

Acute transverse myelitis may be infectious, post-infectious, or autoimmune (associated with or independent of demyelinating disease such as multiple sclerosis or neuromyelitis optica; see "Transverse Myelitis" in Ch. 21).

Viral causes of acute transverse myelitis include VZV (which may or may not be associated with the preceding dermatomal rash of shingles), HSV-1 and HSV-2 (the latter more commonly associated with concurrent radiculitis; see "Infections of Nerve Roots"), CMV, and EBV. CSF analysis in viral myelitis shows elevated protein and lymphocytic pleocytosis. Specific diagnosis is made by CSF viral PCR for all except VZV, for which CSF IgG is more sensitive.

Chronic Viral Myelitis

Causes of subacute to chronic onset viral myelitis include HIV (**vacuolar myelopathy**) and human T-cell lymphocytic virus 1 (HTLV-1) (**tropical spastic paraparesis**). HIV vacuolar myelopathy is a progressive myelopathy (usually thoracic) seen in advanced AIDS. The time of emergence in the disease and time course parallel that of HIV dementia. The dorsal columns and corticospinal tracts are selectively affected, similar to subacute combined degeneration caused by vitamin B12 deficiency. MRI typically shows cord atrophy (see "HIV-associated Vacuolar Myelopathy").

HTLV-1 myelopathy (tropical spastic paraparesis) is seen in a small percentage of the large number of patients infected with the virus, which is endemic throughout the Caribbean, Africa, Central/South America, and Japan. Transmission is by the same modes as for HIV (i.e., blood and sexual fluids). Diagnosis is made by detecting serum or CSF antibodies to HTLV-1. Unfortunately, there are no known effective treatments, although steroids and/or antiretroviral agents are sometimes used empirically.

Tuberculosis of the Spine

Tuberculosis can affect the spine in three ways: involvement of the vertebrae (**Pott's disease**), spinal arachnoiditis/meningitis, or spinal cord tuberculoma. As in tuberculous meningitis, history and/or signs of prior or concurrent pulmonary tuberculosis may be absent. In Pott's disease, tuberculous involvement of the vertebral bodies and discs leads to vertebral destruction, which can ultimately result in vertebral collapse (Fig. 20–9). This most commonly occurs in the thoracic or lumbar spine, leading to paraplegia, bowel/bladder dysfunction, and back pain. Irregularity of the spine

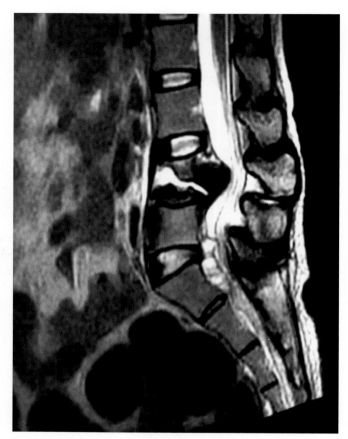

FIGURE 20–9 **Pott's disease (tuberculosis of the spine).** Sagittal T2-weighted MRI of the lumbar spine demonstrating collapse of the L4 vertebra with compression of the roots of the cauda equina.

may be palpated on examination (**gibbus deformity**). Neuroimaging reveals vertebral collapse, which is often apparent on plain film or CT if MRI is unavailable.

Tuberculous spinal meningitis, spinal tuberculoma, and arachnoiditis can present with either a myelopathy or a polyradiculopathy depending on the site(s) of involvement. Arachnoiditis commonly affects the cauda equina. Prolonged treatment with a multidrug regimen is used for spinal tuberculosis just as in tuberculous meningitis. Steroids may be considered. Surgery may be indicated in cases of Pott's disease with unstable fracture and/or cord compression, although is unfortunately often unavailable in many regions of the world with high incidence.

Infections of the Spinal Cord Gray Matter: Acute Flaccid Paralysis & Tetanus

Acute Flaccid Paralysis

Arboviruses (e.g., West Nile virus) and enteroviruses (e.g., poliovirus, enterovirus D-68) can selectively affect the anterior horn cells of the spinal gray matter (**poliomyelitis**), causing acute flaccid paralysis.

Tetanus

Tetanus is caused by the toxin produced by *Clostridium tetani*. It can occur in neonates born to unvaccinated mothers (due to infection of the umbilical stump), in unvaccinated pregnant mothers (due to unhygienic birth or abortion practices), or via wound infection (open wound, injection drug use, surgery) in unvaccinated patients. Tetanus is rare where vaccination rates are high, but still occurs in many parts of the world. The tetanus toxin impedes spinal interneuron inhibitory transmission, leading to disinhibition—and hence increased activation—of alpha motor neurons. This causes excess muscle contraction leading to spasm and rigidity of the muscles of the jaw (**trismus**), face (**risus sardonicus**), extremities, and torso (which can lead to **opisthotonic** posturing). Autonomic dysfunction is common. Diagnosis is clinical. Electromyography (EMG), if performed, shows evidence of continuous motor activity. Treatment is with antitoxin, toxoid vaccine, metronidazole, wound debridement, benzodiazepines for muscular spasm (neuromuscular blockade may be needed), respiratory support (intubation is often necessary), and management of autonomic instability (magnesium and labetalol are often used; note that unopposed beta-blockade can lead to worsening of dysautonomia).

Other Infectious Conditions of the Spine

Mycoplasma can cause an acute infectious or postinfectious myelitis.

The "dorsalis" in tabes dorsalis caused by late-stage syphilis refers to involvement of the dorsal columns and dorsal roots, leading to radicular pain, sensory loss, sensory ataxia, and bladder/bowel dysfunction. By this point in the disease, Argyll-Robertson pupil and/or dementia may be present. Diagnosis and treatment of neurosyphilis are discussed above (see "Syphilitic Meningitis Other Manifestations of Neurosyphilis").

Although NCC most commonly affects the brain, it can also affect the spinal cord. In most cases, patients have concurrent racemose (subarachnoid) disease in the brain (see "Neurocysticercosis").

Schistosomiasis, acquired by swimming in freshwater in endemic regions (Africa, Central/South America), can cause an acute myelitis. Treatment of schistosomiasis of the spine is with praziquantel and steroids.

INFECTIONS OF NERVE ROOTS

Infectious causes of radiculitis include Lyme disease, CMV (if CD4 <50), HSV-2 (most commonly affecting lumbosacral roots of the cauda equina, called **Elsberg's syndrome**), tuberculous arachnoiditis (most commonly affecting the cauda equina), and schistosomiasis. As with any disease process affecting nerve roots (see "Diseases of Nerve Roots" in Ch. 15), infectious radiculitis leads to pain radiating through affected dermatomes, and can also cause weakness, sensory loss, and/or decreased/absent reflexes in the region(s) supplied by the affected root(s). If the roots of the cauda equina are affected,

there can also be bowel and bladder dysfunction. Clues to an underlying infectious etiology of radiculopathy may be found in accompanying or preceding systemic and/or neurologic manifestations of the infectious agent, such as rash, fever, cranial nerve 7 palsy, and/or meningitis in Lyme disease; retinitis, colitis, and/or encephalitis in CMV; or genital rash in HSV-2.

INFECTIOUS PERIPHERAL NEUROPATHIES

Peripheral neuropathy is one of the principal features of leprosy, but can also occur in Lyme disease, diphtheria, hepatitis C (associated with cryoglobulinemia), and HIV.

Leprosy

Leprosy is one of the most common causes of neuropathy worldwide, and is endemic in Africa and Asia. The typical presentation is with mononeuropathy multiplex affecting nerves in the coolest regions of the body (i.e., where nerves are closest to the skin): ulnar, peroneal, posterior auricular, and superficial radial. Nerves may be palpably enlarged, especially the great auricular nerve (behind the ear) and the ulnar nerve (at the elbow). Accompanying hypopigmented patches on the skin or other skin changes are seen in most (but not all) patients. Cranial neuropathies (most commonly cranial nerves 5 and 7) may be seen. Treatment is with rifampicin, clofazimine, and dapsone; the combination of medications and the length of treatment depends on the clinical subtype.

Diphtheric Neuropathy

Corynebacterium diphtheriae causes diphtheria, which most commonly causes pharyngitis characterized by gray pseudomembranes that bleed if disturbed. This condition is rare due to widespread vaccination, but still occurs in lower-income countries. Rarely, diphtheria infection can cause a postinfectious neuropathy with a unique biphasic clinical pattern: Several weeks after pharyngitis, patients present with lower cranial neuropathies (causing dysphagia and dysarthria), followed several weeks later by neuropathy affecting the extremities (usually as cranial neuropathies are resolving). CSF analysis demonstrates albuminocytologic dissociation, and EMG/NCS shows changes consistent with demyelinating polyneuropathy. Treatment of pharyngeal diphtheria is with antibiotics and antitoxin, though the benefit of antitoxin in diphtheric neuropathy is uncertain.

INFECTION AT THE NEUROMUSCULAR JUNCTION: BOTULISM

In botulism, the botulinum toxin produced by *Clostridium botulinum* impedes transmission at the neuromuscular junction through interference with presynaptic acetylcholine vesicle fusion. Patients can be infected through food exposure (e.g., canned, fermented, and/or nonrefrigerated food; honey in infants), a wound (most commonly through intravenous drug use and subcutaneous drug injection [aka skin popping]), or rarely, adult intestinal colonization (usually in patients with history of GI disease). Botulism presents as descending flaccid paralysis beginning with the extraocular muscles and pupils (which may be dilated and poorly reactive, though pupillary changes are not universally present), and progressing to involve additional cranial nerves, respiratory muscles, and the extremities. Foodborne botulism often causes GI symptoms in addition to neurologic symptoms.

The main differential diagnosis for botulism is Guillain-Barré syndrome (e.g., Miller Fisher syndrome or pharyngeal-cervical-brachial variant), but botulism is distinct in that symptoms descend (rather than ascend as they most commonly do in Guillain-Barré syndrome), there are no sensory symptoms (pure motor Guillain-Barré syndrome occurs but is not common), pupils are commonly involved (does not usually occur in Guillain-Barré syndrome), and CSF is typically normal (albuminocytologic dissociation is usually seen in the CSF in Guillain-Barré syndrome) (see "Guillain-Barré Syndrome" in Ch. 27).

EMG in botulism shows diminished CMAP (compound motor action potential) amplitudes that increase with high-frequency repetitive stimulation as in Lambert-Eaton myasthenic syndrome, another presynaptic neuromuscular junction disorder (see "Repetitive Nerve Stimulation in Lambert-Eaton Myasthenic Syndrome" in Ch. 29); sensory nerve conduction study findings are normal. Diagnosis can be made by detecting toxin in serum, stool, or contaminated food source, and treatment is with antitoxin. Although antibiotic treatment is used for wound botulism, antibiotics should not be used for other types of botulism (infant, foodborne, adult intestinal colonization), since this may lead to increased toxin burden in the gastrointestinal tract.

INFECTIOUS MYOSITIS

Infections of the muscle can be caused by:

- Bacteria: muscle abscess, pyomyositis, gangrene due to *Clostridium*
- Parasites: trichinosis, cysticercosis (usually asymptomatic infection), toxoplasmosis
- Viruses: myalgias are common with many viral infections, but true myositis may also be seen

Bacterial muscle infection is usually limited to one muscle (e.g., psoas abscess), viral myositis is usually diffuse, and distribution of symptoms in parasitic myositis depends on the pathogen: Trichinosis most commonly affects the muscles of the eyes and face, whereas cysticercosis and toxoplasmosis cause more diffuse muscle involvement. Treatment is directed against the infectious pathogen.

TABLE 20–3 Neurologic Manifestations of HIV.

Direct Effects of HIV	Opportunistic Infections	Treatment Effects
At time of seroconversion • Aseptic meningitis • Cranial nerve 7 palsy • Guillain-Barré syndrome **Chronic HIV infection** • Distal symmetric polyneuropathy • Vacuolar myelopathy • Neurocognitive disorders/dementia	**CNS: Focal deficits** • Toxoplasmosis • Primary CNS lymphoma (EBV) • Progressive multifocal leukoencephalopathy (PML) **CNS: Global dysfunction** • CMV encephalitis **CNS: Meningitis** • Cryptococcal meningitis **PNS** • CMV radiculitis	**CNS toxicity** • Efavirenz (acute neuropsychiatric symptoms) **PNS toxicity** • Neuropathy (didanosine, stavudine, zalcitabine) • HIV-associated neuromuscular weakness syndrome (stavudine) **Immune reconstitution inflammatory syndrome (IRIS)**

Abbreviations: CMV: cytomegalovirus; CNS: central nervous system; EBV: Epstein-Barr virus; IRIS: immune reconstitution inflammatory syndrome; PML: progressive multifocal leukoencephalopathy; PNS: peripheral nervous system.

NEUROLOGIC MANIFESTATIONS OF HIV

HIV infection and its sequelae can affect any part of the nervous system from the time of seroconversion to advanced AIDS. The neurologic manifestations of HIV can be caused by (Table 20–3):

- HIV itself
- Opportunistic infections
- Toxicities of antiretroviral therapy, including direct toxicity and immune reconstitution inflammatory syndrome (IRIS) triggered by initiation of antiretroviral therapy

Direct Effects of HIV on the Nervous System

The nervous system complications directly related to HIV can be divided into those that occur at the time of seroconversion and those that emerge with advanced illness.

HIV Seroconversion Syndromes Involving the Nervous System

Shortly after HIV infection at the time of seroconversion, the patient may experience a flu-like illness. Neurologic manifestations of HIV seroconversion can occur simultaneously with or independently of this flu-like syndrome. The three most common neurologic manifestations of HIV seroconversion are:

- Aseptic meningitis
- Guillain-Barré syndrome
- Unilateral or bilateral cranial nerve 7 palsies

The aseptic meningitis of HIV seroconversion is characterized by headache and neck stiffness, and the CSF shows moderate protein elevation (typically <100 mg/dl) and mild lymphocytic pleocytosis (typically <30 cells/µL) with normal glucose (a typical viral pattern).

The Guillain-Barré syndrome of acute HIV seroconversion clinically resembles classic Guillain-Barré syndrome, but the CSF will demonstrate a lymphocytic pleocytosis (although generally <50 cells/µL), distinguishing it from postinfectious Guillain-Barré syndrome (in which there are generally fewer or no cells).

The diagnosis and differential diagnosis of cranial nerve 7 palsy is discussed in Chapter 13 (see "Lower Motor Neuron Facial Weakness").

It should be noted that since these three syndromes occur at the time of seroconversion, there will not yet be antibodies to HIV, and so the antibody test will be negative. If suspicion is high for HIV seroconversion, viral load should be obtained.

Neurologic Complications of Advanced HIV Infection

Neurologic complications of advanced HIV infection include:

- Neuropathy
- Dementia
- Vacuolar myelopathy

HIV-associated distal symmetric neuropathy—HIV can cause various different types of neuropathy. The most common is a symmetric length-dependent distal sensory polyneuropathy. Painful small fiber neuropathy, mononeuritis multiplex, and Guillain-Barré syndrome can also occur. The differential diagnosis for HIV-associated distal symmetric polyneuropathy is primarily an antiretroviral treatment-associated neuropathy (see "Antiretroviral-associated Neuropathy").

HIV dementia and HIV-associated neurocognitive disorders—HIV dementia is the extreme condition in a spectrum of neurocognitive disorders observed in HIV patients referred to as **HIV-associated neurocognitive disorders** (HAND). HIV dementia is characterized by severe cognitive deficits often accompanied by incontinence and symmetric motor deficits, with MRI evidence of atrophy and diffuse white matter abnormalities. The incidence of HIV dementia has decreased with widespread use of antiretroviral therapy, but minor cognitive impairment and asymptomatic/subclinical cognitive impairment (i.e., noted only during neuropsychological testing) are not uncommon. The time course of these cognitive changes is chronic and slowly progressive in comparison to the acuity of cognitive changes seen in CNS opportunistic infections (see "Opportunistic Infections of the Nervous System in HIV/AIDS").

HIV-associated vacuolar myelopathy—Just as AIDS may cause progressive cerebral dysfunction, progressive myelopathy may also occur, referred to as **HIV-associated vacuolar myelopathy**. The clinical syndrome is a slowly progressive

myelopathy, most commonly thoracic, and typically without back pain. The chronic time course and absence of back pain distinguish vacuolar myelopathy from most infectious myelitides that can present more acutely in HIV patients, with the exception of HTLV-1 (tropical spastic paraparesis), which can present insidiously as does vacuolar myelopathy.

Opportunistic Infections of the Nervous System in HIV/AIDS

Opportunistic infections in patients with HIV can affect any level of the nervous system:

- Meningitis can be caused by *Cryptococcus*
- Encephalitis can be caused by CMV
- Focal brain lesions can be caused by toxoplasmosis, JC virus (PML), and primary CNS lymphoma (an opportunistic malignancy arising from EBV infection in immunocompromised patients)
- Myelitis can be caused by CMV, VZV, HSV, HTLV-1
- Radiculitis can be caused by CMV

The differential diagnosis of altered mental status and/or focal neurologic deficits in HIV-infected patients depends in part on the CD4 count. Cryptococcal meningitis and PML are only seen in patients with CD4 count less than 200 cells/mm^3, toxoplasmosis and primary CNS lymphoma with CD4 less than 100 cells/mm^3, and CMV encephalitis and radiculitis are only seen in patients with a CD4 count less than 50 cells/mm^3. Global encephalopathy in an HIV-positive patient with a low CD4 count could be due to CMV encephalitis, cryptococcal meningitis, or HIV dementia. An encephalopathy may also be seen if there is a high burden of primary CNS lymphoma or toxoplasmosis lesions, although focal signs are generally seen as well. Focal neurologic signs/symptoms are characteristic of toxoplasmosis, primary CNS lymphoma, and PML. Although PML can easily be distinguished from the other two by neuroimaging (see "Viral Focal Brain Lesions"), toxoplasmosis and primary CNS lymphoma are challenging to distinguish from each other (see "Toxoplasmosis" for further discussion).

Antiretroviral Treatment–Related Complications

Antiretroviral treatment complications fall into two broad categories: direct neurotoxicity of the antiretroviral medications themselves and immune reconstitution inflammatory syndrome (IRIS).

Neurotoxicity of Antiretrovirals

Neurologic toxicities of antiretrovirals include:

- Axonal sensory-predominant peripheral neuropathy caused by nucleoside reverse transcriptase inhibitors didanosine, stavudine, and zalcitabine (mnemonic: **DiSt**(z)**al** neuropathy in HIV can be caused by **di**danosine, **st**avudine, and **zal**citabine)

- HIV-associated neuromuscular weakness syndrome (HANWS) associated with stavudine
- Acute neuropsychiatric symptoms with efavirenz

Antiretroviral-associated neuropathy—Antiretroviral-associated neuropathy emerges within weeks to up to a few months after initiation of antiretroviral treatment with didanosine, stavudine, or zalcitabine. Onset is generally more rapid than in HIV-associated neuropathy, and generally requires a change in antiretroviral regimen to prevent further progression of neuropathy. As with many drug-induced neuropathies, the neuropathy may initially worsen after removal of the offending drug before improving, a phenomenon called "coasting."

HIV-associated neuromuscular weakness syndrome—HIV-associated neuromuscular weakness syndrome (HANWS) is a syndrome of diffuse extremity weakness accompanied by nausea/vomiting, lactic acidosis, and/or hepatomegaly that comes on subacutely within days to weeks after starting (or stopping) stavudine.

Immune Reconstitution Inflammatory Syndrome

Immune reconstitution inflammatory syndrome (IRIS) is a clinical deterioration that can occur when the immune system is reconstituted (e.g., patient with HIV after initiation of antiretroviral therapy). IRIS can be due to a fulminant response of the immune system against an existing active opportunistic infection (paradoxical IRIS), against an undiagnosed subclinical infection (unmasking IRIS), or against HIV itself. The principal risk factors for development of IRIS are the patient's lowest CD4 count (nadir) and the rapidity with which the CD4 count rises after initiation of antiretroviral therapy. IRIS can be prevented if antiretrovirals are initiated before the CD4 count falls too low, but some patients may present initially with a low CD4 count or develop a low CD4 count after a period without treatment. A clinical dilemma occurs when a patient's initial presentation of HIV infection is with an AIDS-defining opportunistic infection, such that initiating antiretrovirals increases the risk of provoking IRIS against the active infection. For many CNS opportunistic infections, it is recommended that the opportunistic infection be treated before initiation of antiretrovirals so as to prevent IRIS. If IRIS occurs, it is generally treated with steroids.

REFERENCES

Armangue T, Leypolt F, Malaga I, Raspall-Chaure M, Marti I, Nichter C, et al., Herpes simplex virus encephalitis is a trigger of brain autoimmunity. *Ann Neurol* 2014;75:317–323.

Attia J, Hatala R, Cook DJ, Wong JG. The rational clinical examination. Does this adult patient have acute meningitis? *JAMA* 1999;282:175–181.

Brouwer MC, McIntyre P, Prasad K, van de Beek D. Corticosteroids for acute bacterial meningitis. *Cochrane Database Syst Rev* 2015(9):CD004405.

Cortese I, Muranski P, Enose-Akahata Y, Ha SK, Smith B, Monaco MC, et al. Pembrolizumab treatment for progressive multifocal leukoencephalopathy. *N Engl J Med* 2019;380:1597–1605.

de Gans J, van de Beek D, European Dexamethasone in Adulthood Bacterial Meningitis Study Investigators. Dexamethasone in adults with bacterial meningitis. *N Engl J Med* 2002;347:1549–1556.

Hasbun R, Abrahams J, Jekel J, Quagliarello VJ. Computed tomography of the head before lumbar puncture in adults with suspected meningitis. *N Engl J Med* 2001;345:1727–1733

Lantos PM, Rumbaugh J, Bockenstedt LK, Falck-Ytter YT, Aguero-Rosenfeld ME, Auwaerter PG, et al. Clinical practice guidelines by the Infectious Diseases Society of America (IDSA), American Academy of Neurology (AAN), and American College of Rheumatology (ACR): 2020 guidelines for the prevention, diagnosis, and treatment of Lyme disease. *Clin Infect Dis* 2020 Nov 30.

Muftuoglu M, Olson A, Marin D, Ahmed S, Mulanovich V, Tummala S, et al. Allogeneic BK virus–specific T cells for progressive multifocal leukoencephalopathy. *N Engl J Med* 2018;379:1443–1451.

Nguyen TH, Tran TH, Thwaites G, Ly VC, Dinh XS, Ho Dang TN, et al. Dexamethasone in Vietnamese adolescents and adults with bacterial meningitis. *N Engl J Med* 2007;357:2431–2440.

Scarborough M, Gordon SB, Whitty CJ, French N, Njalale Y, Chitani A, et al. Corticosteroids for bacterial meningitis in adults in sub-Saharan Africa. *N Engl J Med* 2007;357:2441–2450.

Demyelinating Diseases of the Central Nervous System

This chapter focuses on the following central nervous system demyelinating diseases:

- Multiple sclerosis (MS)
- Neuromyelitis optica spectrum disorder (NMOSD)
- Myelin oligodendrocyte glycoprotein-antibody disease (MOG-antibody disease)
- Acute disseminated encephalomyelitis (ADEM)
- Optic neuritis
- Transverse myelitis

Optic neuritis and transverse myelitis may be caused by a primary central nervous system (CNS) demyelinating disease (e.g., MS, NMOSD, MOG), systemic autoimmune disease, or may occur in the setting of infection, following infection, or as paraneoplastic conditions.

Demyelinating diseases of the peripheral nervous system (e.g., acute inflammatory demyelinating polyradiculoneuropathy [AIDP] and chronic inflammatory demyelinating polyradiculoneuropathy [CIDP]) are discussed in Chapter 27.

MULTIPLE SCLEROSIS

Clinical Features of Multiple Sclerosis

Multiple sclerosis (MS) is a demyelinating disease of the CNS that occurs more commonly in young women and is more prevalent further from the equator. In its most common clinical course, patients have multiple flares of symptoms at multiple time points, and recover from these attacks to varying degrees (**relapsing-remitting** MS). On average, relapses occur approximately every 1–2 years, though some patients have a

more aggressive disease course and others have milder disease. Later in the disease, patients with a relapsing-remitting course may enter a period of progressive decline, a scenario referred to as **secondary progressive** MS. **Primary progressive** MS is the least common clinical phenotype of MS, and is typically a spinal cord predominant illness with steady clinical decline from the time of onset rather than relapses and remissions. Even more rarely, the disease may present fulminantly with large tumor-like lesions (**Marburg variant**, **tumefactive demyelination**, or **Balo's concentric sclerosis**).

Flares of MS present as focal neurologic deficits that emerge and evolve over hours to days and usually resolve completely or near completely in subsequent weeks to months. Relapses in MS cause symptoms referable to central nervous system sites (brain, brainstem, optic nerve, cerebellum, and/or spinal cord). Some of the most common presenting symptoms of relapse or first presentation of MS include:

- **Monocular visual loss** due to optic neuritis (see "Optic Neuritis")
- **Diplopia** due to internuclear ophthalmoplegia caused by a lesion in the MLF (see "Internuclear Ophthalmoplegia" in Ch. 11)
- **Weakness, numbness, and/or urinary urgency/retention** most commonly due to spinal cord lesion(s)
- **Ataxia** most commonly due to a lesion in one of the cerebellar peduncles
- **Vertigo** due to demyelination of the cranial nerve 8 entry zone or the cerebellum

Between flares of MS, the accumulation of subclinical lesions may cause cognitive symptoms, neuropsychiatric symptoms, and/or fatigue. On neurologic examination,

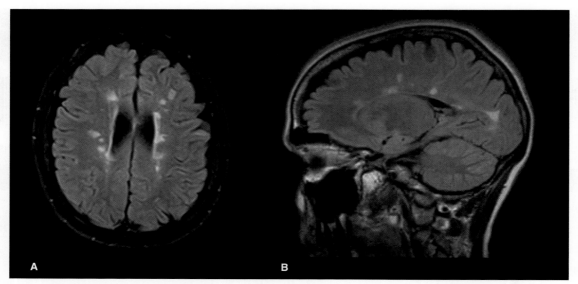

FIGURE 21-1 **MRI of brain lesions in multiple sclerosis.** Axial (**A**) and sagittal (**B**) FLAIR MRI demonstrating periventricular hyperintensities oriented perpendicular to the ventricles (Dawson's fingers).

patients may demonstrate signs outside of regions of new or prior clinical symptoms due to subclinical lesions that have caused CNS damage without having caused clinical flares (e.g., upper motor neuron signs [see "Upper Motor Neuron Lesions Versus Lower Motor Neuron Lesions" in Ch. 4]; relative afferent pupillary defect; see "Impaired Pupillary Constriction" in Ch. 10.)

Other symptoms and signs that may be seen in MS include:

- **Uthoff's phenomenon:** recurrence or emergence of neurologic symptoms with heat (due to environmental temperature in the summer, hot bath, or exercise).
- **L'hermitte's sign:** electrical sensation down the spine with forward flexion of the neck. This can occur in any type of cervical myelopathy and is not specific to MS.
- **Trigeminal neuralgia** (see "Trigeminal Neuralgia" in Ch. 13). Trigeminal neuralgia in MS occurs due to demyelination at the trigeminal entry zone in the pons (the trigeminal nerve itself is peripheral and so not affected in MS). Although MS is not a common cause of trigeminal neuralgia, unilateral or bilateral trigeminal neuralgia in a young patient should lead to consideration of and evaluation for MS.
- **Paroxysmal tonic spasms.** These brief, unilateral, often dystonic-appearing spasms may be provoked by hyperventilation and may respond to carbamazepine (though they are not epileptic). These are caused by lesions in the contralateral corticospinal tract and thought to be due to ephaptic transmission (inappropriate activation of nerve fibers adjacent to demyelinated fibers).

Neuroimaging in Multiple Sclerosis

Neuroimaging is critical in the diagnosis of MS. Lesions of MS have a characteristic morphology and distribution, and imaging characteristics can help to determine whether lesions are acute or chronic. The classic radiologic appearance of MS on brain MRI is several small (but still >3 mm) ovoid T2 hyperintensities perpendicularly oriented to the lateral ventricles and within the corpus callosum. Viewed on a sagittal image, the white matter lesions radiating outward from the corpus callosum have been referred to as **Dawson's fingers** (Fig. 21–1). Other common locations are juxtacortical (adjacent to the cortex), brainstem, cerebellar white matter, and spinal cord. Acute or active lesions may demonstrate enhancement with gadolinium, often in an **open ring** (as compared to the complete ring of contrast enhancement seen with tumor and abscess; see Fig. 21–4). The damage caused by lesions over time can lead to T1 hypointensities at sites of prior demyelination (**T1 black holes**). Lesions in the brainstem, cerebellar white matter, and spinal cord are common. In the spinal cord, MS lesions are typically small and peripherally located (Fig. 21–2) (as compared to the longitudinally extensive lesions of neuromyelitis optica, see "Neuromyelitis Optica Spectrum Disorder" and Fig. 21–3).

A first attack of a classic MS relapse syndrome (e.g., optic neuritis, etc.; see above) is referred to as *clinically isolated syndrome.* Previously, multiple clinical attacks "disseminated in space and time" were required for diagnosis of relapsing remitting MS. Now, the ability of MRI to demonstrate evidence of both *acute* (enhancing) and *chronic* (nonenhancing T2-hyperintense) demyelination allows for the diagnosis of MS to be made at the time of a first attack of a classic MS presenting syndrome (i.e., clinically isolated syndrome). This is important because earlier diagnosis allows for earlier initiation of disease-modifying treatment. According to the 2017 McDonald Criteria (Thompson et al., 2018):

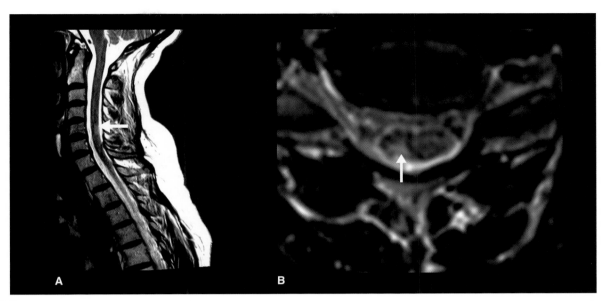

FIGURE 21–2 **MRI of spinal cord lesions in multiple sclerosis.** Sagittal (**A**) and axial (**B**) T2-weighted MRI demonstrating a small, peripherally located T2 hyperintensity in the cervical spinal cord (compare to longitudinally extensive lesion in neuromyelitis optica in Fig. 21–3).

- **Dissemination** in space can be demonstrated:
  - Clinically by history of two or more clinical demyelinating events affecting two different sites *or*
  - In a patient with a single attack (clinically isolated syndrome) by:
    - MRI demonstrating at least one T2-hyperintense lesion in at least two of the following four regions of the CNS:
      - Periventricular
      - Cortical or juxtacortical
      - Infratentorial
      - Spinal cord

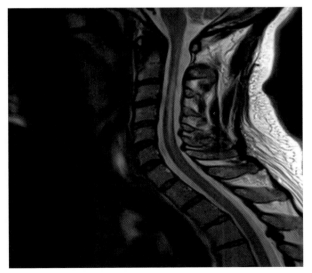

FIGURE 21–3 **MRI of spinal cord lesion in neuromyelitis optica.** Sagittal T2-weighted MRI demonstrating longitudinally extensive hyperintense lesion spanning more than three levels of the cervical spine in a patient with neuromyelitis optica.

- **Dissemination** in time can be demonstrated:
  - Clinically by history of two or more clinical demyelinating events, or
  - In a patient with a single attack (clinically isolated syndrome) by:
    - MRI:
      - New lesion on MRI compared to a prior MRI *or*
      - Simultaneous presence of both enhancing and non-enhancing lesions

    Or
    - CSF oligoclonal bands (see "Oligoclonal Bands") without atypical CSF findings (atypical findings would include protein > 100 mg/dL, pleocytosis > 50 cells/mm3 or nonlymphocyte predominance [e.g., neutrophil, eosinophil, atypical cell])

Primary progressive MS has separate diagnostic criteria:

- 1 year of disability progression not caused by relapse and two of the following:
  - ≥1 T2-hyperintense lesion on MRI in periventricular, cortical or juxtacortical, or infratentorial
  - ≥2 T2-hyperintense lesions on MRI of the spinal cord
  - CSF oligoclonal bands

Note that the McDonald criteria specify that the criteria are to be applied in patients with a typical presentation of MS, *not* to distinguish MS from other diagnoses that may also be characterized by white matter lesions. Other causes of subcortical white matter lesions include chronic microvascular white matter changes, leukodystrophies (see Ch. 31), CNS vasculitis, demyelinating lesions in systemic autoimmune disease (e.g., Sjögren's syndrome), and CADASIL (cerebral autosomal dominant arteriopathy with subcortical infarcts and leukocencephalopathy; see "Cerebral Autosomal Dominant Arteriopathy With Subcortical Infarcts and Leukocencephalopathy (CADASIL) & Cerebral Autosomal Recessive Arteriopathy With Subcortical Infarcts and Leukocencephalopathy (CARASIL)" in Ch. 19). However, in most cases the clinical context in these entities is distinct from that of a patient with MS.

Oligoclonal Bands

The presence of oligoclonal bands in the CSF that are not present in the serum indicates intrathecal IgG synthesis. CSF oligoclonal bands are present in the large majority of patients with MS, but are nonspecific and can be seen in CNS infections and other CNS inflammatory conditions. If oligoclonal bands are present in a patient with clinically isolated syndrome, this finding can be used to satisfy criteria for dissemination in time as per the 2017 revision of the McDonald criteria as long as no atypical CSF findings are present (see above).

Visual Evoked Potentials and Optical Coherence Tomography

Visual evoked potentials (VEP) examine a particular EEG correlate of visual stimulation (P100) to evaluate conduction along the visual pathway. If the latency of P100 is substantially prolonged or is significantly different between the two eyes, this suggests slowed conduction in the optic nerve(s), a sign of optic nerve dysfunction. The optic nerve head can also be examined by optical coherence tomography (OCT) to look for prior damage to the nerve. Abnormal VEP or OCT can suggest prior optic neuritis when history is unclear, but cannot be used to fulfill criteria for dissemination in space or time per McDonald criteria.

Radiologically Isolated Syndrome

Occasionally, an MRI performed for another reason (e.g., headache) may demonstrate what appears to be a "textbook" appearance of MS, but the patient has had no clinical attacks and has a normal neurologic examination. This is called **radiologically isolated syndrome (RIS)**. Such patients should be evaluated for other evidence of possible MS (e.g., spinal cord lesions on MRI, oligoclonal bands) and other causes of CNS white matter disease (e.g., systemic inflammatory disorders, cerebrovascular disease). However, even if ancillary laboratory or radiologic evidence suggestive of MS is discovered, it is unclear how this should be interpreted if the patient has no clinical history suggestive of demyelinating disease. Therefore, such patients are typically followed clinically and with serial imaging. About 50% of patients with RIS will develop MS over 10 years, with younger age at onset, positive CSF oligoclonal bands, infratentorial lesions, spinal cord lesions, and development of enhancing lesions on serial imaging associated with increased risk of developing a clinical demyelinating event (Lebrun-Frenay et al., 2020). As in patients with a clinically isolated syndrome who do not meet criteria for MS,

many practitioners initiate empiric vitamin D supplementation in patients with RIS.

Fulminant Demyelinating Disease

Rarely, fulminant demyelination can occur as a first attack of MS, in a patient with established MS, or as an isolated demyelinating phenomenon. Marburg variant MS, tumefactive demyelination, and Balo's concentric sclerosis are names given to differing radiologic and pathologic appearances of these entities, which may be difficult to distinguish from tumor or other inflammatory condition of the CNS (e.g., CNS vasculitis, sarcoidosis, neuromyelitis optica). Biopsy is necessary for diagnosis. If steroids are ineffective in treating fulminant demyelination, patients may be treated with IVIg or plasma exchange. If these are ineffective, cyclophosphamide and/or rituximab may be considered.

Treatment of Multiple Sclerosis
Acute Treatment of Flares of Multiple Sclerosis

Disabling acute relapses of multiple sclerosis are typically treated with a 3–5 day course of IV or oral corticosteroids. This same treatment is utilized whether it is the first attack or a relapse in a patient with known MS. Corticosteroids shorten relapse duration but do not alter the level of recovery. If symptoms from a very severe relapse do not begin to improve after 2 weeks, plasma exchange may be considered. Relapse should be distinguished from pseudo-relapse, in which symptoms of a prior flare re-emerge in the setting of systemic infection, a phenomenon similar to recrudescence in stroke (see "Recrudescence" in Ch. 19). This distinction can be challenging, since infection can also be a trigger of relapse. When it is unclear, MRI to evaluate for an enhancing lesion that correlates with the patient's symptoms can be obtained.

Long-term Treatment of Relapsing-Remitting MS

The goal of disease-modifying treatment for relapsing-remitting MS is to reduce the risk of relapses and slow the progression of disability. Treatment is generally indicated in all patients with MS unless they have clinically isolated syndrome not meeting criteria for MS, or have not had relapses for two or more years off treatment. The number of medications found to be effective toward these endpoints for relapsing-remitting MS continues to increase (Table 21–1).

There are three categories of disease-modifying therapy: injectables, oral agents, and monoclonal antibody infusions. Injectable agents (interferon beta and glatiramer acetate) have been in use the longest and have the best-established long-term safety, but are considered less effective than oral agents. Oral agents, however, have greater risk of toxicity. Monoclonal antibodies are even more effective but also hold greater risk and so are generally reserved for patients with highly aggressive disease (determined by frequency of relapses and MRI lesion burden).

TABLE 21–1 Disease Modifying Treatments for Relapsing-Remitting Multiple Sclerosis.

	Side Effects/Toxicities	Infections	Monitoring	Mechanism
Injectables				
Interferon beta	Flu-like syndrome Injection site reaction Depression Leukopenia Hepatotoxicity	None	CBC LFTs	Diverse immunomodulatory effects
Glatiramer acetate	Injection site reaction Flushing/anxiety with injection may occur	None	None	Multiple effects on T cells
Orals				
Teriflunomide	Hair loss GI symptoms Hepatotoxicity Pregnancy category X		CBC LFTs	Blocks pyrimidine synthesis → decreases division of inflammatory cells
Dimethyl fumarate/ Monomethyl fumarate	Lymphopenia Flushing GI symptoms	PML	CBC LFTs	Diverse immunomodulatory effects
Fingolimod/Siponimod/ Ozanimod/Ponesimod	Bradycardia Macular edema Skin cancer	Zoster PML Cryptococcus	Cardiac monitoring with first dose Ophthalmologic surveillance Skin examinations CBC, LFTs	Sphingosine receptor modulator → decreases migration of lymphocytes from lymph nodes
Cladribine	Lymphopenia	Zoster PML	CBC	Purine analogue → alters DNA repair mechanism leading to cell death of lymphocytes
Mitoxantrone	Cardiac toxicity AML (use therefore rare)		Echocardiography	Blocks topoisomerase → alters DNA repair mechanism leading to cell death of lymphocytes
Monoclonal antibodies				
Natalizumab	PML	PML	JCV antibody index every 6 months CBC LFTs	Monoclonal antibody against α₄ integrin, decreases lymphocyte entry into CNS
Ocrelizumab/ Ofatumumab/ Rituximab (off label)	Infusion reaction	URI Zoster HSV	Screen for Hep B prior to initiation No live immunization during treatment CBC	Monoclonal antibody CD20 → targets B cells for destruction
Alemtuzumab	Infusion reaction Autoimmune disease Malignancy	URI UTI HSV Opportunistic infections	CBC TFTs	Monoclonal antibody against CD52 → targets lymphocytes for destruction

Abbreviations: CBC: complete blood count; CNS: central nervous system; LFTs: liver function tests; PML: progressive multifocal; HSV: herpes simplex virus; TFTs: thyroid function tests; URI: upper respiratory infection; UTI: urinary tract infection.

Although data on switching agents are limited, patients are generally escalated to a more aggressive therapy if they have clinical or MRI evidence of active disease on their initial treatment regimen.

MS therapies should be discontinued prior to conception in women seeking to become pregnant to avoid risks to the fetus (though some practitioners continue glatiramer acetate during pregnancy). Relapse rates are generally lower during pregnancy.

Notable toxicities and adverse reactions with disease-modifying treatments of which to be aware include:

- Fingolimod: bradycardia and macular edema. Baseline electrocardiogram (ECG) and cardiac monitoring are required with the first dose (due to risk of first-dose bradycardia). Baseline ophthalmologic examination and subsequent periodic ophthalmologic monitoring are also necessary.
- Teriflunomide: hepatotoxicity and teratogenicity (pregnancy category X). Liver function monitoring is required, and women planning to conceive require elimination of teriflunomide with cholestyramine.
- Natalizumab: progressive multifocal leukoencephalopathy (PML) (PML occurs less commonly with fingolimod and dimethyl fumarate). PML is an opportunistic CNS viral infection caused by the JC virus (see "Viral Focal Brain Lesions" in Ch. 20). The risk of developing PML with natalizumab treatment is related to three factors:
  - Whether the patient has antibodies to the JC virus
  - Whether the patient has received prior immunosuppressive therapy
  - Length of treatment with natalizumab beyond 2 years

Any patient being considered for natalizumab treatment must be screened for serum JC virus antibodies, which are the main determinant of risk of developing PML (Schwab et al., 2017). The risk of PML is lowest in patients with negative JC virus antibodies and no prior history of immunosuppression—less than 1 in 10,000 (0.01%).

In patients with positive JC virus antibodies, the overall risk increases to just below 1%, but this risk is dependent on exposure to prior immunosuppression and length of natalizumab treatment. In patients with positive JC virus antibodies and a history of prior immunosuppression, the risk of PML is about 0.3% in the first 2 years of natalizumab treatment, and about 3% after 2 years of treatment. In patients with positive JC virus antibodies and no prior history of immunosuppression, the risk of PML is lower: just under 0.1% in the first 2 years of treatment with natalizumab, and just under 1% after 2 years of treatment. In such patients (JC virus positive with no prior history of immunosuppression), risk of PML can be further stratified by **JC virus antibody index,** which measures JC virus antibody levels. A JC virus antibody index less than 0.9 in a patient with no prior immunosuppression yields a PML risk of 0.01% in the first 2 years of natalizumab treatment, and about 0.1% after 2 years; a JC virus antibody index greater than 0.9 in a patient with no prior immunosuppression yields a PML risk of about 0.1% in the first 2 years of natalizumab treatment, and about 1% after 2 years (all data in this paragraph are from Schwab et al., 2017).

Given these risks, JC virus antibody-negative patients on natalizumab therapy must be screened for JC virus antibody every 6 months to evaluate for seroconversion. If PML develops during natalizumab treatment, natalizumab is discontinued, and plasma exchange is used to remove natalizumab.

Treatment of Progressive Multiple Sclerosis

The only FDA-approved medication for primary progressive MS is ocrelizumab (ORATORIO trial), and the only approved medication for secondary progressive MS is siponimod (EXPAND trial). Other treatments for progressive MS include rituximab, methotrexate, steroids, cyclophosphamide, and mitoxantrone. Supportive treatment to manage symptoms is also essential (see next section).

Symptomatic Management in Multiple Sclerosis

In addition to trying to modify the disease course of MS, many symptoms of MS can be effectively treated:

- Fatigue: amantadine, modafinil
- Gait: dalfampridine (contraindicated if seizures or renal failure)
- Spasticity: baclofen, tizanidine, botulinum toxin
- Bladder dysfunction: anticholinergics (e.g., oxybutynin), alpha-blockers (e.g., terazosin)
- Depression: psychiatric/psychological care, selective serotonin reuptake inhibitors (SSRIs)

NEUROMYELITIS OPTICA SPECTRUM DISORDER

Neuromyelitis optica spectrum disorder (NMOSD or Devic's disease) is an autoimmune disease of the CNS associated with an antibody against aquaporin-4 (AQP4-IgG). Similar to MS, NMOSD most commonly presents with acute flares/attacks. NMOSD predominantly affects the optic nerves and the spinal cord as the name suggests. Another common site of involvement is the area postrema (located in the medulla, posterior and adjacent to the fourth ventricle), leading to intractable nausea, vomiting, and/or hiccups; this may be the first presentation in some cases. The optic neuritis is often severe, commonly bilateral (simultaneously or sequentially), and associated enhancement on MRI often extends posteriorly to the optic chiasm. The myelitis is distinct from that seen in MS in that it is longitudinally extensive: usually longer than three spinal cord levels (Fig. 21–3). Less commonly, narcolepsy (due to hypothalamic involvement), PRES (see

TABLE 21–2 Summary of Differences Between Multiple Sclerosis & Neuromyelitis Optica.

	Multiple Sclerosis (MS)	Neuromyelitis Optica (NMO)
Geographic distribution	More common further from the equator	No particular geographic distribution, but NMO is more common than MS in patients of African and Asian origin
Female predominance	Yes	Yes
MRI findings:		
Periventricular lesions	Adjacent to lateral ventricles	Adjacent to third and fourth ventricles
Spinal cord lesions	Small, radially oriented	Longitudinally extensive
Oligoclonal bands	Common	Uncommon
Disease course	Relapsing remitting Primary progressive Secondary progressive	Nearly always relapsing
Treatment	Acute: Steroids Chronic: See Table 21–1	Acute: Steroids Chronic: Immunomodulatory therapies including rituximab, eculizumab, inebilizumab, satralizumab, tocilizumab, azathioprine, and mycophenolate mofetil

Ch. 19), elevated serum CK, and diffuse cerebral edema may be seen.

Although the optic nerves, spinal cord, and area postrema are the main sites of involvement in NMOSD, lesions elsewhere in the brain are common as well. These are less often symptomatic than in MS, and often differ in location and appearance compared to the classic locations in MS. Lesions in NMOSD may be found in the hypothalamus, around the third and fourth ventricles, and, in rare cases, may form large confluent lesions. Enhancement of the ependyma (lining of the ventricles) can also occur. Although women are more commonly affected than men (similar to MS), the geographic distribution in NMO is uniform (as opposed to the latitude gradient seen in MS). In patients of Asian and African origin, NMO may be more common than MS.

Anti-aquaporin-4 antibody (AQP4-IgG) is highly sensitive and specific for the disease. Serum AQP4-IgG should be part of the evaluation of atypical white matter lesions in the brain, brainstem, and/or spinal cord, since the specificity of the antibody is expanding the spectrum of what is considered NMOSD (and so may even be positive in patients with brain lesions who have neither myelitis nor optic neuritis). Seronegative cases do occur, and a subset of such patients have antibodies to myelin oligodendrocyte glycoprotein (MOG; see "Myelin Oligodendrocyte Glycoprotein (MOG) Antibody Disease".

Oligoclonal bands are less commonly present in NMOSD compared to MS. The CSF is usually inflammatory, and a lymphocytic pleocytosis is common.

When lupus or Sjögren's syndrome causes a myelitis it also tends to be longitudinally extensive. The majority of patients with lupus or Sjögren's syndrome who develop longitudinally extensive transverse myelitis are positive for AQP4-IgG and appear to have NMOSD in addition to the underlying systemic autoimmune disease.

Acute attacks of NMO are treated with IV corticosteroids, with plasma exchange added for fulminant attacks. Long-term immunomodulatory therapies to reduce the risk of subsequent relapses include rituximab (monoclonal antibody against CD20 that depletes B cells), eculizumab (monoclonal antibody against C5 that inhibits complement-induced membrane attack complex), inebilizumab (monoclonal antibody against CD19 that depletes B cells), satralizumab (monoclonal antibody against Il-6), tocilizumab (monoclonal antibody against Il-6), azathioprine, and mycophenolate mofetil. As with all immunomodulatory therapies, there are associated risks of infection with these treatments (of particular note, *N. meningitidis* meningitis with eculizumab).

A comparison of the features of MS and NMOSD is presented in Table 21–2.

MYELIN OLIGODENDROCYTE GLYCOPROTEIN (MOG) ANTIBODY DISEASE

MOG-IgG can be associated with optic neuritis (frequently bilateral; may be monophasic or relapsing), transverse myelitis (which often involves the central cord creating an H sign of signal abnormality in the gray matter on axial MRI, and may also involve the conus medullaris), NMOSD, ADEM (see below), cerebral cortical encephalitis (usually unilateral), and brainstem encephalitis. Patients whose MOG-IgG seropositivity persists after the first attack appear to be at higher risk for a relapsing course, whereas those with transient seropositivity appear to be more likely to have a monophasic course (Lopez-Chiriboga, 2018). Acute attacks are treated with steroids, with escalation to IVIg or plasma exchange if severe. Long-term therapy options for relapse

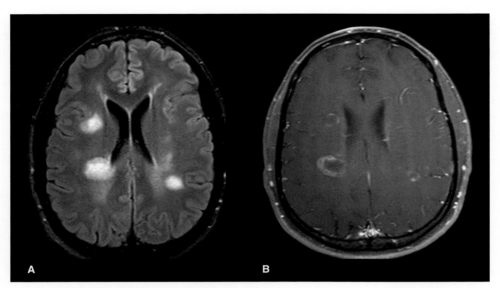

FIGURE 21–4 **MRI in acute disseminated encephalomyelitis (ADEM). A:** Axial FLAIR image showing multiple large hyperintensities in the periventricular white matter. Note that the lesions in ADEM tend to be larger than those seen in MS (see Fig. 21–1). **B:** Axial postcontrast T1-weighted image demonstrating that the lesions in **A** exhibit incomplete (open) rings of enhancement.

prevention include IVIg, rituximab, azathioprine, and myco-phenolate mofetil.

ACUTE DISSEMINATED ENCEPHALOMYELITIS

Acute disseminated encephalomyelitis (ADEM) is a multi-focal CNS demyelinating syndrome more common in children and young adults. ADEM can be thought of as the CNS analogue to Guillain-Barré syndrome in the peripheral nervous system: both are acute inflammatory conditions commonly preceded by infection. Given the multifocal nature of brain lesions in ADEM, the patient can have multifocal neurologic deficits and/or an encephalopathy. The neuroimaging pattern consists of multifocal large T2 hyperintensities in the white matter that may have an incomplete ring of contrast enhancement (Fig. 21–4). CSF is inflammatory with elevated protein and a mild lymphocytic pleocytosis. CSF oligoclonal bands may be present, and do not necessarily predict future development of MS since they can be seen in isolated monophasic ADEM.

Serum MOG-IgG should be checked in patients with ADEM. When elevated transiently at the time of ADEM attack, this may be correlated with a monophasic course, whereas persistent seropositivity several months after the acute attack may predict a relapsing course.

Treatment of ADEM is with IV steroids. IVIg or plasma exchange may be considered in severe cases that do not respond to steroids. Most patients recover entirely. Rarely, ADEM represents a fulminant first presentation of MS. Most patients undergo neuroimaging 6–12 months after presentation to evaluate for any new lesions to suggest the development of MS. The disease may continue to evolve radiographically over the first few months, and the emergence of new radiographic

lesions in the short-term can still be seen in what ultimately turns out to be a monophasic course of the illness.

A fulminant hemorrhagic variant of ADEM known as **Weston-Hurst syndrome** can be fatal.

OPTIC NEURITIS

Optic neuritis is inflammation of the optic nerve. It presents with painful visual loss over days. It is most commonly unilateral, although it can occur bilaterally. The pain is typically worse when the patient moves the affected eye. On examination, decreased acuity, decreased color vision, and an afferent pupillary defect may be observed (see "Impaired Pupillary Constriction due to a Lesion of Cranial Nerve 2" in Ch. 10). Although an inflamed optic nerve head on fundoscopy confirms the diagnosis in the appropriate clinical context, inflammation of the optic nerve may be retrobulbar with no visible abnormality of the optic nerve head itself. Optic nerve enhancement can often be seen on contrast-enhanced MRI of the orbit.

The time course of optic nerve dysfunction is key to the differential diagnosis: A more insidious progression of monocular visual loss may suggest a mass lesion (e.g., optic nerve glioma, optic nerve sheath meningioma), whereas a more acute presentation may suggest a vascular etiology (e.g., ischemic optic neuropathy) (see "Monocular Visual Loss" in Ch. 6).

Although optic neuritis is commonly associated with MS and NMO, other potential etiologies include:

• Systemic inflammatory disease (e.g., sarcoid, lupus)

• Infections (e.g., *Bartonella*, syphilis)

• Paraneoplastic optic neuritis (associated with antibodies against CRMP-5 [collapsing response mediator protein 5])

Most patients with optic neuritis recover significantly over the first 2–4 weeks, although continued recovery may occur over subsequent months. Treatment with IV steroids leads to quicker recovery but does not change the long-term outcome with respect to recovery of visual acuity.

Optic neuritis may be the first flare of MS. Overall, 15 years after an episode of optic neuritis, approximately half of patients will develop MS. The risk is strongly modulated by whether or not there are MRI lesions suggestive of MS at the time of optic neuritis. Patients with zero MRI lesions have a 15-year risk of 25% of developing MS, whereas patients with one or more MRI lesions have a 15-year risk of 72% of developing MS (Optic Neuritis Study Group, 2008). A patient with isolated optic neuritis who does not have MRI evidence of dissemination in space and time is an example of a clinically isolated syndrome, the management of which is discussed above.

If optic neuritis occurs sequentially in one optic nerve and then the other within a short period of time, NMO should be considered.

TRANSVERSE MYELITIS

Transverse myelitis (TM) refers to inflammation of the spinal cord. Like optic neuritis, TM can occur as an isolated monophasic condition (i.e., idiopathic, infectious, or postinfectious), as a flare in a patient with MS or NMO (or as a clinically isolated syndrome), in the setting of systemic autoimmune disease (e.g., lupus, Sjögren's syndrome, sarcoid), or as a paraneoplastic syndrome (antibodies are most commonly against CRMP-5; see "Paraneoplastic Syndromes of the Nervous System" in Ch. 24). The presentation is one of a rapidly evolving myelopathy that leads to weakness and sensory changes in the extremities and bowel and/or bladder dysfunction. The clinical presentation may be symmetric or asymmetric depending on the extent of the lesion. Reflexes may be decreased or absent initially, but hyperreflexia typically emerges over time.

The differential diagnosis for myelitis is broad. If onset of myelopathic symptoms is sudden, vascular etiology (spinal infarct or hemorrhage) or acute spinal cord compression should be considered. Acute-onset myelopathy raises concern for epidural abscess or schistosomiasis (in endemic regions or in patients from them) (see "Infections of the Spine" in Ch. 20). A more subacute progression of myelopathic symptoms suggests malignancy, vascular malformation (e.g., dural arteriovenous fistula [see "Spinal Dural Arteriovenous Fistula" in Ch. 19]), cervical spondylosis, vitamin B12 or copper deficiency, radiation-induced myelopathy (see "Radiation Therapy-Induced Myelopathy" in Ch. 24), or indolent infection (e.g., vacuolar myelopathy of HIV/AIDS, HTLV-1, tuberculosis of the spine, syphilis, neurocysticercosis; see "Infections of the Spine" in Ch. 19). (See also "Causes of Myelopathy" in Ch. 5.)

The main localization-based differential diagnosis for transverse myelitis is Guillain-Barré syndrome (GBS) (see "Guillain-Barré Syndrome" in Ch. 27), since both may cause hyporeflexia or areflexia in the acute setting (upper motor neuron signs take time to emerge after acute spinal cord insult). Bowel/bladder dysfunction is extremely uncommon in GBS, but is common in transverse myelitis. A spinal level to pinprick is common in transverse myelitis but would be atypical in GBS, although confluent sensory loss in GBS may make it difficult to determine if a spinal level is present. Continued progression of symptoms in the legs with no symptoms or signs in the arms would make a lumbar or thoracic spinal lesion more likely than GBS. An acute cervical myelopathy (e.g., cervical transverse myelitis or epidural abscess) may be harder to distinguish from GBS in the acute phase. MRI of the spine should be performed in any case of suspected myelopathy.

MRI in transverse myelitis will generally reveal a T2-hyperintense spinal cord lesion that may enhance. If the lesion is longitudinally extensive (>3 levels), evaluation for NMO, lupus, and Sjögren's syndrome should be pursued.

Lumbar puncture in transverse myelitis typically reveals a nonspecific inflammatory pattern: elevated protein and a mild pleocytosis (usually lymphocytic). A significant pleocytosis (>100 cells) should raise concern for an infectious myelitis.

If there is no antecedent history of infection or vaccination, the question emerges as to whether an episode of transverse myelitis represents the first flare of MS (i.e., a clinically isolated syndrome). As with optic neuritis, if there are brain MRI lesions suggestive of MS, the risk of conversion to MS is far higher than if there are no such lesions (80% vs approximately 10%) (Scott et al., 2011). Transverse myelitis associated with later conversion to MS is typically less severe, with spinal cord lesions that only partially transect the axial diameter of the cord rather than a full-thickness transverse lesion. Postinfectious or infectious myelitis and NMO are typically more severe and the lesions are typically more fully transverse. If oligoclonal bands are present in a patient with transverse myelitis, this is also predictive of later development of MS. As with optic neuritis and clinically isolated syndrome in general, decisions must be individualized about whether or not to begin treatment to reduce the risk of further flares when concern for MS is high in a patient with isolated transverse myelitis.

Treatment of immune-mediated/idiopathic transverse myelitis is with IV steroids. Plasma exchange may be considered in severe cases.

REFERENCES

EXPAND trial Kappos L, Bar-Or A, Cree BAC, Fox RJ, Giovannoni G, Gold R, et al. Siponimod versus placebo in secondary progressive multiple sclerosis (EXPAND): a double-blind, randomised, phase 3 study. *Lancet* 2018;391(10127):1263–1273.

Fox RJ, Ruddick RA. Risk stratification and patient counseling for natalizumab in multiple sclerosis. *Neurol* 2012;78:436–437.

Lebrun-Frenay, Kantarci O, Siva A, Sormani MP, Pelletier D, Okuda DT, et al. Radiologically isolated syndrome: 10-year risk estimate of a clinical event. *Ann Neurol* 2020;88: 407–417.

López-Chiriboga SA et al. Association of MOG-IgG Serostatus With Relapse After Acute Disseminated Encephalomyelitis and Proposed Diagnostic Criteria for MOG-IgG–Associated Disorders. JAMA *Neurol* 2018; 75(11):1355–1363.

ORATORIO *trial* Montalban X, Hauser SL, Kappos L, Arnold DL, Bar-Or A, Comi G, et al. Ocrelizumab versus placebo in primary progressive multiple sclerosis. *N Engl J Med* 2017; 376: 209–220.

Schwab N, Schneider-Hohendorf T, Melzer N, Cutter G, Wiendl H. Natalizumab-associated PML challenges with incidence, resulting risk, and risk stratification. *Neurol* 2017;88:1197–1205.

Scott TF, Frohman EM, De Seze J, Gronseth GS, Weinshenker BG. Evidence-based guideline: clinical evaluation and treatment of transverse myelitis. *Neurol* 2011;77:2128–2134.

The Optic Neuritis Study Group. Multiple Sclerosis Risk after Optic Neuritis: Final Optic Neuritis Treatment Trial Follow-Up. *Arch Neurol* 2008;65:727–732.

Thompson AJ, Banwell BL, Barkhof F, Carroll WM, Coetzee T, Comi G, et al. Diagnosis of multiple sclerosis: 2017 revisions of the McDonald criteria. *Lancet Neurol* 2018;17(2):162–173.

Delirium, Dementia, & Rapidly Progressive Dementia

APPROACH TO ALTERED COGNITION

When assessing patients with acute or chronic changes in cognition, two interrelated questions should be pursued during the history and examination:

- Is the presentation focal or global?
- Is the problem arising from primary brain pathology or a systemic process that is affecting the brain?

Focal deficits suggest focal brain pathology (e.g., stroke, tumor, abscess), although focal findings can occur with systemic disease in the absence of focal central nervous system pathology (e.g., focal seizures or hemichorea caused by hyperglycemia or aphasia caused by cefepime toxicity). Global dysfunction is often due to systemic pathology affecting the brain, although diffuse intrinsic brain pathology can also cause a global encephalopathy (e.g., multiple strokes, multiple metastases, a diffuse infiltrating malignant lesion, acute disseminated encephalomyelitis).

Focal cognitive deficits may give the initial misleading impression that there is a global encephalopathy. Examples of focal deficits that can initially appear to be global encephalopathic states unless examined in detail include Wernicke's aphasia producing lack of comprehension and abnormal speech, and transient global amnesia causing isolated short-term memory impairment. On the other hand, global cognitive dysfunction may make it challenging to elicit coexisting focal deficits on examination since a core feature of global cognitive dysfunction is inattention, which can make it difficult to examine cognitive functions that rely on attention such as language, memory, and ability to follow commands.

DELIRIUM

Delirium is characterized by acute onset of altered mental status with fluctuations in both symptoms and level of arousal. Delirium causes a global encephalopathy, with inattention as the core feature. The differential diagnosis for acutely altered mental status is as broad as the differential diagnosis for any condition in medicine. Delirium can be caused by intrinsic brain pathology (see "Neurologic Causes of Acutely Altered Mental Status"), systemic disease affecting the brain (e.g., renal or hepatic failure, systemic infections, electrolyte disturbances, hypoglycemia or hyperglycemia, hyperammonemia, hypothyroidism or hyperthyroidism), medications, toxins, drugs, or drug withdrawal. Primary psychiatric etiologies may also be causative or contributory. Although new changes in cognition or personality in patients with psychiatric disease may be due to the underlying psychiatric disease, potential reversible medical causes should be sought.

Patients who are older or have baseline neurologic dysfunction (e.g., dementia) are at increased risk of delirium due to any of the above etiologies (as well as due to the disorienting environment of the hospital if the patient is hospitalized).

Neurologic Causes of Acutely Altered Mental Status

Neurologic etiologies of *acute-onset* altered mental status include seizures, stroke and cerebrovascular disease, CNS infections, and transient global amnesia.

Seizures as a Cause of Acutely Altered Mental Status

Nonconvulsive seizures can cause alterations in cognition and level of consciousness ranging from encephalopathy to coma. Diagnosis of nonconvulsive seizures may require continuous EEG monitoring (see "Nonconvulsive Status Epilepticus" in Ch. 18). A postictal state following a seizure can also lead to changes in mental status ranging from confusion to coma. An unwitnessed seizure with subsequent postictal state should be considered as a potential etiology of altered mental status, especially in patients who improve spontaneously from their altered state without any specific medical intervention.

Stroke and Cerebrovascular Disease as Causes of Acutely Altered Mental Status

Although stroke as a cause of acute alteration in mental status is generally easily recognized when focal features are present, certain regions of infarction may lead to global cognitive dysfunction without obvious focal signs. Additionally, focal signs such as subtle visual field deficits or neglect may be hard to elicit in confused patients. Sites of infarction that can lead to changes in mental status without obvious focal features include the thalamus (especially bilateral thalamic strokes due to artery of Percheron territory infarct; see "Posterior Cerebral Artery Territory Infarction" in Ch. 7), inferior division of the right middle cerebral artery (MCA), anterior cerebral artery (ACA) territory (if motor fibers to the leg are spared), posterior cerebral artery (PCA) territory (affecting the hippocampus/medial temporal lobe), and diffuse emboli.

Subacute development of a subdural hematoma can lead to subacute development of altered mental status (see "Subdural Hematoma" in Ch. 19).

CNS Infections as a Cause of Acutely Altered Mental Status

Fever and altered mental status should raise concern for meningitis, encephalitis, or intracranial abscess (see Ch. 20). Although a systemic infection can cause alteration in mental status without direct CNS involvement, lumbar puncture should be considered in patients with fever and altered mental status if there is no obvious systemic source of infection.

Transient Global Amnesia

Transient global amnesia (TGA) is a discrete episode (usually lasting 12 hours or less) during which the ability to form new memories is lost (**anterograde amnesia**). This inability to form new memories leads to repetitive questioning ("Where

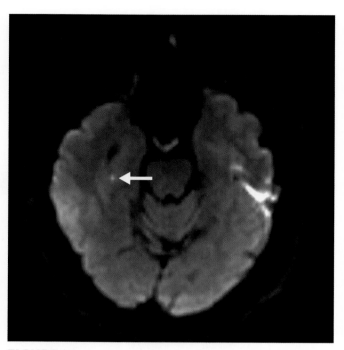

FIGURE 22–1 **MRI in transient global amnesia.** Axial diffusion-weighted imaging (DWI) MRI showing a punctate region of diffusion restriction in the right hippocampus (arrow).

am I?", "How did I get here?") since the short-term memory buffer is essentially erased every few minutes. Patients with TGA may be disoriented with respect to time and place and forget events of the preceding day(s) but do not forget their name or other personal information. If personal information is forgotten, this is highly suggestive of a psychogenic etiology of amnesia (e.g., fugue state) rather than a neurologic etiology.

A trigger commonly precedes TGA such as an emotionally intense situation (e.g., stressful event, sexual intercourse), vigorous exercise, or exposure to cold water. TGA is often idiopathic, but may be the presentation of an infarct (e.g., medial temporal or thalamic), and so neuroimaging should be performed. In some patients with TGA, a punctate region of diffusion restriction can be seen in the hippocampus (Fig. 22–1), leading some to hypothesize that all TGA is a vascular phenomenon, although the pathophysiology of the condition is unknown. Although seizures can produce ictal or postictal amnesia, the period of amnesia with seizures is generally shorter than that in TGA, and seizures are often recurrent, whereas TGA usually lasts for hours and only very rarely recurs.

Medical Causes of Acutely Altered Mental Status

"Toxic-Metabolic" Etiologies of Altered Mental Status

"Toxic-metabolic" encephalopathy refers to altered mental status due to medications, toxins, and/or metabolic abnormalities (e.g., uremia, hepatic failure). When faced with a case of potential toxic-metabolic encephalopathy, the consultant neurologist should try to determine which "toxic" and/or "metabolic" factor(s) may account for the patient's altered state: Does the degree of renal or hepatic failure differ significantly from the patient's baseline? Has a potentially deliriogenic medication been recently added? Has a chronic medication changed in dose or could it be reaching toxic levels at its previously tolerated dose due to new renal or hepatic dysfunction? Applying the catch-all "toxic-metabolic" term to encephalopathies without careful consideration can lead to premature closure and missed diagnoses. By thinking critically through any and all potential neurologic and systemic etiologies of altered mental status, reversible etiologies may be uncovered.

An important example of this is the case of medications. Nearly any medication can cause altered mental status. Neurologists are in the unique position of having seen and diagnosed cases of medication-induced neurotoxicity from medications that only rarely cause neurotoxicity. Other practitioners may have used a medication countless times without seeing neurologic side effects, and thus may not associate a particular drug with the potential to cause delirium. For example, many commonly used antibiotics can rarely cause encephalopathy, including cephalosporins (in particular cefepime and ceftazidime), fluoroquinolones, macrolides, metronidazole, and isoniazid (Bhattacharyya et al., 2016). Cephalosporin-associated encephalopathy is often associated with nonconvulsive seizures, fluoroquinolone- and macrolide-associated encephalopathy with hallucinations and psychotic symptoms, and metronidazole-associated encephalopathy with ataxia and characteristic MRI findings in the cerebellar white matter. Patients who develop alterations in mental status of unclear etiology on any of these medications should generally have these medications replaced with alternative antibiotics given the possibility of antibiotic-associated encephalopathy.

Wernicke's Encephalopathy

Wernicke's encephalopathy is characterized by the triad of encephalopathy, ataxia, and eye movement abnormalities (nystagmus and/or gaze palsies), and is caused by thiamine (vitamin B1) deficiency that occurs in the setting of malnutrition (e.g., in patients with alcohol use disorder, anorexia, gastric bypass surgery, or hyperemesis gravidarum). In many cases of Wernicke's encephalopathy, the complete triad is not present, requiring a high index of suspicion for the condition. Wernicke's encephalopathy can be precipitated acutely by giving glucose to a thiamine-deficient patient without giving thiamine simultaneously. Therefore, thiamine should always be given with glucose infusions in the setting of acutely altered mental status to prevent this complication in patients whose history may be unknown. Serum thiamine levels take a long time to return and may be unreliable, so empiric treatment with intravenous thiamine should be provided if there is any concern for Wernicke's encephalopathy. MRI in Wernicke's encephalopathy can demonstrate signal abnormalities in

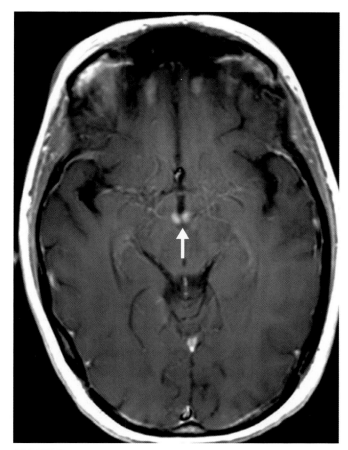

FIGURE 22–2 MRI in Wernicke's encephalopathy. Axial post-contrast T1-weighted image showing enhancement of the mamillary bodies (arrow).

the mammillary bodies, thalamus, and around the third and fourth ventricles (Fig. 22–2).

Not treating Wernicke's encephalopathy can result in **Korsakoff's syndrome**, characterized by anterograde amnesia and confabulation.

If the cause of acute altered mental status is unclear after careful review of the patient's medications and active medical issues, EEG should be considered to look for nonconvulsive seizures, brain imaging should be considered to look for a causative lesion, and lumbar puncture should be considered (if there is concern for CNS infection or inflammation).

DEMENTIA

Dementia is defined as cognitive decline in one or more domains (e.g., memory, language, attention, visuospatial processing, social behavior) sufficient to impair independent daily function.

Causes of Dementia

Insidious onset and gradual progression of cognitive impairment over months to years may be secondary to neurodegenerative diseases (Alzheimer's disease, dementia with Lewy bodies, and frontotemporal dementia being the most common), chronic cerebrovascular disease (vascular dementia), repeated head trauma (chronic traumatic encephalopathy), or due to potentially treatable causes such as:

- Systemic diseases:
  - Metabolic deficiency: vitamin B12 deficiency
  - Endocrine disease: Hypothyroidism
  - Chronic infection: AIDS, syphilis
  - Obstructive sleep apnea
- Medications, such as psychotropic medications in older adults
- Toxins, such as alcohol or drug use, heavy metal poisoning
- Intracranial pathology, such as tumor, chronic subdural hematoma, normal pressure hydrocephalus
- Psychiatric disease, such as depression

Neurodegenerative disease is progressive with no disease-modifying medications, and treatment is limited to symptomatic management and supportive care. Therefore, part of the initial evaluation of patients with dementia is to assess for potentially treatable causes. The history should evaluate for depression, medication history, and sleep apnea. Examination should assess for focal findings that might suggest focal underlying pathology. Mental status testing should be performed to assess for the type and extent of impairment(s), for example with the Mini-Mental State Examination (MMSE) or the Montreal Cognitive Assessment (MOCA).

Frontal release signs may be present on physical examination in patients with dementia, but are not universally present and some of these signs can be seen in non-demented older patients (and occur normally in infants as does Babinski's sign). Frontal release signs include:

- **Snout reflex**: The patient purses the lips when the examiner taps at the center of the lips.
- **Grasp reflex**: The patient cannot inhibit grasping the examiner's hand or an object when placed into the patient's hand.
- **Suck reflex**: The patient will attempt to suck any object (such as a pen) moved toward the mouth.
- **Rooting reflex**: Lightly touching the patient's cheek causes the patient to turn the head toward that side.
- **Palmomental reflex**: Briskly scratching the patient's palm causes a twitch of the ipsilateral chin.

Laboratory evaluation for dementia should include vitamin B12, thyroid-stimulating hormone (TSH), comprehensive metabolic panel, CBC, HIV, syphilis testing, and neuroimaging (ideally MRI). Neuroimaging may reveal an etiology of altered cognition such as malignancy (primary or metastatic), subdural hematoma, normal pressure hydrocephalus, or a characteristic pattern of atrophy associated with a particular neurodegenerative etiology. Formal neuropsychological testing can help to better characterize the nature and degree of cognitive impairment, which may be helpful both in making a diagnosis and in guiding cognitive therapy.

The core features of the most common dementia syndromes are presented in Table 22–1. Terminology related to neurodegenerative diseases can be confusing, since overlapping terms are used for clinical conditions and neuropathological diagnoses at autopsy. For example, different variants of the clinical syndrome of primary progressive aphasia may have underlying frontotemporal lobar dementia pathology or Alzheimer pathology on autopsy; a patient with clinically diagnosed corticobasal syndrome (see Ch. 23) may be found at autopsy to have corticobasal degeneration pathology, Alzheimer pathology, frontotemporal lobar dementia pathology, or progressive supranuclear palsy pathology; and some pathologic findings such as argyrophilic grain disease do not have a clearly defined clinical phenotype. To make matters more complicated, at autopsy, many patients may have more than one pathology (e.g., Alzheimer's pathology and vascular disease, or Alzheimer's and Lewy Body pathology).

Here the focus will be on clinical diagnoses, acknowledging that these are imperfect predictors of underlying pathology. This mismatch between clinical diagnosis and neuropathological diagnosis is one challenge in designing effective clinical trials for neurodegenerative disease, though advances in neuroimaging and CSF biomarkers are improving earlier more precise diagnosis of underlying pathology in patients with neurodegenerative dementia. Some ask why it is important to distinguish between types of dementia clinically/radiologically when there are currently no specific disease-modifying therapies. A precise diagnosis allows for tailoring of symptomatic therapy and also aids in discussion of prognosis. In addition, clinical-radiologic diagnosis is essential to characterizing these diseases in order to improve early identification toward the goal of developing disease-modifying therapies.

Mild Cognitive Impairment

Mild cognitive impairment (MCI) refers to cognitive decline with preserved ability to function independently. Patients with MCI often present for evaluation due to awareness of their deficits, whereas patients with dementia are commonly brought for evaluation by family members and may be less aware of their deficits. MCI is estimated to have a risk of progression to dementia of approximately 10% per year. The most common form of MCI is amnestic MCI in which the patient has isolated memory loss, although patients may have deficits in another individual cognitive domain or multiple domains. In patients with MCI, there does not appear to be a clear benefit to using the cholinesterase inhibitors used in patients with Alzheimer's disease (see "Treatment of Alzheimer's Disease"), although some practitioners will consider their use in patients in whom MCI is thought likely to be due to underlying Alzheimer's pathology.

TABLE 22–1 Clinical Features of Dementia Syndromes.

	Alzheimer's Disease (AD)	Dementia With Lewy Bodies (DLB)	Frontotemporal Dementia (FTD)		Vascular Dementia
			Behavioral Variant FTD (bvFTD)	Primary Progressive Aphasia (PPA)	
Most common initial cognitive deficits	Memory	Visuospatial dysfunction Executive dysfunction	Behavior/personality change	Language deficits	Executive dysfunction Cognitive slowing
Additional features	Visuospatial dysfunction Executive dysfunction Word-finding difficulties	Parkinsonism Hallucinations Fluctuations	Executive dysfunction		May have focal findings
Most common age of onset	>60	>60	50s–60s		>60
Locations of atrophy	Medial temporal Parietal	Variable, may be minimal	Frontotemporal	Language areas	Sites of prior strokes
Locations of hypometabolism/hypoperfusion on nuclear imaging	Temporoparietal Posterior cingulate Precuneus	Occipital Temporoparietal	Frontotemporal	Language areas	N/A
Cerebrospinal fluid findings	$A\beta42\downarrow$ Tau$\uparrow$	N/A	N/A	N/A	N/A
Pathology/Proteinopathy	Aβ42 plaques and tau neurofibrillary tangles	Alpha-synuclein	Tau TDP-43 FUS	Alzheimer pathology in logopenic variant PPA	N/A
Response to cholinesterase inhibitors and memantine	Yes	Yes	No		Yes

Alzheimer's Disease

Clinical Features of Alzheimer's Disease

Alzheimer's disease (AD) is the most common neurodegenerative cause of dementia. AD most commonly presents after age 65, with the first and most prominent cognitive deficit being in memory, specifically memory for recent events (**episodic memory**). Patients may forget to do things they had planned to do (e.g., miss appointments), forget having done something, or forget a conversation. Other symptoms that may also be present initially or may emerge as the disease progresses include getting lost, decreased performance at work, word-finding difficulties, and neuropsychiatric changes such as depression and anxiety. The disease progresses inexorably toward a state of global dementia with patients generally losing an average of 3 points per year on the MMSE.

A small proportion of patients with Alzheimer's disease present before age 65, and these patients with early-onset Alzheimer's disease can have a different clinical phenotype than late-onset AD. Rather than memory impairment, prominent presenting symptoms can include deficits in language (e.g., logopenic primary progressive aphasia; see below), executive dysfunction, higher-order visual processing (including posterior cortical atrophy; see below), and/or behavioral changes (frontal variant AD, also known as behavioral dysexecutive variant AD). Patients with early-onset AD tend to present with a more rapidly progressive disease course and have more widespread cortical atrophy on MRI (often sparing the medial temporal lobe, which is predominantly affected in AD presenting after age 65; see below).

Most cases of AD are sporadic, although some are familial. Familial cases of AD usually begin at a younger age than sporadic cases. Inheritance of familial AD is autosomal dominant due to mutations in the amyloid precursor protein (APP), presenilin 1, or presenilin 2 genes that lead to overproduction of amyloid. Risk of development of Alzheimer's disease is increased in patients with the ε4 allele of apolipoprotein E (APOE). Patients with Down's syndrome also develop early AD since amyloid precursor protein is found on chromosome 21, and so it is present in triplicate in patients with trisomy 21.

Posterior cortical atrophy—In posterior cortical atrophy (also called the visual variant of AD and Benson syndrome), neurodegeneration occurs specifically in parieto-occipital regions, leading to visual cognitive deficits (e.g., elements of Balint syndrome and/or Gerstmann syndrome; see "Balint syndrome" in Ch. 6 and "Gerstmann syndrome" in Ch. 7). The underlying pathology is most commonly Alzheimer pathology, although posterior cortical atrophy can also be caused by other types of neurodegenerative pathology.

Neuroimaging and Laboratory Features of Alzheimer's Disease

MRI in AD usually demonstrates bilateral atrophy in medial temporal regions (hippocampus and entorhinal cortex) and the superior parietal lobe (Fig. 22–3). Nuclear medicine studies in AD show hypometabolism on positron emission tomography (PET) and reduced perfusion on single photon emission computed tomography (SPECT) in bilateral temporoparietal cortex, posterior cingulate cortex, and precuneus. Amyloid PET imaging to identify amyloid burden in the brain is currently mostly used in research settings (e.g., to determine eligibility for clinical trials).

In the cerebrospinal fluid (CSF), low Aβ42 and increased tau (leading to decreased Aβ42/tau ratio) can predict underlying Alzheimer pathology (plaques composed of amyloid and tangles composed of tau) in the appropriate clinical setting. Amyloid is presumably low in the CSF because it has accumulated in plaques in the brain.

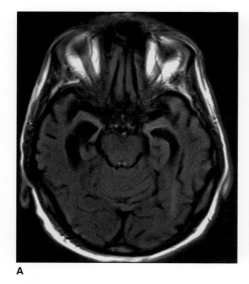 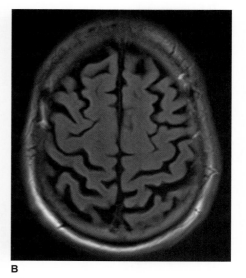

A   B

FIGURE 22–3 Alzheimer's disease. Axial MRI images showing marked bilateral hippocampal atrophy (**A**) and bilateral parietal more so than frontal cortical atrophy (**B**) in a patient with Alzheimer's disease.

Treatment of Alzheimer's Disease

Cholinesterase inhibitors (donepezil, rivastigmine, galantamine) and the N-methyl-D-aspartate (NMDA) antagonist memantine may provide modest symptomatic benefit in cognition in patients with AD. Gastrointestinal side effects can occur with the cholinesterase inhibitors. A common treatment strategy in patients with AD is to use a cholinesterase inhibitor initially (if tolerated), and to add memantine as patients progress to moderate/severe dementia. Otherwise, care of patients with AD is supportive. It should be noted that antipsychotics carry a boxed (black box) warning for increased risk of death when used in patients with dementia, so risks and benefits of utilizing antipsychotics for treatment of psychosis in patients with dementia must be carefully considered and discussed with the patient and their family/caretaker.

Dementia With Lewy Bodies

Clinical Features of Dementia With Lewy Bodies

Dementia with Lewy bodies (DLB) is one of the Parkinson-plus syndromes along with multiple systems atrophy, progressive supranuclear palsy, and corticobasal degeneration (see Ch. 23). These are all diseases in which there are parkinsonian symptoms along with other types of neurologic dysfunction. In addition to dementia characterized by initial deficits in visuospatial and executive function, patients with DLB develop parkinsonism, visual hallucinations (usually nonthreatening hallucinations of people or animals), and fluctuations in attention and level of arousal. History of rapid eye movement (REM) sleep behavior disorder is common (as in other synucleinopathies; see "Nonmotor Symptoms in Parkinson's Disease" in Ch. 23), and neuroleptic sensitivity (worsened parkinsonism and/or cognition with administration of neuroleptics) and autonomic dysfunction (orthostasis, constipation, incontinence, sexual dysfunction) are frequently present.

Patients with Parkinson's disease (see "Parkinson's Disease" in Ch. 23) can develop dementia over the course of the disease. DLB is generally distinguished from Parkinson's disease dementia by the following clinical features: Patients with DLB develop symptoms and signs of dementia before or simultaneously with features of parkinsonism (in Parkinson's disease dementia, parkinsonism usually precedes dementia by years), parkinsonism in DLB is usually symmetric (in Parkinson's disease, parkinsonism usually begins asymmetrically), parkinsonism in DLB is usually less responsive to levodopa (or may not respond at all) compared to patients with Parkinson's disease (whose parkinsonism generally responds to levodopa).

Neuroimaging Features of Dementia With Lewy Bodies

There is no characteristic pattern of atrophy on structural imaging in DLB, but nuclear imaging may show hypometabolism/hypoperfusion in occipital and temporoparietal regions (compared to just temporoparietal hypometabolism/hypoperfusion in AD). Dopamine transporter scanning in DLB shows decreased uptake in the basal ganglia, which confirms a degenerative parkinsonian disease but does not distinguish between DLB and other parkinsonian conditions (e.g., Parkinson's disease, Parkinson's-plus syndromes; see Ch. 23). Reduced uptake on MIBG myocardial scintigraphy is supportive of the diagnosis of DLB (demonstrating autonomic involvement in the heart).

Treatment of Dementia With Lewy Bodies

As in AD, cholinesterase inhibitors and memantine may be useful in symptomatic management of cognitive dysfunction in DLB. As in the other Parkinson-plus syndromes, there is usually little or no response to dopaminergic therapies (in contrast to Parkinson's disease), but if parkinsonism is a prominent disabling feature in a patient with DLB, a trial of levodopa can be considered. Symptomatic treatment can be considered for mood, REM sleep behavior disorder (melatonin or clonazepam), and autonomic dysfunction (fludrocortisone, midodrine, droxidopa). Pimavanserin or other antipsychotics (quetiapine, clozapine) may be considered for hallucinations and psychosis, but note the boxed (black box) warning regarding antipsychotic use increasing mortality in patients with dementia, requiring careful consideration and discussion of risk and benefit.

Frontotemporal Dementia

Frontotemporal dementia (FTD) includes two categories of dementia syndromes: behavioral variant FTD (bvFTD) and primary progressive aphasia (PPA). As the names suggest, bvFTD is characterized by personality changes and neuropsychiatric dysfunction, and PPA is characterized by language deficits. Behavioral and personality changes in bvFTD can include anything from apathy to disinhibition, and from social withdrawal to socially deviant behavior. Patients generally lack insight into the changes in their personality and behavior. Other common features include loss of empathy, obsessive compulsive or perseverative behaviors, and executive dysfunction. PPA has three variants with particular language deficits: nonfluent/agrammatic, semantic, and logopenic (Table 22–2). Neuroimaging in FTD shows selective frontotemporal atrophy (Fig. 22–4) that may be very focal within language areas in PPA.

The most common underlying pathologic findings in FTD are tau, TDP-43, and FUS, with the exception of the logopenic variant of PPA, in which Alzheimer's pathology is most common. Most cases of FTD are sporadic, although inherited cases occur (due to mutations in C9orf72, GRN, or MAPT genes). bvFTD was previously referred to as Pick disease, but this term now refers to a specific pathological subtype (Pick bodies comprised of tau inclusions). Some patients develop syndromes of overlap of FTD with motor neuron disease, corticobasal degeneration, or progressive supranuclear palsy. Treatment is symptomatic/supportive. Selective serotonin reuptake inhibitors (SSRIs) may be helpful in managing the psychiatric symptoms of bvFTD. Unlike patients with AD or

TABLE 22–2 Clinical Features of the Primary Progressive Aphasias.[a]

	Agrammatic (Nonfluent)	Semantic	Logopenic
Expression	*Agrammatic* *Effortful* Errors in sound production	Fluent	*Slow, impaired word retrieval* *Preserved grammar* *Phonologic errors*
Comprehension	*Impaired for phrases with complex syntax*	*Impaired for single words*	Impaired (worse for longer phrases)
Repetition	Impaired	Preserved	*Impaired for sentences (single word repetition may be preserved)*
Naming	Can be impaired	*Severely impaired*	Impaired
Reading/Writing	May be preserved relative to spontaneous speech early	Surface dyslexia/dysgraphia (difficulty reading/writing irregular words [e.g., brought])	Preserved but may make phonologic errors
Region of atrophy/ hypometabolism	Broca's area/left insula	Anterior temporal (left > right)	Left temporoparietal
Most common pathology	Tau, TDP-43	TDP-43	Alzheimer pathology

[a]Core findings for each condition are italicized.

DLB, patients with FTD do not appear to benefit from cholinesterase inhibitors.

Vascular Dementia

Vascular dementia refers to impaired cognitive function due to cerebral infarction. This may be due to accumulation of cognitive deficits from serial strokes in a stepwise manner, more insidious with chronic accumulation of subcortical microvascular disease, sudden after single infarction that impairs cognition (referred to as **strategic infarction;** e.g., thalamic, PCA (affecting medial temporal lobe), ACA), or some combination of these. Clinical signs depend upon site(s) of prior infarction, but executive dysfunction and cognitive slowing are common, and focal features, upper motor neuron signs, parkinsonism, and/or pseudobulbar affect may be

present. In cases of insidious cognitive decline and evidence of both atrophy and subcortical white matter disease on neuroimaging, the differentiation between AD, vascular dementia, and overlap of the two may not be possible. There may be some benefit of cholinesterase inhibitors and memantine in vascular dementia as in AD, so a medication trial may be attempted in ambiguous or presumed overlap cases. Secondary stroke prevention is of course important as in any patient with prior stroke (see "Secondary Prevention of Ischemic Stroke" in Ch. 19).

Normal Pressure Hydrocephalus

Although not a neurodegenerative disease, normal pressure hydrocephalus (NPH) is discussed here since it should be considered in the differential diagnosis of patients presenting

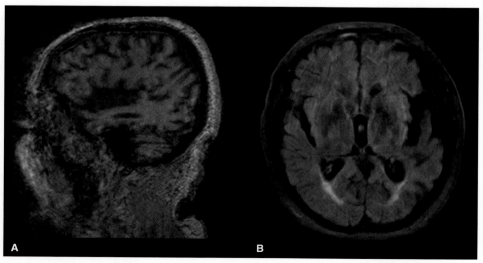

FIGURE 22–4 MRI in frontotemporal dementia. Sagittal (**A**) and axial (**B**) T1-weighted images demonstrating marked left frontotemporal atrophy. Note the widening of the insula (**A**) and the "knife edge" atrophy of the left temporal lobe (**B**).

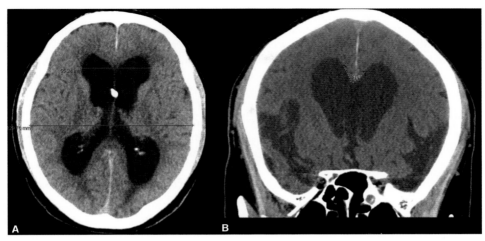

FIGURE 22–5 **Neuroimaging in normal pressure hydrocephalus. A.** Axial CT demonstrating ventriculomegaly with an Evans ratio of 55.24/129.76 = 0.43. **B.** Coronal CT demonstrating a decreased callosal angle, enlarged Sylvian fissures, and crowding of the superior frontal gyri (DESH; see text).

with dementia. The predominant symptoms of NPH are gait dysfunction, urinary urgency/incontinence, and dementia. In this condition, ventricular enlargement leads to frontal lobe dysfunction, and CSF diversion by ventriculoperitoneal (VP) shunt can lead to improvement. NPH may be idiopathic or can be caused by impaired CSF circulation due to prior subarachnoid hemorrhage or meningitis.

In most patients with NPH, gait dysfunction is the first sign of the disorder, and dementia and urinary urgency/incontinence emerge later in the course of the condition. The classic gait pattern in NPH is wide based and "magnetic": The feet appear to be magnetically drawn back to the floor as soon as they are lifted. (Note that severe proprioceptive dysfunction due to large-fiber neuropathy, sensory ganglionopathy, or posterior column dysfunction can also cause a magnetic gait). The walking problem in NPH is due to dysfunction of higher order control of gait, and is not due to weakness or incoordination. This can be demonstrated by having the patient bicycle the legs in bed. Bicycling movements require strength and coordination and are usually normal in NPH in marked contrast to the very impaired gait.

The diagnosis of NPH is suggested by the clinical picture in conjunction with radiologic evidence of ventriculomegaly out of proportion to cerebral atrophy. With aging and/or dementia, there is cerebral atrophy and subsequent *ex vacuo* dilatation of the ventricles to fill the remaining space. This must be distinguished from ventricular enlargement due to hydrocephalus. One way to quantify ventriculomegaly is to calculate the **Evans ratio**, calculated by measurements on axial neuroimaging. The Evans ratio is calculated by dividing the largest "wingspan" of the frontal horns of the lateral ventricles by the maximum horizontal width between the left and right inner table of the skull on the same axial slice (Fig. 22–5A). An Evans ratio greater than 0.3 demonstrates ventriculomegaly, but is nonspecific and must be interpreted in relation to cerebral atrophy causing ex vacuo ventricular dilatation.

A useful radiologic pattern that distinguishes NPH from ex vacuo ventricular dilatation due to atrophy is the finding of **disproportionately enlarged subarachnoid space hydrocephalus (DESH):** In NPH, the Sylvian fissures are enlarged, but the high convexity gyri are tightly crowded medially/superiorly (best noted on coronal sections; see Fig. 22–5B). The finding of gyral crowding superiorly in NPH contrasts with expected sulcal widening due to atrophy. Another radiologic measure to assess for NPH is the callosal angle, which is the angle between the frontal horns of the lateral ventricles on a coronal image at the level of the posterior commissure (normal is ~110°; in patients with NPH, the angle is generally less than 90° as hydrocephalic enlargement of the ventricles "squeezes" them closer together).

Diagnosis of NPH is made by noting improvement of gait and/or cognitive function after a large-volume lumbar puncture or continuous lumbar drainage of spinal fluid. Improvement with one of these tests suggests a likely response to placement of a VP shunt, although even some patients who do not improve with lumbar puncture or lumbar drain may still improve with a VP shunt. This leads to challenging clinical decision making since the differential diagnosis may be between AD with no disease-modifying treatment and the possibility of NPH that could respond to VP shunt (but with the inherent risks of complications of shunt placement; see "Ventriculoperitoneal Shunt" in Ch. 25). In NPH, gait dysfunction is generally more likely to improve with a VP shunt than cognitive impairment, and improvement may be transient (for insightful discussion of challenges related to NPH diagnosis, see: Espay et al., 2017).

RAPIDLY PROGRESSIVE DEMENTIA

Dementia usually arises gradually and is ongoing for months to years by the time patients present for evaluation. When onset and evolution of dementia are more rapid, the condition is referred to as rapidly progressive dementia. Creutzfeldt-Jakob disease is the quintessential rapidly progressive dementia, but the differential diagnosis for this condition is broad and includes many treatable etiologies (Geschwind et al., 2008; Chitravas et al., 2011):

- Inflammatory conditions:
  - Antibody-mediated/paraneoplastic limbic encephalitis (see "Autoimmune Limbic Encephalitis" in Ch. 24)
  - Hashimoto encephalopathy (see "Hashimoto Encephalopathy")
  - CNS vasculitis (see "Cerebral Vasculitis" in Ch. 19)
  - Demyelinating disease (see Ch. 21)
  - Neurosarcoidosis
- Atypically rapid courses of neurodegenerative diseases such as Alzheimer's disease, frontotemporal dementia, dementia with Lewy bodies, corticobasal syndrome
- Malignancy
  - Multiple parenchymal metastases or leptomeningeal metastases (see "Brain Metastases" and "Leptomeningeal Metastases" in Ch. 24)
  - Frontal lobe tumor
  - Diffusely infiltrating tumor (e.g., gliomatosis cerebri; see "Gliomas" in Ch. 24)
  - Intravascular lymphoma (see "Intravascular Lymphoma" in Ch. 19)
- Chronic infections
  - AIDS (see "HIV Dementia and Hiv-Associated Neurocognitive Disorders" in Ch. 20)
  - Neurosyphilis
- Toxins
  - Heavy metal poisoning
  - Chronic alcohol use
- Metabolic etiologies
  - Hepatic dysfunction
  - Chronic renal failure
  - Hyperammonemia (e.g., due to valproic acid or urea cycle disorder)
- Vascular etiologies:
  - Subclinical infarctions leading to accumulated burden of infarcted tissue as can occur in hypercoagulable states, CNS vasculitis, intravascular lymphoma, cerebral autosomal dominant arteriopathy with subcortical infarcts and leukoencephalopathy (CADASIL) (see Ch. 19)
- Adult-onset leukodystrophies (see Ch. 31)

Many of these potential etiologies of rapidly progressive dementia can be discovered (or exonerated) by neuroimaging studies. A normal contrast-enhanced MRI requires extensive evaluation for potentially treatable systemic causes including complete metabolic panel, complete blood count, vitamin B12, HIV, rapid plasma reagin (RPR), erythrocyte sedimentation rate (ESR), C-reactive protein

(CRP), autoimmune studies (antinuclear antibodies [ANA], anti-Ro, anti-La), paraneoplastic antibodies, and antithyroid peroxidase (anti-TPO) and antithyroglobulin (anti-TG) (for Hashimoto's encephalopathy; see "Hashimoto's Encephalopathy"), as well as consideration of lumbar puncture to evaluate for inflammation, infection, and/or antibodies in the CSF. When MRI abnormalities are present but nonspecific (e.g., white matter lesions that could represent inflammatory disease versus neoplasm), brain biopsy may be necessary to make a diagnosis.

Creutzfeldt-Jakob Disease

Creutzfeldt-Jakob disease (CJD) is caused by accumulation of prions in the brain, leading to rapidly progressive dementia. Most cases are sporadic (sCJD) (i.e., no clear cause), although some cases are familial (familial CJD [fCJD], fatal familial insomnia, Gerstmann-Straussler-Scheinker syndrome), and some have been caused by consumption of infected beef (variant CJD [vCJD]) or by iatrogenic transmission (iCJD) from infected neurosurgical instruments, corneal transplants, and human growth hormone. Dementia in CJD can affect any/all cognitive domains and may begin with personality/psychiatric changes. Myoclonus (particularly startle-induced myoclonus) is common, but this finding may be absent in CJD and is nonspecific since myoclonus can be seen in other etiologies of progressively altered cognition (e.g., renal failure, Alzheimer's disease, corticobasal syndrome, or medication-induced encephalopathy; see "Myoclonus" in Ch. 23). Some cases of CJD begin with isolated visual symptoms (**Heidenhain variant**).

MRI in sCJD demonstrates diffusion restriction in the cortical ribbon and basal ganglia, and this finding is highly sensitive and specific for sCJD in the context of rapidly progressive dementia (Vitali et al., 2011) (Fig. 22–6). (These findings are not seen in vCJD, which classically shows abnormalities in the pulvinar of the thalamus on FLAIR sequence.) The MRI features of CJD may not be present early in the disease, and may emerge only on subsequent repeat imaging as the disease progresses. Diffusion restriction in the cortical ribbon can also be seen in status epilepticus and hypoxic-ischemic injury, but both are usually easily distinguished from CJD by history. Limbic regions are rarely affected in isolation in CJD, and if signal changes isolated to limbic regions are seen on MRI in a patient with rapidly progressive dementia, the possibility of an autoimmune or paraneoplastic limbic encephalitis should be pursued (see "Autoimmune Limbic Encephalitis" in Ch. 24).

Definitive diagnosis of sCJD is made by CSF RT-QUIC, an assay that detects misfolded prion protein. CSF RT-QUIC is nearly 100% specific but not 100% sensitive, so false negatives can occur (Hermann et al., 2021). Lumbar puncture is also important to evaluate for potential alternative etiologies of rapidly progressive dementia that might be treatable (e.g., immune-mediated conditions). CSF in sCJD may show elevated protein, but elevated CSF WBC is uncommon and should lead to consideration of alternative diagnoses (e.g., inflammatory or infectious).

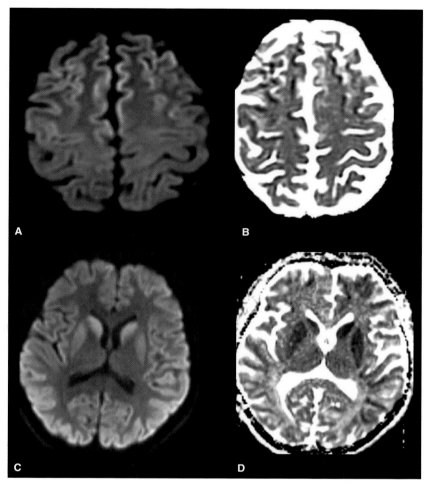

FIGURE 22-6 **MRI in sporadic Creutzfeldt-Jakob disease.** Axial DWI (**A** and **C**) and ADC (**B** and **D**) sequences demonstrating diffusion restriction in the cortical ribbon as well as in the basal ganglia (**C** and **D**).

In sCJD, CSF 14-3-3 protein and periodic sharp-wave complexes on EEG may be present, but both sensitivity and specificity of these findings are much lower than the sensitivity and specificity of RT-QUIC and even MRI, and the presence of CSF 14-3-3 and periodic sharp-wave complexes on EEG may vary over the course of the disease.

Unfortunately, there is currently no effective treatment for CJD, so care is supportive. Patients generally do not survive for more than approximately 1 year from the time of diagnosis.

Hashimoto's Encephalopathy

Hashimoto's encephalopathy is an immune-mediated CNS disorder associated with anti-TPO and/or anti-TG antibodies that responds to immunmodulatory therapy. The condition is also known as steroid-responsive encephalopathy associated with autoimmune thyroiditis (SREAT). Despite the name and the association with anti-thyroid antibodies, there is no clear relationship to thyroid disease, and many patients with Hashimoto's encephalopathy have normal thyroid function. The relationship between the disorder and the antibodies is unclear, especially since healthy older individuals may have elevated titers of these antibodies with no clinical correlate.

Hashimoto's encephalopathy generally presents as a rapidly progressive dementia (over weeks to months). Some cases may present with stroke-like episodes without MRI evidence of stroke. Seizures and myoclonus can occur.

MRI is normal in most cases of Hashimoto's encephalopathy, but may show nonspecific T2/FLAIR hyperintensities. CSF is inflammatory (elevated protein and lymphocytic pleocytosis) in most cases, although it can be normal. Inflammatory CSF in the setting of a rapid decline in cognition and a normal MRI can also occur in autoimmune or paraneoplastic limbic encephalitis (see "Autoimmune Limbic Encephalitis" in Ch. 24).

Many patients with Hashimoto's encephalopathy demonstrate dramatic improvement with steroids. If there is a high index of suspicion for the disorder and no (or minimal) response to steroids, more aggressive immunomodulatory therapy can be considered and may lead to clinical improvement in some patients. With the continued discovery of novel antibodies causing autoimmune encephalitis (see Ch. 24), recent data suggest that Hashimoto encephalopathy may not be a specific entity but a broader term for a heterogeneous group of autoimmune encephalitides with as yet undetermined underlying pathology, and that the antithyroid antibodies may merely reflect concurrent subclinical autoimmune thyroiditis (Mattozzi et al., 2020).

REFERENCES

Bhattacharyya S, Darby RR, Raibagkar P, Gonzalez Castro LN, Berkowitz AL. Antibiotic-associated encephalopathy. *Neurol* 2016;86:963–971.

Chitravas N, Jung RS, Kofskey DM, Blevins JE, Gambetti P, Leigh RJ, et al. Treatable neurologic disorders misdiagnosed as Creutzfeldt-Jakob disease. *Ann Neurol* 2011;70:437–444.

Espay AJ et al. Deconstructing normal pressure hydrocephalus: ventriculomegaly as early sign of neurodegeneration. *Ann Neurol*; 2017;82:503–513.

Geschwind MD, Shu H, Haman A, Sejvar JJ, Miller BL. Rapidly progressive dementia. *Ann Neurol* 2008;64:97–108.

Hermann P, Appleby B, Brandel JP, Caughey B, Collins S, Geschwind MD, et al. Biomarkers and diagnostic guidelines for sporadic Creutzfeldt-Jakob Disease. *Lancet Neurol* 2021; 20:235–246.

Mattozzi S, Sabater L, Escudero D, Arino H, Armangue T, Simabukuro M, et al. Hashimoto encephalopathy in the 21st century. *Neurol* 2020;94(2):e217–e224.

Vitali P, Maccagnano E, Caverzasi E, Henry RG, Haman A, Torres-Chae C, et al. Diffusion-weighted MRI hyperintensity patterns differentiate CJD from other rapid dementias. *Neurology* 2011;76:1711–1719.

Movement Disorders

INTRODUCTION TO MOVEMENT DISORDERS

In most realms of neurologic disease, localization is the first step toward differential diagnosis. In assessing movement disorders, however, the first step is to accurately characterize the type of abnormal movement(s) present, each of which has its own differential diagnosis. The differential diagnosis for movement disorders can generally be divided into the following four broad categories, with each movement disorder having particular etiologies in each category (Table 23–1):

- Primary neurologic diseases
- Structural neurologic lesions
- Systemic conditions
- Medication/drug-induced

Any category of movement disorder can also have a functional etiology, meaning it cannot be explained by a known underlying neurologic disease (previously called "psychogenic" movement disorders; see "Functional Movement Disorders").

Movement disorders are broadly classified as either **hyperkinetic** (increased movement: tremor, chorea, myoclonus, dystonia, tics) or **hypokinetic** (decreased movement: bradykinesia as is seen in parkinsonism). In general, a unilateral movement disorder suggests a structural lesion, whereas a bilateral movement disorder suggests a systemic, toxic, or degenerative cause, but there are many exceptions: hyperglycemic chorea is often unilateral; Parkinson's disease and corticobasal syndrome are often unilateral at onset and remain asymmetric throughout the disease course.

TABLE 23–1 Characteristics & Common Differential Diagnoses of Movement Disorders.

	Movement	Causes			
		Primary Neurologic Diseases	Structural or Vascular Lesions	Medications/Drugs	Systemic Conditions
Tremor	Oscillating movements	Essential tremor Parkinson's disease Wilson's disease	Red nucleus Cerebellum	Lithium Antiepileptics SSRIs Beta-agonists Tacrolimus Alcohol withdrawl	Hyperthyroidism
Parkinsonism	Resting tremor Bradykinesia Rigidity	Parkinson's disease Multiple systems atrophy Progressive supra-nuclear palsy Corticobasal syndrome	Basal ganglia	Antipsychotics Dopamine-blocking antiemetics	Extrapontine myelinolysis
Myoclonus	Lightening-like jerks	Myoclonic epilepsies Corticobasal degeneration Creutzfeldt-Jakob disease DRPLA (juvenile-onset form) Any neurodegenerative disease	Diffuse cortical injury Spinal cord injury Guillain-Mollaret triangle for palatal myoclonus	Dopamine agonists and levodopa Amantadine Antiepileptics SSRIs Opiates Cephalosporins Lithium Benzodiazepine withdrawal	Renal failure Hypoxic-ischemic insult (e.g., cardiac arrest)
Chorea/ athetosis/ ballism	Sinuous dance-like movements (chorea), erratic large-amplitude movements (ballism)	Huntington's disease Neuroacanthocytosis PKAN DRPLA (adult-onset form)	Subthalamic nucleus (for hemiballismus) Basal ganglia for chorea	Dopamine agonists and levodopa Oral contraceptives Antiepileptics Cocaine	Sydenham's chorea Lupus Antiphospholipid antibody syndrome Polycythemia vera Hyperthyroidism Hyperglycemia (often unilateral) Post-cardiac surgery (post-pump chorea)
Dystonia	Sustained, often twisted postures	Cervical dystonia Focal dystonia Dystonia syndromes (DYT1 through DYT25)	Basal ganglia	Antipsychotics Dopamine-blocking antiemetics	
Tics	Brief fully formed movements or vocalizations	Tourette's syndrome Transient tics Neuroacanthocytosis		Cocaine Antipsychotics	

Abbreviations: DRPLA: dentatorubral-pallidoluysian atrophy; PKAN: pantothenate kinase–associated neurodegeneration; SSRIs: selective serotonin reuptake inhibitors.

TABLE 23-2 Characteristics of Tremors.

	Frequency	Amplitude	State(s)	Body Part(s) Affected	Associated Features
Physiologic tremor	High	Low	Postural/action	Hands	Possible trigger such as anxiety, caffeine, hypoglycemia, hyperthyroidism
Essential tremor	Variable	Variable	Postural/action (Can have intentional component)	Hands Head Voice	May improve with alcohol
Parkinsonian tremor	Moderate	Moderate	Rest predominantly, but can reemerge w/posture	Hands Jaw/chin	Bradykinesia Rigidity Postural instability
Cerebellar tremor	Moderate	Moderate	Action/intention	Limbs Sometimes head at rest (titubation)	Nystagmus Ataxia Dysdiadochokinesia
Rubral (Holmes) tremor	Low	Moderate	Rest/postural/action	Limbs	Ipsilateral ataxia and/or Weakness and/or Contralateral cranial nerve 3 palsy
Orthostatic tremor	High	Low	Standing	Legs	None

TREMOR (TABLE 23-2)

Tremor refers to rhythmic oscillation (i.e., shaking) of one or more parts of the body. Tremor can be characterized by:

- Body part(s) affected by tremor
- Frequency: speed of oscillation of tremor
- Amplitude: distance of excursion of tremor
- The state(s) of the body part in which the tremor is observed—rest, posture, and/or action:
  - **Rest tremor** emerges when the affected body part is inactive
  - **Postural tremor** is observed when a posture is sustained against gravity (e.g., the arms and hands outstretched)
  - **Kinetic** or **action tremor** occurs with movement, and can be further characterized by whether the tremor is the same throughout the range of movement or worsens as the affected limb approaches a target (**intention tremor**).

Enhanced Physiologic Tremor

Enhanced physiologic tremor is the augmentation of a baseline tremor that is present in everyone but usually not apparent. This can be brought out or accentuated by emotional states (e.g., anxiety, fear), metabolic states (e.g., hypoglycemia), endocrine conditions (e.g., hyperthyroidism), or caffeine.

Essential Tremor

Essential tremor is a condition that causes tremor in isolation without associated symptoms (i.e., no bradykinesia or rigidity

as seen in Parkinson's disease), and can be either familial or sporadic. Essential tremor almost always involves the hands, is most often symmetric (although may begin asymmetrically and remain asymmetric in some patients), and can also involve the voice and/or head (nodding "yes," "no," or side-to-side). The tremor is typically present with sustained posture and with action, but is typically absent at rest except in very severe cases. The tremulous movement of the hands in essential tremor is most commonly flexion-extension, as opposed to supination-pronation in Parkinson's disease. The frequency and amplitude may differ between patients but are generally constant within an individual patient, although the severity of tremor may worsen over time. Some patients report amelioration with alcohol. There are two peaks in age of onset in the 20s and 60s.

Symptomatic treatment for disabling essential tremor is with beta blockers (commonly propranolol) and/or primidone. Propranolol should be avoided if the patient has asthma or is already on other cardiac medications. Primidone can be sedating. Benzodiazepines, topiramate, gabapentin, and/or botulinum toxin can be considered if first-line medications are ineffective or not tolerated. In patients who have disabling essential tremor refractory to medical therapy, deep brain stimulation (of the ventral intermediate [VIM] nucleus of the thalamus) may be considered.

Parkinsonian Tremor

The tremor of Parkinson's disease or other parkinsonian syndromes is generally present at rest and resolves with intentional action. The tremor may also reemerge with sustained posture of the affected limb(s) (see "Tremor in Parkinson's Disease"). The most common site of tremor is in the hands, causing supination-pronation ("pill rolling") as opposed to the flexion-extension tremor of essential tremor. Tremor in Parkinson's disease can also involve the legs and jaw. Parkinsonian tremor is often associated with rigidity and bradykinesia in the tremulous limb(s).

Cerebellar Tremor

Cerebellar tremor is an oscillating action tremor that is generally absent at rest and emerges with action (intention tremor), most commonly oscillating perpendicular to the plane of intended movement. Associated cerebellar signs such as dysmetria, dysdiadochokinesia, nystagmus, dysarthria may also be present (see Ch. 8).

Rubral (Holmes) Tremor

Rubral (Holmes) tremor is a tremor caused by a lesion that disrupts the pathway involving the superior cerebellar peduncle, red nucleus of the midbrain, and ventrolateral (VL) nucleus of the thalamus (see "Superior Cerebellar Peduncles: Output Back to the Brain" in Ch. 8). Rubral tremor is typically a slow tremor present at rest that augments with posture and movement. The most common lesion location is in the midbrain where the superior cerebellar peduncle meets the red nucleus. Given this localization in the midbrain, associated contralateral hemiparesis, contralateral ataxia, and/or ipsilateral cranial nerve 3 palsy may be present (see "CN 3: The Oculomotor Nerve" in Ch. 11). Treatment options include carbidopa-levodopa, beta blockers, and antiepileptics; in severe refractory cases, deep brain stimulation may be considered.

Orthostatic Tremor

Orthostatic tremor is a rapid tremor of the legs that occurs only with standing and resolves upon sitting or walking. The tremor can be auscultated with a stethoscope on the thigh or calf, where a helicopter-like sound will be heard. Orthostatic tremor can be seen in isolation or may accompany Parkinson's disease or atypical parkinsonian syndromes (e.g., MSA, PSP, DLB, see below). Clonazepam is the most commonly used treatment, but if ineffective, gabapentin may be considered.

Functional Tremor

A functional tremor can be challenging to distinguish from the types of tremor discussed above. Clues to the diagnosis on history include sudden onset, maximal severity at onset, and a fluctuating course rather than the progressive course seen in degenerative causes of tremor or static course seen with a fixed structural lesion. On examination, the tremor may be variable in amplitude or frequency, disappear with distraction, and entrain to the rhythm of other movements (e.g., finger tapping in contralateral hand). Treatment is with cognitive behavioral therapy (see "Functional Movement Disorders").

Other Causes of Tremor

Other neurologic conditions associated with tremor include dystonia (see "Dystonia"), Wilson's disease (see "Wilson's Disease"), tardive tremor (see "Tardive Dyskinesia"), fragile X associated tremor ataxia syndrome (see Ch. 8), and peripheral neuropathy (e.g., CIDP).

As with all movement disorders, medications and systemic conditions must also be considered (Table 23–1). Tremors caused by medications and systemic conditions are most commonly symmetric, high-frequency, and worse with posture and action with the exception of tremors caused by antidopaminergic treatments, which are generally more parkinsonian in phenomenology.

MYOCLONUS

Myoclonus refers to rapid jerking movements. Myoclonus should not be confused with clonus, which is rhythmic contraction–relaxation seen in association with hyperreflexia with upper motor neuron lesions (see "Upper Motor Neuron Lesions Versus Lower Motor Neuron Lesions" in Ch. 4). Myoclonus generally affects a whole muscle, leading to obvious movement of a part of the body (distinguishing myoclonus from fasciculations, which are twitches of a few muscle fibers visible as movements beneath the skin). Asterixis is sometimes referred to as negative myoclonus, a sudden loss of tone causing a jerking movement.

Myoclonus can occur normally (physiologic myoclonus, e.g., when falling asleep [hypnic jerks]), or due to a range of neurologic diseases, systemic conditions, and medications (see Table 23–1). In practice, myoclonus is most commonly seen due to systemic conditions (e.g., renal failure, hypoxic-ischemic injury), medications, and toxins (e.g., bismuth). Primary neurologic conditions in which myoclonus can occur include:

- Essential myoclonus
- Epileptic conditions
  - Juvenile myoclonic epilepsy (JME)
  - Myoclonic epilepsy with ragged red fibers (MERRF)
  - Storage diseases (Lafora body disease, neuronal ceroid lipofuscinosis, sialidosis)
  - Unverricht-Lundborg syndrome
- Degenerative dementias
  - Creutzfeldt-Jackob disease (CJD)
  - Corticobasal syndrome (CBS)
  - While myoclonus is a common feature of CJD and CBS it can be seen in any neurodegenerative dementia (AD, DLB, etc.)
- Immune-mediated
  - Opsoclonus-myoclonus associated with neuroblastoma in children and anti-Ri antibodies in adults (most commonly seen with breast and lung cancers in adults) (see "Opsoclonus-Myoclonus" in Ch. 24)
  - Hashimoto encephalopathy

- Infectious (herpes simplex virus, subacute sclerosing panencephalitis)
- Myoclonus-dystonia (DYT11)
- Structural lesions
  - Guillain-Mollaret triangle leading to palatal myoclonus (see below)
  - Spinal lesions
    - **Segmental** (affecting a particular muscle or muscle group)
    - **Propriospinal** (causing axial myoclonus that may lead to torso flexion)
  - Peripheral: For example, hemifacial spasm (see "Hemifacial Spasm")

Myoclonus can be classified by clinical etiology (physiologic, essential, epileptic, secondary/symptomatic) and underlying physiology determined by EEG-EMG correlation (cortical, cortical-subcortical, subcortical-nonsegmental, segmental, peripheral). Cortical myoclonus may be triggered by action or touch whereas subcortical myoclonus may be triggered by startle.

Palatal myoclonus (sometimes referred to as palatal tremor) may be idiopathic (essential palatal myoclonus) or due to a lesion in the **Guillain-Mollaret triangle**: dentate nucleus of cerebellum–(superior cerebellar peduncle)→contralateral red nucleus–(central tegmental tract)→ipsilateral inferior olive–(inferior cerebellar peduncle)→contralateral dentate nucleus (i.e., back to dentate nucleus where the triangle began). In such cases, hypertrophy of the inferior olive in the medulla may be seen on neuroimaging. Palatal myoclonus may be accompanied by rhythmic eye movements (oculopalatal myoclonus/tremor) and the patient may report a persistent clicking sound.

Diffuse myoclonus may be seen in the acute period after anoxic brain injury, and myoclonic status epilepticus is often associated with a poor prognosis in this context. **Lance-Adams syndrome** refers to the delayed emergence of action-induced myoclonus during recovery after anoxic brain injury. In Lance-Adams syndrome, there is no or minimal myoclonus at rest, but attempted action triggers myoclonic jerks of the active limb(s).

Treatment of Myoclonus

When there is a clear reversible underlying cause of myoclonus (e.g., renal failure), this should be treated. Any potentially causative medications should be discontinued if possible. For symptomatic control of myoclonus, levetiracetam, valproate, and clonazepam can be used.

CHOREA

Chorea refers to irregular dance-like movements (same etymologic root as choreography). Chorea exists on a continuum with **athetosis** (slow sinuous movements) and **ballism**

(larger amplitude often more violent-appearing movements). Sometimes choreiform movements may be subtle, appearing as "fidgeting" and disguised by incorporation into voluntary movements (**parakinesia**). Other features seen in patients with chorea include motor impersistence (which can be demonstrated by inability to keep the tongue protruded such that it darts in and out of the mouth, or in milkmaid grip) and hung-up reflexes (delayed relaxation after eliciting tendon reflex). Chorea may be seen in the following conditions:

- Hereditary neurologic diseases
  - Huntington's disease
  - Dentatorubral-pallidoluysian atrophy (DRPLA)
  - Neuroacanthocytosis
  - Pantothenate kinase–associated neurodegeneration (PKAN)
  - Some of the spinocerebellar ataxias (SCA2, SCA3, SCA17)
  - Wilson's disease
- Structural lesion of the basal ganglia
  - Tumor
  - Infection: toxoplasmosis has a predilection for the basal ganglia
  - Stroke: stroke in the subthalamic nucleus is associated with contralateral hemiballismus
- Systemic diseases
  - Immune-mediated
    - Sydenham's chorea (poststreptococcal/rheumatic fever)
    - Lupus
    - Antiphospholipid antibody syndrome
    - Antibody-mediated: anti-CRMP5, anti-NMDA, anti-IGLON5, others (see Ch. 24)
  - Metabolic: hyperglycemia (often unilateral and associated with contralateral T1 hyperintensity in the basal ganglia on MRI), hyperthyroidism
  - Post-cardiac surgery: post-pump chorea (more common in children)
  - Polycythemia vera
- Pregnancy: chorea gravidarum
- Medications: dopaminergic therapy for Parkinson's disease, oral contraceptives
- Drugs: cocaine
- Congenital: choreoathetotic cerebral palsy

Sydenham's Chorea

Sydenham's chorea occurs months following infection with group A beta-hemolytic streptococcus in children. The other features of rheumatic fever (carditis and arthritis) are not always present. Accompanying behavioral changes including obsessive-compulsive disorder are common. Anti-streptolysin O should be checked but can be normal when chorea emerges months after rheumatic fever. Symptoms usually resolve over months, but some practitioners utilize steroids in severe cases. Sydenham's chorea may recur, so penicillin prophylaxis is often administered until adulthood.

Hereditary Causes of Chorea

The most common hereditary cause of chorea is Huntington's disease. Rarer hereditary causes of chorea include neuroacanthocytosis, McLeod syndrome, and pantothenate kinase–associated neurodegeneration.

Huntington's Disease

Huntington's disease is an autosomal dominantly inherited condition causing chorea and neuropsychiatric symptoms (e.g., dementia, depression, psychosis). Chorea is generally widespread throughout the body, but presence of forehead chorea is characteristic. As the illness progresses, chorea can give way to parkinsonism. Additional examination findings include motor impersistence of the tongue (inability to keep the tongue protruded such that it darts in and out of the mouth) and slowed or absent saccades. Neuroimaging may demonstrate caudate atrophy. Definitive diagnosis is made by genetic testing, and requires genetic counseling of the patient and family since the disease is dominantly inherited. Huntington's disease is caused by a CAG repeat in the *huntingtin* gene (chromosome 4), and increasing repeat length leads to the phenomenon of anticipation such that the disease presents at an earlier age of onset in subsequent generations. Treatment is largely supportive and symptomatic. Treatment options for chorea include tetrabenazine and deutetrabenazine (both of which decrease presynaptic dopamine release) and antipsychotics.

A juvenile form of Huntington's disease (**Westphal variant**) is characterized by parkinsonism, dystonia, and seizures rather than chorea.

Dentatorubral-Pallidoluysian Atrophy

Dentatorubral-pallidoluysian atrophy (DRPLA) is an autosomal dominantly inherited condition caused by a CAG repeat in the *atrophin 1* gene (chromosome 12), leading to degeneration of all of the structures listed in the name of the disease: dentate nucleus (dentato), red nucleus (rubral), globus pallidus (pallido), and the subthalamic nucleus (also known as the body of Luys). The adult-onset form of the disease (onset after age 20) is characterized by ataxia, chorea, and dementia. The juvenile-onset form of the disease (onset before age 20) causes seizures, myoclonus, ataxia, and intellectual disability (without chorea). Neuroimaging in DRPLA demonstrates cerebellar atrophy, brainstem atrophy (most prominent in the anterior pons), and subcortical white matter abnormalities. The disease is most common in Japan, although a variant has been described in an African-American family in North Carolina (**Haw River syndrome**).

Neuroacanthocytosis

Neuroacanthocytosis is an autosomal recessively inherited condition characterized by chorea, oral dystonias (causing biting of the tongue and lips as well as swallowing difficulties), neuropsychiatric symptoms, seizures, tics, neuropathy,

and/or parkinsonism with characteristic acanthocytes on blood smear (red cells with "spikes").

McLeod Syndrome

McLeod syndrome is an X-linked condition similar to neuroacanthocytosis, but may also be associated with myopathy and cardiomyopathy, and is less likely to have the oral dystonias characteristic of neuroacanthocytosis.

Pantothenate Kinase–Associated Neurodegeneration

Pantothenate kinase–associated neurodegeneration (PKAN), formerly called Hallervorden-Spatz disease, is an autosomal recessive disorder that is an example of a group of rare disorders classified as neurodegeneration with brain iron accumulation (NBIA). Patients with PKAN demonstrate both extrapyramidal features (dystonia, rigidity, chorea), pyramidal features, dysarthria, and dysphagia, most commonly beginning in childhood. The characteristic MRI signature is the "eye of the tiger sign" on T2-weighted imaging: T2 hyperintensity of the center of the globus pallidus interna surrounded by hypointensity (Fig. 23–1).

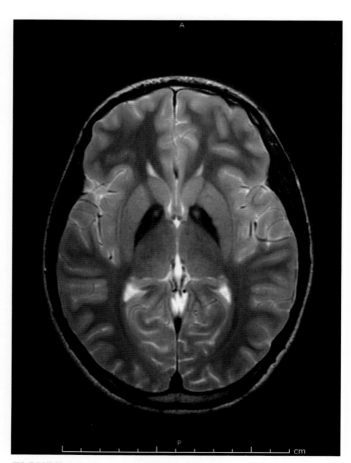

FIGURE 23–1 Pantothenate kinase-associated neurodegeneration. Axial T2-weighted MRI showing "eye of the tiger sign" (globus pallidus hyperintensity surrounded by hypointensity). (Reproduced with permission from Dr. Claudio De Gusmao.).

DYSTONIA

Dystonia refers to involuntary sustained (or paroxysmally sustained) postures of one or more body parts due to muscle contraction that often leads to twisting movements/postures of the affected limb(s). Tremor may accompany dystonia in some cases. Patients may describe maneuvers whereby touching the dystonic region lessens the dystonia, called a **sensory trick** (or **geste antagoniste**).

Dystonia can present in several ways:

- Dystonia may occur in isolation or as part of a syndrome with multiple additional features (e.g., corticobasal syndrome, neuroacanthocytosis, Wilson's disease)
- Dystonia may be focal (confined to one body part), segmental (confined to one limb), multifocal (more than one limb but not generalized), or generalized
- Dystonia may or may not be task-specific (e.g., writer's cramp or musician's dystonia)
- Dystonia may be primary (idiopathic or genetic) or may be secondary to:
  - Structural lesions of the basal ganglia: for example, infarct, trauma, neoplastic, or infectious. (Such lesions often lead to hemidystonia [i.e., dystonia on one side of the body.])
  - Drugs: for example, acute dystonic reaction or tardive dystonia with dopamine-blocking agents

In most cases, dystonia is most effectively treated with botulinum toxin injection, though clonazepam, baclofen, and trihexyphenidyl may be considered. Some dystonias may respond to levodopa. Deep brain stimulation is used in severe cases.

Rarely, patients with dystonia may develop **status dystonicus** (also known as dystonic storm), characterized by rapidly worsening continuous dystonia. This can be triggered by infection, medication change, or surgery/anesthesia. Status dystonicus can be complicated by rhabdomyolysis and respiratory failure, often requiring intubation, mechanical ventilation, sedation, and paralysis. If benzodiazepines and baclofen are ineffective in treating status dystonicus, deep brain stimulation or intrathecal baclofen pump may be considered. The differential diagnosis for status dystonicus includes neuroleptic malignant syndrome and malignant hyperthermia.

Focal Dystonias
Torticollis (Cervical Dystonia)
Torticollis is a common dystonia that causes neck twisting (**torticollis**), forward flexion (**anterocollis**), extension (**retrocollis**), or tilting to one side (**laterocollis**). Sensory tricks that may ameliorate the symptoms include touching the chin or neck. A head tremor may be associated. Botulinum toxin injection is first-line treatment.

Task-Specific Dystonias
Task-specific dystonias emerge only during the provocative activity: for example, writing in writer's cramp or playing a musical instrument in musician's dystonia (which may affect the hands or mouth depending on the instrument).

Blepharospasm
Blepharospasm is dystonia of the periorbital muscles leading to involuntary bilateral closure of the eyes. When disabling, botulinum toxin injected into the orbicularis oculi may be effective.

Laryngeal Dystonia (Spasmodic Dysphonia)
Vocal cord dystonia leads to changes in the voice. If the adductors are affected, patients develop interruptions in speech production particularly affecting vowel sounds. If the abductors are affected, patients develop a whispering, breathiness to their speech. In some patients both adductors and abductors are affected. Treatment is with speech therapy and botulinum toxin injection into affected vocal cord muscles.

Genetic Dystonias

An ever-increasing list of genetic dystonias (numbered DYT[x]; e.g., DYT1, DYT25) is emerging with different gene loci, inheritance patterns, geographic distribution, and clinical phenotype. Some of these syndromes cause an isolated dystonia, while others are accompanied by other movement disorders such as parkinsonism (DYT3, DYT5, DYT 12) or myoclonus (DYT11, DYT15). Nomenclature is moving away from numerical classification to classification based on the affected gene (e.g., DYT1 referred to as DYT-TOR1A). Some of the more common genetic dystonias include:

- DYT1 (DYT-TOR1A): an autosomal dominantly inherited childhood-onset dystonia that begins in one limb and subsequently generalizes, and is more common in (but not limited to) patients of Ashkenazi Jewish heritage.
- DYT3 (DYT-TAF1 or Lubag): an X-linked syndrome affecting Filipino men in which both dystonia and parkinsonism are present.
- DYT5 (DYT-GCH1 or Segawa syndrome): an autosomal dominantly inherited childhood-onset disorder in which dystonia of the lower extremities arises later in the day and may be absent after rest. Since the condition responds well to levodopa therapy it is sometimes referred to as **dopa-responsive dystonia**.

Acute Dystonic Reactions

Acute dystonic reactions are medication-induced dystonias that can affect any region of the body including the limbs, the eyes (**oculogyric crisis**), the neck (torticollis), the tongue, or the mouth. The most commonly implicated drugs are antidopaminergic agents such as antipsychotics and antiemetics. Acute dystonic reactions may occur after the first dose or within days of initiation of the offending medication. Treatment is with benztropine or diphenhydramine and discontinuation of the medication.

TICS, TOURETTE'S SYNDROME, & STEROTYPIES

Tics

Tics are brief movements (**motor tics**) or vocalizations (called either **phonic** or **vocal tics**), classified as simple or complex. Simple motor tics involve one muscle group (e.g., grimace, eye blink) whereas complex motor tics involve more than one muscle group and/or a sequence of movements, which may be purposeful or nonpurposeful. Simple phonic tics include grunting and throat-clearing, whereas complex phonic tics are words or phrases, including echolalia (repeating what others say) or coprolalia (cursing). Tics are generally preceded by a premonitory urge, able to be suppressed, and accompanied by a sense of relief after they occur. They may diminish with sustained attention on a task and may be aggravated by prolonged voluntary suppression. Tics can occur in the following clinical contexts:

- Tics can occur transiently (<1 year) in children (transient motor tics; transient phonic tics)
- Tics can occur as part of Tourette's syndrome, a primary tic disorder (see "Tourette's Syndrome" below)
- Tics can occur secondary to:
  - Drugs, including cocaine, antipsychotics, antiepileptics
  - Developmental disorders, including autism, fragile X syndrome
  - Neurodegenerative conditions, including neuroacanthocytosis

Tourette's Syndrome

Tourette's syndrome is a disorder in which tics are the primary feature. For diagnosis of Tourette's syndrome, both motor and phonic tics must have occurred for over 1 year beginning before age 18 (although most cases present at a much younger age), with changes in types of tics over time. Obsessive-compulsive disorder and/or attention deficit–hyperactivity disorder may co-occur with Tourette's syndrome, and so these conditions should be screened for and treated. Some cases resolve spontaneously in the transition to adulthood, whereas others persist. Treatment involves cognitive-behavioral therapy, and if severely disabling, medications such as alpha agonists (clonidine, guanfacine; both also effective for comorbid ADHD), antipsychotics (pimozide, haloperidol, aripiprazole, or fluphenazine), or dopamine-depleting agents (tetrabenazine) may be used.

Sterotypies

Sterotypies are repetitive purposeless movements, such as the rocking or spinning seen in patients with autism or the hand wringing seen in patients with Rett syndrome.

PARKINSONISM, PARKINSON'S DISEASE, & PARKINSON-PLUS SYNDROMES

Parkinson's disease (PD) is a neurodegenerative disease with the core features of tremor, bradykinesia, rigidity, and postural instability. Additional motor features include decreased facial expression (**hypomimia**), decreased blink rate, small handwriting (**micrographia**), stooped posture, shuffling gait with reduced arm swing, **festination** (increasingly rapid small steps), difficulty turning when walking, and difficulty turning over in bed. The constellation of some or all of these motor features is referred to as **parkinsonism**. In addition to idiopathic PD, other causes of parkinsonism include:

- Medications: most commonly antipsychotics and antiemetics (see "Drug-Induced Parkinsonism")
- Cerebrovascular disease (vascular parkinsonism)
- Toxins, including manganese and MPTP (1-methyl-4-phenyl-1,2,3,6-tetrahydropyridine) (MPTP may contaminate the illicit synthetic opioid MPPP [1-methyl-4-phenyl-propionoxypiperidine])
- Metabolic conditions such as extrapontine myelinolysis
- Neurodegenerative diseases aside from idiopathic PD, called the Parkinson-plus syndromes (see "Parkinson-Plus Syndromes"):
  - Multiple systems atrophy (MSA)
  - Progressive supranuclear palsy (PSP)
  - Corticobasal syndrome (CBS)
  - Dementia with Lewy bodies (DLB)

Parkinson's Disease

Clinical Features of Parkinson's Disease

Tremor, bradykinesia, and rigidity typically begin unilaterally in patients with idiopathic Parkinson's disease, but usually become bilateral as the disease progresses (although commonly remain asymmetric). Some patients may have a tremor-predominant form of the disease without much rigidity or gait dysfunction, some patients may have no tremor at all and have predominant bradykinesia and rigidity (akinetic-rigid form), and some patients may have predominant postural instability and gait dysfunction. The tremor-predominant form of PD may have a more benign course than other forms of the disease.

Although most cases of Parkinson's disease are idiopathic/sporadic, familial forms are associated with mutations in a growing number of genes including *LRRK2* (autosomal dominant) and *parkin* (*PARK2*; autosomal recessive with onset in youth).

Tremor in Parkinson's disease—The tremor of PD is most commonly a tremor of the hand(s) that is present at rest and resolves with movement, but may also reemerge after sustained posture (e.g., holding the arms and hands out straight). The tremor may be pill-rolling (supination-pronation movements of the fingers and thumb giving the impression that the patient is rolling a pill in the hand), but this is not always the case. Rest tremor may emerge when distracting the patient, for example, by asking the patient to perform serial seven subtractions. The tremor typically presents unilaterally and, although it may become bilateral throughout the course of the disease, it often remains asymmetric in its severity. Tremor of the jaw may also be present, but tremor of the head (as is seen in essential tremor) is not typically a feature of Parkinson's disease.

Bradykinesia in Parkinson's disease—Bradykinesia denotes slowing of movements. This may be evident in observing the patient's normal activities, and can be elicited on examination by testing finger tapping, foot tapping, or repeated pronation–supination movements ("as if screwing in a light bulb"). These movements should be tested one side at a time to avoid entrainment, which may mask asymmetries. Patients with bradykinesia will demonstrate both slowing of these movements and decreased amplitude (**hypokinesia**) of movement.

Rigidity in Parkinson's disease—The limb(s) of the body with tremor and/or bradykinesia may be noted to have **cogwheel rigidity**, whereby a joint appears to "click" through the passive range of motion rather than move smoothly when moved slowly through the range of motion by the examiner. This can be brought out by the technique of reinforcement, asking the patient to make circles or other repeated movements with the hand on the side opposite the limb being evaluated for rigidity. In idiopathic PD, rigidity is commonly asymmetric, affecting the limb(s) with tremor more so than the others. Axial rigidity can be evaluated for by moving the patient's neck passively through its range of motion.

Postural instability in Parkinson's disease—Postural instability tends to emerge later in the course of Parkinson's disease (although it may be present earlier in the course of progressive supranuclear palsy; see "Progressive Supranuclear Palsy"). Postural instability can be assessed using the **pull test** to look for **retropulsion**. The examiner stands behind the patient with the patient's back to the examiner, preferably with a wall behind the examiner to break a fall should one occur. The examiner then explains that she or he will be pulling briskly on the patient's shoulders and that the patient should maintain balance however necessary. After a brisk, forceful tug on the patient's shoulders, the patient's response is observed. Normally, a patient with intact postural stability will maintain balance with no steps or one or two steps backward. In a patient with postural instability due to parkinsonism, the patient will exhibit retropulsion, requiring several (more than three) small steps to regain balance; in severe cases, the patient will simply fall backward.

Gait in Parkinson's disease—Gait in PD is generally slow with small shuffling steps (**marche à petit pas**). Arm swing is usually diminished (usually more prominently on the side of greater tremor and/or rigidity). Turning is often difficult, requiring a number of small steps to turn. Some patients may start walking slowly and then accelerate with increasingly rapid small steps (**festination**). In advanced PD, some patients may develop freezing of gait, freezing in place and unable to proceed. Freezing may be able to be overcome by a visual stimulus (e.g., a line on the ground).

Other signs in Parkinson's disease—When tapping slowly and rhythmically between the eyes, normal individuals will blink several times and then stop blinking. Patient's with Parkinson's disease may not extinguish the blink response and continue to blink with each tap, called **Myerson's sign** or the **glabellar sign**.

Nonmotor symptoms in Parkinson's disease—Nonmotor features of PD include fatigue, pain, depression, anxiety, dementia, autonomic dysfunction (including constipation, orthostatic hypotension, urinary dysfunction), decreased sense of smell, and **REM sleep behavior disorder** (RBD). In RBD, patients act out their dreams, which often involve kicking, punching, and/or running. RBD and olfactory dysfunction may precede the onset of Parkinson's disease by years, and RBD is associated with a high risk of future development of a neurodegenerative disorder (most commonly synucleinopathies such as PD, multiple systems atrophy, and dementia with Lewy bodies). Shoulder pain is another symptom that can precede other features of PD. Dementia is typically not present at onset of parkinsonian symptoms in idiopathic PD. If dementia and parkinsonism arise concurrently, dementia with Lewy bodies should be considered (see "Dementia with Lewy Bodies" in Ch. 22). Autonomic dysfunction is usually a more prominent feature in multiple systems atrophy as compared to in PD.

Diagnosis & Differential Diagnosis of Parkinson's Disease

Parkinson's disease is a clinical diagnosis. A tremor-predominant presentation must be distinguished from essential tremor, drug-induced tremor, physiologic tremor, and hyperthyroidism. Asymmetry of tremor and accompanying bradykinesia and rigidity on the side of tremor are suggestive of PD. Early falls and/or impaired vertical gaze with parkinsonism suggest progressive supranuclear palsy (PSP). Early and severe autonomic dysfunction with parkinsonism suggests multiple system atrophy (MSA). Dementia and hallucinations arising before or concurrently with parkinsonism suggest dementia with Lewy bodies (DLB). Improvement in symptoms with levodopa is also suggestive of PD, although some Parkinson-plus syndromes may have an initial response to levodopa. When there is clinical ambiguity, a dopamine transporter SPECT (single photon emission computed tomography) scan can be used to look for asymmetric decreased activity in the basal ganglia. However, dopamine transporter SPECT only distinguishes a neurodegenerative parkinsonian syndrome from "*not* a neurodegenerative parkinsonian syndrome" (i.e., it does not distinguish *between* PD, multiple systems atrophy, progressive supranuclear palsy, and corticobasal syndrome). Dopamine transporter SPECT can be useful in a patient in whom there is a question of PD versus essential tremor (if the latter presents asymmetrically, as it sometimes does) or PD versus drug-induced parkinsonism (see "Drug-Induced Parkinsonism").

Treatment of Parkinson's Disease

Pharmacologic treatment of PD is symptomatic, and therefore should begin when the disease begins to interfere with activities of daily living. For example, if the patient has a mild tremor in the nondominant hand that the patient does not feel is bothersome, treatment is not necessarily required. The available medications for PD include:

- Levodopa: given combined with carbidopa. Carbidopa inhibits peripheral dopamine breakdown, increasing the amount of levodopa that enters the CNS and decreasing peripheral side effects such as nausea.
- Dopamine agonists: pramipexole and ropinirole are the most commonly used agents in this category (pergolide is no longer in use due to cardiac valvular toxicity).
- Catecholamine *O*-methyl transferase (COMT) inhibitors: entacapone and tolcapone are used with carbidopa-levodopa to potentiate its effect (tolcapone can rarely cause hepatotoxicity and so entacapone is more commonly used).
- Anticholinergics: trihexyphenidyl is used predominantly for tremor.
- Monoamine oxidase B (MAO-B) inhibitors: selegiline and rasagiline.
- Amantadine: particularly useful in the treatment of dopamine replacement–induced dyskinesias (see "Treatment-Induced Dyskinesias in Parkinson's Disease")

In addition, exercise (aerobic and tai chi), speech therapy (for hypophonia if present), and psychiatric care (if depression, anxiety, or psychosis is present) are all important aspects of supportive care for PD.

Dopamine replacement with levodopa or a dopamine agonist is first-line therapy when the disease begins to become disabling. Levodopa is more effective than dopamine agonists and causes fewer initial side effects, but may be associated with a higher risk of subsequent motor complications (**dyskinesias**) than dopamine agonists. Side effects of dopamine agonists include daytime somnolence, peripheral edema, psychosis, hallucinations, and impulse control disorders (including hypersexuality, pathologic gambling). Side effects of levodopa include dizziness and nausea, which may be ameliorated by taking the medication with food (although this can decrease the absorption of the medication if the medication is taken with a high-protein meal).

Some practitioners suggest that younger patients should initially be treated with dopamine agonists, whereas patients who develop the disease later in life should begin immediately on levodopa. Advocates of this strategy prefer dopamine agonists in younger patients since these patients will likely survive longer with the disease and be prone to later treatment-related motor complications with levodopa such as dyskinesias. However, many practitioners prefer to initiate levodopa directly once patients are sufficiently symptomatic to require treatment at any age, since levodopa is more effective than dopamine agonists, causes fewer side effects, and treatment-related dyskinesias in many patients are mild, tolerable, and nondisabling. As the disease progresses, nearly all patients with PD will ultimately require levodopa. Levodopa and dopamine agonists are much more effective for rigidity and bradykinesia and often have less effect on tremor. If tremor is the predominant feature, trihexyphenidyl may be considered (see below).

COMT inhibitors potentiate the effects of carbidopa-levodopa and can be added to this medication as the disease advances and length of response to levodopa decreases, a phenomenon called **wearing off**.

Anticholinergic medications such as trihexyphenidyl are most effective for tremor, and may be used in patients in whom tremor is the predominant disabling feature. Due to anticholinergic side effects such as confusion, this medication is often avoided in older adults.

MAO-B inhibitors and amantadine provide only minor symptomatic benefits and are sometimes used in early disease. Some data suggest a possible neuroprotective effect of rasagiline, but this is debated. Amantadine may also be useful in patients who develop dyskinesias (see "Treatment-Induced Dyskinesias in Parkinson's Disease" below).

Regimens involving multiple agents are inevitably necessary as the disease progresses, and must be individualized for each patient (Fig. 23–2). As the dopaminergic pathways continue to degenerate, the effect of levodopa may wear off quickly between doses (**off states**), requiring higher doses and/or increased dose frequency to maintain symptomatic relief (**on states**). Taking levodopa on an empty stomach may increase efficacy (although may also increase nausea). Additional strategies at this stage include increasing the dose or frequency of levodopa, adding a COMT inhibitor to potentiate the effect of levodopa, adding an MAO-B inhibitor, and/or adding a dopamine agonist. If a COMT inhibitor or a dopamine agonist is added, a dose reduction in levodopa may be necessary.

Treatment-induced dyskinesias and motor fluctuations in Parkinson's disease—Dyskinesias—usually manifesting as involuntary choreoathetoid movements—generally arise after about 5 years of levodopa therapy, though may arise sooner if treatment is initiated at a more advanced stage of the disease. Dyskinesias should be characterized by their timing in relation to levodopa dosing: peak dose (during the on state), wearing off (as the patient approaches the next dose), or diphasic (shortly after taking levodopa and again shortly

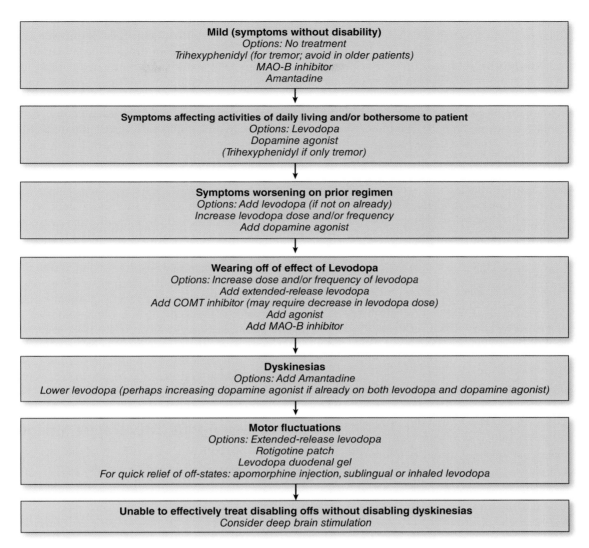

FIGURE 23–2 Algorithm showing possible treatment options in patients with Parkinson's disease at various stages of the disease. See also algorithms in Connolly and Lang, 2014.

before the next dose). Dyskinesias can be treated with addition of amantadine or with lowering of levodopa dose, but this can lead to a "rock and hard place" scenario between the patient being "off" (parkinsonian) and "on" but dyskinetic. Strategies to provide a more constant replacement of dopaminergic therapy to decrease motor fluctuations include adding extended-release levodopa, rotigotine patch, and levodopa duodenal gel (administered via gastrostomy tube). For quick relief of off states, options include apomorphine subcutaneous injection, sublingual or inhaled levodopa preparations, or dissolving levodopa in a carbonated beverage. However, motor fluctuations can be very challenging to manage pharmacologically, requiring consideration of deep brain stimulation.

Deep brain stimulation in the treatment of Parkinson's disease—Deep brain stimulation (DBS) is performed by surgical implantation of stimulating leads in the subthalamic

nucleus (STN) or globus pallidus interna (GPi) connected to a stimulator that is placed in the soft tissue of the chest. The parameters of the stimulator can be adjusted by an external programming device. DBS increases the amount of time the patient spends in the "on" state without dyskinesias. Patients will not improve beyond their best response to levodopa and will still require medications, although often levodopa dosing can be decreased, which may account in part for the reduction in dyskinesias.

DBS only ameliorates motor symptoms, and generally does not lead to improvement in nonmotor aspects of PD. DBS is contraindicated in patients with cognitive impairment or severe psychiatric disease as these can worsen with DBS. Surgical complications of DBS include intracerebral hemorrhage and intracranial infection, although these are not common occurrences. Hardware complications can occur due to lead breakage or migration. In addition to PD, DBS can also be considered in essential tremor and dystonia, although it is not currently used in Parkinson-plus disorders.

Treatment of Nonmotor Symptoms in Parkinson's Disease—Nonmotor symptoms in PD can be as disabling as motor symptoms. Evaluation for and treatment of nonmotor symptoms are therefore essential to improve quality of life and reduce disability in patients with PD. Symptoms to screen for include psychiatric comorbidities (depression, anxiety, psychosis, impulse control disorders), autonomic symptoms (constipation, orthostatic hypotension), drooling, cognitive decline, and sleep disorders (including sleepiness, REM sleep behavior disorder). Treatment modalities include physical therapy, occupational therapy, speech therapy, psychiatry and cognitive behavioral therapy, and pharmacologic therapy. Specific symptoms and their treatment include:

- Depression: SSRI, SNRI
- Anxiety: SSRI, SNRI, buspirone
- Psychosis: decrease antiparkinsonian medications (particularly trihexyphenidyl, amantadine, dopamine agonists [monitoring for symptoms of dopamine withdrawal]); start quetiapine (monitor QT interval), clozapine (monitor CBC), or pimavanserin
- Constipation: dietary modifications, stool softeners
- Orthostatic hypotension: decrease antihypertensives (if taking and if possible), increase hydration; start fludrocortisone, midodrine, droxidopa, or pyridostigmine
- Drooling: sublingual atropine drops, botulinum toxin to salivary glands
- Dementia: rivastigmine, donepezil
- REM sleep disorder: melatonin, clonazepam

Drug-Induced Parkinsonism

Parkinsonism can be induced by dopamine-blocking agents, most commonly:

- Antipsychotics: more common with typical/first-generation antipsychotics, but can occur with atypical/second-generation antipsychotics
- Dopamine antagonist antiemetics: metoclopramide, prochlorperazine
- The rarely used antihypertensives reserpine and alpha-methyldopa

Drug-induced parkinsonism can also be seen rarely with antiepileptics (most commonly valproic acid, although this more commonly causes isolated tremor rather than parkinsonism), antidepressants, and amiodarone.

In drug-induced parkinsonism, bradykinesia and rigidity are typically symmetric but can present asymmetrically as in PD. Tremor may be at rest, postural, or both. Symptoms generally emerge within months of starting the offending medication but can also emerge with change of dosage later in the course of medication treatment. Other associated drug-induced movement disorders such as tardive dyskinesia and akathisia may also be present (see "Tardive Dyskinesia"), although drug-induced parkinsonism may be present in isolation. Treatment is ideally discontinuation of the offending medication when possible. If ongoing antipsychotic treatment is necessary for the underlying disorder, clozapine can be considered (although this requires monitoring of complete blood cell count [CBC] due to risk of developing agranulocytosis with this medication). Most cases of drug-induced parkinsonism are reversible, although this can take months. If a patient requires a particular typical or atypical antipsychotic for the underlying psychiatric condition and cannot be on a lower dose or changed to another medication, anticholinergic medication (e.g., benztropine) may be used as symptomatic treatment. Dopamine replacement is generally ineffective.

An important diagnostic consideration in older patients who develop parkinsonian symptoms while on antipsychotic medications or dopamine-blocking antiemetics is whether idiopathic PD is emerging or being in some way "unmasked" by antidopaminergic therapy. In such patients—especially if there is no improvement with removal of the offending agent—dopamine transporter imaging can be useful since this will be normal in drug-induced parkinsonism but abnormal in PD (or any Parkinson-plus syndrome).

Parkinson-Plus (Atypical Parkinsonism) Syndromes

The **Parkinson-plus syndromes** (also called atypical parkinsonism) are neurodegenerative diseases that cause parkinsonism but also have additional features not seen in Parkinson's disease. The Parkinson-plus syndromes include multiple systems atrophy (MSA), progressive supranuclear palsy (PSP), corticobasal syndrome (CBS), and dementia with Lewy bodies (DLB) (see Table 23–3). With the exception of CBS, parkinsonism is typically symmetric at onset compared to the unilateral onset typically seen in Parkinson's disease.

Multiple Systems Atrophy

Multiple systems atrophy (MSA) is a disease characterized by parkinsonism and/or cerebellar dysfunction accompanied by autonomic dysfunction. Two variants of the disease are recognized, which are named based on their predominant feature: MSA-P (**P** for parkinsonism; formerly called striatonigral degeneration) and MSA-C (**C** for cerebellar; formerly called olivopontocerebellar atrophy). Parkinsonian features, when present, are typically symmetric at onset (as compared to asymmetric in Parkinson's disease), and tend to progress more rapidly than in Parkinson's disease. Tremor is not a predominant feature, and when present is most commonly an action tremor as opposed to the rest tremor typically seen in Parkinson's disease (although rest tremor can occur in MSA). Autonomic dysfunction in MSA can manifest as orthostatic hypotension, urinary incontinence, and/or erectile dysfunction. These autonomic features may also be seen in

TABLE 23–3 Clinical Features of the Parkinsonian Syndromes.

	Parkinson's Disease	Dementia With Lewy Bodies	Multiple Systems Atrophy	Progressive Supranuclear Palsy	Corticobasal Syndrome
Distinguishing feature(s)	Parkinsonism	Dementia Hallucinations Fluctuations	Autonomic dysfunction	Early falls Vertical gaze dysfunction	Alien limb Apraxia Myoclonus
Motor features (in addition to parkinsonism)	Dyskinesias with dopamine replacement therapy	N/A	Cerebellar and/or pyramidal signs	Prominent axial rigidity	Alien limb Apraxia Myoclonus Dystonia Mirror movements
Symmetry of motor features	Typically begins unilaterally, but may become bilateral	Typically bilateral	Typically bilateral	Typically bilateral	Typically unilateral
Dementia	Late	Early (visuospatial dysfunction prominent)	Present in some patients	Early (Executive dysfunction prominent)	Late
Autonomic	Late/mild	Late	Prominent	Unusual	Unusual
Speech	Hypophonic	Not usually impaired	Dysarthric	Dysarthric	Not usually impaired
Other	Treatment-induced dyskinesias	Hallucinations, fluctuations	Stridor	Eye movement abnormalities (see text)	Cortical sensory signs
Average age of onset	60s	50s–80s	50s	60s	60s
Neuroimaging[a]	No findings on structural neuroimaging	Temporo-occipital hypometabolism on PET	Hot cross buns sign in pons (Fig. 23–2)	Humming bird and Mickey Mouse signs due to midbrain atrophy (Fig. 23–3)	Asymmetric parietal/basal ganglia atrophy and hypometabolism
Response to levodopa	Yes	None or minimal/transient	None or minimal/transient	None or minimal/transient	None or minimal/transient
Pathology	Synuclein	Synuclein	Synuclein	Tau	Tau, AD, FTLD/TDP

Abbreviations: AD: Alzheimer's disease; PET: positron emission tomography.

[a]All can have abnormal dopamine transporter imaging.

Parkinson's disease and dementia with Lewy bodies, but are typically milder in those diseases.

Additional features of MSA can include anterocollis (forward flexed posture of the neck), Pisa syndrome (head, neck, and trunk flexion to one side like the leaning tower of Pisa), hyperreflexia and/or Babinski's sign(s), dysarthria and/or dysphagia, nocturnal stridor, pseudobulbar affect (uncontrolled laughing and/or crying), and/or Raynaud's phenomenon. Although parkinsonian features may initially respond to levodopa in some patients with MSA leading to diagnostic consideration of Parkinson's disease, this response is generally not sustained, and levodopa may worsen orthostatic hypotension.

In MSA-C, MRI may reveal the "hot cross bun" sign (resembling a plus sign in a circle) in the pons due to degeneration of the crossing corticopontocerebellar fibers destined for the middle cerebellar peduncles (Fig. 23–3). MRI abnormalities may also be present in the putamen (linear T2 hyperintensity lateral to the putamen is referred to as the putaminal

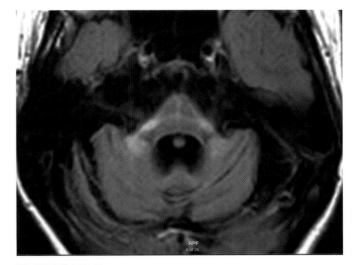

FIGURE 23–3 **MRI in multiple systems atrophy.** Axial FLAIR MRI demonstrating the "hot cross buns" sign and middle cerebellar peduncle atrophy in a patient with MSA-C.

rim or putaminal split sign), and atrophy may be seen in the putamen, middle cerebellar peduncle, pons, and/or cerebellum; these structures may also demonstrate hypometabolism on PET. Dopamine transporter imaging may be abnormal (decreased uptake in basal ganglia), but this can occur in any neurodegenerative parkinsonian syndrome and does not distinguish between them. Treatment is supportive.

Progressive Supranuclear Palsy

Progressive supranuclear palsy (PSP) is characterized by gait dysfunction (leading to falls) and oculomotor dysfunction (most commonly problems with vertical gaze). The first symptom is usually falls, commonly backward. The vertical gaze palsy characteristic of the disease may not be present initially, leading to initial diagnostic consideration of Parkinson's disease. However, tremor is rare in PSP, and most of the rigidity in PSP is axial (neck and back) rather than in the extremities as is commonly seen in Parkinson's disease. Patients have difficulty looking up and down voluntarily, but since the problem is supranuclear (hence the name of the disease), vertical eye movements can be elicited with vertical oculocephalic maneuvers (since the cranial nerve 8—medial longitudinal fasciculus [MLF]—cranial nerves 3, 4, and 6 pathways are intact; see "Supranuclear Versus Nuclear Lesions Affecting Eye Movements" in Ch. 11). Before vertical gaze palsy develops, slowing of vertical saccades compared to horizontal saccades may be noted. Downgaze palsy is more specific for the disease, since decreased upward gaze can be seen in many neurodegenerative disorders as well as in otherwise healthy older patients. Cognitive and behavioral changes are often present early in the disease.

Other features of PSP include dysarthria and/or dysphagia, a startled/surprised appearance of the face, retrocollis,

and ocular motor findings including square-wave jerks (saccadic intrusions away from the point of focus), eyelid opening apraxia (difficulty reopening the eyes after closure), and failure to suppress the vestibulo-ocular reflex (see "The Vestibulo-Ocular Reflex" in Ch. 12). The **applause sign** (inability to clap only three times and then stop; i.e., patient keeps clapping due to motor perseveration) is often associated with PSP, but can be present in any neurodegenerative disease.

Neuroimaging can reveal midbrain atrophy without pontine atrophy, resulting in a "hummingbird" appearance of the brainstem in midsagittal view (Fig. 23–4A). However, the brainstem in this view looks like a bird even in normal patients, and the pattern of midbrain atrophy in PSP may be more easily identifiable in the axial plane as a "carving out" of the space between the cerebral peduncles creating a "Mickey Mouse" appearance (Fig. 23–4B). More precise than relying on the appearance is calculation of the midbrain anteroposterior diameter and midbrain-pons ratio on sagittal section; midbrain anteroposterior length less than 9.35 mm and midbrain-pons ratio less than 0.52 are highly predictive of PSP, distinguishing it from PD, MSA, and normal controls (Massey et al., 2013). As in MSA, levodopa may be helpful initially but often is not, and any response is often mild and transient compared to Parkinson's disease. Therefore, treatment is supportive.

The classic PSP syndrome described here is also known as Richardson syndrome (PSP-RS). Variants of PSP include those with isolated or predominant: parkinsonism (PSP-P), progressive gait freezing (PSP-PGF), cerebellar features (PSP-C), symptoms of behavioral variant frontotemporal dementia (PSP-F), speech and language disorder (PSP-SL; most commonly nonfluent primary progressive aphasia, see Ch. 23), and corticobasal syndrome (PSP-CBS). Many of these

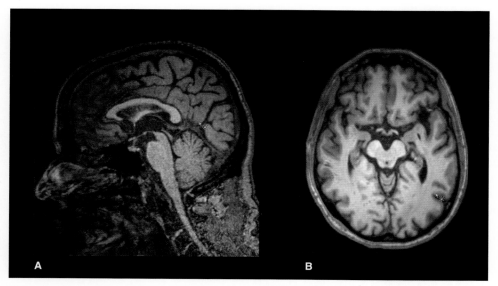

FIGURE 23–4 **MRI in progressive supranuclear palsy. A:** Sagittal T1-weighted MRI demonstrating the hummingbird sign (midbrain atrophy with spared pons). **B:** Axial T1-weighted MRI demonstrating the Mickey Mouse sign (decreased anteroposterior size of the midbrain when measured from between the cerebral peduncles to the superior colliculi, leading to a "carved out" appearance between the cerebral peduncles).

presentations may initially be very challenging to distinguish from other neurodegenerative diseases, but generally evolve into classic PSP over time. Rarely, a PSP-like syndrome may emerge after thoracic aortic surgery with induced hypothermia (**Mokri syndrome**).

Corticobasal Syndrome & Corticobasal Degeneration

Corticobasal syndrome (CBS) refers to a clinical phenotype, and **corticobasal degeneration** (CBD) refers to a pathologic diagnosis (based on a specific anatomic distribution of tau pathology). The clinical phenotype of CBS can be caused by CBD pathology, but also by Alzheimer's disease (AD) pathology, progressive supranuclear palsy (PSP) pathology, frontotemporal dementia (FTD) pathology, or mixed pathology. CBD pathology can give rise to clinical syndromes of CBS, PSP, FTD, an AD-like picture, or a mixed phenotype.

Symptoms of CBS are typically asymmetric (like Parkinson's disease, but unlike MSA and PSP), and the affected side may demonstrate both cortical findings (such as myoclonus, apraxia, sensory neglect, and/or the alien limb phenomenon [involuntary purposeful limb movements]) and subcortical findings (such as parkinsonism, dystonia). Dementia, dysarthria, and eye movement abnormalities (saccadic breakdown of smooth pursuit and/or slowed saccades) may be present. Neuroimaging may reveal asymmetric parietal cortical atrophy (most pronounced contralateral to the affected limb) and PET may demonstrate asymmetric decreased cortical and basal ganglia metabolism. Treatment is supportive.

Dementia With Lewy Bodies

In **dementia with Lewy bodies** (DLB), parkinsonism (usually symmetric) is accompanied by dementia, hallucinations, and fluctuations in level of arousal/mental state. Unlike Parkinson's disease dementia, in which the motor features of parkinsonism precede the development of dementia by years, in DLB, dementia and parkinsonism usually arise concurrently. (For further discussion of DLB, see "Dementia With Lewy bodies" in Ch. 22.)

FUNCTIONAL MOVEMENT DISORDERS

Functional movement disorders are movement disorders believed to be due to abnormal nervous system function rather than an underlying structural cause (previously called psychogenic movement disorders). Clues to a functional movement disorder in the history include: abrupt onset with maximal severity at onset (while many movement disorders emerge gradually, stroke-induced movement disorders can also present abruptly with maximal deficit), fluctuating course, and precipitating psychological or physical trauma (though this may not be present). Clues to a functional etiology on examination

include: inconsistency, distractibility (many movement disorders actually worsen with distraction and diminish with focus on the movement, e.g., the tremor of PD), entrainment (see "Functional Tremor"), and other functional signs (give-way weakness, disability beyond what would be expected for examination findings). Treatment involves explaining the diagnosis to the patient (see neurosymptoms.org) and multidisciplinary management including physical and occupational therapy, cognitive-behavioral therapy, and treatment of any coexisting psychiatric condition.

OTHER MOVEMENT DISORDERS

Tardive Dyskinesia

Long-term use of dopamine blocking agents over months to years can lead to **tardive dyskinesias**: involuntary choreoathetotic movements most commonly involving the mouth and/or tongue (although they can occur in any part of the body). Tardive tremors, dystonias, and akathisia (restlessness) can also occur. The typical (first-generation) antipsychotics are the most common culprits, although tardive dyskinesia can be caused by atypical (second-generation) antipsychotics. Tardive dyskinesia can also occur after discontinuation of antipsychotics, especially when stopped abruptly. Prolonged metoclopramide use can also cause tardive syndromes.

Treatment of tardive dyskinesia is by withdrawing the offending agent by slow taper, although symptoms may persist for months or even years. However, in many patients, antipsychotic drug withdrawal may be contraindicated from a psychiatric perspective. Ideally, such patients should be switched to an atypical antipsychotic, or if already on one, to clozapine or quetiapine, which carry the lowest risk of tardive dyskinesia. Clozapine requires regular monitoring of CBC due to risk of agranulocytosis. When a patient requires ongoing antipsychotic medications that cannot be changed or lowered in dose from the psychiatric perspective, dopamine depleting agents (tetrabenazine, deutetrabenazine, valbenazine), a benzodiazepine, propranolol, or amantadine may be initiated; trihexyphenidyl can be considered for the treatment of tardive tremor, and botulinum toxin injection may be used for tardive dystonia. Deep brain stimulation may be used in severe cases not responsive to medications. Ideally, tardive dyskinesia can be prevented by avoiding long-term use of typical antipsychotic agents when possible.

Restless Leg Syndrome

In **restless leg syndrome** (RLS), patients feel unpleasant sensations in the legs (such as crawling, aching) causing a desire to move, and moving the legs relieves the sensation. This typically occurs at night in bed, or when resting late in the day. RLS should not be confused with periodic limb movements of sleep (PLMS), which are actual movements of the limbs during sleep. PLMS are commonly present in patients with RLS, but many people have PLMS without RLS. PLMS is more likely to be noted by the bed partner (since the patient is asleep), whereas RLS is noted by the patient.

Most cases of RLS are idiopathic, but an important reversible cause for which to evaluate is iron deficiency anemia. When RLS is due to iron deficiency anemia, symptoms often respond to iron replacement. Pregnancy, renal failure, and peripheral neuropathy are predisposing factors to RLS (although evaluation for iron deficiency should be performed in such patients as well). It is also important to evaluate for an underlying neuropathy, which may produce similar symptoms or coexist with RLS.

Treatment for disabling RLS symptoms is with a dopamine agonist (pramipexole or ropinirole) or alpha-2-delta calcium channel ligand (gabapentin enacarbil, gabapentin, or pregabalin). With long-term dopamine agonist use, symptoms may worsen in severity and timing (i.e., beginning earlier in the day), a phenomenon called **augmentation.** Levodopa carries greater risk of augmentation than dopamine agonists, and so it should not be the initial agent used for treatment of RLS. If augmentation occurs, patients can be switched from one agonist to another or from dopamine agonists to gabapentin or pregabalin. In patients who do not respond to any of these drug classes, opioids may be effective.

Stiff Person Syndrome

In **stiff person syndrome,** patients develop muscle stiffness and spasm, first in the axial muscles and later in the proximal extremity muscles. Stiffness is generally apparent in how the patient walks, and palpable paraspinal muscle rigidity is present on examination. EMG, if performed, will reveal continuous muscle activity. The syndrome may be a sporadic autoimmune syndrome (associated with anti-glutamic acid decarboxylase [GAD] antibodies and often accompanied by other autoimmune diseases such as type 1 diabetes) or paraneoplastic (associated with anti-amphiphysin antibodies and anti-glycine receptor antibodies; anti-glycine receptor antibodies may also be associated with the related, more severe condition **progressive encephalomyelitis with rigidity and myoclonus [PERM]**). Therefore, patients with stiff person syndrome should be evaluated for underlying malignancy. Treatment is with diazepam, baclofen, and immunomodulatory therapy (most commonly intravenous immunoglobulin [IVIg], but other agents may be considered if IVIg is ineffective or contraindicated).

Hemifacial Spasm

Hemifacial spasm is a condition in which there are paroxysmal contractions of half of the face. Neuroimaging may reveal a vascular loop contacting the facial nerve. Botulinum toxin is the most effective treatment, but patients may respond to carbamazepine. Microvascular decompression of the facial nerve may be considered in refractory cases.

Faciobrachial Dystonic Seizures

An important differential diagnosis to consider in patients with hemifacial spasm is **faciobrachial dystonic seizures.** These are very brief episodes in which there is momentary dystonic posturing of one side of the face and the ipsilateral arm, which may occur many times per day (or even per hour) after onset. This entity is important to recognize as it is associated with anti-LGI1 (leucine-rich, glioma inactivated 1) antibodies. Faciobrachial dystonic seizures often precede the development of limbic encephalitis associated with anti-LGI1 antibodies, and development of limbic encephalitis may be prevented by early treatment with steroids upon recognition of faciobrachial dystonic seizures (Irani et al., 2011; Irani et al., 2013). This is one of the autoimmune encephalitides that is most commonly not associated with an underlying malignancy, although it may rarely be associated with thymoma or small cell lung cancer (see "Paraneoplastic/Antibody-mediated Syndromes of the Nervous System" in Ch. 24).

Anti-LGI1 encephalitis is often accompanied by hyponatremia. MRI may show signal change in the basal ganglia and/or limbic regions (though can be normal). Unlike most other antibody-mediated CNS syndromes, CSF is often normal and serum antibodies may be more sensitive for the diagnosis than CSF antibodies. Treatment is with immunomodulatory therapy.

Wilson's Disease

Wilson's disease is an autosomal recessive disease that affects the liver and brain, presenting in childhood or early adulthood. Many of the neurologic manifestations are movement disorders, which can include parkinsonism, tremor, dystonia, ataxia, and/or chorea. The classic tremor of Wilson's disease is a **wing-beating tremor** elicited by having the patient sustain the arms elevated with elbows flexed (like wings). Cognitive and psychiatric symptoms are common. Seizures may occur. A pathognomonic ocular finding, the **Kayser-Fleischer ring** (a dark ring encircling the periphery of the iris), is almost always present in patients with neurologic manifestations of the disease. The diagnosis can usually be made by decreased serum ceruloplasmin and increased urinary copper on 24-hour urine collection, but liver biopsy may be necessary if these tests are inconclusive. MRI may reveal a pattern of signal change in the midbrain called the "face of the giant panda" sign. Treatment with copper chelation (D-penicillamine or trientine) can be highly effective. In cases refractory to such treatments, liver transplantation may be considered.

Fahr Disease and Fahr Syndrome

Although asymptomatic calcification in the basal ganglia is a common nonspecific finding on CT, extensive basal ganglia calcification can cause a syndrome of parkinsonism (and/or other movement disorders), cognitive impairment or neuropsychiatric dysfunction, and/or ataxia (if there is cerebellar involvement). Symptomatic basal ganglia calcification can occur in genetic conditions such as Fahr disease (which can

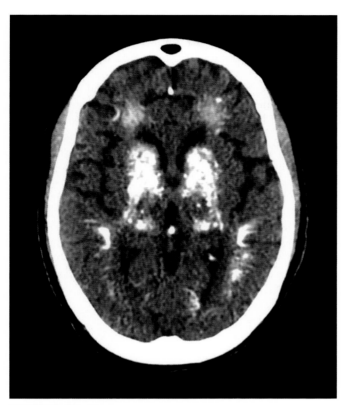

FIGURE 23–5. **Fahr syndrome.** Extensive calcification in the basal ganglia and subcortical white matter in a patient with severe hypoparathyroidism (for differential diagnosis of basal ganglia calcifications, see text).

be inherited in an autosomal dominant fashion [primary familial brain calcification] or occur sporadically [idiopathic basal ganglia calcification]), Cockayne syndrome, Aicardi-Goutières syndrome, and mitochondrial disease. It can also occur secondary to parathyroid disorders (hypoparathyroidism, pseudo-hypoparathyroidism, or pseudopseudohypoparathyroidism) and congenital infections (e.g., TORCH infections). The designation Fahr syndrome is sometimes used to refer to secondary causes of this condition. Calcifications in Fahr disease and Fahr syndrome may extend beyond the basal ganglia into the subcortical white matter and cerebellar white matter (Fig. 23–5). Evaluation of parathyroid function (serum calcium, serum parathyroid hormone level) should be pursued before making a diagnosis of familial or idiopathic basal ganglia calcification (Fahr disease).

REFERENCES

Connolly BS, Lang AE. Pharmacological treatment of Parkinson disease: a review. *JAMA* 2014;311:1670–1683.

Irani SR, Michell AW, Lang B, Pettingill P, Waters P, Johnson MR, et al. Faciobrachial dystonic seizures precede Lgi1 antibody limbic encephalitis. *Ann Neurol* 2011;69:892–900.

Irani SR, Stagg CJ, Schott JM, Rosenthal CR, Schneider SA, Pettingill P, et al. Faciobrachial dystonic seizures: the influence of immunotherapy on seizure control and prevention of cognitive impairment in a broadening phenotype. *Brain* 2013:136; 3151–3162.

Massey LA, Jäger HR, Paviour DC, O'Sullivan SS, Ling H, Williams DR, et al. The midbrain to pons ratio: a simple and specific MRI sign of PSP. *Neurol* 2013;80:1856–1861.

Neoplastic and Paraneoplastic Disorders of the Nervous System & Neurologic Complications of Chemotherapy and Radiation Therapy

The nervous system can be affected in several ways in patients with neoplastic disease:

- Directly due to primary nervous system tumors or metastases to nervous system structures

- Indirectly due to:

  - Tumors of non-neurologic origin impinging upon nervous system structures

  - Toxicities of chemotherapy and radiation therapy

  - Paraneoplastic syndromes affecting the nervous system

Therefore, in patients with a known history of systemic malignancy, the differential diagnosis of new neurologic symptoms includes direct effects of the cancer itself (metastases to or compression of neurologic structures), complications of treatment (radiation or chemotherapy), and paraneoplastic syndromes. Direct (metastases) or indirect (paraneoplastic) effects of systemic malignancy on the nervous system may also be the presenting feature of a systemic cancer.

INTRACRANIAL TUMORS

Primary or metastatic intracranial tumors may present with headaches, seizures, and/or focal neurologic deficits. Progressive focal neurologic deficits can occur if the tumor affects an eloquent area (e.g., affecting motor, speech, visual, or cerebellar pathways). Diffuse infiltrative lesions or diffuse metastases can present with global cognitive dysfunction and/or personality changes without obvious focal deficits. Some patients with intracranial tumors may present first with a seizure with no preceding history of neurologic dysfunction or headache.

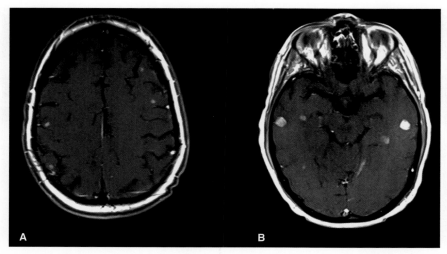

FIGURE 24-1 Cerebral metastases. Axial T1-weighted postcontrast MRI images demonstrating multiple small enhancing lesions at the gray–white junction in a patient with breast cancer.

Brain metastases may also be discovered in the presymptomatic stage as part of a staging evaluation for a known systemic malignancy.

Particular tumors to consider in particular clinical scenarios include:

- Hearing loss, tinnitus, imbalance: cerebellopontine angle tumor (most commonly vestibular schwannoma or meningioma)
- Bitemporal hemianopia: pituitary tumors, craniopharyngioma
- Unilateral visual disturbance: optic glioma, optic nerve sheath meningioma, or olfactory groove meningioma (olfactory groove meningioma may also cause unilateral loss of smell)
- Multiple cranial neuropathies: skull base lesion, brainstem lesion, or leptomeningeal metastases

In general, steroids are often used for the treatment of peritumoral vasogenic edema in patients whose brain tumors are symptomatic (e.g., headache and/or focal deficits) as a result of the location and size of the mass and its surrounding edema. It should be noted that steroids are part of the treatment for primary central nervous system lymphoma and can alter biopsy results if administered prior to biopsy. Therefore, when there is concern for primary central nervous system lymphoma, steroids should ideally be avoided until after biopsy. Antiseizure medications should be initiated if seizures occur due to intracranial tumors, although there is no benefit (and there may be harm) to administering prophylactic antiseizure medications to patients with brain tumors who have not had seizures.

Brain Metastases

Metastases to the brain from systemic cancer are far more common than primary brain tumors. Brain metastases from lung cancer, breast cancer, melanoma, and colon cancer are most common. Metastases are most commonly found at the gray–white junction, appearing as one or more ring-enhancing lesions on contrast-enhanced neuroimaging (Fig. 24–1). Melanoma, renal cell carcinoma, thyroid carcinoma, and choriocarcinoma have the highest propensity for intratumoral hemorrhage. However, given that lung cancer is the most common cause of cerebral metastases, it is the most common cause of hemorrhagic brain metastases.

Gastrointestinal cancer metastases have a predilection for the posterior fossa. Prostate cancer only very rarely metastasizes to the brain, but can metastasize to the skull and/or dura mater, causing neurologic symptoms by impinging upon the brain and/or cranial nerves.

The evaluation of a single brain lesion suspicious for neoplasm requires a search for systemic malignancy including imaging of the chest, abdomen, and pelvis with CT and/or PET. However, even if a systemic malignancy is found, an isolated CNS lesion could still be an independent primary brain tumor rather than a metastasis, so brain tissue may still ultimately be required for diagnosis.

Treatment of brain metastases involves surgical resection (for large, symptomatic metastases), stereotactic radiosurgery, and/or whole brain radiation.

Leptomeningeal Metastases (Carcinomatous Meningitis)

Leptomeningeal metastases (carcinomatous meningitis) can cause headache, nausea/vomiting, cranial nerve involvement, and/or confusion. Spinal leptomeningeal involvement affecting the nerve roots can cause radicular pain with focal or multifocal motor and/or sensory deficits in the limbs. Common causes of leptomeningeal metastases include breast cancer, lung cancer, hematologic malignancies, and melanoma. When Waldenström macroglobulinemia leads to lymphoplasmacytic infiltration of the leptomeninges, this is referred to as

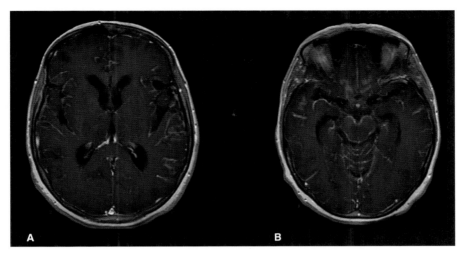

FIGURE 24-2 **Leptomeningeal metastases.** Axial T1-weighted postcontrast MRI images demonstrating enhancement in the cerebral sulci (**A** and **B**) as well as in the cerebellar folia and surrounding the brainstem (**B**) in a patient with breast cancer.

Bing-Neel syndrome (less commonly, Bing-Neel syndrome may affect the brain parenchyma). Leptomeningeal metastases often have no accompanying brain metastases. They may rarely be the presenting feature of a systemic malignancy. Contrast-enhanced brain imaging reveals enhancement of the leptomeninges, which can be noted in the cerebellar folia, surrounding the brainstem, and invaginating the cerebral sulci (Fig. 24-2). Hydrocephalus may also be present. A normal MRI does not exclude the possibility of leptomeningeal metastases, and definitive diagnosis is made by detecting malignant cells in the cerebrospinal fluid (CSF) by cytology/flow cytometry. Treatment of leptomeningeal metastases is directed at the primary underlying cancer, but prognosis is generally poor.

Primary Intracranial Tumors

Primary intracranial tumors can arise from any of the structures and constituent cell types of the central nervous system, including:

- Glial cells: astrocytoma, oligodendroglioma, glioblastoma (Table 24-1)
- Neurons: neurocytoma, ganglioglioma, gangliocytoma
- Neural progenitor cells: medulloblastoma, neuroblastoma
- The meninges: meningioma
- Choroid plexus: choroid plexus papilloma and choroid plexus carcinoma
- Ependyma: ependymoma
- Pineal gland: pineoblastoma, pineocytoma
- Pituitary: pituitary adenoma
- Hematologic system: primary CNS lymphoma, intravascular lymphoma

Meningiomas and glial tumors are the most common primary intracranial tumors, although both are less common than metastases.

Meningiomas

Meningiomas are tumors of the dura mater that enhance uniformly on contrast-enhanced neuroimaging and often have a dural tail of enhancement at the margins of the tumor (Fig. 24-3). Compression of local nervous system structures can cause focal deficits and/or seizures. Treatment of meningiomas is surgical. Postoperative radiation therapy is used for grade 3 (malignant) meningiomas and incompletely resected grade 2 (atypical) meningiomas. Radiation therapy without surgery may be considered for inoperable meningiomas, or in patients who are not good surgical candidates. If a meningioma is discovered incidentally when brain imaging

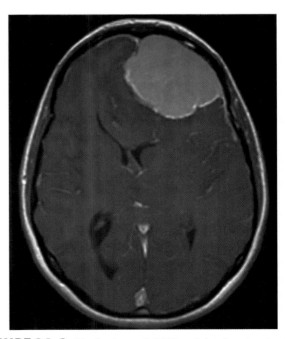

FIGURE 24-3 **Meningioma.** Axial T1-weighted postcontrast MRI image demonstrating a left frontal meningioma that enhances homogenously and has a dural tail extending peripherally on each side.

TABLE 24–1 Grading, Molecular Signatures, & Other Features of Some Common Gliomas.

	Grade	Other mutated genes	Other features
Pilocytic astrocytoma	1	BRAF NF1	Most common in children, often in post. fossa
Subependymal giant cell astrocytoma	1	TSC1 TSC2	Most commonly seen in tuberous sclerosis
Pleomorphic xanthoastrocytoma	2, 3	BRAF CDKN2A/B	Most commonly cortical
Oligodendroglioma, IDH-mutant, and 1p/19qcodeleted	2, 3	TERT promoter CIC FUBP1 NOTCH1	
Astrocytoma, IDH-mutant	2, 3, 4	ATRX TP53 CDKN2A/B	
Glioblastoma, IDH-wildtype	4	TERT promoter Chromosomes 7, 10 EGFR	
Diffuse hemispheric glioma, H3 G34-mutant	4	ATRX TP53	More common in children
Diffuse midline glioma, H3 K27-altered	4	TP53 ACVR1 PDGFRA EGFR EZHIP	More common in children; often occurs in thalamus or brainstem (formerly called diffuse intrinsic pontine glioma)

Data from Louis DN, Perry A, Wesseling P, et al: The 2021 WHO Classification of Tumors of the Central Nervous System: a summary. *Neuro Oncol.* 2021;23(8):1231-1251.

is performed for another reason, it can generally be followed with serial imaging and neurologic examination if it is small and asymptomatic.

Gliomas

The classification of glial neoplasms has moved from exclusively histology-based to categorization that involves histology and molecular/genetic signatures (see Table 24–1), as the latter correlate better with prognosis and may represent treatment targets.

On neuroimaging, lower grade diffuse gliomas are typically T2/FLAIR hyperintense lesions with little or no contrast enhancement (Fig. 24–4). Glioblastoma appears as a contrast-enhancing mass with a necrotic center, and often progresses along white matter tracts such as across the corpus callosum ("butterfly glioma") (Fig. 24–5).

Glioblastoma is usually associated with 18-month survival or less even with treatment, although patients with lower grade tumors can survive for over a decade with treatment.

Treatment regimens for gliomas involve maximal surgical resection (when feasible), fractionated focal radiation therapy,

and chemotherapy (most commonly with temozolomide). Glioblastoma with MGMT promotor methylation responds better to temozolomide and is associated with a better prognosis than glioblastoma without this feature. In glioblastoma, there is also evidence for benefit of tumor treating fields (electrical current applied to the scalp). Recurrent tumors may be treated with bevacizumab (leads to improvement in MRI and progression-free survival but not survival) or lomustine. Regimens may be modified for older adults (e.g., temozolomide only or with hyperfractionated radiation).

Gliomatosis cerebri was a term previously used for infiltrating, usually high-grade, glial cell tumor that appears as diffuse and confluent on neuroimaging studies but generally does not enhance with contrast (Fig. 24–6). Given its inoperability, prognosis is poor. The term was removed from the 2016 WHO classification as its specific molecular signature is variable.

Pilocytic astrocytoma is a grade 1 tumor seen most commonly in children in the posterior fossa, characterized on neuroimaging by a cystic lesion with a mural nodule. Subependymal giant cell astrocytoma is a grade 1 tumor seen most

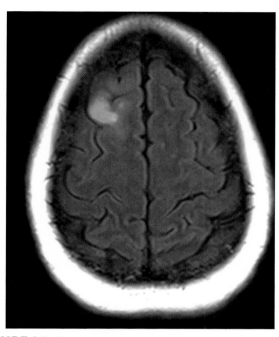

FIGURE 24–4 **Low-grade glioma.** Axial FLAIR MRI image demonstrating T2/FLAIR hyperintensity with gyral expansion in the right frontal lobe. There was no enhancement on postcontrast images (not shown). Pathology revealed oligodendroglioma (grade 2).

commonly in tuberous sclerosis (see "Neurocutaneous Syndromes & Associated Nervous System Neoplasms").

Other Primary CNS Tumors

There are a large number of additional primary parenchymal CNS tumors. Select tumors are listed in Table 24–2. In general, pediatric primary brain tumors are more common in the posterior fossa whereas adult primary brain tumors are more common in the cerebral hemispheres.

Primary CNS Lymphoma

Primary CNS lymphoma (PCNSL) is most commonly a diffuse large B-cell lymphoma. It can occur in immuno-competent patients as well as in patients who are immuno-compromised (commonly associated with Epstein-Barr virus [EBV] in patients who are immunocompromised). Rarely, other non-Hodgkin's lymphomas aside from DLBCL can affect the nervous system in isolation or in association with systemic involvement.

Neuroimaging demonstrates one or more lesions in the supratentorial or infratentorial white matter that are typically hyperdense on CT, homogenously contrast enhancing (compared to ring-enhancement in glioblastoma), and often demonstrate diffusion restriction due to high cellularity (Fig. 24–7). Involvement of the leptomeninges, dura, spine, or posterior chamber of the eye may be seen in isolation or in combination with parenchymal involvement. In patients who are immunocompromised, PCNSL may show ring enhancement and so must be distinguished from toxoplasmosis (see Ch. 20).

Intravascular B-cell lymphoma limited to the lumen of blood vessels is discussed in Chapter 19 (see "Intravascular Lymphoma") and neurolymphomatosis (infiltration of nerve roots and nerves) is discussed below (see "Tumors of the Peripheral Nervous System")

If there is suspicion for PCNSL, lumbar puncture should be obtained with cytology, flow cytometry, and IgH gene rearrangement, although CSF analysis is insensitive (three large-volume lumbar punctures may be required to approach adequate sensitivity), and biopsy is often required to make the diagnosis. If PCNSL is under consideration, steroids should be avoided prior to biopsy as they may alter biopsy results. Evaluation for extent of involvement should include imaging of the entire neuraxis, PET (or CT of chest/abdomen/pelvis) of the body, testicular ultrasound, and slit lamp evaluation of the eye.

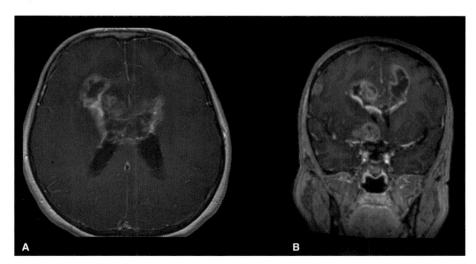

FIGURE 24–5 **Glioblastoma.** Axial (**A**) and Coronal (**B**) T1-weighted postcontrast MRI images demonstrating an enhancing lesion crossing the corpus callosum ("butterfly glioma").

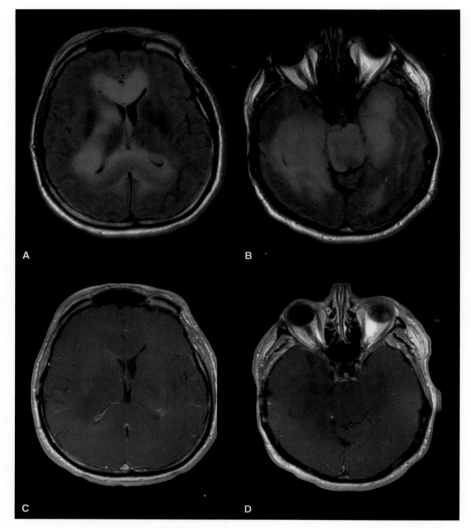

FIGURE 24–6 Gliomatosis cerebri. Axial FLAIR MRI (**A–B**) demonstrating a diffusely infiltrative lesion affecting all lobes of the brain bilaterally, crossing the corpus callosum, with no enhancement on T1 postcontrast sequences (**C–D**).

TABLE 24–2 Additional Tumors of the CNS.

	Grade	Cell of Origin	Imaging	Other Info
Dysembryoplastic neuroepithelial tumor (DNET)	1	Mixed neuronal/glial	Most commonly cortical in temporal lobe; cystic; can enhance (but may not); calcifications often present	Children/young adults; presents w/epilepsy
Ganglioglioma	1 (rarely higher if anaplastic)	Mixed neuronal/glial	Most common in temporal lobe; often cystic; can enhance (but may not); calcifications often present	Children/young adults; presents w/epilepsy
Gangliocytoma	1	Mixed neuronal/glial	Often cystic; can enhance (but may not); calcifications often present	Most common in children/young adults When present in cerebellum, called Lhermitte-Duclos syndrome
Hemangioblastoma	1	Vascular	Cerebellar, (most common) cystic, enhancing, mural nodule	Sporadic or in von Hippel-Lindau (associated with pheochromocytoma and clear cell renal carcinoma)
Central neurocytoma	2	Mixed neuronal/glial	Intraventricular, enhancing, cystic, calcifications	
Medulloblastoma	4	Embryonal	Cerebellar, enhancing	Most common in children

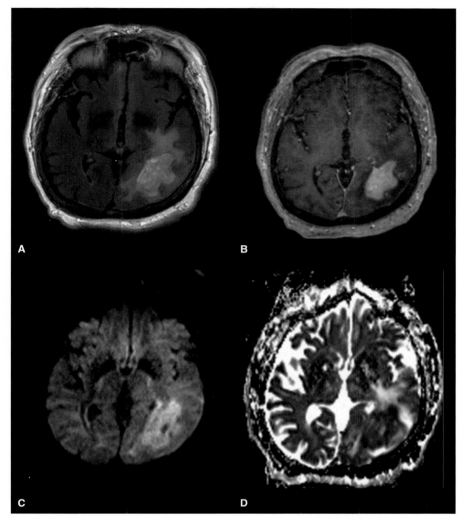

FIGURE 24–7 **Primary CNS Lymphoma.** Axial FLAIR (**A**), T1-postcontrast (**B**), DWI (**C**), and ADC (**D**) MRI images demonstrating a left occipital homogenously enhancing (B), diffusion restricting (C–D) lesion.

Treatment of PCNSL is with chemotherapy (methotrexate + one or more of a variety of agents including rituximab, temozolomide, and others). Surgery is not indicated, and radiation is generally reserved for relapse or patients who cannot tolerate chemotherapy.

TUMORS OF THE SPINE

Spinal tumors generally present with back pain and a subacute myelopathy (see Ch. 5). If the vertebral bodies are the site of involvement, a vertebral fracture may lead to acute myelopathy. The back pain from spinal tumors is often worse when the patient is lying down (compared to benign etiologies of back pain that tend to improve in the supine position). Spinal tumors are generally classified by their compartment: intramedullary, extramedullary intradural, or extramedullary extradural. Just as in the brain, metastases are more common in all of these compartments than primary spinal tumors.

- **Intramedullary** (in the spinal cord itself): intramedullary metastases, ependymoma, astrocytoma, glioblastoma, lymphoma
- **Extramedullary** (outside the spinal cord), further divided into two subcategories:
  - **Extramedullary intradural**: dural metastases, meningioma, schwannoma, neurofibroma
  - **Extramedullary extradural**: bone metastases or primary tumors of bone

Myxopapillary ependymoma is a particular type of ependymoma that arises from the conus medullaris and presents with symptoms referable to the conus medullaris and cauda equina (see "Cauda Equina & Conus Medullaris Syndromes" in Ch. 17).

Depending on the compartment, rapidity of symptom onset, and type of tumor, steroids, chemotherapy, radiation therapy, and/or surgery are treatment options for spinal tumors.

TUMORS OF THE CRANIAL NERVES

The cranial nerves can be affected by:

- Primary tumors of cranial nerves, such as schwannoma, optic nerve glioma, cranial nerve neurofibroma
- Skull base tumors, including olfactory groove meningioma
- Metastases to the orbit, cavernous sinus, skull base, or leptomeninges
- Tumors of facial structures including parotid tumor affecting cranial nerve 7, or nasopharyngeal carcinoma invading the skull base
- Tumors of other intracranial structures, such as glomus jugulare tumor affecting cranial nerves 9, 10, and 11, or pituitary adenoma affecting the optic chiasm
- Perineural spread of head and neck cancers along the branches of the trigeminal and/or facial nerves, which is most commonly caused by squamous cell cancer of the skin

Cranial nerves can be affected individually or together in any of the above scenarios, and a new cranial neuropathy in a patient with known malignancy requires MRI with contrast to look for metastases in any of the sites above. If no lesion is revealed, CT of the skull base may demonstrate bony disease causing cranial neuropathy. As mentioned above, imaging may be normal in patients with leptomeningeal disease, and in such cases, diagnosis requires CSF cytology.

Numb Chin Sign

Numbness of the chin should raise concern for potential metastatic malignancy involving the mental nerve (a branch of the trigeminal nerve). The numb chin sign can be the first sign of cancer in a patient without a known history of cancer, or it can be the first sign of metastatic disease in a patient with known cancer (see "Numb Chin Sign" in Ch. 13).

Primary Cranial Nerve Tumors: Schwannomas

Schwannomas can arise on any peripheral nerve myelinated by Schwann cells. This includes all of the cranial nerves except cranial nerve 2, which is part of the CNS, and so it is not myelinated by Schwann cells.

Vestibular Schwannoma

Schwannoma of the eighth cranial nerve (**vestibular schwannoma**) is the most common cranial nerve schwannoma and one of the most common cerebellopontine angle tumors (meningioma is another common tumor at the cerebellopontine angle). Vestibular schwannoma is also referred to as acoustic neuroma, which is a less accurate term since the tumor arises from Schwann cells (not neurons) and from the vestibular portion of the nerve (not the auditory portion).

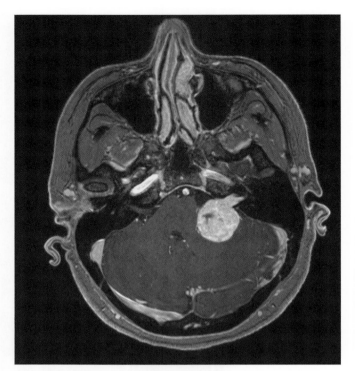

FIGURE 24–8 Vestibular schwannoma. Axial T1-weighted postcontrast MRI image demonstrating a homogenously enhancing mass at the left cerebellopontine angle.

Vestibular schwannoma typically presents with subacute to chronic unilateral sensorineural hearing loss and/or tinnitus. Dizziness/vertigo is less common because the tumor develops slowly, allowing for central compensation for peripheral vestibular dysfunction. The tumor can impinge on the seventh cranial nerve (both cranial nerve 7 and cranial nerve 8 travel in the internal auditory canal), and large tumors can compress the brainstem and/or cerebellum. MRI with contrast is the ideal imaging modality for diagnosing this tumor, which tends to enhance uniformly (Fig. 24–8). Depending on the size and rate of growth, watchful waiting with radiologic surveillance, surgery, or stereotactic radiosurgery may be considered as treatment strategies. Bilateral vestibular schwannomas are a hallmark of neurofibromatosis type 2 (see "Neurocutaneous Syndromes & Associated Nervous System Neoplasms").

TUMORS OF THE PERIPHERAL NERVOUS SYSTEM

Nerve roots, the brachial and lumbar plexus, and peripheral nerves can be compressed or infiltrated by tumor. Any spinal tumor or metastasis can cause root compression. Apical lung tumors and axillary lymph node disease from breast cancer are examples of malignancies that can affect the brachial plexus; colon, urologic, or gynecologic cancers may affect the lumbosacral plexus. Differentiating plexus compression/infiltration from radiation-induced plexopathy is discussed in Chapters 16 and 17.

Neurolymphomatosis refers to infiltration of one or more nerves or nerve roots with lymphoma. This may occur in patients with known lymphoma or it may be the initial presentation of the disease.

Primary tumors of the peripheral nervous system are rare. They can occur in isolation or in the setting of neurofibromatosis (see "Neurocutaneous Syndromes & Associated Nervous System Neoplasms"). Tumors of the peripheral nervous system include schwannomas, neurofibromas, and malignant peripheral nerve sheath tumors. Neurofibromas can affect the small nerve fibers of the skin (**dermal neurofibromas**) or larger nerves (**plexiform neurofibromas**). Plexiform neurofibromas can undergo malignant transformation to become malignant peripheral nerve sheath tumors. The primary symptoms of all of these peripheral nerve tumors are pain and a deficit in the region supplied by the nerve, and a mass may be palpable on examination. MRI is the preferred diagnostic imaging modality, and biopsy is usually necessary to make a definitive diagnosis.

The term **neuroma** refers to thickening of a portion of a nerve, often secondary to trauma (e.g., Morton's neuroma in the foot caused by injury from running). Neuromas are not neoplastic.

NEUROCUTANEOUS SYNDROMES & ASSOCIATED NERVOUS SYSTEM NEOPLASMS

Neurocutaneous syndromes are multiorgan system diseases that involve the nervous system and skin. The neurocutaneous disorders most commonly associated with nervous system tumors are neurofibromatosis type 1 (NF1), neurofibromatosis type 2 (NF2), and tuberous sclerosis (TS). They are all autosomal dominant, though can occur sporadically without family history due to germline mutation. The nervous system tumors, skin findings, systemic findings, and genetics of these conditions are compared in Table 24–3. Mnemonic to remember which skin findings are seen in TS: Tubers are a type of vegetable that grows in the ground, so remember: *Tubers grow in a leafy patch* (leafy: ash leaf spots; patch: shagreen patch).

NEUROTOXICITY OF CHEMOTHERAPY & RADIATION THERAPY

Neurotoxicity of Chemotherapy

Chemotherapeutic agents can cause peripheral and central nervous system complications. Many agents can be associated

TABLE 24–3 Comparison of Neurofibromatosis Type 1, Neurofibromatosis Type 2, & Tuberous Sclerosis.

	Neurofibromatosis Type 1	Neurofibromatosis Type 2	Tuberous Sclerosis
Most common nervous system tumors	Neurofibroma (skin and plexiform) Optic glioma	Bilateral vestibular schwannoma Meningioma Schwannomas of other nerves Spinal ependymoma	Cortical tubers Subependymal giant cell astrocytoma (SEGA) Subependymal nodules
Skin findings	Neurofibromas Café-au-lait spots Axillary freckling	Can have same skin findings as in NF1, although less commonly and usually fewer lesions	Ash leaf spots Shagreen patch Facial angiofibroma Ungual/periungual fibroma
Systemic disease	Bony abnormalities: • Sphenoid wing dysplasia • Thinning of long bones Vascular abnormalities: • Renal artery stenosis • Moyamoya • Aneurysms	Uncommon	Cardiac rhabdomyoma Renal angiomyolipoma
Ocular	Lisch nodules of iris	Cataracts	Retinal hamartoma
Other	Focal areas of signal intensity (FASI): asymptomatic, non-enhancing T2 hyperintensities		Seizures Developmental delay
Chromosome/ Gene	17/*NF1* (Neurofibromin)	22/*NF2* (Merlin)	9/*TSC1* (Hamartin) 16/*TSC2* (Tuberin)

Abbreviations: NF1: Neurofibromatosis 1; SEGA: subependymal giant cell astrocytoma.

TABLE 24–4 Chemotherapeutic Agents Commonly Associated With Neurologic Complications.

Encephalopathy	Seizures	PRES	Cerebellar Syndrome	Vascular Complications	Myelopathy	Neuropathy	Myositis
Acute:	• Busulfan	• Bortezomib	• Cytarabine	• L-asparaginase (venous sinus thrombosis)	Methotrexate (intrathecal)	• Platins	• Immune checkpoint inhibitors
• Ifosfamide	• Ifosfamide	• Combination chemotherapy	• 5-FU			• Vinca alkaloids	
• Methotrexate	• Methotrexate			• Bevacizumab (ischemic stroke and intracerebral hemorrhage)		• Taxanes	
• CAR T-cell therapy						• Thalidomide	
Chronic:						• Bortezomib	
Methotrexate						• Immune checkpoint inhibitors	

Abbreviations: 5-FU: 5-fluorouracil: PRES: posterior reversible encephalopathy syndrome.

with neurotoxicity, some of the most common of which that cause each syndrome are listed in Table 24–4. The unique complications of immunotherapies such as checkpoint inhibitors and CAR T-cell therapy are discussed separately (see "Neurologic Complications of Immunotherapies for Cancer").

Chemotherapy-Induced Peripheral Neuropathy

The most common chemotherapy-induced neurotoxicity is peripheral neuropathy. Common culprits include platins, taxanes, vinca alkaloids, bortezomib, and brentuximab. The neuropathy emerges during treatment, and is most commonly sensory (although motor and autonomic involvement can occur). Oxaliplatin can also cause painful paresthesias at the time of infusion, often worsened by cold temperature.

As with other toxic neuropathies, the symptoms of chemotherapy-induced neuropathy may worsen following termination of therapy (a phenomenon called **coasting**). Although chemotherapy-induced neuropathy improves and often resolves completely in most patients over the months after chemotherapy has been completed, it may persist in some patients. In patients presenting with neuropathy in the setting of chemotherapy, it is prudent to check vitamin B12, hemoglobin A1c, and serum protein electrophoresis (SPEP) with immunofixation to evaluate for any potentially reversible causes of peripheral neuropathy that may have predisposed the patient to chemotherapy-induced neuropathy (see Ch. 27).

For pain associated with chemotherapy-induced neuropathies, current guidelines recommend duloxetine (Hershman et al., 2014). Tricyclic antidepressants, gabapentin, and capsaicin cream may also be considered as for other causes of neuropathic pain.

Chemotherapy-Induced Acute CNS Neurotoxicity

An acute reversible encephalopathy, sometimes accompanied by seizures, can occur within hours to days of administration of methotrexate or ifosfamide. Acute methotrexate-induced encephalopathy may present with focal features and corresponding areas of diffusion restriction on MRI. An acute reversible cerebellar syndrome can be seen with cytarabine and 5-fluorouracil (5-FU).

Chemotherapeutic agents can cause posterior reversible encephalopathy syndrome (PRES; see "Posterior Reversible Encephalopathy Syndrome (PRES)" Ch. 19), especially in combination, although bortezomib can cause PRES on its own.

Methotrexate-Induced Chronic Encephalopathy

In addition to the acute encephalopathy that can be caused by methotrexate, patients can develop a chronic dementing syndrome that develops months to years after treatment. The MRI correlate is a diffuse subcortical leukoencephalopathy (confluent periventricular white matter T2/FLAIR hyperintensities). The risk of development of methotrexate leukoencephalopathy is increased if the patient has undergone whole brain radiation.

Intrathecal chemotherapy (most commonly methotrexate) can cause aseptic meningitis or myelopathy.

Neurologic Complications of Immunotherapies for Cancer
Immune Checkpoint Inhibitors

The immune checkpoint inhibitors include anti-PD-1 antibodies (pembrolizumab and nivolumab), anti-PD-L1 antibodies (e.g., atezolizumab, avelumab, durvalumab), and anti-CTLA-4 antibodies (ipilimumab). Neurotoxicity is most commonly associated with anti-PD-1 therapies, anti-CTLA-4 therapies, and combination therapy. The peripheral nervous system is most commonly affected: Guillain-Barré syndrome, cranial neuropathies, mononeuritis multiplex, myasthenia gravis (sometimes associated with simultaneous myositis and myocarditis), and myositis have been reported. In the central nervous system, encephalitis (often antibody-mediated), aseptic meningitis, hypophysitis, and myelitis can occur. Treatment generally involves stopping the checkpoint inhibitor and initiating steroids; IVIg and plasma exchange are considered in severe cases.

Chimeric Antigen Receptor (CAR) T-Cell therapy

A large proportion of patients undergoing CAR T-cell therapy for hematologic malignancy develop neurotoxicity (immune

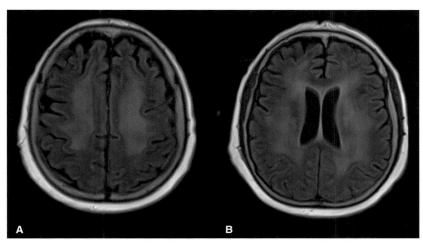

FIGURE 24–9 **Radiation-induced leukoencephalopathy.** Axial FLAIR MRI images demonstrating T2/FLAIR hyperintensity in the subcortical periventricular white matter.

effector cell-associated neurotoxicity syndrome [ICANS]) either concurrently with or following the cytokine release syndrome that occurs in many patients shortly after infusion of CAR T-cells. The most common features are altered mental status (ranging from encephalopathy/delirium to coma), headache, aphasia, and tremulousness. Less commonly, focal deficits, seizures, and cerebral edema can occur. Imaging is typically unremarkable, but ischemic stroke and hemorrhage have been reported (Rubin et al., 2019). Treatment is with steroids; tocilizumab is used for cytokine release syndrome and so is often used if both this and ICANS are present, but is not currently recommended for isolated ICANS.

Neurotoxicity of Radiation Therapy

Radiation therapy can cause neurologic complications affecting the brain, spine, and/or brachial or lumbar plexus.

Neurotoxicity of Radiation Therapy to the Brain

The acute to subacute effects of brain radiation can include headache, nausea, and fatigue. In some patients, worsening of the focal symptoms related to the tumor may occur and the MRI appearance of the lesion may appear to worsen due to radiation necrosis (**pseudoprogression**), although this must be distinguished from actual tumor progression with serial imaging.

Months to years following brain radiation, cognitive deficits can develop subacutely, presenting as a dementing syndrome. The MRI correlate is a severe leukoencephalopathy (Fig. 24–9).

Radiation can also affect the cerebrovascular system (radiation vasculopathy), leading to stenosis or occlusion of the carotid arteries or intracranial vasculature, which can predispose to stroke or the development of moyamoya (see "Moyamoya" in Ch. 19).

Strokelike Migraine Attacks After Radiation Therapy (SMART) Syndrome—SMART syndrome can occur years following brain radiation. It is characterized by transient focal neurologic deficits, headache, and/or seizures. Symptoms may last from hours to days before resolving completely. During the episode, the patient may clinically appear to have had a stroke, although neuroimaging will not reveal one, and EEG does not reveal ongoing seizure activity (both seizure and stroke are in the differential diagnosis for SMART syndrome). Neuroimaging shows a characteristic pattern of gyral enhancement (Fig. 24–10), which also resolves following resolution of symptoms if neuroimaging is repeated.

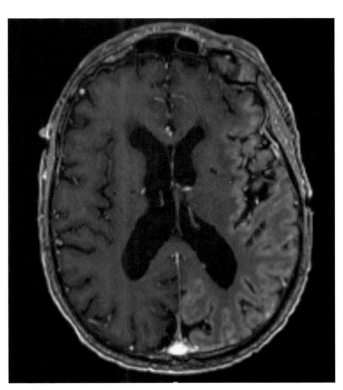

FIGURE 24–10 **SMART syndrome.** Axial T1-weighted postcontrast MRI image demonstrating gyral enhancement of the cortex of the majority of the left hemisphere.

Radiation Therapy–Induced Cranial Nerve Palsies

Radiation can affect any cranial nerve(s) depending on the field of radiation. For example, radiation-induced optic neuropathy can cause painless subacute visual loss months or even years following radiation to the pituitary (differential diagnosis includes radiation-induced cataract).

Radiation Therapy–Induced Myelopathy

The spinal cord can be affected by spinal irradiation for primary tumors or metastases or in the setting of mantle radiation, which includes the neck and chest. Like radiation's effects on the brain, there can be both acute and chronic sequelae of radiation injury to the spinal cord. In the acute setting, transient painful paresthesias can occur, and L'hermitte's sign may be present. Months to years later, a subacute myelopathy may develop, with corresponding T2 hyperintensity in the spinal cord or cord atrophy. Some experts recommend steroids and/or hyperbaric oxygen to treat chronic radiation myelopathy, but data are limited.

Radiation injury to the brachial plexus and lumbar plexus are discussed in Chapters 16 and 17, respectively. Radiation-induced plexopathy is typically painless and demonstrates myokymic discharges on EMG; malignant infiltration of the plexus is typically painful and does not demonstrate myokymic discharges on EMG.

PARANEOPLASTIC/ANTIBODY-MEDIATED SYNDROMES OF THE NERVOUS SYSTEM

Paraneoplastic conditions are cancer-related complications that are not due to direct organ involvement by the tumor or metastasis. The paraneoplastic syndromes that directly affect the nervous system are immune-mediated, associated with antibodies to cell-surface antigens or intracellular antigens (Table 24–5). Note that antibody-mediated neurologic syndromes can also occur without an associated neoplasm, a situation more commonly seen with antibodies to cell-surface antigens.

Antibody-mediated neurologic syndromes can affect any level of the neuraxis or multiple levels simultaneously (Table 24–6). Therefore, it is important to consider an antibody-mediated syndrome in the differential diagnosis of subacute development of neurologic symptoms of any type. When associated with neoplasia, paraneoplastic syndromes often precede the diagnosis of systemic cancer. Some general principles regarding paraneoplastic/antibody-mediated syndromes of the nervous system are as follows:

- Some of the syndromes are unifocal (e.g., limbic encephalitis, cerebellar degeneration), whereas some of the syndromes are multifaceted (e.g., encephalomyelitis, anti-IgLON5, anti-DPPX).
- Some antibodies are associated with a single syndrome (e.g., anti-NMDA receptor antibodies cause limbic encephalitis), while other antibodies can cause a number of different syndromes either independently or simultaneously (e.g., anti-Hu antibody, which can cause encephalitis, myelitis, encephalomyelitis, cerebellar degeneration, sensory ganglionopathy, and peripheral neuropathy).
- Certain neoplasms can be associated with a wide variety of paraneoplastic antibodies/syndromes (e.g., small cell lung cancer), whereas other tumors are associated most commonly with a particular syndrome (e.g., neuroblastoma and opsoclonus-myoclonus; ovarian teratoma and anti-NMDA receptor encephalitis).

Evaluation for a presumed CNS paraneoplastic/antibody-mediated syndrome generally involves obtaining MRI, EEG, and lumbar puncture. Although MRI, EEG, and lumbar puncture may show patterns consistent with specific antibody-mediated syndromes, these studies may be normal or demonstrate only nonspecific findings (e.g., inflammatory CSF). In such cases, the diagnosis may be made by identifying the underlying cancer and/or an associated antibody in the CSF or serum. Since new antibodies are being identified rapidly, not all cases that are presumed to be antibody-mediated can be "proven" since assays may not yet be commercially available for recently described or not-yet described antibodies.

If a paraneoplastic/antibody-mediated syndrome is diagnosed in a patient with no known cancer, an evaluation for cancer should be undertaken based on the most likely site(s) of malignancy associated with the presenting syndrome (e.g., testicular ultrasound, pelvic ultrasound, mammogram, chest CT). If no evidence of malignancy is found, full-body PET may reveal the underlying cancer. In a patient with a paraneoplastic/antibody-mediated neurologic syndrome in whom an exhaustive evaluation for neoplasm is unrevealing, close clinical and radiologic surveillance (with PET) should be continued every 6 months for several years. Some patients may ultimately be found to have an antibody-mediated syndrome with no associated malignancy.

In general, treatment involves treating the underlying malignancy (if present) and immunomodulatory therapy (most commonly steroids, IVIg, plasma exchange, rituximab, cyclophosphamide). Syndromes caused by antibodies against cell surface receptors tend to respond better to immunomodulatory therapy than syndromes caused by antibodies against intracellular targets.

A number of the syndromes listed in Table 24–6 are discussed in other chapters. Here, limbic encephalitis and opsoclonus-myoclonus-ataxia syndromes are discussed.

TABLE 24–5 Comparison of Cell Surface & Intracellular Antibodies Affecting the Nervous System.

	Cell Surface	Intracellular
Association with neoplasia	Less common	Very common
Immunology	Antibody-mediated	T-cell mediated
Response to treatment	Robust	Often minimal

TABLE 24–6 Antibody-Mediated Syndromes Affecting the Nervous System.

Level of Nervous System	Syndrome	Antibody * = less frequently associated with neoplasm (c) = cell surface (i) = intracellular	Most Commonly Associated Neoplasm(s)
Brain	Limbic encephalitis	Anti-NMDA* (c)	Ovarian teratoma
		Anti-AMPA* (c)	Breast, lung, thymoma
		Anti-GABA-A* (c)	Thymoma
			Hodgkin's lymphoma
		Anti-GABA-B* (c)	Small cell lung cancer (SCLC)
		Anti-LGI1* (c) (w/ faciobrachial dystonic seizures; see Ch. 23)	SCLC, thymoma
		Anti-mGlur5	Hodgkin's lymphoma (Ophelia syndrome), SCLC
		Anti-CV2/CRMP5 (c)	SCLC, thymoma
		Anti-Hu (ANNA1) (i)	Small cell lung cancer
		Anti-Ma2 (c)	Testicular cancer
		Anti-GAD65*+ (i)	SCLC, thymoma
Meninges	Meningitis (may be accompanied by encephalitis and/or myelitis; often causes enhancement radiating out from lateral ventricles on MRI)	Anti-GFAP* (i)	Ovarian teratoma
Brainstem (and cerebellum)	Rhomboencephalitis (vertigo, tinnitus, hearing loss, ataxia, diplopia)	Anti-KLHL11 (i)	Testicular cancer (most commonly seminoma)
	Brainstem encephalitis (Gaze palsies, dysarthria/dysphagia) +/or diencephalic encephalitis (sleep disorders) +/or limbic encephalitis	Anti-Ma2 (i)	Testicular cancer, NSCLC
Cerebellum	Cerebellar degeneration	Anti-Yo (i)	Ovarian, breast
		Anti-Hu (ANNA1) (i)	SCLC
		Anti-Ri (ANNA2) (i)	Breast, gynecologic
		Anti-Tr (c)	Hodgkin's lymphoma
		Anti-Ma2 (i)	Testicular
		Anti-mGlur1 (c)	Hodgkin's lymphoma
		Anti-NfL (i)	SCLC, Merkel cell
		Anti-Zic4 (i)	SCLC
		Anti-GAD65*+ (i)	SCLC, thymoma
Optic nerve	Optic neuropathy	Anti-CRMP-5 (i)	SCLC
Retina	Retinopathy	Anti-Recoverin (i)	SCLC
		Anti-Bipolar cell (i)	Melanoma
Spinal cord	Myelitis (often part of an encephalomyelitis but can be isolated)	Anti-Hu (ANNA1) (i)	SCLC
		Anti-CRMP-5 (i)	
	Necrotizing myelopathy	Anti-Hu (ANNA1) (i)	SCLC, hematologic malignancies
		Anti-CRMP-5 (i)	
Dorsal root ganglia	Ganglionopathy/Sensory neuronopathy (see Ch. 15)	Anti-Hu (ANNA1) (i)	SCLC

(Continued)

TABLE 24–6 Antibody-Mediated Syndromes Affecting the Nervous System. (*Continued*)

Level of Nervous System	Syndrome	Antibody * = less frequently associated with neoplasm (c) = cell surface (i) = intracellular	Most Commonly Associated Neoplasm(s)
Peripheral nerves	Sensorimotor neuropathy	Anti-Hu (ANNA1) (i)	SCLC
		Anti-CRMP5 (i)	Thymoma
		Paraprotein-associated; see Ch. 26	Plasma cell disorders (see Ch. 26)
	Autonomic neuropathy (see Ch. 27)	Anti-ganglionic ACh-R (c)	SCLC, thymoma
		Anti-Hu (ANNA1) (i)	SCLC
Motor neurons	ALS-like syndrome	?	Rare case reports of association with hematologic malignancies, breast cancer
Neuromuscular junction	Lambert-Eaton myasthenic syndrome (see Ch. 29)	Voltage-gated calcium channels (VGCC) (c)	Small cell lung cancer
	Myasthenia gravis (see Ch. 29)	ACh-R* (c)	Thymoma
Muscle	Dermatomyositis (see Ch. 30)	Anti-NXP2	Gastrointestinal, breast
		Anti-TIF1-gamma	
Other	Opsoclonus-myoclonus	?	Neuroblastoma
		Anti-Ri (ANNA2) (i)	Breast, gynecologic
	Stiff person syndrome (see Ch. 23)	Anti-amphiphysin (i)	SCLC, breast
		(Anti-GAD65+ in *non*-paraneoplastic)	
	Progressive encephalomyelitis with rigidity and myoclonus (PERM) (see Ch. 23)	Anti-glycine* (c)	Thymoma
		Anti-GAD65*+ (i)	
	Isaac's syndrome (neuromyotonia)	Anti-CASPR2* (c)	SCLC, thymoma
	and		
	Morvan's syndrome (neuromyotonia + encephalitis)		
	Weight loss/diarrhea, dementia, hyperexcitability (hyperekplexia, myoclonus, tremor)	Anti-DPPX*(c)	Lymphoma
	Sleep disorder (sleep apnea, parasomnia, stridor), dysarthria, dysphagia, gait disorder, movement disorder (chorea, tremor), supranuclear gaze palsy, dysautonomia, PSP-like syndrome, and/or cognitive dysfunction; chronic onset	Anti-IgLON5* (c)	-

Abbreviations: AchR: acetylcholine receptor; AMPA: alpha-amino-3-hydroxy-5-methlyl-4-isoxazolepropionic acid receptor; ANNA1 and ANNA2: antineuronal nuclear antibodies 1 and 2; CASPR: contactin-associated protein-like 2; CRMP5: collapsing response mediator protein 5; DPPX: dipeptidyl-peptidase-like protein 6; GABA-B: gamma-aminobutyric acid B; GAD: glutamic acid decarboxylase; KLHL11: kelch-like protein-11; LGI1: leucine-rich, glioma inactivated 1; NfL: neurofilament light chain; NMDA: *N*-methyl-D-aspartate; NSCLC: non-small cell lung cancer; SCLC: small cell lung cancer.

aAsterisk (*) indicates antibodies that also commonly occur independently of a systemic cancer.

+Anti-GAD65 antibodies are seen in patients with diabetes and in low titer in the general population and only high titers in appropriate clinical context should be considered to represent an autoimmune condition related to anti-GAD65 antibodies.

Autoimmune Limbic Encephalitis

Autoimmune limbic encephalitis is an antibody-mediated encephalitis characterized by limbic features: psychiatric symptoms, altered cognition (most commonly short-term memory loss), and seizures. MRI may reveal T2/FLAIR hyperintensities and/or contrast enhancement in limbic structures (but can be normal), EEG may show seizures and/or temporal lobe epileptiform discharges (but can be normal or nonspecific), and CSF is typically inflammatory (but may be normal). A growing list of antibodies have been associated with autoimmune limbic encephalitis, some of which are only rarely associated with malignancy (i.e., autoimmune encephalitis rather than paraneoplastic encephalitis; see Table 24–6). Diagnosis is made by demonstration of the causative antibody in the CSF. Isolated antibodies in the serum only with no CSF antibody should be viewed with skepticism as they are often false positives (except for LGI1 antibodies, for which serum may be more sensitive than CSF). Noting that antibody results can take time to return and the urgency of initiating treatment, recent guidelines suggest that autoimmune limbic encephalitis should be considered if there is subacute development (<3 months) of memory loss, seizures, or psychiatric symptoms; bilateral medial temporal lobe hyperintensity on MRI and CSF pleocytosis (>5 cells/mm^3) or EEG with temporal slowing; and other potential etiologies have been excluded (e.g., infection, prion disease, demyelinating disease, toxic-metabolic, vascular, etc.) (Graus et al., 2016).

Anti-NMDA Receptor Encephalitis

Anti-NMDA receptor encephalitis is characterized by subacute onset (over weeks to months) of neuropsychiatric symptoms (behavioral changes, psychosis, memory loss, language deficits) and seizures followed by development of movement disorders (most commonly orofacial dyskinesias, but can include dystonia, chorea, catatonia), and autonomic instability (cardiovascular and hypoventilation). Patients often experience a preceding prodrome of a viral-like illness. MRI may demonstrate T2/FLAIR hyperintensities in limbic regions or may be normal. EEG can demonstrate seizures, slowing, or the more unique finding of extreme delta brush. CSF is often inflammatory and may demonstrate oligoclonal bands. The diagnosis is confirmed by demonstrating anti-NMDA receptor antibodies in the CSF; positivity in the serum alone without CSF positivity is often a false positive result.

This condition is most commonly seen in young women in the setting of ovarian teratoma, the removal of which (usually accompanied by immunomodulatory therapy) may be curative. Therefore, pelvic ultrasound is an essential part of the evaluation of patients with presumed anti-NMDA receptor encephalitis. However, only about half of patients with anti-NMDA receptor encephalitis have an underlying tumor. Treatment includes removal of the underlying tumor (if present) and immunomodulatory therapy. Anti-NMDA receptor encephalitis can rarely occur following herpes simplex virus encephalitis, presenting as what appears to be a relapse of encephalitis (see "Herpes Simplex Virus Encephalitis" in Ch. 20). Comprehensive reviews of this condition can be found in Dalmau et al., 2011 and Dalmau et al., 2019).

Opsoclonus-Myoclonus/ Opsoclonus-Myoclonus-Ataxia

The combination of opsoclonus and myoclonus in a child warrants a search for an underlying neuroblastoma. In adults, anti-Ri is the antibody that is usually associated with this syndrome,

and the most common malignancies are breast, gynecologic, or lung cancer (most commonly small cell lung cancer).

CEREBROVASCULAR COMPLICATIONS OF CANCER

Systemic cancers can predispose to ischemic stroke or intracranial hemorrhage through a variety of mechanisms. Vascular complications may be the presenting feature of an undiagnosed systemic malignancy or may arise in patients with known cancer. Vascular complications can also be caused by radiation (see "Neurotoxicity of Radiation Therapy to the Brain") and chemotherapy (such as bevacizumab, L-asparaginase). Aside from treatment-related effects:

- Ischemic stroke in the setting of malignancy can be caused by:
  - Hypercoagulability of malignancy (**Trousseau's syndrome**; especially common with adenocarcinomas, particularly GI malignancies)
  - Disseminated intravascular coagulation
  - Tumor embolism from metastatic or primary cardiac tumor such as atrial myxoma or nonbacterial thrombotic endocarditis (formation of thrombus on cardiac valves with subsequent embolism)
- Intracerebral hemorrhage in the setting of malignancy can be caused by:
  - Hemorrhage into brain metastases: most common in melanoma, renal cell carcinoma, thyroid cancer, and choriocarcinoma, although it can occur with any metastatic brain tumor
  - Thrombocytopenia due to hematologic malignancy
  - Coagulopathy: for example, due to disseminated intravascular coagulation
- Venous sinus thrombosis in the setting of malignancy can be caused by:
  - Hypercoagulability of malignancy
  - Tumor compression of the venous sinuses

If ischemic stroke, intracerebral hemorrhage, or venous sinus thrombosis occurs in a patient with cancer, the patient should be evaluated for other potential causes of cerebrovascular disease prior to attributing the cerebrovascular complication directly to the underlying malignancy.

When malignancy is thought to be the cause of ischemic stroke, therapeutic anticoagulation with low molecular weight heparin or direct oral anticoagulant may be considered if there are no contraindications, although this is based on data for venous thromboembolism in the setting of malignancy rather than specific data for stroke in this setting.

REFERENCES

Dalmau J, Armangué T, Planagumà J, Radosevic J, Mannara F, Leypoldt F, et al. An update on anti-NMDA receptor encephalitis for neurologists and psychiatrists: mechanisms and models. *Lancet Neurol* 2019;18:1045–1057.

Dalmau J, Lancaster E, Martinez-Hernandez E, Rosenfeld MR, Balice-Gordon R. Clinical experience and laboratory investigations in patients with anti-NMDAR encephalitis. *Lancet Neurol* 2011;10:63–74.

Graus F, Titulaer MJ, Balu R, Benseler S, Bien CG, Cellucci T, et al. A clinical approach to diagnosis of autoimmune encephalitis. *Lancet Neurol* 2016;15:391–404.

Hershman DL, Lacchetti C, Dworkin RH, Lavoie Smith EM, Bleeker J, Cavaletti G, et al. Prevention and management of chemotherapy-induced peripheral neuropathy in survivors of adult cancers: American Society of Clinical Oncology Clinical Practice Guideline. *J Clin Oncol* 2014;32:1941–1967.

Louis DN, et al. The 2021 WHO Classification of Tumors of the Central Nervous System: a summary. *Neuro-oncology* 2021;23(8):1231–1251.

Rubin DB, Danish HH, Ali AB, Li K, LaRose S, Monk AD, et al. Neurological toxicities associated with chimeric antigen receptor T-cell therapy. *Brain* 2019;142(5):1334–1348.

Disorders of Intracranial Pressure

INCREASED INTRACRANIAL PRESSURE (INTRACRANIAL HYPERTENSION)

General Principles of Intracranial Pressure

Intracranial Contents Contributing to Intracranial Volume & Pressure

The skull contains three components that contribute to intracranial volume: the brain, its blood supply, and the cerebrospinal fluid (CSF). The brain accounts for approximately 80% of the intracranial volume, the arterial and venous blood approximately 10%, and the CSF approximately 10%. The skull is fixed and can only accommodate small changes in intracranial volume before intracranial pressure rises. Increased intracranial pressure can arise due to increased volume of any of the three intracranial contents (brain, blood volume, or CSF).

Increased intracranial pressure due to increased brain volume—Both focal brain lesions and diffuse brain pathology can lead to increased intracranial pressure (ICP). A focal brain lesion (e.g., stroke, tumor, abscess, demyelination) can cause increased ICP either by mass effect or by obstruction of the ventricular system leading to obstruction of CSF flow. Diffuse cerebral edema (e.g., secondary to severe head trauma, hypoxic-ischemic injury, hyponatremia, meningoencephalitis) raises overall brain volume, increasing ICP.

Increased intracranial pressure due to increased blood volume—Increased blood volume can occur either due to decreased venous outflow (e.g., venous sinus thrombosis) or due to increased arterial blood flow (e.g., due to cerebral vasodilation).

Increased intracranial pressure due to increased cerebrospinal fluid volume—Increased CSF volume (**hydrocephalus**) can occur due to obstruction of CSF circulation or rarely due to increased CSF production (e.g., due to choroid plexus papilloma). Obstruction of CSF circulation can be caused by a blockage anywhere within the ventricular system (e.g., tumor, intraventricular hemorrhage, congenital aqueductal stenosis) or a blockage of the arachnoid granulations where CSF is absorbed into the venous circulation (e.g., due to meningitis, subarachnoid hemorrhage). Ventricular obstruction causes **noncommunicating hydrocephalus**: The ventricles cannot communicate with one another to allow for CSF to circulate. In noncommunicating hydrocephalus, only the ventricles proximal to the obstruction will dilate (e.g., obstruction of the third ventricle will lead to dilation of the lateral ventricles but not the fourth ventricle). Obstruction of the arachnoid granulations causes **communicating hydrocephalus**: The ventricles can still communicate with one another, but CSF cannot be reabsorbed. In communicating hydrocephalus, all of the ventricles will dilate.

If brain volume increases, there is the possibility of limited compensation in the other two compartments (CSF and blood) to maintain constant intracranial volume (**Monro-Kellie doctrine**). The compensatory mechanisms include displacing CSF into the spinal column, constriction of arterioles, and collapse of veins. However, if intracranial volume increases beyond a certain point, compensation is no longer possible, and ICP rises.

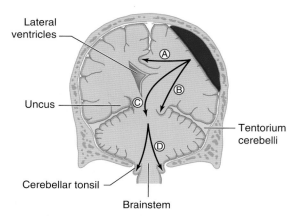

FIGURE 25-1 Schematic depicting different types of brain herniation. A: Subfalcine herniation. **B:** Uncal herniation. **C:** Transtentorial (central) herniation. **D:** Tonsillar herniation. Reproduced with permission from Aminoff M, Greenberg D, Simon R: *Clinical Neurology*, 9th ed. New York, NY: McGraw Hill; 2015.

There are two main potential consequences of increased ICP: brain herniation and decreased cerebral perfusion.

Brain Herniation (Fig. 25–1)

Brain herniation refers to shift of brain tissue beyond its normal location. Types of herniation include subfalcine, uncal, transtentorial (central), upward, and tonsillar.

Subfalcine herniation—In this type of herniation, the cingulate gyrus herniates beneath the falx cerebri (the interhemispheric dura). This can compress the anterior cerebral arteries, leading to stroke.

Uncal herniation—In this type of herniation, the medial temporal lobe compresses the ipsilateral third nerve causing pupillary dilatation. If uncal herniation progresses to the point of compressing the contralateral midbrain against the tentorium, the *contralateral* cerebral peduncle can be affected, leading to motor deficits and upper motor neuron signs *ipsilateral* to the side of uncal herniation (**Kernohan's notch phenomenon**). For example, uncal herniation on the left generally first causes left pupillary dilatation due to compression of the left cranial nerve 3. If uncal herniation progresses, the *right* cerebral peduncle can be compressed against the tentorium, causing hemiparesis contralateral to this peduncle (i.e., on the left) since the corticospinal tract has not yet crossed. Therefore, the hemiparesis is ipsilateral to the side of uncal herniation and the dilated pupil (on the left in this example).

Transtentorial (central) herniation—In this type of herniation, the central components of the brain (thalami, midbrain) herniate downward through the tentorium cerebelli, which can lead to bilateral pupillary dilatation and can ultimately proceed to coma, cardiorespiratory dysfunction, and death.

Upward herniation—With a large cerebellar mass lesion (or diffuse cerebellar pathology), the cerebellum can herniate upward through the tentorium. This causes brainstem compression leading to coma and pupillary abnormalities (the pupils may be small due to pontine distortion or dilated due to midbrain distortion). Upward herniation may be precipitated by CSF drainage via placement of an external ventricular drain (EVD) in patients with increased cerebellar volume (e.g., cerebellar tumor or hemorrhage): An upward pressure vector from the expanded cerebellum leads to upward displacement when pressure from above is decreased.

Tonsillar herniation—In this type of herniation, the cerebellar tonsils descend below the foramen magnum, compressing the medulla (**coning**). This can cause coma, cardiorespiratory dysfunction, and death.

Cerebral Perfusion Pressure

Cerebral perfusion pressure (CPP) is determined by the pressure of the blood reaching the brain (mean arterial pressure [MAP]) and the ICP acting against this blood pressure:

$$CPP = MAP - ICP$$

Therefore, if ICP rises at a constant MAP, cerebral perfusion pressure will fall, which can lead to decreased cerebral perfusion.

Symptoms & Signs of Increased Intracranial Pressure

The symptoms and signs of intracranial hypertension depend on the degree to which ICP is elevated and the rapidity with which ICP rises. Symptoms may include headache, blurred vision, nausea/vomiting, and alteration in mental status ranging from somnolence to coma. Headache due to elevated ICP is classically worse in the supine position and improves with standing. Signs of intracranial hypertension can include:

- **Papilledema.** Papilledema may not be present acutely since it can take hours to days to develop.
- **Unilateral or bilateral sixth nerve palsy.** This is referred to as a "false localizing sign" in this context, since it appears focal but is a sign of a generalized process (elevated ICP) causing pressure on one or both abducens nerves due to the long intracranial course of this cranial nerve (see "Cranial Nerve 6: The Abducens Nerve" in Ch. 11 for discussion of the signs of sixth nerve palsy).
- **Cushing's response:** hypertension, bradycardia, and irregular respiration can result from compression of the medulla.
- **Signs of herniation** related to compression of particular structures may be present depending on the location and cause of the responsible lesion(s) (see "Brain Herniation").

Treatment of Acutely Increased Intracranial Pressure

Basic measures to treat elevated ICP include:

- Elevating the head of the patient's bed to 30 degrees, which allows gravity to help with venous and CSF drainage.
- Hyperventilating the patient if they are mechanically ventilated, although this is only a temporizing measure. Hyperventilation decreases ICP by decreasing arterial CO_2, leading to cerebral arterial vasoconstriction.
- Treatment of any complications of the underlying illness that could lead to further increases in ICP (i.e., treating seizures, fever, agitation, and pain).
- Avoidance of hypotonic IV fluids (i.e., avoiding any IV solution less concentrated than normal saline) since these can worsen cerebral edema.

More definitive treatment strategies rest on the principles discussed above: attempting to decrease the volume of one or more of the intracranial contents in the fixed "box" of the skull (i.e., brain, CSF, and blood supply) or "opening the box" (i.e., hemicraniectomy or suboccipital craniectomy). One cannot decrease blood supply since this could lead to decreased cerebral perfusion. In fact, in the setting of elevated ICP, one must work to maintain an adequate MAP to preserve CPP (see equation on the previous page). However, one can decrease the volume of the brain (using hyperosmolar therapy to pull water out of it) and/or remove CSF (diversion via an EVD or ventriculoperitoneal shunt). If hyperosmolar therapy or CSF drainage are inadequate, one can "open the box" by performing a hemicraniectomy or suboccipital craniectomy to allow room for the brain to expand out of the skull defect rather than herniate intracranially. If ICP cannot be controlled with these treatments, pentobarbitol coma and therapeutic hypothermia can be considered to reduce brain metabolism.

If there is a tumor with surrounding edema, a large demyelinating lesion, or intracranial infection, steroids can decrease inflammation related to these etiologies. However, steroids do *not* appear to be beneficial (and may be harmful) for other causes of elevated intracranial pressure such as stroke and head trauma.

Hyperosmolar Therapy in the Treatment of Acutely Increased Intracranial Pressure

Hypertonic solutions draw water into them. Hypertonic IV fluids increase the tonicity of the serum, pulling water out of the brain into the bloodstream to reduce brain volume. Hyperosmolar therapy is particularly effective in treating cerebral edema. However, even if ICP is elevated due to a large mass without significant edema (e.g., an intraparenchymal hermorrhage), hyperosmolar therapy can shrink the normal regions of the brain, thereby reducing overall brain volume to decrease ICP.

Hyperosmolar therapy is generally utilized to treat edema that is expected to be transient, since hyperosmolar therapy cannot be given indefinitely. Examples include malignant edema from a full-territory middle cerebral artery (MCA) infarct or large cerebellar infarct (stroke-related edema typically peaks within the first several days after stroke and then recedes), diffuse edema from acute encephalitis or meningitis (which should resolve with effective antibiotic treatment), and severe head trauma with diffuse cerebral edema.

Two equations are important in understanding treatments that increase serum tonicity to pull water from the brain:

$$\text{Calculated serum osmolarity} = [2 \times \text{Na}] + [\text{Glu}/18] + [\text{BUN}/2.8]$$

$$\textbf{Osmolar (or osmolal) gap} = \text{measured serum osmolality (a laboratory value) minus the calculated osmolarity (as calculated by the prior equation)}$$

The normal value for the serum osmolar gap is around 10 (since other serum osmoles beyond sodium, glucose, and BUN normally contribute). The gap can be pathologically increased by ethylene glycol, ethanol, and other alcohols.

To treat increased ICP, serum osmolarity can be increased by adding an osmole (mannitol) or increasing one of the osmoles in the above equation (sodium).

Mannitol in the treatment of acutely increased intracranial pressure—Mannitol adds an additional osmole to the serum, increasing the osmolar gap and serum tonicity. Mannitol can be given through a peripheral IV, and the lowest effective dose should be utilized (range generally 0.5–1.0 g/kg). The effect of mannitol occurs within minutes and lasts hours. Mannitol can be given every 6–8 hours, but should not be given if serum osmolarity is greater than 320. Complications of mannitol therapy can include electrolyte abnormalities, increased intravascular volume (which may be poorly tolerated in the setting of congestive heart failure), and hypotension and/or renal dysfunction from diuresis.

Hypertonic saline in the treatment of acutely increased intracranial pressure—23% saline can be given by central line as a bolus (30 mL). Like mannitol, it acts rapidly, has a duration of effect on the order of hours, causes diuresis, and can cause renal and cardiac complications. A serum sodium of up to 160 is generally targeted.

When necessary, mannitol and 23% saline can be given in alternation (e.g., both every 8 hours staggered by 4-hour intervals so the patient gets one or the other every 4 hours). Hyperosmolar therapy should not be stopped abruptly, but rather weaned by progressively increasing the time interval between doses as tolerated.

A continuous infusion of 3% saline may be used to achieve eunatremia in patients with cerebral edema who are hyponatremic. Some practitioners set a sodium goal (i.e., maintain a hypernatremic state) even in patients who are not hyponatremic; others prefer eunatremia, reserving the possibility of rapidly creating an osmotic gradient with a bolus of hypertonic saline if there is an acute rise in ICP.

CSF Diversion in the Treatment of Acutely Increased Intracranial Pressure

An external ventricular drain (EVD) is a temporary catheter that allows for CSF drainage directly from the ventricles. An EVD is similar to a ventriculoperitoneal (VP) shunt except that rather than shunting CSF to another location in the body, CSF is shunted directly to the outside world. An EVD serves two purposes:

- CSF drainage to reduce ICP without requiring lumbar puncture (since lumbar puncture may precipitate herniation in cases of increased ICP)
- Measurement of ICP to allow for targeted therapy for elevated ICP

Treatment of Chronically Increased Intracranial Pressure: Ventriculoperitoneal Shunt & Endoscopic Third Ventriculostomy

Ventriculoperitoneal Shunt

Chronic hydrocephalus may be treated by insertion of a ventriculoperitoneal (VP) shunt. VP shunts are placed in the lateral ventricle, and pass under the skin to the peritoneal cavity. Some shunts have a programmable valve so that settings for drainage can be adjusted by an external magnetic device (and so must be reprogrammed after being subjected to the magnetism of an MRI).

Complications of VP shunts include shunt failure (leading to reemergence of hydrocephalus), overshunting (leading to intracranial hypotension; see "Decreased Intracranial Pressure: Intracranial Hypotension"), and shunt infection. Shunt infection can present with fever and/or shunt failure. Diagnosis of shunt infection is by shunt puncture (direct puncture of the shunt reservoir rather than lumbar puncture), and treatment is with antibiotics and shunt replacement. A shunt series refers to a series of radiographs of the head, neck, chest, and abdomen to look for any discontinuities in the shunt.

Endoscopic Third Ventriculostomy

An alternative to shunting in obstructive hydrocephalus is endoscopic third ventriculostomy. In this procedure, an endoscope is passed through the skull into the ventricular system and a hole is made in the third ventricle to allow CSF to pass directly into the subarachnoid space. This procedure is most commonly used to treat congenital aqueductal stenosis.

Pseudotumor Cerebri

Causes of Pseudotumor Cerebri

Pseudotumor cerebri is a condition in which symptoms and signs of elevated ICP develop without a structural lesion, hydrocephalus, or other apparent etiology on neuroimaging. The syndrome is most commonly an idiopathic condition in young women with elevated body mass index (**idiopathic intracranial hypertension**), although it can also be caused by medications (e.g., tetracycline, vitamin A, and medications derived from vitamin A [e.g., retinoids]), endocrine disease, treatment of endocrine disease, or withdrawal of treatment for endocrine disease (e.g., thyroid medications, growth hormone, steroids).

Symptoms & Signs of Pseudotumor Cerebri

Symptoms and signs of pseudotumor cerebri include:

- Headache
- Pulsatile tinnitus (usually described as a "whooshing" in the ears)
- Visual changes including:
  - Transient blacking out of vision after bending forward.
  - Double vision from unilateral or bilateral cranial nerve 6 palsy due to elevated ICP.
- Enlargement of the blind spot and restricted peripheral vision due to papilledema. Importantly, these visual field deficits may not be noted by the patient or on bedside visual field testing. Therefore, all patients with pseudotumor cerebri should be followed with formal visual field testing (e.g., automated perimetry).
- Papilledema, most commonly bilateral.

Diagnosis of Pseudotumor Cerebri

In any patient with symptoms and signs of elevated ICP, neuroimaging must be performed to evaluate for a mass lesion, hydrocephalus, or venous sinus thrombosis. MRI features suggestive of idiopathic intracranial hypertension include flattening of one or both optic discs and/or an empty sella. Diagnosis is confirmed by elevated opening pressure on lumbar puncture, and lumbar puncture may lead to temporary symptom relief.

Treatment of Pseudotumor Cerebri

In patients with medication-induced pseudotumor cerebri, offending medications should be discontinued. In patients with an endocrine cause of pseudotumor cerebri, the underlying disease must be treated. In patients with obesity-associated idiopathic intracranial hypertension, weight loss and acetazolamide are the mainstays of treatment. Acetazolamide works by decreasing CSF production. If acetazolamide is not tolerated, topiramate or furosemide may be considered. Patients' visual fields must be followed closely with formal testing, and any clinical worsening or worsening in visual fields may warrant surgical intervention to prevent permanent visual loss.

Surgical options for the treatment of pseudotumor cerebri include VP shunt and optic nerve sheath fenestration. Optic nerve sheath fenestration decompresses the optic nerve, which can improve vision or prevent further visual loss, but it may be less effective than VP shunt for the treatment of headache. In patients who present with a rapidly progressive course of pseudotumor cerebri, frequent lumbar punctures may be needed as a bridge to surgical intervention if surgery is not immediately available.

DECREASED INTRACRANIAL PRESSURE (INTRACRANIAL HYPOTENSION)

Causes of Intracranial Hypotension

Decreased intracranial pressure (**intracranial hypotension**) can occur if there is any break in the meninges allowing for leakage of CSF. Causes include:

- Lumbar puncture: diagnostic, for epidural anesthesia, or for intrathecal chemotherapy
- Head, neck, or back trauma leading to a dural tear
- Cranial or spinal surgery
- Local spinal pathology (e.g., meningeal diverticula, local bony disease)
- In some cases, no clear cause of intracranial hypotension is determined (**spontaneous intracranial hypotension**)

Symptoms & Signs of Intracranial Hypotension

Reduced CSF results in reduced buoyancy for the brain, causing it to sag. The sagging brain tugs on the dura, causing headache. The headache associated with intracranial hypotension worsens when standing and improves when supine, the opposite pattern of that seen in intracranial hypertension. Patients may also report neck pain and/or dizziness. Hearing loss, tinnitus, diplopia, and symptoms/signs of other cranial neuropathies may be present, caused by traction on cranial nerves due to the sag of the brain. In the most severe cases, distortion of the sagging frontal lobes and brainstem can cause alterations in consciousness and cognition—anything from a sense of "fogginess" to dementia (frontotemporal brain sagging syndrome; Wicklund et al., 2011) to coma.

Diagnosis of Intracranial Hypotension

The characteristic neuroimaging findings of intracranial hypotension are logical based on the pathophysiology (Fig. 25–2). As CSF leaks, the ventricles collapse, the brain sags, and the subdural spaces become prominent, which can cause subdural hematomas or subdural fluid collections to form. Since CSF volume is low, the venous system dilates to maintain intracranial volume, which leads to enlargement of the venous sinuses, pachymeningeal enhancement due to dilation of dural veins, and pituitary hyperemia.

Not all of these features are always seen, but uniform diffuse pachymeningeal enhancement on neuroimaging is a common clue to the diagnosis. Note that pachymeningeal enhancement can also be seen as an incidental asymptomatic finding after lumbar puncture in patients without symptoms of intracranial hypotension. The differential diagnosis of pachymeningeal enhancement also includes dural metastases, inflammatory meningitis, and less commonly infectious meningitis, though dural enhancement tends to be less smooth and symmetric in these scenarios compared to the enhancement pattern seen with intracranial hypotension.

A mnemonic to remember the radiologic signs of intracranial hypotension is provided in a review of the topic (Schievink, 2006): **SEEPS**

Subdural fluid collections

Enhancement of the pachymeninges

Engorgement of venous structures

Pituitary hyperemia

Sag of the brain

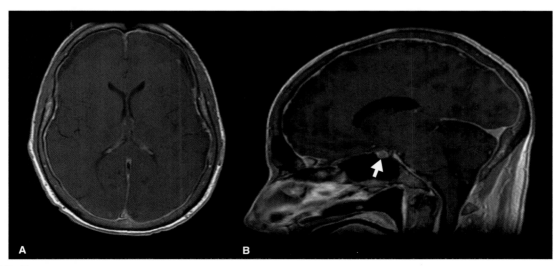

FIGURE 25–2 **MRI findings in intracranial hypotension.** Axial (**A**) and sagittal (**B**) T1-weighted postcontrast images demonstrating smooth diffuse pachymeningeal enhancement, bilateral frontal subdural fluid collections (**A**), pituitary hyperemia (**B**, arrow), and sag of the frontal lobe and brainstem (**B**).

The diagnosis of intracranial hypotension can generally be made by MRI findings, but if lumbar puncture is obtained, CSF pressure will be low and there may be elevated protein and pleocyotosis. MRI of the spine is not sufficiently sensitive to find small tears in the dura, and myelography or radionuclide cisternography may be necessary. However, these tests are generally only pursued if patients fail conservative management (see "Treatment of Intracranial Hypotension"). When the classic symptoms and radiologic features are present and there is no clear etiology (i.e., spontaneous intracranial hypotension), empiric treatment may be successful even if the site of the leak is not localized.

Treatment of Intracranial Hypotension

Conservative management of intracranial hypotension includes bed rest, caffeine (oral and/or IV), and aggressive hydration. If these do not lead to symptom amelioration, intracranial hypotension can be treated with an epidural blood patch. This involves injecting a small amount of the patient's own blood into the epidural space. It is unclear exactly how this works; it may "patch" the leak, or may lead to an alteration in CSF flow dynamics resulting in reequilibration of the system. An epidural blood patch often leads to rapid improvement in headache. If a blood patch is ineffective or its effects are transient, it can be repeated after a few days. If patients do not improve after several attempted blood patches, myelography or radionuclide cisternography should be performed with the goal of localizing the leak so as to surgically repair it.

REFERENCES

Schievink WI. Spontaneous spinal cerebrospinal fluid leaks and intracranial hypotension. *JAMA* 2006;295:2286–2296.
Wicklund MR et al. Frontotemporal brain sagging syndrome: An SIH-like presentation mimicking FTD. *Neurology* 2011;76(16): 1377–1382.

Headache

APPROACH TO HEADACHE

When a patient presents for evaluation of headache(s), the goal of the history and examination is to answer two questions:

- Is there an underlying cause of headache(s) in need of further laboratory/neuroimaging evaluation (i.e., **secondary headache**)?
- If there is no underlying cause of headache(s), which **primary headache syndrome** best describes the headache (e.g., migraine, tension, cluster)?

When headaches are determined to be primary rather than secondary, although they may be benign with respect to etiology, such headaches can be extremely disabling. Proper recognition of the precise primary headache syndrome is important because different headache syndromes respond to different abortive and prophylactic medications.

Importantly, a headache syndrome that perfectly fits the description of one of the primary headache syndromes does not always signify that there is no underlying cause. Acute stroke or a structural lesion can produce headaches that meet clinical criteria for primary headache syndromes such as migraine (**symptomatic migraine**), so clinical context is important in determining the need for further evaluation.

SECONDARY CAUSES OF HEADACHE

The causes of secondary headache range from benign (e.g., eye strain due to need for prescription glasses) to life threatening (e.g., aneurysmal rupture, bacterial meningitis).

Causes of secondary headache can be broadly classified as related to:

- Intracranial structures: meninges, brain, and/or cerebral blood vessels
- Head and neck structures: eyes, ears, nose, sinuses, jaw/teeth, neck, cervical/extracranial vasculature
- Systemic causes: hypertension, systemic infection, medications

In some patients in whom a cause for headache cannot be found, headache may be a symptom of an underlying psychiatric disorder (e.g., somatization disorder).

Red flags in a patient's history that should raise concern for a serious underlying etiology of headache can be divided into (Table 26–1):

- **Characteristics** of the headache itself:
  - **Onset:** concerning if acute and maximal in intensity at or shortly after onset (**thunderclap headache**)
  - **Evolution:** concerning if increasing in frequency and/or severity
  - **Timing:** concerning if wakes from sleep or worse in morning
  - **Relation to prior headaches:** concerning if different in quality, severity, and/or timing
- **Provoking factors:** concerning if worsens with coughing, straining, sneezing, supine position
- **Accompanying symptoms/signs:** concerning if fever, seizure, focal neurologic signs, and/or papilledema present

- **Context/patient history:** concerning if:
  - New headache in an older adult with no prior history of headache
  - History of cancer
  - History of immunosuppression (e.g., medications or HIV)

TABLE 26–1 Headache Red Flags & Their Clinical Significance.

	Underlying Potentially Concerning Pathophysiology	Not-to-Miss Diagnoses
Thunderclap onset	Vascular	Intracranial hemorrhage
		Hypertensive emergency
		Venous sinus thrombosis
		RCVS
		Cervical artery dissection
		Pituitary apoplexy
Wakes from sleep **Worse with coughing/ sneezing/ straining** **Increasing in frequency and/ or severity**	Elevated intracranial pressure	Intracranial tumor Hydrocephalus Idiopathic intracranial hypertension
New headache in older adult with no prior history of headache	Mass lesion Inflammatory disease	Intracranial tumor Giant cell arteritis Primary CNS vasculitis
New headache in patient with history of cancer	Metastasis	Metastasis
New headache in patient with history of immunosup- pression	Opportunistic infection	Toxoplasmosis Primary CNS lymphoma Cryptococcal meningitis
Headache and fever	Intracranial infection	Meningitis Cerebral abscess
Headache and seizures	Focal lesion	Intracranial tumor Intracranial infection Intracranial hemorrhage
Headache and focal neurologic signs	Focal lesion	Intracranial tumor Intracranial infection Intracranial hemorrhage Ischemic stroke

Abbreviations: CNS: central nervous system; RCVS: reversible cerebral vasoconstriction syndrome.

Any of these features warrant evaluation with neuroimaging to look for an underlying cause.

In addition to these classic red flags, other patterns of headache that require particular evaluation include:

- New headache in a patient ≥60 years old with scalp tenderness, jaw claudication, myalgias, and/or visual loss should raise concern for **giant cell (temporal) arteritis**. This diagnosis should be pursued by checking erythrocyte sedimentation rate (ESR), C-reactive protein (CRP), and considering temporal artery ultrasound and/or biopsy. If caught early and treated with steroids, visual loss can be prevented.
- Headache that is worse with standing and improves in the supine position (**orthostatic headache**) should raise concern for **intracranial hypotension**. This can be caused by cerebrospinal fluid (CSF) leak due to prior trauma or prior lumbar puncture, or may be spontaneous (see "Decreased Intracranial Pressure (Intracranial Hypotension)" in Ch. 25).
- Headaches with visual changes and/or pulsatile tinnitus in a patient with obesity, endocrine disease, or in a child taking tetracycline should raise concern for **pseudotumor cerebri (idiopathic intracranial hypertension)**. Early intervention with weight loss and/or acetazolamide can prevent visual loss (see "Pseudotumor Cerebri" in Ch. 25).

PRIMARY HEADACHE DISORDERS

Migraine

Clinical Features of Migraine

The classic migraine headache is unilateral, pulsating/throbbing, sufficiently severe to impede daily activities, lasts hours to a few days, is accompanied by photophobia, phonophobia, nausea, and/or vomiting, and causes the patient to seek a dark, quiet, relaxing space. An aura accompanies migraine headache in only about 20%–25% of patients.

Migraine aura is most commonly visual or somatosensory. The visual aura is often described as bright spots or wavy lines that move through the visual field (**scintillating scotoma**), though other types of visual distortions may also occur. The somatosensory aura that may accompany migraine is generally unilateral tingling that slowly spreads over minutes across one side of the body. Although somatosensory seizures can produce similar spreading tingling symptoms, the spread of symptoms in migraine is generally slower as compared to the rapid spread of symptoms with somatosensory seizures. Migraines and seizures both generally cause positive symptoms (e.g., tingling, scintillating scotoma) as compared to transient ischemic attack (TIA) and ischemic stroke, which typically cause negative symptoms (e.g., numbness or visual field deficit), though there can be exceptions.

Migraine aura typically emerges over minutes and precedes the headache. However, the aura and headache may occur concurrently. Some patients experience migraine aura without headache (**acephalgic migraine**). Less common auras include:

- Speech disturbance or confusion
- Vertigo (**vestibular migraine**)
- Monocular visual changes (**ocular migraine**, also called **retinal migraine**)
- Ophthalmoplegia (**ophthalmoplegic migraine**)
- Brainstem and/or cerebellar symptoms (**migraine with brainstem aura**; formerly called **basilar migraine**)
- Hemiplegia. **Hemiplegic migraine** occurs in association with inherited mutations in sodium channels (SCN1A), calcium channels (CACNA1A), or sodium-potassium pump (ATP1A2).

Migraine may be preceded by a prodrome of fatigue, irritability, decreased concentration, and/or yawning hours to days before headache onset, and may be followed by a postdrome of fatigue, GI symptoms, and head/neck pain following a migraine.

A clinical diagnosis of migraine does not necessarily exclude the possibility of an underlying etiology: Tumors or strokes can cause migraine-type headaches that may be accompanied by migraine-type aura. Therefore, neuroimaging is warranted when migraines occur for the first time in older adults, although a first migraine can occur at any age including in older adults. In patients with migraine with no underlying cause who undergo neuroimaging, nonspecific T2/FLAIR hyperintensities in the subcortical white matter may be observed. These are generally easily distinguished from the lesions of multiple sclerosis in that they are smaller and fewer in number, and tend not to involve the corpus callosum as do the white matter lesions of multiple sclerosis.

Some patients with **episodic migraine** can develop daily or near-daily headaches (**chronic migraine**, also called **transformed migraine**). This is more common in patients with psychiatric comorbidities, poorly controlled migraines, and/or overuse of caffeine and/or analgesics (see "Medication Overuse Headache" below).

Treatment of Migraine

When evaluating a patient with suspected migraines, it is important to help the patient determine potential triggers. These may be related to dietary factors (e.g., particular foods, beverages, irregular eating schedule, alcohol, caffeine), irregular sleep patterns, stress, and/or the menstrual cycle. It is helpful to ask patients to keep a headache diary documenting headache occurrence in relation to such factors in order to determine potential triggers that can be eliminated or at least modified. Excessive or irregular use of caffeine is a common trigger of migraine, and patients should be counseled to reduce caffeine intake and avoid variability in amount of caffeine consumed from day to day. It must be explained to patients that their headaches may worsen during the period of caffeine withdrawal, but that they will ultimately feel better with respect to headache frequency and severity after this period.

Treatment of migraine requires a plan for both acute headaches (abortive treatment) and, if headaches are sufficiently frequent (≥4 days/month) or incapacitating, consideration of a prophylactic agent.

Acute treatment of migraine—Categories of acute migraine therapies include:

- Migraine-specific therapies: triptans, ergotamine, CGRP antagonists (gepants), 5-HT1F agonists (ditans)
- Anti-inflammatory medications: nonsteroidal anti-inflammatory drugs (NSAIDs), acetaminophen, steroids
- Antiemetics: metoclopramide, prochlorperazine, chlorpromazine
- Supportive treatment: IV fluids, IV magnesium

In patients whose acute migraine does not respond to the above medications, a single dose of intravenous steroids and/or valproate can be considered. A brief steroid taper over several days can also be considered.

The abortive medications may be given individually or in combination, except for ergots and triptans, which cannot be given together due to the risk of coronary vasoconstriction. When patients are self-administering abortive regimens at home, they must take the medication(s) early in the course of a migraine to effectively abort it. For patients in whom nausea/vomiting is prominent, injectable or nasal spray formulations of triptans may be used instead of oral formulations. Triptans and ergots should be avoided in patients with coronary artery disease, and are also generally avoided in hemiplegic and basilar migraines due to concern for increased risk of stroke (see "Migraine & Stroke" below). Gepants and ditans are considered safe in patients with cardiovascular disease. It is imperative to explain to patients that acute treatment agents must be used only for the most severe headaches and generally no more than twice per week. If acute abortive agents or analgesics are used more than 10–15 days per month (i.e., more than two to three times per week), they can induce medication overuse headache (see "Medication Overuse Headache" below).

Preventive treatment of migraine—A prophylactic agent can be considered if a patient experiences four or more migraine headaches per month or disabling migraines of any frequency that interfere with the patient's lifestyle. With prophylactic agents, it must be clearly explained to the patient that the medication must be taken daily (i.e., not just when the patient has a headache), and that the benefit may take several months to emerge.

Categories of prophylactic agents include:

- Antihypertensives: beta blockers, calcium channel blockers
- Antidepressants: tricyclic antidepressants, serotonin-norepinephrine reuptake inhibitors
- Alternative agents: riboflavin, magnesium, feverfew
- Antiepileptics: valproate and topiramate
- Migraine-specific: anti-CGRP monoclonal antibodies

Different patients may respond better to one particular agent, although this is often unpredictable. Selection of a prophylactic agent should take patient context and comorbidities into account. Child-bearing age would preclude use of valproate or topiramate due to the increased risk of teratogenic effects (unless one of these is the only effective agent and the patient is strictly adherent to contraception). Tricyclic antidepressants may be ideal in a patient with depression and/or insomnia. Beta blockers may not be tolerated in patients with low blood pressure, orthostasis, or asthma. Any individual agent should be slowly uptitrated over several months before deciding whether or not it is effective.

In patients with chronic migraine who do not respond to prophylactic agents, botulinum toxin injections or CGRP monoclonal antibodies may be considered.

Migraine & Stroke

Migraine with aura is considered an independent risk factor for stroke, especially in young women. This risk is augmented by smoking and the use of oral contraceptives. Therefore, patients with migraine should be counseled on the risks of smoking, and any comorbid stroke risk factors should be aggressively treated. WHO and ACOG guidelines recommend that estrogen-containing oral contraceptive pills should be avoided in women with migraine with aura, as well as in women with migraine without aura after age 35; however, data are limited and some recommend risk/benefit assessment on a case-by-case basis (for review and discussion, see Sheikh et al., 2018).

Migrainous infarction refers to stroke that occurs in the setting of migraine. The most common presentation of migrainous infarction is persistence of migraine aura beyond the migraine headache. Migrainous infarction most commonly occurs in the posterior circulation. In patients with a history of migrainous infarction, triptans and ergotamines are generally not used since they may increase the risk of vascular complications such as stroke.

Tension Headache

Tension headaches are typically holocephalic, "squeezing" in quality, mild to moderate in intensity (i.e., not impeding daily activities as migraine does), and generally have no associated features aside from possible phonophobia or photophobia (but not both). Stress is a common provoking factor. Treatment involves stress reduction and NSAIDs for acute headaches. In patients for whom a prophylactic agent is needed due to tension headache frequency and/or severity, a tricyclic antidepressant is generally used.

The Trigeminal Autonomic Cephalalgias: Cluster Headache, Hemicrania Continua, Paroxysmal Hemicrania, SUNCT, & SUNA

The trigeminal autonomic cephalalgias are characterized by unilaterality, sharp stabbing severe facial/periorbital pain, and associated autonomic features: lacrimation, rhinorrhea, conjunctival injection, facial sweating, pupillary abnormalities, ptosis, and/or eyelid edema. Ipsilateral photophobia and nausea/vomiting may also be present. The five described trigeminal autonomic cephalalgias, from shortest length of headache to longest, are short-lasting unilateral neuralgiform headache attacks with conjunctival injection and tearing (SUNCT) and short-lasting unilateral neuralgiform headache attacks with cranial autonomic symptoms (SUNA), paroxysmal hemicrania, cluster headache, and hemicrania continua (Table 26–2). These headache syndromes can lead to agitation during headaches (especially cluster headache and hemicrania continua), which is in contrast to the desire for a calm environment that patients describe during migraine.

Hemicrania continua presents as a continuous unilateral headache with associated episodic exacerbations with unilateral autonomic features, while the other four trigeminal autonomic cephalalgias are entirely episodic.

Attacks of SUNCT and SUNA can occur up to 100 times per day but last less than 10 minutes. SUNCT and SUNA differ in that SUNCT typically has multiple autonomic symptoms including conjunctival injection and lacrimation, whereas SUNA only has one of those two features (although it may have additional autonomic features among those listed above). Attacks of paroxysmal hemicrania occur around 10 times per day, lasting less than 30 minutes. Cluster headache occurs in clusters over a particular period of the year (usually weeks), and can last from 15 minutes to 3 hours.

Unlike migraine (which is more common in women), cluster headache is more common in men, and paroxysmal hemicrania is equally common in both sexes. The other trigeminal autonomic cephalalgias (SUNCT, SUNA, hemicrania continua) are all more common in women.

Given the focality and rarity of these headache syndromes, brain imaging with vascular imaging is usually obtained to evaluate for an underlying cause. Particular attention should be paid to the pituitary on neuroimaging studies, since trigeminal autonomic cephalalgias may be associated with pituitary pathology.

Hemicrania continua and paroxysmal hemicrania are treated with indomethacin, and response to indomethacin can confirm the diagnosis of these headache disorders. Cluster headache is treated acutely with 100% oxygen or a triptan; verapamil or lithium can be used for prophylaxis. SUNCT/SUNA are rare with limited data on treatment; antiepileptics (specifically lamotrigine, topiramate, or gabapentin) may be effective.

Chronic Daily Headache

Daily headaches can occur in patients with a prior history of episodic migraines (transformed/chronic migraine) or tension headaches (chronic tension headache). When a new daily

TABLE 26–2 Clinical Characteristics of the Primary Headache Disorders.

	Migraine	Tension	Cluster	SUNCT	SUNA	Paroxysmal Hemicrania	Hemicrania Continua
SYMPTOMS							
Quality	Throbbing	Squeezing	Sharp, stabbing				
Severity	Severe	Mild–moderate	Severe				
Laterality	Unilateral	Holocephalic	Unilateral				
Frequency	Variable	Variable	Every other day up to 8/day	Up to 100/day		~10/day	Continuous with superimposed exacerbations
Length	Hours to days	Hours to days	15–180 minutes	<10 min		<30 min	Continuous for days
Nausea/vomiting	Common	No	Rare	Can occur		Uncommon	
Phonophobia/ photophobia	Common	May have one or other, not both	Common	Can occur		Common	
Aura	20%–25%	No	No				
Trigeminal autonomic features	Can occur	No	Yes				
TREATMENT							
Acute	NSAIDs Acetaminophen Triptans Ergots Antiemetics CGRP receptor antagonists (gepants) 5-HT1F agonists (ditans)	NSAIDs	Oxygen Triptans	N/A (Too brief for acute treatment)			
Prophylactic	TCAs SNRIs Antihypertensives (beta blockers) Antiepileptics (valproate and topiramate) Magnesium, riboflavin CGRP monoclonal antibodies	TCAs	Verapamil Galcanezumab (CGRP monoclonal antibody) Lithium Occipital nerve block Short course of oral steroids during cluster period	Lamotrigine Topiramate Gabapentin		Indomethacin	

Abbreviations: NSAIDs: nonsteroidal anti-inflammatory drugs; SNRIs: serotonin-norepinephrine reuptake inhibitors; SUNA: short-lasting unilateral neuralgiform headache attacks with cranial autonomic symptoms; SUNCT: short-lasting unilateral neuralgiform headache attacks with conjunctival injection and tearing; TCAs: tricyclic antidepressants.

headache arises suddenly in a patient with no prior history of episodic headaches, this generally necessitates brain imaging to evaluate for an underlying cause. If none is found, the designation **new daily persistent headache** may be applied. New daily persistent headache arises suddenly and may appear to have characteristics resembling migraine or tension headache. A prophylactic agent should be chosen based on which primary headache syndrome the predominant clinical features of the daily headache most closely resemble. In all patients who

develop daily headache, a detailed medication history should be obtained to evaluate for whether there is analgesic overuse, which itself can lead to headache (see "Medication Overuse Headache" below).

Other Primary Headache Disorders

There are number of rarer primary headaches listed by the International Headache Society Classification of Headache

Disorders, criteria for which can be found on their website. These are characterized as:

- *Headaches associated with physical exertion:* primary cough headache, primary exercise headache, primary headache associated with sexual activity, primary thunderclap headache
- *Headaches caused by external stimuli:* cold stimulus headache, external pressure headache
- *Epicranial headaches:* primary stabbing headache, nummular headache (nummular means coin-shaped)
- *Miscellaneous:* hypnic headache (awakens patient from sleep), new daily persistent headache

Evaluation for secondary causes is recommended for these entities given their rarity and since many are associated with potential red flags for vascular causes (thunderclap, association with exercise and sexual activity), elevated intracranial pressure (primary cough headache, hypnic headache), or other conditions (scalp pain [as in nummular headache] can occur in giant cell arteritis).

OTHER CAUSES OF HEADACHE

Medication Overuse Headache

A common scenario is one in which a patient with a prior history of episodic headache presents with daily headaches, and history reveals that the patient is taking analgesic medications on a daily or near-daily basis. Analgesic overuse can result in daily headaches if analgesics are taken more than 10–15 days per month for 3 or more months (10 or more days per month for opiates, triptans, combination pills, or a combination of any analgesic and one of these; 15 or more days per month for NSAIDs or acetaminophen alone). Patients with medication overuse headache will only improve if they wean off of analgesic medications. This can be done slowly or rapidly depending on patient preference except in the case of opioids or butalbital-containing medications, which must be weaned slowly to avoid withdrawal. Patients should be warned that they may feel worse during the weaning period. Therefore, a clear plan for abortive treatment (without return to analgesic overuse) is important, and some patients tolerate weaning from analgesics better with initiation of a prophylactic agent during the period of weaning.

All patients with headaches of any type for whom an abortive regimen is prescribed should be given clear guidance about when and how often to use abortive agents and warned about the possibility of developing medication overuse headache if analgesic medications are used more frequently than recommended.

Occipital Neuralgia

Occipital neuralgia presents with episodic shock-like pain radiating from the occiput over the crown of the head (in the distribution of the C2 nerve root or the greater occipital

nerve that originates from it). On examination, the pain may be reproduced with percussion over the occipital condyle, but this sign is not always present. MRI of the brain and upper cervical spine should be performed to look for a structural etiology causing compression of upper cervical roots, although usually none is found. Occipital nerve block with lidocaine injection can be highly effective, and confirms the diagnosis if it is effective. If this is ineffective or does not provide lasting benefit, antiepileptics (e.g., gabapentin, carbamazepine) can be considered.

Other neuralgias discussed elsewhere in this book are **trigeminal neuralgia** (Ch. 13) and **glossopharyngeal neuralgia** (Ch. 14).

Headache & Neurologic Deficits With Cerebrospinal Fluid Lymphocytosis (HaNDL)

Headache and neurologic deficits with cerebrospinal fluid lymphocytosis **(HaNDL)** is a syndrome in which there is a headache (typically migrainous in character and episode length) accompanied by transient focal neurologic deficits (commonly somatosensory disturbances) and a lymphocytic pleocystosis in the CSF (generally hundreds of cells per cubic millimeter). Given that these clinical and laboratory features could represent meningitis (although there is typically no nuchal rigidity or fever), encephalitis, or central nervous system vasculitis, the diagnosis is generally made only as a diagnosis of exclusion after these entities are excluded by neuroimaging (which is normal in HaNDL) and negative CSF viral and bacterial studies. The headache, focal deficit, and pleocystosis often recur within a few weeks after the original attack, but typically do not recur after that. The initial and subsequent episodes resolve spontaneously, so there is no particular treatment indicated. However, since the initial attack may raise concern for meningitis or encephalitis, these conditions are often treated empirically with antibiotic and/or antiviral therapy while awaiting results of CSF analysis.

Chiari Malformation

Chiari malformations are congenital abnormalities of the posterior fossa. Type 1 is characterized by the cerebellar tonsils lying greater than 5 mm below the foramen magnum, which may be accompanied by a syrinx (see Ch. 5) (Fig. 26–1). Type 2 is characterized by more extensive abnormalities including inferior displacement of the brainstem and cerebellum causing hydrocephalus and an associated myelomeningocele. Type 3 has similar brainstem and cerebellar abnormalities and displacement as in type 2, but is accompanied by an occipital encephalocele. Type 2 and type 3 cause extensive neurologic dysfunction and are typically clinically apparent in infancy. Type 1 is mentioned here because it may be clinically inapparent in childhood, but patients may present with headaches in adulthood. Chiari type 1 is sometimes also noted incidentally on neuroimaging in a patient with (or without) headache.

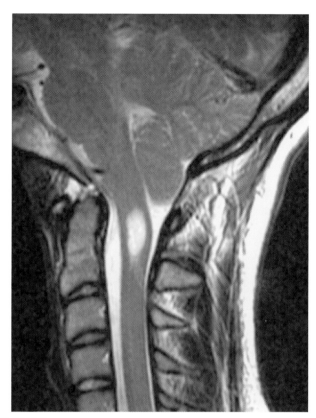

FIGURE 26–1 **Chiari Type 1 malformation.** T2-weighted sagittal MRI image demonstrating low-lying cerebellar tonsils and syrinx of the cervical spine. (Reproduced with permission from Ropper A, Samuels M, Klein J: *Adams and Victor's Principles of Neurology*, 10th ed. New York, NY: McGraw Hill; 2014.)

Chiari type 1 can present with progressive headache that is typically occipital, and is commonly associated with neck pain. The headache typically worsens with activities that elevate intracranial pressure (e.g., laughing, coughing, the Valsalva maneuver). Due to crowding of posterior fossa structures, patients may present with cranial neuropathies, cerebellar symptoms/signs (downbeat nystagmus is a classic finding), and/or upper motor neuron signs. If there is progressive neurologic dysfunction, decompressive surgery should be considered.

The more challenging cases are patients with a Chiari type 1 malformation diagnosed by neuroimaging who present with isolated headache and no neurologic deficits. In such cases, clinical history is of utmost importance to determine if the headache is consistent with the features typically seen in headaches caused by a Chiari malformation (i.e., posterior and exacerbated by laughing, coughing, and/or the Valsalva maneuver). If the patient's clinical history is consistent with migraine or another primary headache syndrome, the finding of a Chiari type 1 malformation may be incidental, and surgical intervention in such cases often fails to improve headaches (or may even worsen them).

If an isolated headache in a patient with Chari type 1 is consistent with the type of headache associated with Chiari type 1, but the pain is not intractable and there are no other neurologic findings, patients may be treated symptomatically and followed clinically and with serial imaging. Such patients are generally referred for consideration of decompressive surgery only if there is clinical and/or radiologic progression.

REFERENCE

Sheikh HU, Pavlovic J, Loder E, Burch R. Risk of stroke associated with use of estrogen containing contraceptives in women with migraine: a systematic review. *Headache* 2018;58(1):5–21.

Peripheral Neuropathy

Peripheral neuropathies can be classified as **mononeuropathy** (affecting one nerve), **mononeuropathy multiplex** (affecting multiple individual nerves), and **polyneuropathy** (affecting peripheral nerves diffusely). Mononeuropathies of the upper and lower extremities are discussed in Chapters 16 and 17, and mononeuropathy multiplex is discussed in Chapter 15. This chapter focuses on polyneuropathy.

CLASSIFICATION & DIFFERENTIAL DIAGNOSIS OF PERIPHERAL POLYNEUROPATHY

Polyneuropathies can be classified by:

- **Modality affected**: sensory, motor, sensorimotor, autonomic
- **Fiber type affected**: large fiber (proprioception/vibration) versus small fiber (pain/temperature)
- **Pathophysiology**: axonal versus demyelinating

Sensory symptoms can include negative symptoms (numbness), positive symptoms (paresthesias, pain), and/or sensory ataxia due to impaired proprioception (see "Distinguishing Cerebellar Ataxia From Sensory Ataxia" in Ch. 8). Neuropathies affecting motor fibers lead to weakness with lower motor neuron features (see "Upper Motor Neuron Lesions Versus Lower Motor Neuron Lesions" in Ch. 4). Autonomic neuropathy can lead to orthostatic hypotension, bowel/bladder dysfunction, impaired sweating, erectile dysfunction, and/or pupillary abnormalities.

The etiologies of peripheral polyneuropathy include:

- **Metabolic causes**: diabetes, metabolic syndrome, uremia, vitamin B12 (cobalamin) deficiency, vitamin B1 (thiamine) deficiency (dry beriberi)
- **Medications**:
  - Chemotherapy: platins, taxanes, bortezomib, immune checkpoint inhibitors (see "Chemotherapy-Induced Peripheral Neuropathy" in Ch. 24)
  - Antiretrovirals: didanosine, stavudine, zalcitabine (see "Antiretroviral-Associated Neuropathy" in Ch. 20)
  - Antibiotics: metronidazole, linezolid, quinolones, nitrofurantoin
  - Antimycobacterials: isoniazid, dapsone
  - Amiodarone
- **Toxins**: heavy metals (e.g., mercury, arsenic, lead), alcohol
- **Inflammatory processes**:
  - Primary neurologic inflammatory disorders: acute inflammatory demyelinating polyradiculoneuropathy (AIDP) and chronic inflammatory demyelinating polyneuropathy (CIDP)
  - Inflammatory neuropathies secondary to systemic inflammatory disease: Sjögren's syndrome, lupus, sarcoidosis
- **Malignancy**:
  - Paraprotein-associated neuropathies: myeloma, POEMS syndrome (polyneuropathy, organomegaly, endocrinopathy, monoclonal gammopathy, and skin changes), secondary amyloidosis (see Table 27–1)
  - Paraneoplastic (see "Paraneoplastic Syndromes of the Nervous System" in Ch. 24)

- **Infections**: HIV, leprosy (see "HIV-Associated Distal Symmetric Neuropathy" and "Leprosy" in Ch. 20)
- **Hereditary diseases:** Neuropathy may be the only (or predominant) feature of hereditary conditions (e.g., Charcot-Marie-Tooth disease) or may be one component in a multisystem hereditary disease (e.g., Tangier disease, Fabry's disease, acute intermittent porphyria) (see Table 27–3)

Axonal versus Demyelinating Neuropathies

Axonal neuropathies affect the longest nerves first since these are the most sensitive to dysfunction in axonal physiology.

This causes symptoms in a **length-dependent** pattern. The longest nerves are those that lead from the spinal cord to the toes. Therefore, patients with axonal neuropathies typically present first with sensory changes and/or weakness in the feet and loss of the ankle reflexes, but with preserved reflexes and sensorimotor function elsewhere. As an axonal neuropathy progresses, the symptoms and signs can ascend the legs and ultimately begin to involve the distal upper extremities over time. The hands are generally not affected in axonal neuropathies until the neuropathy has progressed to the level of the mid-shins in the lower extremities.

In contrast, demyelinating neuropathies affect myelin throughout the peripheral nervous system, so short and long nerves can be affected simultaneously. This causes both

TABLE 27–1 **Paraprotein-Associated Neuropathies.**

	Paraprotein		Neuropathy Type(s)	Neuropathy Clinical Phenotype(s)	Systemic Features	Associated Hematologic Malignancy
	Heavy Chain	Light Chain				
MGUS	IgM (most common; can be anti-MAG) IgG IgA	Kappa	Demyelinating (IgM) Axonal (IgG, IgA, IgM)	Sensory Sensorimotor DADS	None	1%/year risk of developing multiple myeloma
Multiple myeloma	IgG IgM	Kappa	Axonal	Sensorimotor	Hypercalcemia Anemia Renal disease Fatigue Bone pain	Plasma cell tumor of bone
Waldenström's macroglobulinemia	IgM (can be anti-MAG)	Kappa	Demyelinating Axonal	Sensory-predominant with sensory ataxia	Hepatosplenomegaly Adenopathy	Lymphoplasmacytic lymphoma
POEMS syndrome	IgG IgA	Lambda	Demyelinating	Sensorimotor with predominant weakness and pain	Polyneuropathy Organomegaly Endocrinopathy M spike Skin changes Elevated VEGF Elevated platelets Papilledema	Osteosclerotic myeloma
AL amyloidosis[a]	IgG IgA IgM	Lambda	Autonomic Painful small fiber Axonal	Sensory Sensorimotor Small fiber Autonomic Can be associated with carpal tunnel syndrome	Nephrotic syndrome Restrictive cardiomyopathy Hepatomegaly Macroglossia Facial purpura	Multiple myeloma Waldenström's macroglobulinemia Lymphoma Idiopathic (no malignancy identified)

Abbreviations: DADS: distal acquired demyelinating symmetric neuropathy; MGUS: monoclonal gammopathy of undetermined significance; POEMS: polyneuropathy, organomegaly, endocrinopathy, monoclonal gammopathy, and skin changes; VEGF: vascular endothelial growth factor.

[a]Familial amyloidosis (most commonly due to mutations in transthyretin) also causes painful small fiber and autonomic neuropathy, but is not associated with a paraprotein.

proximal and distal symptoms and signs, and can lead to involvement of both the hands and the feet simultaneously at presentation, a **non–length-dependent** pattern. Since the longest nerves have the most myelin, they have the most possible territory to be demyelinated by a demyelinating process, so symptoms may still begin in the distal extremities. However, the hands and feet may be affected simultaneously at presentation, and diminution or loss of tendon reflexes may be more diffuse at presentation than in axonal neuropathies.

The clinical distinction between axonal and demyelinating neuropathies is important because it guides the differential diagnosis: The majority of axonal neuropathies are caused by toxins, medications, or metabolic etiologies, whereas the majority of demyelinating neuropathies are caused by immune/inflammatory etiologies, although exceptions exist in all categories. This broad pathophysiologic distinction is logical because toxins, medications, and metabolic dysfunction alter axonal metabolism, leading to axonal dysfunction (axonal neuropathy), whereas myelin is affected in most immune-mediated inflammatory neuropathies (e.g., acute inflammatory demyelinating polyradiculoneuropathy [AIDP] and chronic inflammatory demyelinating polyneuropathy [CIDP]).

Nerve conduction studies in axonal neuropathies primarily demonstrate *decreased amplitudes*, whereas demyelinating neuropathies primarily demonstrate *slowing of conduction velocities* (and prolonged distal latencies). In most inherited demyelinating neuropathies, slowing of conduction velocity tends to be diffuse; in most acquired demyelinating neuropathies (e.g., compressive or inflammatory), demyelination causes focal/multifocal conduction block (see "Nerve Conduction Studies" in Ch. 15 for further discussion). Additionally, evaluation of multiple nerves with EMG/nerve conduction studies can demonstrate whether longer nerves are preferentially affected (length dependence, suggestive of axonal neuropathy) or whether shorter nerves are affected alongside longer nerves that are not affected (non–length dependence, suggestive of demyelinating neuropathy, but can also be seen in other conditions such as mononeuropathy multiplex and ganglionopathy [see Ch. 15]).

Small Fiber Neuropathy

The small unmyelinated nerve fibers that carry pain/temperature sensation and transmit autonomic signals may be affected in isolation or in conjunction with large fiber involvement. Small fiber neuropathy is characterized by pain that is typically burning in character with allodynia (pain response to a nonpainful stimulus; e.g., the bedsheets touching the feet). Symptoms are most commonly length-dependent, beginning in the feet.

Examination of patients with small fiber neuropathy demonstrates diminished pain and temperature sensation in affected areas, allodynia, and/or hyperalgesia (disproportionate response to painful stimulus). If there is isolated small fiber neuropathy with no concurrent large fiber involvement, reflexes will be normal.

EMG/nerve conduction studies are usually normal in small fiber neuropathy (unless large fibers are also affected), since small unmyelinated fibers cannot be assessed by EMG/nerve conduction studies. The diagnosis can be confirmed by skin biopsy to evaluate the density of nerve fibers in the epidermis, but if the clinical picture is clear, an evaluation for an underlying cause may be pursued without biopsy. Etiologies of small fiber neuropathy include:

- **Metabolic**: diabetes
- **Toxic**: alcohol
- **Infectious**: HIV, hepatitis C
- **Inherited**: Fabry's disease, hereditary sensory and autonomic neuropathy (HSAN), amyloidosis
- **Inflammatory**: Sjögren's syndrome, sarcoid, celiac disease, paraneoplastic (most commonly associated with anti-Hu antibodies)

Some cases of small fiber neuropathy are idiopathic.

As with any cause of neuropathic pain, symptomatic management includes antidepressants (amitriptyline, nortriptyline, duloxetine), antiepileptics (gabapentin, pregabalin), and topical treatments (lidocaine patch, capsaicin cream).

Autonomic Neuropathy

The autonomic nervous system includes the sympathetic pathways and parasympathetic pathways. Dysfunction of the autonomic pathways can cause orthostatic hypotension, bowel and/or bladder dysfunction, impaired sweating, and/or erectile dysfunction. Autonomic neuropathy can occur concurrently with neuropathy affecting other modalities (i.e., sensory, motor, small fiber) such as in diabetes, Guillain-Barré syndrome, hereditary sensory and autonomic neuropathy (HSAN), Sjögren's syndrome, amyloidosis, and paraneoplastic neuropathy. Autonomic neuropathy may also occur in isolation in any of these conditions, as well as in Chagas' disease and autoimmune autonomic neuropathy. Autoimmune autonomic neuropathy is commonly postinfectious with antibodies against ganglionic nicotinic acetylcholine receptors.

Diagnosis of autonomic neuropathy can be made by evaluating autonomic function with tests of sweating and tests of the cardiovascular response to provocative maneuvers (e.g., Valsalva maneuver, tilt table). Treatment is directed at the underlying cause. Orthostatic symptoms may be managed with education of the patient not to move from supine to seated to standing too rapidly, compression stockings or abdominal binder, and/or fludrocortisone or midodrine.

ACUTE POLYNEUROPATHY

Most polyneuropathies arise subacutely or chronically. The differential diagnosis for the etiology of an acute-onset polyneuropathy includes:

- Guillain-Barré syndrome: acute inflammatory demyelinating polyradiculoneuropathy (AIDP) or acute axonal forms (see "Guillain-Barré Syndrome")
- Toxins
  - Organophosphates (often accompanied by cholinergic [parasympathetic] symptoms)
  - Thallium (may be accompanied by hair loss)
  - Arsenic (other heavy metals more often cause subacute neuropathy, but arsenic may cause an acute or subacute neuropathy)
- Acute intermittent porphyria causes a recurrent acute motor-predominant neuropathy with abdominal pain, psychiatric disturbances, and/or seizures. Triggers include barbiturates, antiepileptics, sulfonamides, alcohol, and fasting. Diagnosis is by urine porphobilinogen, and treatment is with glucose and hematin.

Botulism presents similarly to an acute polyneuropathy, but is actually a disorder of the neuromuscular junction (see "Infection at the Neuromuscular Junction: Botulism" in Ch. 20). Viral poliomyelitis affects the anterior horn cells (acute flaccid paralysis) and can also present similarly to an acute polyneuropathy (e.g., West Nile virus, enterovirus; see "Acute Flaccid Paralysis" in Ch. 20)

An acute-onset myelopathy (e.g., transverse myelitis) can be difficult to distinguish from an acute polyneuropathy, since upper motor neuron signs may not yet be present at the time of onset of a myelopathy (see "Transverse Myelitis" in Ch. 21). The presence of bowel/bladder dysfunction and/or a spinal level on examination with acute-onset weakness is more suggestive of myelopathy than polyneuropathy. If symptoms progress in the lower extremities without any involvement of the upper extremities, this also suggests a spinal cord process (because a generalized polyneuropathy would not be expected to remain isolated to the legs).

Guillain-Barré Syndrome
Clinical Features of Guillain-Barré Syndrome

Guillain-Barré Syndrome (GBS) is the overarching term for acute-onset and rapidly progressive immune-mediated polyneuropathy. The underlying pathophysiology can be either demyelinating (acute inflammatory demyelinating polyradiculoneuropathy [AIDP]) or axonal (acute motor axonal neuropathy [AMAN] and acute motor and sensory axonal neuropathy [AMSAN]). AIDP is more common, with AMAN being most commonly seen in Asia and Central/South America. Axonal variants can be associated with anti-ganglioside antibodies.

The core features of GBS are the development and rapid progression of symmetric paresthesias and/or weakness in the extremities and loss of reflexes, often following a diarrheal (commonly *Campylobacter jejuni*) or respiratory illness, or more rarely after vaccination or surgery. The notion of "ascending paralysis" in GBS is often misunderstood—it does *not* mean that the symptoms start in the hands and feet and progresses proximally, but rather that the symptoms typically begin in the lower extremities and progress to the upper extremities.

Since AIDP is a demyelinating neuropathy, symptoms and signs are non–length-dependent, and patients can present with distal paresthesias and proximal weakness (e.g., gluteal and/or hip flexor causing gait abnormalities) simultaneously. Pain in the back and/or feet may be an early feature. The pattern of a slightly abnormal gait due to proximal weakness and nonspecific sensory symptoms and/or pain in the feet may lead initial examiners to miss the diagnosis (often invoking a functional disorder), especially since reflexes may still be present early in the disease. With progression of deficits and loss of reflexes, the diagnosis becomes clearer. Maximal disability is usually reached at 2–3 weeks into the illness.

Facial weakness is common in GBS, occurring in over half of patients and usually bilateral (facial weakness is in a lower motor neuron pattern since GBS affects peripheral nerves, including the cranial nerves). Autonomic instability is also common, mostly commonly manifesting as fluctuations in heart rate and blood pressure. Hyponatremia may occur and is likely due to the syndrome of inappropriate antidiuretic hormone secretion (SIADH). Bladder involvement in GBS is rare, and if present, should prompt consideration of spinal cord pathology (e.g., epidural abscess, transverse myelitis), which is the main differential diagnosis for rapidly progressive symmetric weakness and sensory changes.

Beyond the core features of areflexia and symmetric sensory and motor deficits, there is considerable variation in the spectrum and severity of GBS. Pure sensory, pure motor, and pure autonomic variants exist. The **Miller Fisher variant** presents with ophthalmoplegia, ataxia, and areflexia but with no or minimal weakness, and is associated with anti-GQ1B antibodies.[*] A variant of Miller Fisher syndrome with ophthalmoplegia, ataxia, hyperreflexia, and encephalopathy is called **Bickerstaff encephalitis**, and is also associated with anti-GQ1B antibodies. In a GBS variant referred to as **facial diplegia with acral paresthesias,** patients present with isolated bilateral lower motor neuron-pattern facial weakness accompanied by paresthesias in the distal extremities and decreased or absent reflexes, but without extremity weakness. The **pharyngeal-cervical-brachial** variant causes dysphagia, neck weakness, proximal upper extremity weakness, and areflexia that is often limited to the upper extremities, and may also cause ptosis; anti-GT1a antibodies may be seen with this variant.

Severity of GBS may be mild with patients remaining ambulatory throughout the illness, or may be severe with progression to complete quadriplegia with respiratory failure requiring intubation and mechanical ventilation.

---

[*]If ophthalmoplegia and sensory ataxia develop chronically, CANOMAD (**c**hronic **at**axic **n**europathy, **o**phthalomoplegia, Ig**M** Paraprotein, cold **a**gglutinins, **d**isialosyl antibodies [anti-GD1b or anti-GQ1b]), should be considered; this is a paraprotein-associated neuropathy, not a GBS variant.

Diagnosis of Guillain-Barré Syndrome

Cerebrospinal fluid (CSF) analysis in GBS demonstrates elevated protein and no or few white blood cells (although CSF can be normal early in the disease). This dissociation between elevated protein and minimal or no elevation in white blood cells is referred to as **albuminocytologic dissociation**. Although this pattern of CSF findings is usually taught/learned in the context of GBS, it is a nonspecific pattern seen in inflammatory disorders of the nervous system. If there is a CSF pleocytosis in a patient with GBS, the possibilities of HIV seroconversion (see "HIV Seroconversion Syndromes Involving the Nervous System" in Ch. 20), Lyme disease, and neurolymphomatosis as the cause of an acute polyneuropathy should be considered. Lumbar puncture may be normal early in the course of GBS.

In AIDP, nerve conduction studies show a demyelinating pattern with slowed velocities/increased latencies, conduction block, and absent F waves (reflecting proximal demyelination in the roots; see "F Wave" in Ch. 15). Diminished amplitudes are observed in axonal variants. A commonly observed early pattern in GBS is **sural sparing**: normal (or relatively normal) sensory amplitudes in the sural nerve despite decreased sensory amplitudes in upper extremity nerves (this pattern can also be seen in CIDP). It should be noted that very early in the disease course, EMG/nerve conduction studies may be normal.

MRI in GBS, if obtained due to clinical concern for spinal cord pathology, may show enhancement of nerve roots.

Management of Guillain-Barré Syndrome

Vital capacity and negative inspiratory force should be assessed upon presentation and monitored serially. This should be done even in patients with no respiratory symptoms, so early respiratory weakness can be detected by these measures before it becomes clinically apparent. In patients with significant facial weakness, there may be difficulty making a seal on the instruments used to test respiratory parameters, leading to falsely alarming values. A rough bedside measure of vital capacity can be obtained and followed serially by asking the patient to inhale maximally and then count as high as possible while exhaling on one breath—every 10 accounts for roughly 1 liter of vital capacity (i.e., patient counts to 20 on one breath—equivalent to about 2 liters of vital capacity, 30 approximately 3 liters). Neck flexion and extension musculature is supplied by C3-C5 as is the phrenic nerve, so evaluating for neck flexion/extension weakness can serve as a measure of muscles innervated by the same roots as the diaphragm. Patients with clinically apparent respiratory failure or a trajectory of worsening respiratory parameters generally require intubation.

GBS that progresses rapidly and/or causes gait impairment is treated with IV immunoglobulin (IVIg) or plasmapheresis, which appear to be equivalent in efficacy. Treatment usually does not lead to any noticeable improvement in the acute setting, but can lessen the ultimate severity of the disease and shorten the time to recovery. Treatment requires intensive supportive care, usually in an intensive care setting except in mild cases. The prognosis is related to the severity of the disease, but the majority of patients without respiratory failure will recover completely or with minor sensorimotor deficits.

Critical Illness Polyneuropathy & Critical Illness Myopathy

Patients hospitalized in intensive care units for sepsis or other critical illnesses can develop an axonal sensorimotor polyneuropathy and/or a myopathy over an acute to subacute period. Critical illness polyneuropathy and myopathy are part of the differential diagnosis for unexplained failure to wean from a ventilator (the differential diagnosis also includes myasthenia gravis and prolonged neuromuscular blockade).

Critical illness polyneuropathy and myopathy both cause diffuse symmetric weakness of the extremities. Facial weakness may be present in some cases, but extraocular weakness usually does not occur. Critical illness polyneuropathy will cause impaired sensation in addition to weakness. Although sensation is spared in critical illness myopathy, sensation can be difficult to assess in critically ill patients, and patients may have preexisting sensory loss from an underlying preexisting neuropathy. Reflexes may be spared in critical illness myopathy, but are typically absent in critical illness polyneuropathy. Serum creatine kinase (CK) may be elevated in critical illness myopathy. If EMG/nerve conduction studies are performed, both conditions show diminished compound motor action potentials (CMAPs) (due to axonal loss in critical illness neuropathy; due to muscle fiber loss in critical illness myopathy). However, sensory nerve action potentials (SNAPs) are only diminished in critical illness polyneuropathy as opposed to critical illness myopathy, in which they should be normal. Neuromuscular blockade and high-dose steroids used to treat the underlying critical illness may increase the risk of the development of critical illness myopathy.

Although a distinction can sometimes be made clinically/electrophysiologically between critical illness polyneuropathy and critical illness myopathy, patients may have both, and there is no treatment for either aside from rehabilitation. Medication-induced causes of neuropathy or myopathy should be searched for before making the diagnosis of critical illness myopathy or polyneuropathy. Many patients who recover from the underlying critical illness will recover to some degree from critical illness neuropathy/myopathy over subsequent months.

CHRONIC POLYNEUROPATHY

Causes of Peripheral Polyneuropathy

The differential diagnosis for chronic symmetric polyneuropathy is extensive, as noted at the beginning of the chapter. The most common cause in higher-income countries is diabetes mellitus, and neuropathy may be the presenting feature of the disease. Leprosy is one of the most common causes of poly-neuropathy worldwide (see "Leprosy" in Ch. 20).

When evaluating a patient with a suspected polyneuropathy, the history should assess for:

- Types of symptoms: pain, paresthesia, numbness, weakness, incoordination
- Distribution of symptoms: non–length-dependent (demyelinating) versus length-dependent (axonal)
- Medication exposures: chemotherapy, antibiotics, antiretrovirals, antimycobacterials, amiodarone
- Toxic exposures: alcohol, heavy metals
- HIV risk factors
- Diet: vegetarian diet can cause vitamin B12 deficiency; history of gastric bypass can cause multiple vitamin and mineral deficiencies if patients are not taking supplementation

The most common pattern of peripheral neuropathy is **distal symmetric polyneuropathy**. The American Academy of Neurology guidelines (England et al., 2009) recommend the following initial laboratory tests for the evaluation of distal symmetric polyneuropathy:

1. Fasting blood glucose or hemoglobin A1c to evaluate for diabetes
2. Vitamin B12 and methylmalonic acid (MMA) levels to assess for vitamin B12 deficiency
3. Serum protein electrophoresis/immunofixation (SPEP/IFE) to evaluate for a monoclonal gammopathy as a cause of paraprotein-associated neuropathy

Even in patients with a clear potential cause of neuropathy (e.g., exposure to chemotherapy known to cause neuropathy), it can be useful to check serum vitamin B12, hemoglobin A1c, and SPEP with immunofixation to evaluate for additional common and potentially reversible underlying etiologies as possible contributors to the patient's neuropathy. In a patient with known diabetes, vitamin B12 deficiency, or myeloma, one should consider sending laboratory tests to evaluate for the other two potentially contributing causes.

If no etiology is determined with this first-pass laboratory screening, additional testing depends on the clinical context and can include EMG/nerve conduction studies to further characterize the neuropathy, autoimmune serologies (ANA, Ro, La), cryoglobulins, HIV, celiac antibodies, paraneoplastic antibodies (anti-Hu), heavy metals, and genetic testing for Charcot-Marie-Tooth disease (see "Charcot-Marie-Tooth Disease" below).

Diabetes most commonly causes a distal symmetric sensory or sensorimotor polyneuropathy, but can also cause painful small fiber neuropathy, autonomic neuropathy, lumbosacral radiculoplexus neuropathy (see Ch. 17), mononeuropathy (see Chs. 16–17), and mononeuropathy multiplex (see Ch. 15). Small fiber neuropathy is usually chronic in onset and evolution, but rarely an acute small fiber neuropathy can

occur in diabetic patients whose diabetes rapidly comes under control after long-standing hyperglycemia. This condition is called treatment-induced neuropathy of diabetes (or insulin neuritis) and presents with symmetric, neuropathic pain in the extremities and autonomic dysfunction.

Vitamin B12 deficiency can cause myelopathy and/or cognitive changes in addition to peripheral neuropathy. A mixed picture of myeloneuropathy can be seen (e.g., absent reflexes with Babinski sign; absent reflexes in one region with brisk reflexes in another). The differential diagnosis for myeloneuropathy also includes copper deficiency, adrenomyeloneuropathy (see Ch. 31), and the combination of myelopathy and neuropathy caused by different etiologies (e.g., cervical stenosis and diabetic neuropathy). Myelopathy and neuropathy can also occur concurrently in HIV (see "Neurologic Complications of Advanced HIV Infection" in Ch. 20).

The type of neuropathy and systemic features of paraprotein-associated neuropathies vary based on the underlying condition (Table 27–1). Screening for monoclonal gammopathy (SPEP/immunofixation) is part of the initial evaluation for patients with peripheral neuropathy so as not to miss the opportunity for potential early detection of a hematologic malignancy. If a monoclonal gammopathy is discovered by a neurologist in the evaluation of a peripheral neuropathy, further evaluation and management is best undertaken in collaboration with a hematologist/oncologist.

Chronic Inflammatory Demyelinating Polyradiculoneuropathy (CIDP) & Its Variants

Like acute inflammatory demyelinating polyradiculoneuropathy (AIDP), chronic inflammatory demyelinating polyradiculoneuropathy (CIDP) is an immune-mediated, symmetric, non–length-dependent polyradiculoneuropathy with demyelinating features on nerve conduction studies and albuminocytologic dissociation in the CSF. However, CIDP usually presents insidiously over months (compared to the acute presentation of AIDP), and is not usually preceded by an antecedent infection (as is common in AIDP). The course can be either slowly progressive or relapsing. Some patients present acutely/subacutely and initially may appear to have AIDP, but either relapse or continue to progress beyond the usual course expected with AIDP. There are sensory, motor, and sensorimotor variants of CIDP (Table 27–2). Postural and action tremor may be seen. Cranial nerve involvement in CIDP is uncommon, but can occur. Nerve conduction studies show demyelinating features (increased latencies, decreased velocities) with conduction block, CSF shows albuminocytologic dissociation, and MRI (if obtained) can show nerve root enlargement and enhancement. For the treatment of CIDP, steroids (daily or pulsed), IVIg or subcutaneous Ig, or plasma exchange may be used, depending on the variant (see Table 27–2).

TABLE 27-2 **Variants of CIDP.**

		Clinical		Treatment	Associated Antibody
"Classic" CIDP	Sensorimotor	Symmetric	Proximal and distal	Steroids IVIg Plasma exchange	N/A
MADSAM (Lewis-Sumner syndrome)	Sensorimotor	Asymmetric	Multifocal	Steroids IVIg	N/A
DADS	Sensorimotor	Symmetric	Distal	Responds poorly when associated with anti-MAG	Anti-MAG
MMN	Motor	Asymmetric	Multifocal	IVIg	Anti-GM1
CISP	Sensory	Symmetric	Proximal and distal	IVIg Steroids	N/A

Abbreviations: CIDP: chronic immune demyelinating polyradiculoneuropathy; CISP: chronic immune sensory polyradiculoneuropathy; DADS: distal acquired demyelinating symmetric neuropathy; MADSAM: multifocal acquired demyelinating sensory and motor neuropathy; MMN: multifocal acquired demyelinating sensory and motor neuropathy.

Variants of CIDP (Table 27-2)

A symmetric but distal-predominant variant of CIDP known as **distal acquired demyelinating symmetric (DADS)** neuropathy is important to recognize since it can be associated with a monoclonal protein (typically IgM) and a specific autoantibody (anti-myelin associated glycoprotein [anti-MAG]), and generally responds poorly to immunotherapy (Table 27–2). A rare purely sensory form of CIDP called **chronic immune sensory polyradiculoneuropathy (CISP)** presents similarly to sensory ganglionopathy (sensory deficits including sensory ataxia with preserved strength; see "Diseases of Dorsal Root Ganglia: Ganglionopathy (Sensory Neuronopathy)" in Ch. 15).

Two CIDP variants of asymmetric onset are **multifocal acquired demyelinating sensory and motor neuropathy (MADSAM;** also called **Lewis-Sumner syndrome)** and **multifocal motor neuropathy (MMN).** The "multifocal" aspect of these names refers to the fact that these variants tend to present asymmetrically, with multiple focal neuropathies as opposed to the more confluent symmetric presentation of classic CIDP. MADSAM affects both sensory and motor nerve fibers as the name suggests. MMN is purely motor and should be considered in the differential diagnosis for motor neuron disease (e.g., amyotrophic lateral sclerosis [ALS]; see "Amyotrophic Lateral Sclerosis (ALS) & Its Variants" in Ch. 28) and vice versa. MMN can be associated with anti-GM1 antibodies. MMN does not respond to treatment with steroids (and may worsen when steroids are administered), but usually responds to treatment with IVIg.

Hereditary Neuropathies (Table 27-3)

Neuropathy can occur as the primary or only feature of a genetic disease (e.g., some variants of Charcot-Marie-Tooth disease), or may be one component of a genetic syndrome affecting multiple levels of the nervous system (e.g., Fabry's disease, familial amyloidosis, porphyria, some of the spinocerebellar ataxias, some of the leukodystrophies) .

Charcot-Marie-Tooth Disease (Hereditary Motor & Sensory Neuropathies)

The most common presentation of Charcot-Marie-Tooth disease (CMT) is a slowly progressive distal-predominant sensorimotor neuropathy with hammer toes and high arches of the feet. These classic features occur in the most common variants of CMT1 and CMT2. Most patients present in adolescence or early adulthood but may have noted clumsiness and poor performance in sports in childhood. Rarer forms of CMT may have diverse features in addition to neuropathy. Many of the most common forms of CMT are dominantly inherited, so there is typically a family history of the disease. Nerve conduction studies in CMT may reveal a demyelinating (CMT1, CMT3, CMT4) or an axonal (CMT2) pattern. If genetic testing is performed, it is targeted based on the most common mutations seen for the electrophysiologic/pathologic subtype (demyelinating versus axonal), and the inheritance pattern (dominant, recessive, or X-linked). The most common mutations are:

- Demyelinating CMT: *PMP22* and *MPZ*
- Axonal CMT: *MFN2*
- X-linked CMT: *GJB1*

Dejerine-Sottas disease (CMT3) is a rare infantile-onset severe form of the disease, and should be included in the differential of the "floppy (hypotonic) baby."

Treatment of CMT is supportive, aimed at maintenance of ambulation with orthoses and physical therapy.

Hereditary Sensory & Autonomic Neuropathies

The hereditary sensory and autonomic neuropathies (HSAN) are a group of very rare diseases that cause sensory loss (most

TABLE 27–3 Hereditary Neuropathies.

	Clinical Features		Onset	EMG/NCS	Inheritance	Gene
	Type of Neuropathy	Other Features				
CMT						
CMT1	Distal sensorimotor	Nerve enlargement	Teens–20s	Demyelinating	Autosomal dominant	Most common: • *PMP22* duplication (*CMT1A*) • *MPZ* (*CMT1B*)
CMT2	Distal sensorimotor		20s–30s	Axonal	Autosomal dominant	Various; *MFN2* most common
CMT3 (Dejerrine-Sottas)	Distal sensorimotor & proximal weakness	Nerve enlargement	Infantile	Demyelinating	Autosomal recessive or dominant	*PMP22* *MPZ* *EGR2*
CMT4	Distal sensorimotor		Childhood	Demyelinating	Autosomal recessive	Various
CMTX	Distal sensorimotor	Transient CNS events	Childhood	Demyelinating	X-linked	*GJB1*
HSAN						
HSAN1	Loss of pain/temperature sensation	Weakness	20s and older	Axonal	Autosomal dominant	*SPTLC1*
HSAN2	Loss of sensation in all modalities		Infantile	Axonal	Autosomal recessive	*WNK1*
HSAN3	Autonomic Loss of pain/temperature sensation		Infantile	Axonal	Autosomal recessive	*IKBKAP*
HSAN4	Complete pain insensitivity Anhidrosis	Intellectual disability	Infantile	Axonal	Autosomal recessive	*NKRT1*
HSAN 5	Complete pain insensitivity		Infantile	Axonal	Autosomal recessive	*NGFB*
Others						
HNPP	Focal neuropathies at sites of compression		20s or older	Demyelinating	Autosomal dominant	*PMP22* deletion
Fabry's disease	Painful small fiber neuropathy	Cardiac disease Stroke Renal dysfunction Angiokeratomas on abdomen	Childhood or older	Small fiber	X-linked	Alpha-galactosidase
Refsum's disease	Sensorimotor	Retinitis pigmentosa Deafness	Infantile or older	Demyelinating or axonal	Autosomal recessive	Phytanoyl–CoA alpha hydroxlase
Tangier disease	Painful small fiber neuropathy or Recurrent mononeuropathy multiplex	Large, orange tonsils Low HDL/elevated triglycerides	Childhood or older	Small fiber Demyelinating or axonal	Autosomal recessive	*ABCA1*
Familial amyloid polyneuropathy	Small fiber Sensorimotor Autonomic	Cardiac Renal Ocular	30s–80s	Axonal	Autosomal dominant	Transthyretin (TTR) Apolipoprotein A1 Gelsolin

Abbreviations: CNS: central nervous system; CMT: Charcot-Marie tooth disease; EMG/NC: electromyography/nerve conduction studies; HDL: high-density lipoprotein; HNPP: hereditary neuropathy with liability to pressure palsies; HSAN: hereditary sensory and autonomic neuropathies.

commonly loss of pain and temperature sensation) and/or autonomic dysfunction, as the name suggests. Most subtypes of HSAN are infantile-onset and autosomal recessive, with the exception of HSAN1, which is adult-onset and autosomal dominant. Most subtypes of HSAN cause profound loss of pain and temperature sensation, which can result in unnoticed injuries and subsequent complications such as skin ulceration leading to infection. Supportive management therefore focuses on prevention and treatment of these complications.

Hereditary Neuropathy With Liability to Pressure Palsies

Caused by a deletion in the same gene that is duplicated in CMT1A (*PMP22*), hereditary neuropathy with liability to pressure palsies **(HNPP)** is a dominantly inherited condition that causes increased risk of focal neuropathies at common sites of compression (median at carpal tunnel, ulnar at medial elbow, peroneal at fibular head; see Chs. 16–17). A symmetric polyneuropathy may also be present.

Other causes of polyneuropathy discussed elsewhere in this book include infections (HIV, leprosy; see "HIV-Associated Distal Symmetric Neuropathy" and "Leprosy" in Ch. 20), chemotherapy-induced neuropathy (see "Chemotherapy-Induced Peripheral Neuropathy" in Ch. 24), and paraneoplastic neuropathy (see Paraneoplastic Syndromes of the Nervous System" in Ch. 24).

REFERENCE

England JD, Gronseth GS, Franklin G, Carter GT, Kinsella LJ, Cohen JA, et al. Practice Parameter: evaluation of distal symmetric polyneuropathy: role of laboratory and genetic testing (an evidence-based review). *Neurol* 2009;72:185–192.

Motor Neuron Disease

OVERVIEW OF MOTOR NEURON DISEASE

This chapter discusses a group of diseases that affect motor neurons in isolation, collectively referred to as **motor neuron disease**. Motor neuron disease can affect upper motor neurons (motor neurons of the central nervous system), lower motor neurons (motor neurons of the peripheral nervous system), or both (Table 28–1). The primary symptom of motor neuron disease is weakness. The distribution of weakness, associated signs (upper motor neuron vs lower motor neuron vs both; see "Upper Motor Neuron Lesions Versus Lower Motor Neuron Lesions" in Ch. 4), and pace of progression differ depending on the disease. Just as there are upper and lower motor neurons for the muscles of the extremities, the motor cranial nerves contain lower motor neurons under the control of upper motor neuron cortical input (**corticobulbar tract**). The muscles of the face, larynx, and pharynx (**bulbar muscles**) are affected in many motor neuron diseases.

AMYOTROPHIC LATERAL SCLEROSIS (ALS) & ITS VARIANTS

Clinical Features of Amyotrophic Lateral Sclerosis (ALS)

The most common motor neuron disease is **amyotrophic lateral sclerosis** (**ALS**). ALS affects the motor system both centrally and peripherally leading to weakness in the limbs and bulbar and respiratory muscles, with both upper motor neuron signs and lower motor neuron signs on examination.

ALS has a pure central nervous system/upper motor neuron variant known as **primary lateral sclerosis**, a pure peripheral nervous system/lower motor neuron variant called **progressive muscular atrophy**, and a pure brainstem variant known as **progressive bulbar atrophy**. These variants are less common and may accumulate additional features over time, developing into ALS (i.e., lower motor neuron signs emerge in primary lateral sclerosis, upper motor neuron signs develop in progressive muscular atrophy, extremity weakness arises in progressive bulbar atrophy).

ALS typically begins after the age of 50, but can affect younger patients. Early-onset cases are often familial. Slowly progressive weakness most commonly begins in one limb and progresses over time to involve the other limbs, the tongue, the larynx, the pharynx, and the respiratory muscles. In the flail arm (brachial amyotrophic diplegia) variant, patients present with bilateral, predominantly proximal arm weakness that may be asymmetric; in the flail leg variant, patients present with bilateral predominantly distal leg weakness that may be asymmetric. Both flail arm and flail leg presentations have predominantly lower motor neuron signs and may have a slower progression to other regions and a better prognosis. ALS can also begin in the bulbar muscles and spread to the limbs. Pseudobulbar affect (laughing and/or crying out of proportion to the emotion felt) can occur in later stages of the disease. Eye movements and bowel/bladder control are usually normal until the very latest stages of the disease (bladder control is normal due to sparing of Onuf's nucleus in the sacral spinal cord).

Examination reveals a combination of both upper motor neuron signs (hyperreflexia, clonus, Babinski's sign, increased jaw jerk reflex) and lower motor neuron signs (atrophy, fasciculations), and both types of findings may be present in the same limb. A characteristic pattern of atrophy of the muscles of the hand in ALS called the **split hand** may be seen in which the thenar muscles (first dorsal interosseous, abductor

TABLE 28-1 Clinical Features of Motor Neuron Disease.

	Lower Motor Neuron Involvement	Upper Motor Neuron Involvement	Bulbar Muscle Involvement
Amyotrophic lateral sclerosis	✓	✓	✓
• **Primary lateral sclerosis**		✓	✓ (late)
• **Progressive muscular atrophy**	✓		✓ (late)
• **Progressive bulbar atrophy**			✓
Spinal muscular atrophy (see Table 28–2)	✓		✓ (types 1 and 2)
Spinal bulbar muscular atrophy (Kennedy's disease)	✓		✓

pollicis brevis) are atrophied whereas the hypothenar muscles (abductor digiti minimi) are spared. Tongue fasciculations are a classic finding but are not always present, especially if the bulbar muscles are not involved. In some patients, ALS and frontotemporal dementia (see Ch. 22) occur together, but cognition may be affected even in patients with ALS without frontotemporal dementia. ALS typically progresses to respiratory failure and death within 2–3 years of diagnosis, but progressive lateral sclerosis and progressive muscular atrophy can have a much more indolent course and far longer survival.

Although most cases of ALS are sporadic, a minority of cases are familial. The most commonly associated mutations are in the genes *C9orf72* and *SOD1*. Mutations in these genes can be inherited in an autosomal dominant pattern, but can also occur sporadically.

Diagnosis & Differential Diagnosis of Amyotrophic Lateral Sclerosis (ALS)

Per the El Escorial criteria (Brooks et al., 2000), a definite diagnosis of ALS can be made if there are both upper motor neuron and lower motor neuron signs in three of four regions of the body (defined as bulbar, cervical, thoracic, and lumbar). A probable diagnosis of ALS can be made if there are upper motor neuron and lower motor neuron signs in two regions with one affected upper motor neuron region superior to involved lower motor neuron regions. For probable diagnosis, lower motor neuron features may be determined by EMG or clinical examination.

Nerve conduction studies in ALS demonstrate decreased compound motor action potentials (CMAPs) (from motor axon loss) with normal sensory nerve action potentials (SNAPs). EMG demonstrates evidence of motor nerve irritability (fasciculation potentials), muscle fiber denervation (fibrillation potentials), and muscle fiber reinnervation (increased amplitude and duration of motor unit action potentials ([MUAPs] with polyphasia). (For explanation of interpretation of EMG findings, see "Introduction to Electromyography and Nerve Conduction Studies" in Ch. 15.)

The diagnosis of motor neuron disease requires that other potential etiologies of motor system pathology have been excluded such as cervical spine disease for upper motor neuron dysfunction and neuropathy for lower motor

neuron disease. Therefore, in the evaluation of suspected ALS, MRI of the cervical spine should be performed to evaluate for cervical myelopathy, and MRI of the brain should be considered if there are isolated bulbar features at the time of initial evaluation. In patients with both upper and lower motor neuron signs at presentation, additional causes of combined myelopathy and neuropathy (**myeloneuropathy**) that should be considered include vitamin B12 deficiency, copper deficiency, and adrenomyeloneuropathy (see Ch. 31). Isolated paraplegia with upper motor neuron signs can occur in hereditary spastic paraplegia (see "Hereditary Spastic Paraplegia" in Ch. 5).

Although myopathies and neuromuscular junction disorders affect the motor system in isolation, their presentation is generally distinct from that of motor neuron disease. Myopathies and neuromuscular junction disorders are generally symmetric and do not cause upper or lower motor neuron signs. Myasthenia gravis (the most common neuromuscular junction disorder) causes fatigable weakness and often involves the eyelids and/or extraocular muscles at presentation (see Ch. 29), both of which are not generally involved at presentation in ALS (although eye movements may be affected late in the course of ALS). Multifocal motor neuropathy (see Ch. 27) can closely imitate motor neuron disease, causing asymmetric lower motor neuron-pattern weakness involving multiple extremities over time, but no upper motor neuron signs occur in multifocal motor neuropathy. The possibility of multifocal motor neuropathy is assessed for by looking for conduction block on nerve conduction studies (see Chs. 15 and 27).

When a patient develops weakness and atrophy in one or both upper extremities in isolation suggestive of flail arm variant ALS, **Hirayama disease (monomelic amyotrophy)** should be considered in the differential diagnosis. In Hirayama disease, an anatomic abnormality of the spine causes the anterior horn cells of the cervical spinal cord to be compressed when the neck is flexed. This leads to chronic development of unilateral or bilateral forearm weakness and atrophy, usually sparing the brachioradialis. Hirayama disease is more common in young men. MRI of the cervical spine in Hirayama disease may be normal unless performed with the neck in flexion, which will demonstrate anterior shift of the posterior dura leading to compression of the anterior spinal cord against the vertebral bodies. Hirayama disease is treated with

TABLE 28–2 Clinical Features of Spinal Muscular Atrophy (SMA).

	Age of Onset	Motor Ability	Survival Without Treatment
Type 1 (Werdnig-Hoffman)	In the first months of life (decreased fetal movements may be noted)	Cannot lift head	Generally <2 years
Type 2	Before 18 months	Can sit but cannot stand without assistance	Young adulthood
Type 3 (Kugelberg-Welander)	By 3 years (Type 3A) After 3 years (Type 3B)	Can walk independently (although may lose that ability)	Can be normal
Type 4	Adult-onset	Proximal weakness	Can be normal

a cervical collar for several months, and surgical intervention if this measure fails to stop progression of the condition.

Treatment of Amyotrophic Lateral Sclerosis (ALS)

The only medications found to have a disease modifying effect in ALS are riluzole (an oral medication that decreases glutamate-mediated excitotoxicity) and edaravone (an infusion that reduces oxidative stress by acting as a free radical scavenger). Riluzole can increase the time to development of respiratory failure and can prolong survival by several months. Edaravone has been shown to slow disease progression in patients with early ALS. Care is otherwise supportive, addressing symptoms such as spasticity (baclofen, tizanidine), pseudobulbar affect (dextromethorphan-quinidine), respiratory muscle weakness (bilevel positive airway pressure [BiPAP]), and nutrition (enteral feeding via percutaneous endoscopic gastrostomy [PEG] tube). Patients must be counseled early on end-of-life decision making to begin a discussion of whether or not they will ultimately want to be placed on a ventilator. (For a thoughtful and poignant discussion of patients' choices in ALS, see Chs. 8 and 9 in Ropper and Burrell, 2014.)

SPINAL MUSCULAR ATROPHY (SMA) & SPINAL BULBAR MUSCULAR ATROPHY (KENNEDY'S DISEASE)

Spinal muscular atrophy (SMA) is an autosomal recessively inherited purely lower motor neuron disease caused by mutations in the survival motor neuron (SMN) gene. In contrast to ALS and its variants, SMA usually presents symmetrically, with proximal muscles affected predominantly. SMA types 1–4 differ in age of onset and severity, with the lower numbers

signifying earlier onset and more severe and rapid progression (Table 28–2). Nusinersin (an intrathecally administered antisense oligonucleotide), onasemnogene abeparvovec (an intravenously administered viral vector gene therapy), and risdiplam (an oral small molecule that modifies SMN gene splicing) are novel therapeutic agents that have dramatically altered the landscape of SMA, leading to newborn screening for early identification and treatment.

Kennedy's disease (spinal bulbar muscular atrophy) is an X-linked adult-onset disease of lower motor neurons that predominantly affects the proximal upper extremities and bulbar muscles. The genetic mutation is in the androgen receptor, and gynecomastia and infertility are usually present.

Other diseases that can affect motor neurons exclusively discussed elsewhere in this book include viral infections of the anterior horn cells (polio, enterovirus D68, West Nile virus; see "Acute Flaccid Paralysis" in Ch. 20), multifocal motor neuropathy (a demyelinating neuropathy affecting motor nerves in isolation; see "Variants of CIDP" in Ch. 27), and hereditary spastic paraplegia (see "Hereditary Spastic Paraplegia" in Ch. 5).

REFERENCES

Brooks BR, Miller RG, Swash M, Munsat TL, World Federation of Neurology Research Group on Motor Neuron Diseases. El Escorial revisited: revised criteria for the diagnosis of amyotrophic lateral sclerosis. *Amyotroph Lateral Scler Other Motor Neuron Disord* 2000;1:293–299.

Ropper AH, Burrell BD. Endgame: facing down Lou Gehrig's disease. In: *Reaching Down the Rabbit Hole.* New York, NY: St. Martin's Press; 2014.

Ropper AH, Burrell BD. The examined life: what it takes to survive a motor-neuron death sentence. In: *Reaching Down the Rabbit Hole.* New York, NY: St. Martin's Press; 2014.

Diseases of the Neuromuscular Junction

C H A P T E R

29

CHAPTER CONTENTS

MYASTHENIA GRAVIS

Clinical Features of Myasthenia Gravis

Myasthenic Crisis

Diagnostic Testing in Myasthenia Gravis

Screening for Thymoma in Myasthenia Gravis

Treatment of Myasthenia Gravis

CONGENITAL MYASTHENIC SYNDROMES & NEONATAL MYASTHENIA GRAVIS

Congenital Myasthenic Syndromes

Neonatal Myasthenia Gravis

LAMBERT-EATON MYASTHENIC SYNDROME

Clinical Features of Lambert-Eaton Myasthenic Syndrome

Diagnosis of Lambert-Eaton Myasthenic Syndrome

Evaluation for Malignancy in Lambert-Eaton Myasthenic Syndrome

Treatment of Lambert-Eaton Myasthenic Syndrome

At the neuromuscular junction, motor neurons release acetylcholine that binds to acetylcholine receptors on the postsynaptic muscle fibers, causing them to contract. Diseases of the neuromuscular junction can be classified as either presynaptic (e.g., Lambert-Eaton syndrome, botulism) or postsynaptic (e.g., myasthenia gravis) (Fig. 29–1). Congenital myasthenia gravis can be caused by mutations in either presynaptic or postsynaptic neuromuscular junction structures.

MYASTHENIA GRAVIS

Clinical Features of Myasthenia Gravis

Myasthenia gravis is a postsynaptic disorder of the neuromuscular junction in which antibodies are produced against components of the acetylcholine receptors on muscle. These antibodies are most commonly against the acetylcholine receptor itself, leading to blocking and destruction of these receptors.

Weakness in myasthenia fluctuates and is fatigable: It emerges or worsens with exertion and late in the day, and resolves with rest. Imagine acetylcholine rushing across the

neuromuscular junction to synapse on its receptors on the muscles. If these receptors are blocked or diminished in number due to antibody-mediated destruction, the available receptors will quickly be saturated, and no further response to acetylcholine can be elicited. This leads to initial muscular force but subsequent fatigue.

In most patients with myasthenia gravis, one or both eyes are involved at presentation with fluctuating/fatigable ptosis and/or diplopia (due to extraocular muscle weakness). The pupils are not affected. The disease may remain limited to the eyes in a small proportion of patients (**ocular myasthenia**). In patients whose symptoms are initially isolated to the eyes, about half will ultimately develop signs of generalized myasthenia gravis beyond the eyes over subsequent years. Beyond the eyes, facial weakness, dysphagia, laryngeal weakness leading to a hypophonic and/or nasal voice, jaw weakness, and neck weakness are common, and extremity weakness and respiratory weakness also occur.

Myasthenia gravis has a bimodal distribution in its age of presentation, most commonly presenting in younger women (20s–30s) and older men (≥60). There are several bedside maneuvers that can be used to evaluate for fatigability on clinical examination.

329

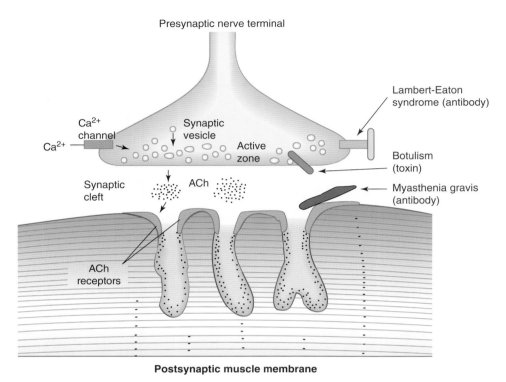

FIGURE 29–1 **Schematic of the neuromuscular junction and sites of "lesions" in neuromuscular disease.** (Reproduced with permission from Aminoff M, Greenberg D, Simon R: *Clinical Neurology*, 9th ed. New York, NY: McGraw Hill; 2015.)

For the eyes:

- **Ptosis time** assesses the amount of time a patient can sustain upgaze. In patients with myasthenia, one or both eyelids may start to slowly fall like descending curtains due to fatigue of the levator palpebrae muscles.
- Ptosis may improve after applying ice to the eyelids (**icepack test**), since cold temperatures may facilitate neuromuscular transmission.
- With attempted sustained eye closure, the eyes may start to open (**peek sign**) due to fatigable weakness of the orbicularis oculi.
- If the examiner lifts the eyelid on one side to relieve ptosis, ptosis may emerge on the other side. This is because the eyelids are controlled to move conjugately, so the force to attempt to overcome a ptotic lid is distributed to both lids. When the examiner relieves the ptotic lid of the force being required to lift it, the other lid also has less force directed toward it and may droop.
- After asking the patient to close the eyes gently and then look up rapidly, the affected eyelid may move rapidly upward and then fall back to a ptotic position (**Cogan's lid twitch**). Resting the lid presumably allows for a "rebound" of the lid before it again fatigues.
- Saccades may undershoot their goal (**hypometric saccades**), but may be more rapid than normal. The increased rapidity of saccades presumably reflects some sort of central adaptation attempting to overcome the weakened extraocular muscles: An extra burst of energy makes the eye move quickly over a small distance rather than at normal speed over the intended distance.

Fatigable weakness can also be elicited in the extremities. After testing bilateral deltoid strength to assure that it is symmetric at baseline, the patient is asked to abduct one arm 100 times ("like a flapping wing"). The examiner then retests the deltoids to look for whether exercise has caused weakening of one side, leading to asymmetric strength.

Myasthenic Crisis

The most feared complication of myasthenia gravis is **myasthenic crisis**. This is an acute exacerbation in myasthenia causing respiratory failure requiring intubation. Myasthenic crisis can be triggered by any physiologic stress (e.g., infection, surgery) or by medications including:

- Antibiotics: quinolones, macrolides, aminoglycosides
- Cardiac medications: beta blockers, calcium channel blockers, quinidine, procainamide
- Magnesium
- Anesthetic agents
- Neuromuscular blocking agents

Rarely, myasthenic crisis may occur as the first presentation of myasthenia gravis. It should also be considered in the differential diagnosis of failure to extubate a patient following surgery.

Treatment of myasthenic crisis is with steroids and immunomodulatory therapy (IVIg or plasma exchange), treatment of any potential triggers (e.g., treating infection, discontinuing any potential medication triggers), and mechanical respiratory support until respiratory muscle weakness improves with treatment.

Diagnostic Testing in Myasthenia Gravis

Electrodiagnostics in the Diagnosis of Myasthenia Gravis: Repetitive Nerve Stimulation & Jitter

Just as the muscles fatigue with exertion in myasthenia gravis, repetitive electrical stimulation leads to a diminution in muscle activity. When a motor nerve is stimulated at 2–3 Hz in patients with myasthenia gravis, a decrement in compound motor action potential (CMAP) is observed (See "Low-Frequency & High-Frequency Repetitive Nerve Stimulation in Myasthenia Gravis & Lambert-Eaton Myasthenic Syndrome" below).

A more sensitive test for disorders of the neuromuscular junction is to evaluate for **jitter** on single-fiber EMG. Jitter is a measure of the variability of firing of pairs of muscle fibers within the same motor unit. Due to abnormalities of neuromuscular transmission in neuromuscular junction disorders, this variability is increased (increased jitter). Increased jitter is the single most sensitive test for myasthenia, but is a nonspecific finding that does not distinguish between diseases of the neuromuscular junction (e.g., myasthenia vs Lambert-Eaton syndrome), and can also be seen in motor neuron disease and myopathy.

Antibody Testing in the Diagnosis of Myasthenia Gravis

The most common antibodies seen in myasthenia gravis are against the acetycholine receptor (**AChR**), present in about 80% of patients with generalized myasthenia. Approximately one third to one half of the patients with myasthenia gravis who do not have AChR antibodies have antibodies against muscle-specific tyrosine kinase (**MuSK**). Patients with MuSK antibodies are most commonly women, and compared to patients with AChR antibody-associated myasthenia gravis, they tend to have less ocular involvement, more prominent facial and bulbar weakness with dysarthria, and are more likely to have respiratory compromise; they are less likely to have thymomas, and are less likely to respond to acetylcholinesterase inhibitors (their symptoms may worsen on them) or thymectomy. Patients without AChR or MuSK antibodies are considered to be seronegative, although some such patients do have antibodies to other postsynaptic components of the neuromuscular junction (e.g., LRP4).

The Tensilon Test in the Diagnosis of Myasthenia Gravis

The Tensilon test uses edrophonium (Tensilon is the brand name), an acetylcholinesterase inhibitor that inhibits the breakdown of acetylcholine in the neuromuscular junction. Edrophonium increases the availability of acetylcholine in the synapse to activate muscle. Therefore, administering edrophonium can lead to rapid improvement in myasthenic symptoms.

Edrophonium is not specific to nicotinic acetylcholine transmission and can increase parasympathetic (muscarinic) transmission as well, causing bradycardia and/or bronchoconstriction. Therefore, if the test is performed, it should be with cardiac monitoring, and atropine should be readily available in case of a cardiac complication. However, this test is only rarely used since there is easier access to safer tests listed above.

Screening for Thymoma in Myasthenia Gravis

Patients with myasthenia are frequently found to have an associated thymoma or thymic hyperplasia (most common with AChR antibodies; rare in patients with MuSK antibodies). Therefore, all patients with myasthenia should undergo CT or MRI of the chest for evaluation of the mediastinum. Thymectomy is indicated if a thymoma is detected, and is also beneficial in patients with myasthenia who do not have thymoma (MGTX trial 2016, 2019), though does not appear to be beneficial in patients with MuSK antibodies. In myasthenic patients with severe respiratory and/or bulbar weakness who are going to undergo thymectomy, a course of IVIg or plasma exchange is generally performed preoperatively to reduce the risk of perioperative complications.

Treatment of Myasthenia Gravis

Treatments for myasthenia can be divided into symptomatic (acetylcholinesterase inhibitor) and disease-modifying therapies (immunomodulatory therapy and thymectomy). Pyridostigmine is the most commonly used acetylcholinesterase inhibitor. Pyridostigmine acts by inhibiting breakdown of acetylcholine to increase the amount available in the neuromuscular junction to activate the reduced postsynaptic acetylcholine receptors on muscle cells. The medication can take effect quickly, but the effects only last for several hours, requiring dosing at regular intervals throughout the day. This medication only treats symptoms and does not modify disease activity or progression. Side effects are due to acetylcholine excess, which can result in increased parasympathetic activity: drooling, diarrhea, and abdominal cramps. As noted above, patients with MuSK antibodies may not improve or may even worsen with acetylcholinesterase inhibitors.

When pyridostigmine is taken in excess, **cholinergic crisis** can occur, causing muscle weakness and respiratory distress due to bronchoconstriction. This must be differentiated from myasthenic crisis in patients with worsening weakness and respiratory symptoms, although cholinergic crisis occurs less commonly than myasthenic crisis. Pupillary constriction, excessive drooling, and/or diarrhea may be clues to cholinergic excess rather than myasthenia exacerbation as the cause of an acute change in symptoms in a patient with myasthenia.

If a patient does not respond to pyridostigmine or responds only transiently, immunomodulatory treatment is generally required. Oral steroids are used commonly, although azathioprine and mycophenolate are the most commonly used steroid-sparing agents in patients who cannot tolerate steroids or who will need prolonged immunomodulatory treatment. Refractory cases may require more aggressive immunomodulatory therapy (e.g., IVIg, plasma exchange, eculizumab, rituximab, cyclophosphamide). When steroids are used, they are generally started at a low dose and uptitrated slowly since myasthenia can transiently worsen with high-dose steroids. Once a therapeutic dose of steroids is reached, it is generally maintained for at least 1 month and then slowly tapered to the lowest dose that adequately treats the patient's symptoms, which is maintained.

For acute worsening of symptoms or myasthenic crisis, IVIg or plasma exchange is generally used with steroids, as discussed above.

CONGENITAL MYASTHENIC SYNDROMES & NEONATAL MYASTHENIA GRAVIS

Congenital Myasthenic Syndromes

Congenital myasthenic syndromes are a group of disorders in which symptoms of myasthenia gravis develop in infancy due to mutations in either presynaptic or postsynaptic neuromuscular junction proteins. Like the adult form of the disease, symptoms include fluctuating ptosis, extraocular muscle weakness, bulbar weakness, and respiratory muscle weakness. Some patients respond to acetylcholinesterase inhibitors, which may be both diagnostic and therapeutic, but definitive diagnosis is made by genetic testing.

Neonatal Myasthenia Gravis

Neonatal myasthenia gravis occurs when a woman with immune-mediated myasthenia gravis passes AChR antibodies to the fetus during pregnancy. This causes the infant to be hypotonic with bulbar weakness at birth, leading to impaired feeding and weak cry. Most infants recover within 1–2 months. Treatment during this period is supportive with respect to nutritional and ventilatory support, and the acetylcholinesterase inhibitor neostigmine may be used.

LAMBERT-EATON MYASTHENIC SYNDROME

Clinical Features of Lambert-Eaton Myasthenic Syndrome

Lambert-Eaton myasthenic syndrome (LEMS) is a disorder that affects the neuromuscular junction presynaptically. Antibodies are produced against the presynaptic voltage-gated calcium channels (VGCC) involved in acetylcholine release.

LEMS may be a paraneoplastic syndrome (most commonly associated with small cell lung cancer) or may occur without associated malignancy. Patients present with proximal weakness more prominent in the lower extremities and autonomic features such as dry eyes, dry mouth, orthostasis, constipation, erectile dysfunction, and decreased sweating. Reflexes are typically diminished or absent.

Just as myasthenia gravis and LEMS affect opposite sides of the neuromuscular junction, their clinical and electrophysiologic features also contrast (Table 29–1). Ocular muscles are

TABLE 29–1 Clinical Features of Myasthenia Gravis & Lambert-Eaton Myasthenic Syndrome.

		Myasthenia Gravis	Lambert-Eaton Myasthenic Syndrome
Presenting site of weakness		Most commonly ocular	Predominantly proximal lower extremities
Response to exercise		Fatigues	Weakness improves initially then fatigues
Ocular symptoms		Prominent, often presenting feature	Mild if present, and rarely the presenting symptom
Dysarthria, dysphagia, respiratory weakness		Common	Rare
Autonomic features		Do not occur	Common (decreased salivation and sweating, constipation)
Repetitive stimulation	**Low frequency**	CMAP decrement	CMAP decrement
	High frequency	CMAP decrement or no change	CMAP increment
CMAPs		Normal	Decreased
Single-fiber jitter		Increased	Increased
Autoantibodies		AChR & MuSK most common	VGCC
Site of autoantibody interaction		Postsynaptic	Presynaptic
Associated malignancy		Can be associated with thymoma	Small cell lung cancer most common, although can occur with others or with no malignancy
Symptomatic treatment		Pyridostigimine (acetylcholinesterase inhibitor)	3,4-Diaminopyridine (potassium channel blocker)

Abbreviations: AChR: acetylcholine receptor; CMAP: compound motor action potential; MuSK: muscle-specific tyrosine kinase; VGCC: voltage-gated calcium channels.

rarely involved in LEMS, and when they are, involvement is usually mild and not commonly present at onset as in myasthenia gravis. In contrast to the fatigable weakness seen in myasthenia gravis, patients with LEMS may actually improve initially when exercising, but they then ultimately fatigue. Exercise-induced facilitation in LEMS can be noted in two ways on examination: After repeated actions (such as repeated hand grip), an action may become stronger, and diminished reflexes may improve after sustained contraction of the muscle involved in the reflex (e.g., quadriceps for knee reflex). This phenomenon of facilitation can also be noted on EMG: CMAP is typically reduced at baseline in LEMS, but with high-frequency repetitive stimulation or exercise, the CMAP actually increases (compared to the decrease with repetitive stimulation in myasthenia gravis; see below).

The diagnosis of LEMS can generally be made by repetitive nerve stimulation, and can be confirmed by the detection of serum antibodies against voltage-gated calcium channels (VGCC).

Diagnosis of Lambert-Eaton Myasthenic Syndrome

Low-Frequency & High-Frequency Repetitive Nerve Stimulation in Myasthenia Gravis & Lambert-Eaton Myasthenic Syndrome

Repetitive Nerve Stimulation in Myasthenia Gravis—In myasthenia gravis, the problem is at the postsynaptic acetylcholine receptors. Low-frequency repetitive stimulation leads to initial release of acetylcholine, but subsequently leads to less acetylcholine release since ample time has not been provided to allow presynaptic acetylcholine to replenish. Therefore, reduced acetylcholine release with low-frequency repetitive

stimulation leads to decrease in muscle activation, leading to a decrement in CMAPs (Fig. 29–2A).

Repetitive nerve stimulation in Lambert-Eaton myasthenic syndrome—In LEMS, there is impaired presynaptic release of acetylcholine. With decreased acetylcholine release, CMAPs are low at baseline since less acetylcholine is released per stimulus than normally would be. Low-frequency stimulation leads to a decremental response in LEMS as it does in myasthenia, since only a little acetylcholine is released to begin with, and less is released with additional low-frequency stimulation. With high-frequency stimulation, however, presynaptic release of acetylcholine is increased because high-frequency stimulation leads to increased calcium entry into the presynaptic neurons, overcoming the electrophysiologic "lesion" in LEMS. This leads to incremental increase in CMAPs with high-frequency stimulation (Fig. 29–2B).

Why doesn't high-frequency stimulation improve CMAPs in myasthenia gravis? Because there is no problem with release of acetylcholine but rather a problem with the response to it: Even with increasing acetylcholine release with high-frequency stimulation, there is an insufficient amount of available postsynaptic acetylcholine receptors to respond to the increase in synaptic acetylcholine.

Why don't high-frequency or low-frequency stimulation affect neuromuscular transmission in people *without* neuromuscular junction disorders? Normally, more acetylcholine is released into the synapse in than is necessary to depolarize the postsynaptic muscle (called the **safety factor**). So normal individuals already have ample acetylcholine to activate postsynaptic muscle fibers at baseline, and so there is no change in CMAPs with increasing acetylcholine release in repetitive stimulation.

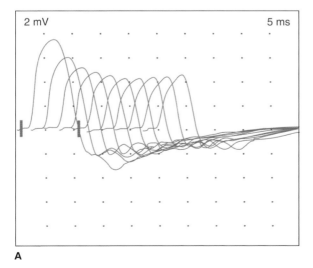

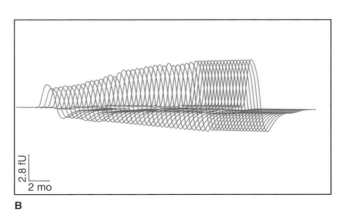

FIGURE 29–2 **EMG findings in repetitive stimulation in myasthenia gravis and Lambert-Eaton myasthenic syndrome. A:** CMAP decrement with low-frequency (3 Hz) repetitive stimulation in a patient with myasthenia gravis. **B:** Incremental CMAP increase with high-frequency (20 Hz) repetitive stimulation in a patient with Lambert-Eaton myasthenic syndrome. (Reproduced with permission from Amato A, Russell J: *Neuromuscular Disorders*, 2nd ed. New York, NY: McGraw Hill; 2015.)

Evaluation for Malignancy in Lambert-Eaton Myasthenic Syndrome

In all patients with LEMS, a chest CT should be performed to evaluate for lung cancer, and if none is found, a PET scan should be considered. Although some cases do occur with no associated malignancy, screening for an underlying malignancy should be performed every 6 months for several years since the syndrome may precede the radiologic appearance of the underlying cancer.

Treatment of Lambert-Eaton Myasthenic Syndrome

In malignancy-associated LEMS, the syndrome can improve with treatment of the underlying cancer. Pyridostigmine is less effective for symptomatic management than with myasthenia gravis, but the potassium channel blocker 3,4-diaminopyridine (amifampridine) may be effective.

Immunomodulatory treatment is often used in cases not associated with malignancy, and may also be used in malignancy-associated disease.

Botulism, an infectious condition that affects the neuromuscular junction, is discussed in Chapter 20 ("Infection at the Neuromuscular Junction: Botulism").

REFERENCES

MGTX trial 2016. Wolfe GI, Kaminski HJ, Aban IB, Minisman G, Kuo HC, Marx A, et al. Randomized trial of thymectomy in myasthenia gravis. *N Engl J Med* 2016;375:511–522.

MGTX trial 2019. Wolfe GI, Kaminski HJ, Aban IB, Minisman G, Kuo HC, Marx A, et al. Long-term effect of thymectomy plus prednisone versus prednisone alone in patients with non-thymomatous myasthenia gravis: 2-year extension of the MGTX randomised trial. *Lancet Neurol* 2019;18(3):259–268.

Diseases of Muscle

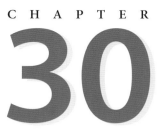

CAUSES OF MUSCLE DISEASE

Muscle disease can be caused by:

- **Inflammatory diseases**: polymyositis, dermatomyositis, inclusion body myositis, immune-mediated necrotizing myopathy
- **Medications**: most commonly statins and corticosteroids, but other immunosuppressive agents in addition to steroids (e.g., cyclosporine, tacrolimus), zidovudine, colchicine, chloroquine, immune checkpoint inhibitors, and amiodarone can also cause myopathy
- **Systemic diseases**: HIV, endocrine disease, rheumatologic disease, critical illness
- **Genetic disorders**, which can be further divided into genetic defects in:
  - **Structural muscle proteins**: muscular dystrophies, congenital myopathies
  - **Metabolic pathways**: glycogen storage diseases, disorders of lipid metabolism
  - **Mitochondria**: mitochondrial myopathies such as myoclonic epilepsy with ragged red fibers (MERRF)
  - **Ion channels**: periodic paralyses

CLINICAL FEATURES OF MUSCLE DISEASE

The hallmark of muscle disease is weakness. Diseases of muscle are distinguished from central nervous system or peripheral nervous system causes of weakness by lack of upper or lower motor neuron signs (although severe weakness can cause decreased reflexes), lack of sensory changes, and by the pattern and distribution of weakness. The most common pattern of weakness in diseases of muscle is symmetric proximal weakness, although there are myopathies that specifically affect particular distal muscle groups in isolation (e.g., distal myopathies) or in addition to proximal muscles (e.g., inclusion body myositis), and some muscle diseases can begin (and/or remain) asymmetric in some patients (e.g., inclusion body myositis, fascioscapulohumeral muscular dystrophy). Weakness in some muscle diseases develops insidiously (e.g., dermatomyositis, polymyositis, muscular dystrophies), but in others it can be rapidly progressive (e.g., immune-mediated necrotizing myopathy). In some muscle diseases weakness occurs only with particular precipitants (e.g., exercise in metabolic myopathies, potassium level in periodic paralyses). When weakness is exercise–induced, diseases of the neuromuscular junction must also be considered (see Ch. 29).

LABORATORY TESTING IN MUSCLE DISEASE

An elevated serum creatine kinase (CK) is seen in many muscle diseases, but may not necessarily be elevated in all muscle diseases. CK elevation can also be caused by muscle injury, exercise, and generalized tonic-clonic seizures. Aspartate aminotransferase (AST) and alanine aminotransferase (ALT) ("liver enzymes") do not just rise in liver disease, but may also be elevated due to muscle breakdown. Aldolase elevation can also be caused by either liver or muscle disease. An increase in gamma-glutamyl transferase (GGT) with elevated AST/ALT can help to distinguish liver injury as the cause of the rise in AST/ALT because GGT is present only in the liver and not in muscle. Myoglobinuria suggests muscle breakdown, which can occur due to primary muscle disease or in the setting of muscle injury (e.g., extreme exercise, toxins, trauma).

In nerve conduction studies in muscle diseases, compound motor action potential (CMAP) amplitudes may be reduced due to loss of muscle fibers, but sensory nerve action potentials (SNAPs) and conduction velocities should be normal (unless there is concurrent neuropathy). Electromyography (EMG) in muscle diseases can reveal increased insertional activity, spontaneous discharges (including fibrillation potentials, positive sharp waves, complex repetitive discharges), and early recruitment and rapid firing of motor unit action potentials (MUAPs) with decreased amplitude, decreased duration, and polyphasia (see "Electromyography" in Ch. 15). Myotonia on EMG may be seen in the myotonic dystrophies, myotonia congenita, and paramyotonia congenita. EMG can be normal in some myopathies (e.g., steroid myopathy).

Muscle MRI can demonstrate inflammatory changes in muscle in inflammatory myopathies. Muscle biopsy can reveal characteristic specific histologic patterns of the various myopathies, and also allows for immunostaining for particular enzymes in order to diagnose metabolic myopathies.

INFLAMMATORY MYOPATHIES

The inflammatory myopathies include dermatomyositis, polymyositis, inclusion body myositis, and immune-mediated necrotizing myopathy. Details of these diseases are compared in Table 30–1, and some general points are noted below.

TABLE 30–1 Clinical Features of the Inflammatory Myopathies.

	Polymyositis	Dermatomyositis	Inclusion Body Myositis	Immune-Mediated Necrotizing Myopathy
Weakness	Proximal, symmetric		Quadriceps Finger flexors Ankle dorsiflexors Face can be involved Can begin asymmetrically	Proximal, symmetric
Associated features	Rash Interstitial lung disease Cardiac involvement Association with malignancy Overlap with systemic autoimmune disease		Dysphagia	Statin use Malignancy Systemic autoimmune disease
Gender predominance	Women		Men	None
Age of onset	Usually <50		Usually >50	Usually >50 when statin-associated
Site of inflammatory involvement on biopsy	Endomysial	Perimysial/perivascular	Endomysial	Minimal (muscle necrosis is the prominent feature)
Associated autoantibodies	ANA	Anti-MDA-5, Mi-2, NXP-2, TIF-1, SAE	Anti–cytoplasmic 5'-nucleotidase 1A	Anti-HMG-CoA reductase Anti-SRP
Treatment	Immunomodulatory treatment: • Steroids (first line) • Azathioprine, IVIg, methotrexate, mycophenolate mofetil, rituximab		None available	Immunomodulatory treatment

Abbreviations: ANA: antinuclear antibody; HMG-CoA: 3-hydroxy-3-methylglutaryl coenzyme A; SRP: signal recognition particle; TIF: transcriptional intermediary factor; tRNA: transfer RNA.

Dermatomyositis, Polymyositis, Anti-Synthetase Syndrome, & Overlap Myositis

Dermatomyositis and polymyositis both cause proximal symmetric weakness of subacute to chronic onset, are more common in women, tend to present prior to age 50, may be associated with interstitial lung disease and/or cardiomyopathy, may be associated with underlying malignancy (more common with dermatomyositis), may have overlapping features with systemic autoimmune diseases, often have elevations in serum CK (although not always), and generally respond to immunomodulatory therapy. Dermatomyositis and polymyositis are distinguished from one another predominantly by the presence of skin findings in dermatomyositis and differing pathologic findings on muscle biopsy. The dermatologic features of dermatomyositis may precede, co-occur with, or follow the muscle symptoms, and can include findings on the knuckles (**Gottron's papules**), neck (called the **V sign** due to its V shape), back (**shawl sign**), and eyelids (**heliotrope rash**).

A growing number of antibodies have been found in affected patients. Particular antibodies correlate with severity of myositis, severity of skin involvement, presence of interstitial lung disease, and association with underlying malignancy (e.g., anti-TIF1 and anti-NXP-2 are associated with increased risk of malignancy in dermatomyositis).

Anti-synthetase antibodies (most commonly anti-Jo-1; also anti-PL-7, anti-PL-12, others) are associated with a unique syndrome called **anti-synthetase syndrome**, which causes myositis, mechanic's hands, Raynaud phenomenon, arthritis, and interstitial lung disease.

In patients with systemic autoimmune conditions (e.g., lupus, systemic sclerosis) who develop concurrent myopathy, this is called **overlap myositis**. Antibodies include anti-Ku, anti-PMScl, and anti-U1 RNP (with lupus or systemic sclerosis).

Inclusion Body Myositis

Inclusion body myositis differs from dermatomyositis and polymyositis in several ways: It is more common in men, onset is generally after age 50, it causes distal weakness (finger flexion and foot dorsiflexion) in addition to proximal weakness (particularly in the quadriceps), it may present asymmetrically, and there is no response to immunomodulatory therapy. Dysphagia is common and facial weakness can also occur. IBM is associated with anti-cytoplasmic 5′-nucleotidase 1A antibodies, and a significant proportion of patients have concurrent T-cell large granular lymphocytic leukemia.

Immune-Mediated Necrotizing Myopathy

Immune-mediated necrotizing myopathy can occur in the context of statin use, malignancy, or associated autoimmune disease (most commonly mixed connective tissue disease or scleroderma). The course is generally more rapid in onset than the other inflammatory myopathies, and the CK is often extremely elevated. When associated with statin use, antibodies to HMG-CoA reductase may be present; in non–statin-associated cases, anti–signal recognition particle (SRP) antibodies may be present, though in some cases of non–statin-associated immune-mediated necrotizing myopathy anti-HMG-CoA reductase antibodies may be seen.

MUSCULAR DYSTROPHIES

The muscular dystrophies are diseases caused by genetic defects in muscle proteins. They differ in the pattern of muscles affected, age of onset, associated nonmuscular features (e.g., cardiac disease), and pattern of inheritance. Diagnosis is made by targeted genetic testing based on clinical phenotype and family history. Treatment of the muscular dystrophies is largely supportive. Duchenne muscular dystrophy is the only muscular dystrophy for which a disease-modifying treatment is available (steroids). Details of the muscular dystrophies are compared in Table 30–2, and some general points are noted below.

Duchenne & Becker Muscular Dystrophy

Duchenne muscular dystrophy (DMD) and Becker muscular dystrophy (BMD) are X-linked disorders arising from a mutation in the protein dystrophin. In DMD, there is absence or near absence of the protein, whereas in BMD, there is marked reduction in the amount of the protein leading to a milder form of the disease.

DMD presents in early childhood with difficulty walking and falls due to proximal leg weakness. Classic signs include a waddling gait, calf pseudohypertrophy (prominent calves due to replacement of muscle with fat), and Gower's sign (inability to rise from being seated on the ground without use of the arms). Weakness is progressive, with most patients requiring a wheelchair by age 12, and few surviving beyond their 20s. Cardiac and pulmonary dysfunction inevitably develop, so regular screening for these manifestations is necessary. Cognitive dysfunction is present in many patients. Treatment with steroids (prednisone or deflazacort) increases the time that patients remain ambulatory and slows the progression of the disease. Genetic therapy with antisense oligonucleotides is under active investigation. Otherwise, care is supportive.

BMD is milder in severity and rate of progression, with patients presenting in later childhood or even in adulthood in the mildest cases. Patients remain ambulatory beyond age 16. Respiratory dysfunction, if present, is less severe than in DMD, although cardiac dysfunction may be similar in severity to DMD. Steroids are not typically used in BMD.

Diagnosis of both DMD and BMD is made by genetic testing. CK is usually elevated.

TABLE 30–2 Clinical Features of the Muscular Dystrophies.

	Duchenne (DMD)	Becker (BMD)	Emery-Dreifuss (EDMD)	Limb Girdle (LGMD)	Facioscapulohumeral (FSHD)	Oculopharyngeal (OPMD)	Myotonic Dystrophy Type 1 (DM1)	Myotonic Dystrophy Type 2 (DM2)
Pattern of weakness	Proximal followed by distal	Same as DMD but milder	Biceps Triceps Ankle dorsiflexors	Proximal limbs & varied	Face Shoulder girdle Pectorals Biceps/triceps Abdominal Ankle dorsiflexors Can begin asymmetrically	Ptosis Dysphagia Extraocular muscles	Face Neck Finger flexors Ankle dorsiflexors	Proximal limbs Neck Finger flexors
Cardiac involvement	Yes	Yes	Yes	Varies	Rare (usually asymptomatic arrhythmias)	No	Yes	Yes (milder than in DM1)
Other	Pulmonary Cognitive	Pulmonary (although milder)	Contractures (elbows, Achilles tendon)	Varies	Hearing loss Retinal vascular changes	Extremity weakness More common in French Canadians	Myotonia Pain Cataracts GI dysfunction Endocrine dysfunction (hypogonadism) Cognitive dysfunction Frontal balding, "hatchet face," "fish mouth" Subcortical white matter changes in anterior temporal lobes	Any features of DM1 can be present but are generally milder
Age of onset	Early childhood (Non-ambulatory by age 12)	Later childhood (Ambulation beyond age 16)	10–20s	Varies	10–20s	50s–60s	Congenital, childhood, and adult-onset variants	Adulthood (after age 30)
Inheritance	X-linked	X-linked	XL or AD or AR	AD (type 1) AR (type 2)	AD	AD	AD	AD
Gene	Dystrophin Absent (or nearly absent)	Dystrophin Reduced	*Emerin* (XL) or *Lamin* (AD or AR)	Calpain, Dysferlin, Sarcoglycan, others	*DUX4* (FSHD1) *SMCHD1* (FSHD2)	*PABPN1*	*DMPK*	*CNBP (ZNF9)*

Abbreviations: AD: autosomal dominant; AR: autosomal recessive: GI: gastrointestinal; XL: X-linked.

Emery-Dreifuss Muscular Dystrophy

Emery-Dreifuss muscular dystrophy (EDMD) causes weakness of the biceps, triceps, and ankle dorsiflexors, contractures at the elbows and ankles, and severe cardiac disease. Onset is usually in the teens or 20s. Treatment centers mostly on management of cardiac complications (cardiomyopathy and arrhythmias), and is otherwise supportive.

Limb Girdle Muscular Dystrophy

There are over 30 subtypes of limb girdle muscular dystrophy (LGMD), sharing the core feature of proximal weakness of the arms, legs, or both. Type 1 LGMDs are autosomal dominantly inherited, while type 2 LGMDs are autosomal recessively inherited. The LGMDs vary with respect to age of onset, whether or not distal musculature is affected in addition to limb girdle musculature, and whether there is cardiac involvement.

Facioscapulohumeral Muscular Dystrophy

As the name suggests, facioscapulohumeral muscular dystrophy (FSHD) affects the muscles of the face, scapula, and humerus. In spite of not being included in the name, ankle dorsiflexion weakness and abdominal muscle weakness may be seen in some cases. Weakness of shoulder muscles leads to scapular winging, and weakness of biceps, triceps, and pectorals with sparing of the deltoid and forearm musculature leads to a characteristic appearance of the shoulder and arm ("Popeye arm"). In contrast to many other genetic diseases of muscle, FSHD can present asymmetrically.

Oculopharyngeal Muscular Dystrophy

As the name suggests, oculopharyngeal muscular dystrophy (OPMD) causes ptosis and dysphagia. Extraocular muscle weakness may also be present. Although not included in the name, mild proximal extremity weakness can also occur in OPMD. The disease is more common in French Canadians. Unlike the other dystrophies discussed here, OPMD tends to present much later in life. Myasthenia gravis (see Ch. 29) should be considered in the differential diagnosis.

Myotonic Dystrophy

Myotonic dystrophy is characterized by weakness, **myotonia** (impaired relaxation after muscle activation), and a large number of systemic comorbidities including cataracts, gastrointestinal dysfunction, endocrine dysfunction (most commonly hypogonadism), and cardiac dysfunction. Myotonia can be elicited by engaging the patient in a handshake and noting impaired release of the patient's grip, or by percussing the base of the patient's thumb and noting thumb abduction followed by delayed relaxation (**percussion myotonia**). Myotonia can be treated with mexiletine.

Type 1 myotonic dystrophy (DM1) is the more severe form of the disease. DM1 can present in adulthood, in childhood, or congenitally due to genetic anticipation of a CTG repeat. DM1 has a characteristic facial appearance due to frontal balding, ptosis, temporal and jaw muscle wasting leading to a "hatchet"-shaped face, and perioral and jaw muscle weakness causing a "fish mouth" appearance of the mouth. Extremity weakness is more prominent distally (finger flexion, ankle dorsiflexion).

Type 2 myotonic dystrophy (DM2) does not typically share the facial features of DM1, often has more prominent proximal weakness, and has fewer and milder systemic manifestations.

Myotonic dystrophy is one of the few classes of muscular dystrophy with abnormal findings on brain MRI: T2/FLAIR hyperintensity in the anterior temporal subcortical white matter (a region also affected in CADASIL [cerebral autosomal dominant arteriopathy with subcortical infarcts and leukoencephalopathy], although white matter changes are far more extensive in CADASIL; see Ch. 19).

Myotonia can also be seen in **myotonia congenita** (caused by a chloride channel mutation) and **paramyotonia congenita** (caused by a sodium channel mutation). In these diseases, patients experience stiffness rather than weakness and have myotonia on examination and EMG.

In summary for the muscular dystrophies:

- The muscular dystrophies are a diverse group of genetic disorders characterized by progressive weakness.
- Most muscular dystrophies are autosomal dominantly inherited, except DMD and BMD (which are X-linked), Emery-Dreifuss muscular dystrophy (which can be X-linked, autosomal dominant, or autosomal recessive), and Type 2 LGMD (which is autosomal recessive; Type 1 LGMD is autosomal dominant).
- Most muscular dystrophies begin in early adulthood, except OPMD (which begins in later adulthood), and DMD, BMD, and congenital DM1 (which begin in childhood).
- Many muscular dystrophies also have cardiac manifestations that must be screened for and managed (in collaboration with a cardiologist).
- DMD is the only muscular dystrophy for which there is a disease-modifying treatment (steroids).

DISTAL MYOPATHIES (DISTAL MUSCULAR DYSTROPHIES)

The distal myopathies (also called distal muscular dystrophies) are distinct from most adult-onset muscle disorders in that they predominantly affect distal rather than proximal muscles. Details of the distal myopathies are compared in Table 30–3, and some general points are noted below.

Most of the distal myopathies primarily cause weakness in ankle dorsiflexion, which is usually the presenting feature. Exceptions are Miyoshi myopathy, which predominantly affects plantar flexion; Welander myopathy, which typically begins in the hands (before affecting dorsiflexion); and Laing

TABLE 30–3 Clinical Features of the Distal Myopathies (Distal Muscular Dystrophies).

	Udd	Markesbury-Griggs	Nonaka	Miyoshi	Laing	Welander
Most commonly affected muscles	Dorsiflexion	Dorsiflexion	Dorsiflexion	Plantarflexion	Neck Dorsiflexion	Hands Dorsiflexion
Cardiac involvement	Occurs	Occurs	No	No	Occurs	No
Age of onset	>30	>30	>30	>30	<30	>30
Inheritance	AD	AD	AR	AR	AD	AD
Geography (or geography of origin)	Finland	Europe	Japan	Japan and Europe	Europe	Scandinavia
Gene/protein	*Titin*	*ZASP*	*GNE*	*Dysferlin*	*MYH7*	*TIA1*

Abbreviations: AD: autosomal dominant; AR: autosomal recessive.

myopathy, which also involves the neck (in addition to ankle dorsiflexion). Most distal myopathies present in adulthood and can arise quite late in adulthood, although Laing myopathy typically presents earlier. Most have a particular geographic distribution (or region of origin) that can be inferred from the name of the disease. Given the distal onset, peripheral neuropathy is the main differential diagnosis, particularly hereditary neuropathies (e.g., Charcot-Marie-Tooth disease; see Ch. 27) given the inherited nature of these diseases.

CONGENITAL MUSCULAR DYSTROPHIES & CONGENITAL MYOPATHIES

Muscle disease is one of many potential etiologies of infantile hypotonia ("floppy baby"), which can localize anywhere along the neuraxis. In addition to considering spinal muscular atrophy (see Ch. 29), congenital muscular dystrophies and myopathies are rare conditions that present with hypotonia at birth or in early infancy and delayed motor development. Details of these diseases are compared in Table 30–4, and some general points are noted below.

Brain (e.g., cortical anomalies) and/or ocular abnormalities (e.g., cataracts, retinal detachment) occur in addition to muscle involvement in several of the congenital muscular dystrophies (muscle-eye-brain disease, Fukuyama congenital muscular dystrophy, Walker-Warburg syndrome), although these do not occur in the congenital myopathies. Contractures at birth (**arthrogryposis**) are common in the congenital muscular dystrophies but not in the congenital myopathies. The congenital muscular dystrophies are classified by the protein affected (e.g., fukutin, merosin, collagen, dystroglycan), whereas the congenital myopathies are classified by their histologic appearance on muscle biopsy (e.g., central core, centronuclear, nemaline rod). Each histologic pattern in congenital myopathies can be caused by mutations in a number of genes coding muscle proteins, so classification of these diseases is also moving in the direction of gene/protein-based. Of note, central core myopathies are caused by mutations of the ryanodine receptor, placing patients at risk for malignant hyperthermia if exposed to general anesthesia.

METABOLIC MYOPATHIES

Myopathies due to genetic defects in metabolic pathways should be considered when patients present with muscle cramps, pain, and/or myoglobinuria provoked by exercise, cold, fasting, and/or metabolic stress (e.g., infection, general anesthesia). Notably,

TABLE 30–4 Clinical Features of the Congenital Muscular Dystrophies & Myopathies.

	Congenital Muscular Dystrophies	Congenital Myopathies
Arthrogryposis (contractures at birth)	Common	Uncommon
Facial weakness	Uncommon	Common
Brain involvement	Occurs in several syndromes	Does not occur
Course	Usually progressive	Often static, but may be slowly progressive
CK	Usually elevated	Usually normal
Classified by	Gene/protein affected	Histologic appearance on muscle biopsy and gene/protein affected
Examples	Muscle-eye-brain disease Ullrich muscular dystrophy/Bethlem myopathy Fukuyama congenital muscular dystrophy Walker-Warburg syndrome	Central core Centronuclear Nemaline rod

however, some of the metabolic myopathies can present with progressive proximal weakness rather than exercise-induced symptoms, mimicking inflammatory myopathies or adult-onset limb girdle muscular dystrophies. This is particularly important for acid maltase deficiency (also known as adult-onset Pompe disease), which can present this way, and is the only metabolic myopathy treatable with enzyme replacement (alpha-glucosidase). The metabolic myopathies that are symptomatic with exertion are referred to as **dynamic**, whereas those with nonexertional progressive symptoms are referred to as **static**. Details of the metabolic myopathies are compared in Table 30–5, and some general points are noted below.

The metabolic myopathies due to glycogenic pathway dysfunction that cause exercise-induced symptoms do so early in the course of exercise, whereas those due to disorders in lipid metabolism pathways tend to cause symptoms after sustained exercise. This is because glucose is consumed first in muscle metabolism, followed by lipids. Patients with glycogen storage diseases may also report that they get a "second wind" if they rest and then resume exercise, whereas this does not occur with disorders of lipid metabolism.

Most myopathies caused by defects in metabolic pathways can present either as a severe infantile disorder (with hypotonia, hepatosplenomegaly, and/or cardiopulmonary dysfunction) or in adulthood (with dynamic or static muscle symptoms as described above).

All of the metabolic myopathies are autosomal recessive, all cause CK elevation, and many can be diagnosed by muscle biopsy with immunohistochemical stains for metabolic enzymes. Diagnosis can also be made by genetic testing.

Forearm Exercise Test in Metabolic Myopathies

The **forearm exercise test** is a bedside test that may distinguish between different defects in the muscle metabolic pathways. To perform the forearm exercise test, a baseline blood draw for lactate, pyruvate, and ammonia is obtained, and then a second blood draw is obtained from the same arm after repetitive muscle contraction (opening-closing of the hand) to examine changes in the quantities of these three metabolites. This test is done by some practitioners with a blood pressure cuff inflated around the arm to induce ischemia of the arm, but some believe that this is dangerous and not necessary. Normally, lactate, pyruvate, and ammonia all rise after exercise. Depending on the enzyme defect, different patterns in these three metabolites may be observed after exercise. In many (but not all) glycogen metabolism disorders, lactate and pyruvate do not rise as much as expected (since the pathway producing them is deficient). In the one metabolic myopathy caused by impaired purine metabolism (myoadenylate deaminase deficiency), lactate and pyruvate rise normally, but ammonia (a product of purine metabolism) does not. The test is generally normal in disorders of lipid metabolism.

MITOCHONDRIAL MYOPATHIES

Like the metabolic myopathies, mitochondrial myopathies can also cause exercise intolerance. Mitochondrial disease can rarely cause an isolated myopathy. More commonly, myopathy occurs as a component of a multisystem mitochondrial disorder, and myopathy may be asymptomatic, mild, or a major component. One mitochondrial disorder in which myopathy is a prominent feature is myoclonic epilepsy with ragged red fibers (MERRF). The gene mutation in MERRF, *A8344G*, can be recalled by the resemblance of the double 4 in A8**344**G to the double R in ME**RR**F (see Ch. 31 for more on mitochondrial diseases).

The combination of muscle and brain disease (e.g., myopathy accompanied by encephalopathy and/or seizures) should lead to consideration of mitochondrial disease. Elevated serum lactate is a common finding in mitochondrial disease but is nonspecific. Muscle biopsy in mitochondrial myopathies demonstrates ragged red fibers (on modified Gomori trichrome stain), absence of staining for cytochrome oxidase (COX), and intense staining for succinic dehydrogenase (SDH) and nicotinamide adenine dinulceotide dehydrogenase (NADH). Definitive diagnosis can be made by genetic testing.

HYPERKALEMIC & HYPOKALEMIC PERIODIC PARALYSIS

The periodic paralyses are rare autosomal dominantly inherited conditions in which patients episodically develop flaccid paralysis in response to a variety of triggers: rest after exercise, cold, or dietary factors. Patients generally have normal strength between episodes. The dietary triggers of hyperkalemic and hypokalemic periodic paralyses can be remembered by the effects of insulin on potassium: *in*sulin drives potassium *in*to cells (the same effect insulin has on glucose). Therefore, a high carbohydrate meal will lead to insulin secretion and movement of potassium into cells, resulting in decreased serum potassium (which can provoke an episode of weakness in hypokalemic periodic paralysis). Fasting will decrease insulin secretion, resulting in increased serum potassium (which can provoke an episode of weakness in hyperkalemic periodic paralysis). Details of hyperkalemic and hypokalemic periodic paralysis are compared in Table 30–6, and some general points are noted below.

EMG in periodic paralysis may demonstrate reduced CMAP amplitude after exercise.

If a patient is in the midst of an acute attack and potassium is particularly low or high, cardiac monitoring is recommended.

Hypokalemic periodic paralysis can also be caused by hyperthyroidism, and so additional clinical and laboratory features of hyperthyroidism should be sought in patients with hypokalemic periodic paralysis, especially when there is no family history of the condition.

TABLE 30–5 Clinical Features of the Metabolic Myopathies.

	Disorders of Glycogen Storage					Disorders of Lipid Metabolism			Disorders of Purine Metabolism
	Type 2 Pompe	Type 3 Cori	Type 4 Andersen	Type 5 McArdle	Type 7 Tarui	Carnitine Transport Deficiencies	Carnitine Metabolism Disorders	Fatty Acid Dehydrogenase Deficiencies	Myoadenylate Deaminase Deficiency
Dynamic/ static	Static	Static	Static	Dynamic	Dynamic	Static and dynamic	Dynamic	Dynamic	Dynamic
Enzyme	Acid maltase	Glycogen debrancher enzyme	Glycogen branching	Muscle phosphorylase	Phosphofruc-tokinase	Carnitine transporter	Carnitine palmitoyl transferase 2	Very long, long, medium, and short-chain acyl-coenzyme A dehydrogenase	Myoadenylate deaminase
Exercise onset		N/A		Early in exertion				With sustained exercise	
Second wind		N/A		Yes				No	
Forearm exercise test	Normal			Decreased lactate/pyruvate rise			Normal		Decreased ammo-nia rise
Treatment	Alpha glucosidase		Liver transplant			Carnitine	Low-fat diet/ avoidance of prolonged exercise	Avoid fasts	
Other						Can be unmasked by valproate			

342

TABLE 30–6 Clinical Features of Hyperkalemic & Hypokalemic Periodic Paralysis.

	Hyperkalemic Periodic Paralysis	Hypokalemic Periodic Paralysis
Provoking factors		
Food	Fasting	Large carbohydrate-rich meal
	High-potassium intake	Alcohol
Exercise	Rest after exercise	
Other	Cold	
Attack length	Hours	Hours – 1 day
Channel	Sodium channel (SCN4A)	Calcium channel (CACNA1S)
		Sodium channel (SCN4A)
Inheritance	Autosomal dominant	
Treatment		
Acute	Inhaled beta agonist, IV calcium	Potassium (oral or IV)
Chronic		
Diet	High carbohydrate/Low potassium	Low carbohydrate/Low sodium
Diuretic	K+-wasting (e.g., thiazide)	K+-sparing (e.g., spironolactone)
	Acetazolamide/Dichlorphenamide	Acetazolamide/Dichlorphenamide

A rare cause of periodic paralysis is **Andersen-Tawil syndrome**, in which paralysis can be triggered by hypokalemia, hyperkalemia, or occur in the setting of normal potassium. Other features of the condition include cardiac arrhythmias (ventricular arrhythmias and prolonged QT interval), short stature, and dysmorphic facial features. The disease is caused by a mutation in a potassium channel (*KCNJ2*).

MUSCLE DISEASE DUE TO SYSTEMIC DISEASES & MEDICATIONS

A number of systemic diseases can cause myopathy including:

- Infections: HIV, trichinosis, bacterial pyomyositis (see "Infectious Myositis" in Ch. 20)
- Endocrine disease: hyperthyroidism or hypothyroidism, hyperparathyroidism, Cushing's syndrome

- Critical illness: critical illness myopathy (see "Critical Illness Polyneuropathy & Critical Illness Myopathy" in Ch. 27)
- Rheumatologic disease: lupus, Sjögren's syndrome, scleroderma, and overlap syndromes with dermatomyositis and polymyositis

Medication-induced myopathy can be seen with a large number of medications, but common culprits include:

- Cholesterol-lowering medications (statins and fibrates)
- Immunomodulatory therapy (steroids, chloroquine, cyclosporine, tacrolimus, immune checkpoint inhibitors)
- Amiodarone
- Zidovudine
- Colchicine

Valproate can cause or unmask an underlying myopathy due to interference with the carnitine pathway.

Statin-Induced Myopathy

Statins can cause mild muscle symptoms (pain and cramps), a myopathy (weakness), or severe muscle damage (rhabdomyolysis or necrosis). Risk factors for statin-induced myopathy include:

- Statin dose: higher dose associated with higher risk of myopathy
- Patient age: older age associated with higher risk of myopathy
- Genetic factors: *SLCO1B1* gene associated with higher risk of myopathy
- Other concurrent medications: concurrent fibrates and statins associated with higher risk of myopathy
- Which statin is being used: atorvastatin and simvastatin appear to have a higher risk of myopathy than other statins

Statin-induced myopathy should be considered when a patient develops muscle-related symptoms after initiating the medication and serum creatine kinase (CK) is found to be elevated. Treatment is generally to stop the statin and trend the serum CK until it returns to normal (treating rhabdomyolysis if present). If the patient requires statin therapy, a different statin can be tried. Rarely, patients will continue to get worse after statin discontinuation due to a statin-induced immune-mediated necrotizing myopathy associated with anti–HMG CoA reductase antibodies (see "Immune-Mediated Necrotizing Myopathies" above). This entity is diagnosed by biopsy and treated with immunomodulatory therapy.

Leukodystrophies & Mitochondrial Diseases

CHAPTER CONTENTS

LEUKODYSTROPHIES

MITOCHONDRIAL DISEASES

LEUKODYSTROPHIES (TABLE 31–1)

The leukodystrophies are diseases that affect the white matter of the CNS. These diseases can begin in infancy, childhood, or adulthood. Infantile-onset leukodystrophies are generally characterized by initial hypotonia followed by spasticity and intellectual disability. Seizures may also occur. In childhood-onset leukodystrophies, there is typically developmental and motor regression. Adult-onset leukodystrophies are characterized by dementia, psychiatric symptoms, and development of spasticity.

Many individual leukodystrophies have particular clinical hallmarks (e.g., neuropathy in Krabbe disease and metachromatic leukodystrophy) and particular distributions of white matter changes on MRI (involving or sparing the juxtacortical U fibers; frontal vs posterior predominant). Adrenoleukodystrophy, Krabbe disease, and metachromatic leukodystrophy can be treated with bone marrow transplantation, but the other leukodystrophies are treated supportively. Distinctive clinical and imaging features (beyond core features listed above) and genetics of the leukodystrophies are listed in Table 31–1.

Adrenomyeloneuropathy is a subtype of adrenoleukodystrophy that presents in adulthood with myelopathy, neuropathy, and adrenal insufficiency (the brain can be involved, but often is not, unlike the other leukodystrophies). Therefore, adrenomyeloneuropathy should be considered in the differential diagnosis for combined myelopathy and neuropathy (myeloneuropathy), as can also be seen with vitamin B12 deficiency and copper deficiency. As with adrenoleukodystrophy, inheritance of adrenomyeloneuropathy is X-linked, and diagnosis is made by elevated serum very long-chain fatty acids (VLCFAs) and genetic testing. Treatment for the condition is limited to the treatment of the adrenal insufficiency.

MITOCHONDRIAL DISEASES (TABLE 31–2)

Mitochondrial diseases arise from mutations in mitochondrial genes (either in mitochondrial DNA or in nuclear DNA encoding mitochondrial proteins). All mitochondria are inherited maternally so mitochondrial disorders most often follow a pattern of maternal inheritance (i.e., only passed from a mother to her children), although nuclear mutations in mitochondrial genes can be autosomally inherited, and some cases of mitochondrial disease are due to sporadic de novo mutations.

Mitochondrial disorders are generally characterized by multiorgan system dysfunction (deafness, diabetes, short stature, cardiac disease, and myopathy are common features), exercise intolerance, exacerbation with systemic illness, and elevated serum lactate. The most common characteristic features of five mitochondrial syndromes that affect the nervous system (beyond the general features just listed) are presented in Table 31–2. MELAS (mitochondrial encephalopathy with lactic acidosis and stroke) is also discussed in Chapter 19 and mitochondrial myopathy in Chapter 30.

TABLE 31–1 Clinical & Laboratory Features of the Leukodystrophies.

	Age of Onset	Unique Clinical Features	Neuroimaging White Matter Changes	Neuroimaging U Fibers	Gene Mutation	Inheritance	Diagnosis	Other
Adrenoleuko-dystrophy	Childhood (most commonly 4–8 years old) or adulthood	Visual and/or behavioral problems in children; Adrenal insufficiency; Adrenomyelo-neuropathy can occur in adults	Posterior predominance	Spared	*ABCD1*	XL	Plasma very long chain fatty acids	Treatments: Bone marrow transplant; Lorenzo's oil
Alexander disease	Any age	Macrocephaly; Seizures	Frontal predominance	Involved	*GFAP*	Sporadic or AD	Genetic testing	Pathology: Rosenthal's fibers
Canavan disease	Infancy	Macrocephaly	Diffuse	Involved	Aspartoacylase	AR	Urine NAA; Decreased aspartoacylase activity in skin fibroblasts	Increased NAA peak on MR-spectroscopy
Krabbe disease	Any age (but most commonly infancy)	Irritability; Peripheral neuropathy	Posterior predominance	Spared	Galactocerebrosidase	AR	Decreased galactocerebrosidase activity in skin fibroblasts	Globoid cells on pathology; Treatment with bone marrow transplant
Metachromatic leukodystrophy	Any age	Peripheral neuropathy	Frontal predominance	Spared	Arylsulfatase A	AR	Decreased arylsulfatase A activity in skin fibroblasts	Treatment with bone marrow transplant
Pelizaeus-Merzbacher disease	Infancy or childhood	Eye movement abnormalities	Diffuse	Spared	*PLP1*	XL	Genetic testing	Pathology: tigroid appearance of white matter
Vanishing white matter disease	Any age	Ataxia and/or spasticity; Spared cognition; Ovarian failure may be seen in affected women	White matter hypointense ("vanished") rather than hyperintense as in other leukodystrophies	Involved	*eIF2B*	AR	Genetic testing	

Abbreviations: AD: autosomal dominant; AR: autosomal recessive; MR: magnetic resonance; NAA: *N*-acetylaspartate; XL: X-linked.

TABLE 31–2 Clinical & Laboratory Features of Mitochondrial Diseases Affecting the Nervous System.

	Brain	Eyes	Other	Neuroimaging	Gene
MELAS	Strokelike episodes Seizures Migraine			Stroke-like cortical lesions that do not correspond to vascular territories	*A3243G*
MERRF	Myoclonic epilepsy		Myopathy (ragged red fibers on muscle biopsy)		*A8344G*
Leigh syndrome	Seizures Cognitive dysfunction (developmental delay or regression)	Ophthalmoplegia		Signal changes in brainstem on MRI	Multiple
Kearns-Sayre syndrome	Ataxia	Progressive ophthalmoplegia Pigmentary retinopathy	Cardiac disease	Signal changes in basal ganglia and brainstem on MRI	Multiple
Leber hereditary optic neuropathy		Bilateral optic neuropathy			*G1178A*

Abbreviations: MELAS: mitochondrial encephalopathy with lactic acidosis and stroke; MERRF: myoclonic epilepsy with ragged red fibers; MRI: magnetic resonance imaging.

Index

Note: Page numbers followed by *f* and *t* indicate figures and tables, respectively.